Jong's

COMMUNITY DENTAL HEALTH

FIFTH EDITION

Jong's

COMMUNITY DENTAL HEALTH

FIFTH EDITION

George M. Gluck, DDS, MPH
Associate Professor
Division of Reconstructive and Comprehensive Care
New York University
College of Dentistry
New York, New York

Warren M. Morganstein, DDS, MPH
Senior Associate Dean and Professor
Department of Oral Health Care Delivery
Baltimore College of Dental Surgery
Dental School
University of Maryland
Baltimore, Maryland

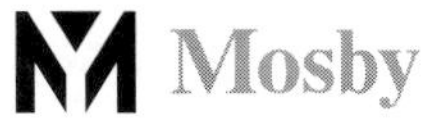

An Affiliate of Elsevier Science
St. Louis London Philadelphia Sydney Toronto

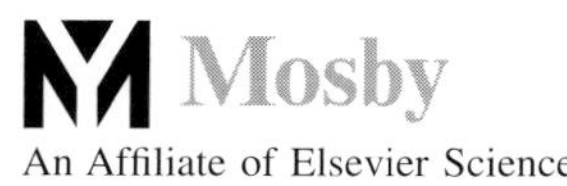

An Affiliate of Elsevier Science

11830 Westline Industrial Drive
St. Louis, Missouri 63146

JONG'S COMMUNITY DENTAL HEALTH ISBN 0-323-01467-4

FIFTH EDITION
Previous editions copyrighted 1981, 1988, 1993, 1998

Library of Congress Cataloging-in-Publication Data

Jong's community dental health / [edited by] George M. Gluck, Warren M. Morganstein—5th ed.
p. cm.
Includes bibliographical references and index.
ISBN 0-323-01467-4
1. Dental public health. 2. Community dental services. I. Title: Community dental health. II. Gluck, George M. III. Morganstein, Warren M.
RK52 .J66 2002
362.1'976'00973—dc21 2002066049

Publishing Director: Linda L. Duncan
Senior Acquisitions Editor: Penny Rudolph
Developmental Editor: Jaime Pendill
Project Manager: Linda McKinley
Production Editor: Jim Rygelski
Designer: Julia Dummitt

GW/FF

Printed in China

Last digit is the print number: 9 8 7 6 5 4 3 2

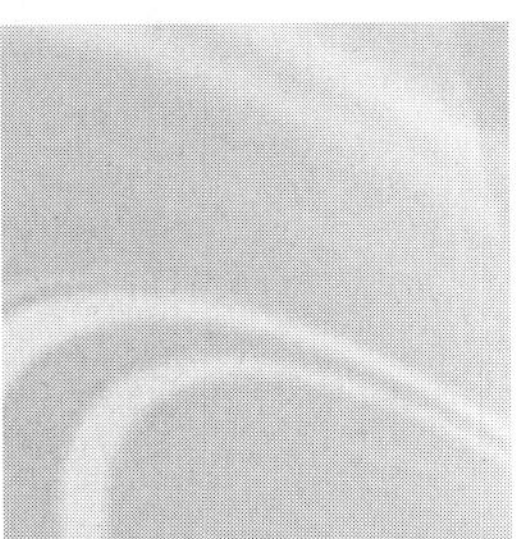

CONTRIBUTORS

Van B. Afes, MS, MA
Assistant Professor and Curator, New York University School of Medicine; Adjunct Associate Professor and Director of the Library, New York University College of Dentistry, New York

Myron Allukian, Jr., DDS, MPH
Director of Oral Health, Boston Public Health Commission, Boston, Massachusetts

Howard L. Bailit, DMD, PhD
Professor and Director, Health Policy and Primary Care Research Center, University of Connecticut Health Center, Farmington, Connecticut

Tryfon Beazoglou, PhD
Associate Professor, Department of Pediatric Dentistry, School of Dental Medicine, University of Connecticut, Farmington, Connecticut

Muriel J. Bebeau, PhD
Professor, Department of Preventive Sciences, School of Dentistry; Executive Director, Center for the Study of Ethical Development; Faculty Associate, Center for Bioethics, University of Minnesota, Minneapolis

Helene Bednarsh, BS, RDH, MPH
Clinical Instructor, Health Policy and Health Services, Boston University Goldman School of Dental Medicine; Director, HIV Dental, Boston Public Health Commission, Boston, Massachusetts

Lester E. Block, DDS, MPH
Director of Graduate Studies in Public Health, Division of Health Services Research and Policy, School of Public Health, University of Minnesota, Minneapolis

David O. Born, PhD
Professor and Director, Division of Health Ecology, University of Minnesota School of Dentistry, Minneapolis

Hillary L. Broder, PhD, MED
Professor, Department of Community Health, University of Medicine and Dentistry of New Jersey—NJ Dental School, Newark, New Jersey

James Crall, DDS, ScD
Division of Community Health, Columbia University School of Dental and Oral Surgery, New York

Marianne B. De Souza, RDH, BA, MS
Director, Greater New Bedford Tobacco Control Program, New Bedford Department of Public Health, New Bedford, Massachusetts

Eliezer Eidelman, DrOdont, MSD
Professor and Chairman, Department of Pediatric Dentistry, Hadassah School of Dental Medicine, The Hebrew University, Jerusalem, Israel

James R. Freed, DDS, MPH
Clinical Professor of Dentistry, School of Dentistry, University of California at Los Angeles

Eugene Hittelman, MA, EdD
Associate Professor, Epidemiology and Health Promotion, New York University College of Dentistry, New York

Alice M. Horowitz, PhD
Senior Scientist, National Institute of Dental and Craniofacial Research, National Institutes of Health, Bethesda, Maryland

Jeffrey P. Kahn, PhD, MPH
Director, Center for Bioethics; Professor of Medicine, University of Minnesota, Minneapolis

Bennett Klein, Esq., BA, JD
Director, AIDS Law Project, Gay and Lesbian Advocates and Defenders, Boston, Massachusetts

Nancy R. Kressin, PhD
Research Health Psychologist, Center for Health Quality, Outcomes, and Economic Research, Bedford VA Medical Center; Associate Professor, Health Services Department, Boston University School of Public Health, Bedford, Massachusetts

Mark D. Macek, DDS, Dr PH
Assistant Professor, Department of Oral Health Care Delivery, Baltimore College of Dental Surgery Dental School, University of Maryland, Baltimore

Madalyn L. Mann, BS, RDH, MS
Director of Extramural Programs, General Dentistry, Boston University Goldman School of Dental Medicine, Boston, Massachusetts

David G. Pendrys, DDS, PhD
Associate Professor, Department of Behavioral Sciences and Community Health, School of Dental Medicine, University of Connecticut, Farmington, Connecticut

Benjamin Peretz, DMD
Clinical Associate Professor, Department of Pediatric Dentistry, Hadassah School of Dental Medicine, The Hebrew University, Jerusalem, Israel

Burton R. Pollack, DDS, JD, MPH
Professor and Dean Emeritus, Dental Medicine (Health Law), School of Dental Medicine, State University of New York at Stony Brook

Lynda Rose, MS
Senior Programmer/Statistical Analyst, Division of Preventive Medicine, Brigham and Women's Hospital, Harvard Medical School; Adjunct Faculty, Boston University School of Medicine, School of Public Health, Boston University, Boston, Massachusetts

Yvette R. Schlussel, PhD
Epidemiologist, Department of Family Practice and Community Medicine, St. Vincent's Catholic Medical Center, Jamaica, New York

Rima Bachiman Sehl, DDS, MPA
Associate Professor, Epidemiology and Health Promotion, New York University College of Dentistry, New York

Michael Skolnick, BS
University of Medicine and Dentistry of New Jersey–New Jersey Dental School, Newark, New Jersey

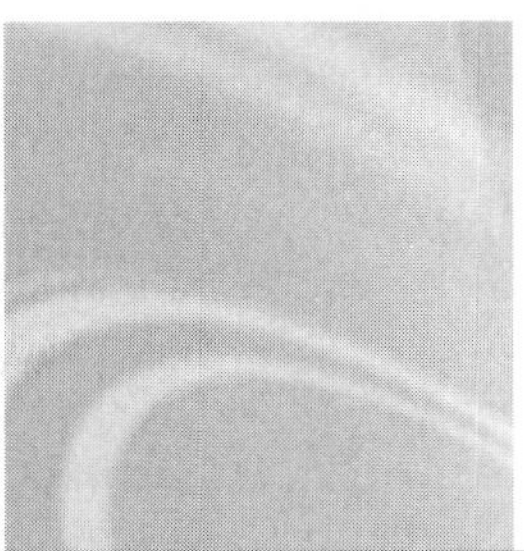

PREFACE

The fifth edition of *Jong's Community Dental Health* is keenly aware of its historical perspective. The new century, coupled with the rapid emergence of new technology, promises a rapidly changing dental public health landscape. This edition begins with a discussion of the organizational evolution of public health during the last century and launches us into the future through the first Surgeon General's Report devoted to dentistry.

A brief summary of public health over the last two hundred years reflects an accelerating pace of change and suggests an important role for dentistry. Public health during the nineteenth century was marked by urbanization and need for better sanitation. Key functions included the organization of health departments and dealing with the epidemiologic conundrum of the nature of disease.

The twentieth century saw the application of the germ theory and implementation of the scientific method. Also during this period one of the most exquisite of public health discoveries was made: the relationship between dental caries and the fluoride ion. Frederick McKay, a Colorado dentist, observed that his patients had chocolate-like stains on their teeth. However, few of his patients had tooth decay. H. Trendley Dean, director of dental research at the National Institutes of Health, collected water samples. He examined children's teeth and ultimately established the relationship between fluoride and the reduction in dental caries. Today the scope of public health has broadened to include social, political, economic and cultural factors that affect all aspects of health. Finally, affecting all of these areas is the discussion of bioethics.

Part I (Dental Care Delivery) includes Chapters 1 through 4. Chapter 1 defines public health, describes the public health process, and explains the impact of public health on public policy. The author has compiled an appendix that describes government structure and interrelationships of agencies that affect public health activities. Chapter 2 summarizes the first Surgeon General's Report on dentistry and underscores the reasons why dentistry has assumed such an important role in the health of the U.S. population. The next two chapters describe the make-up of the dental care delivery system: from managed care to care for the indigent. The poorly understood Medicaid program is brought up to date, and the role of dentistry within the Medicaid program is brought into perspective.

Part II (Demographic Shifts and Dental Health) comprises Chapters 5 through 7. Chapter 5 anticipates the increasing diversity of the U.S. population. The social and cultural health behaviors of these populations are considered. Strategies for communication between providers and individuals from diverse population groups are suggested, and culturally determined attitudes are described. Chapter 6 describes demographic shifts and focuses on the aging population and the special needs of the elderly. Chapter 7, at the other end of the aging continuum, discusses the nature of caries in children and some elements of prevention.

Part III (Distribution of Dental Disease and Prevention) consists of Chapters 8 through 13. Chapter 8 describes the distribution of dental disease. An updated epidemiologic version of the nature and distribution of oral disease, oral disease trends, and changes in the manner in which certain diseases are described is presented. Chapter 9 summarizes the status of the human immunodeficiency virus (HIV) and describes current infectious-disease challenges. The authors also review current infectious-disease–related litigation and describe its impact on the practice of dentistry. Chapter 10 describes community programs that are designed to alleviate and prevent dental disease. In tandem, the authors of Chapter 11 (two dental hygienists) continue the discussion of prevention, comparing recent health promotion programs with previous approaches and strategies and commenting on recent innovations. Chapter 12 introduces and emphasizes the importance of planning, and lists the steps that comprise the initial and subsequent stages of successful planning. Chapter 13 contrasts program evaluation and conventional research design. The discussion includes a definition and an explanation of outcomes assessment. The process of outcomes assessment has become the core process for the development of dental education curriculum.

Part IV (Research in Dental Public Health) describes two interdependent approaches to the analysis of public health research, behavioral research, and community-based research: (1) biostatistics and (2) evidenced-based research. The chapter on biostatistics (Chapter 14) confronts the notion that the researcher may manipulate statistical data to support a biased position. The author then develops the concept of biostatistics to demonstrate how bias becomes less likely through the application of statistical concepts and discipline. Chapter 15, through a discussion of the basic tenets of research design and a discussion of evidence-based dentistry, explains how "evidenced-based" provides a powerful tool for an analysis of the scientific literature.

Part V (Ethics and the Law in Community Dental Health) deals with public health and community-based issues from a bioethical and legal perspective. Chapter 16 defines some basic principles of bioethics. The authors conclude that bioethics is about dilemmas that arise in individual cases. They spend the bulk of the chapter presenting ethical dilemmas that arise in reality-based dental cases. They subsequently provide analysis from an ethical-philosophic perspective. Among the several cases, the authors lay out an in-depth portrayal of third-party dentistry, sketch out dilemmas derived from third party scenarios, and demonstrate how dentists and dental hygienists are involved. Chapter 17, which provides a description of the basics of the U.S. legal system, comments on contemporary issues and how they affect the future of dental public health. The author suggests that the new technology is bound to bring about a burst of malpractice cases.

The first edition of *Jong's Community Dental Health* was created for the purpose of supporting the educational curriculum of dental and allied health students. The fifth edition, however, includes matters that all those interested in the nature of dental delivery in the United States will find edifying.

George M. Gluck
Warren M. Morganstein

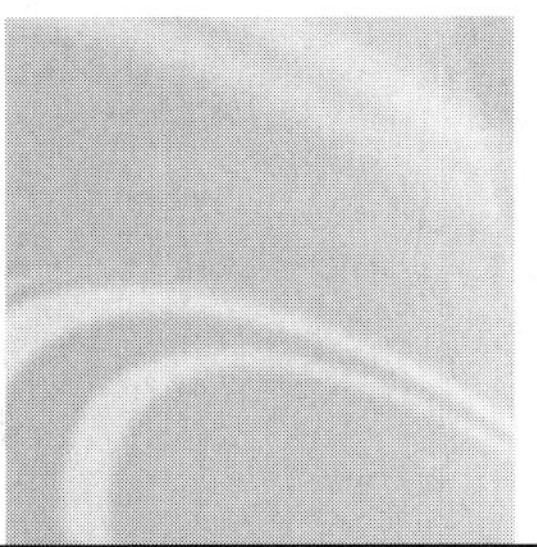

ACKNOWLEDGMENTS

Any book is a collaborative enterprise. Certainly a book such as this one, which integrates the works of various contributors, owes much to the work of many individuals. The co-editors are responsible for the selection of topics and contributors. At times, the editors have felt like the organizers of a community dental health symposium.

This book has benefited from the inspiration, cooperation, assistance, wisdom, and generosity of many people. Our acquisitions editor, Penny Rudolph, and the staff at Mosby have been especially helpful. However, most of all, the book owes its theme, its organization, and the commitment of many of the contributors to the early work of Dr. Anthony Jong. At the time of his death, Dr. Jong was an associate dean and chairman of the department of dental public health at the Boston University dental school. He forged this book out of his dual interests: providing dental care for the underserved and inspiring dental students and dental hygiene students to pursue their interest, if not their career, in the field of dental public health.

George M. Gluck
Warren M. Morganstein

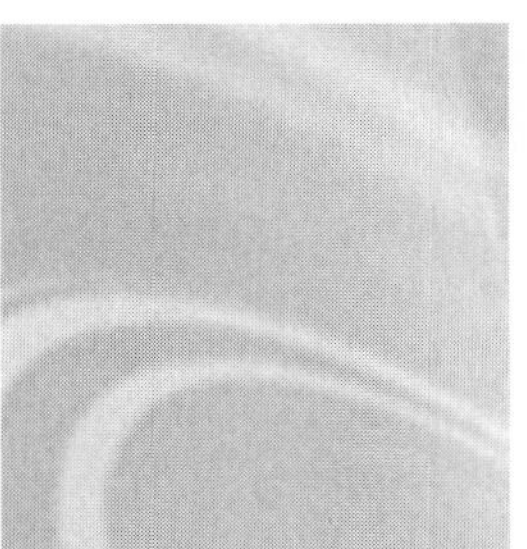

PERSPECTIVE

AN EXPANDING ROLE FOR DENTAL PUBLIC HEALTH

The September 11, 2001, terrorist attack has had an important impact on the nation's economy, and both national and local governments have had to focus on security issues and the reallocation of scarce resources. Leading up to September the nation was once again locked in debate over the increasing costs of health care, and greater attention was being drawn to a burgeoning crisis in dental care delivery. Reports from various states and at the national level focus on an impending shortage of dentists across the country. This shortage is multifaceted but is chiefly the result of the fact that large numbers of dentists trained during the 1970s and into the 1980s are rapidly reaching retirement age. With the cutbacks in enrollments and the closures of dental schools that occurred from the early 1980s into the late 1990s, diminishing numbers of dentists have been trained, and current production will not keep up with retirement and mortality losses to the profession over the next decade or two. With the flattening of the stock market, some have speculated that many planned dental retirements may be delayed several years while dentists wait for their retirement portfolios to recover. Should that speculation prove accurate, the projected shortage of dentists would be forestalled but will nonetheless affect dental care delivery within the decade.

Additionally, population demographics suggest that workers who might normally enter dental paraprofessional fields will have expanded opportunities in other sectors of the economy, and many states will be forced to rely on immigration as a workforce resource if they are to maintain levels of economic growth. These shortages will, of course, have an impact on dentists and their practices, driving up employee wages and indirect costs; productive capacity of practices could easily be compromised. Then, too, although few persons expect large-scale military drafts such as those seen during World War II, the Korean War, or the Vietnam War, the direct impact of a prolonged military conflict on the dental workforce is uncertain but could have a compounding negative effect.

In addition to a very real workforce crisis in dentistry, managed care, health care financing pressures, stagnating rural economies, fewer social and health service resources, an aging population, student indebtedness, minority health disparities, new challenges from an array of diverse ethnic communities, and a multitude of other factors are converging, putting enormous pressure on the dental care delivery system. The impact of these forces is yet to be felt; however, major, indeed revolutionary, changes face the profession over the next 10 to 25 years. Among the changes that seem most certain is that of the role of dental public health: as a field of study and as a career, dental public health seems destined to expand its influence and its realm of responsibility. Dental educators, professional associations, and governmental bodies will find it necessary to expand the role of public health agencies, to explore new avenues of preventive dental education and care, to evaluate alternative methods of outreach and care delivery, and, ultimately, to rethink the entire system of dental education and dental care delivery.

DAVID O. BORN, PHD

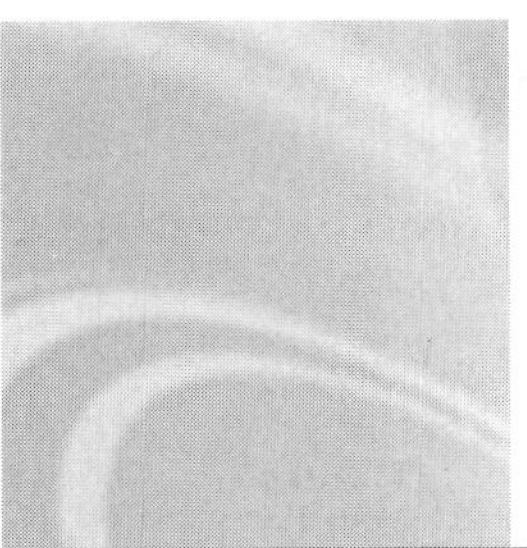

CONTENTS

PART

I

DENTAL CARE DELIVERY

CHAPTER

1

DENTAL PUBLIC HEALTH: AN OVERVIEW

Lester E. Block • James R. Freed

The goal of the dental profession is to protect and preserve the oral health of the public. Each dentist, dental hygienist, dental assistant, and dental laboratory technician is a member of a team of health care workers combating diseases that jeopardize the health of the public. As with any good team, each member has an important role to play for the team to be successful. The purpose of this chapter is to examine the discipline of dental public health and the contribution that dental public health practitioners make to protect and preserve the oral health of the public. Perhaps most importantly, this chapter seeks to emphasize the importance of teamwork among dental health professionals to achieve the goal of optimal oral health for the public and the importance of teamwork between them and other health professionals because dental public health is an integral component of public health and is directly affected by public health programs and policies.

WHAT IS PUBLIC HEALTH?

Mission of Public Health

"Public health is a coalition of professions united by their shared mission," states the Institute of Medicine of the National Academy of Sciences.[1] The phrase "coalition of professions" stresses that the achievement of better public health requires more than the participation of the various health professions. It includes contributions from engineers, educators, statisticians, political scientists, policy analysts, and administrators, among many others. So one distinguishing aspect of public health is individuals and groups banding together to achieve a common goal.

The next distinguishing characteristic of public health is the "shared mission" that this coalition of professions seeks to achieve. The public health mission statement developed by the Institute of Medicine is "fulfilling society's interest in assuring conditions in which people can be healthy."[1] In 1995 a blue ribbon committee convened by the Public Health Service published both a vision and a mission statement for public health: "Vision: Healthy People in Healthy Communities" and "Mission: Promote Physical and Mental Health and Prevent Disease, Injury, and Disability."[2] These mission statements are similar to those of the American Dental Association (ADA) and American Dental Hygienists' Association (ADHA). The "History and Mission Statement" of the ADA calls for the protection, enhancement, improvement, and promotion of the public's oral and general health and well-being.[3] The ADHA mission statement begins with, "To improve the public's total health."[4]

The primary public health mission, however, differs from those of the ADA and ADHA in that its primary focus is on "society's interest." Public health is concerned with communitywide concerns and the overall public interest, rather than the health interests of particular individuals or groups (which is not to negate the important part that individual health care concerns have in public health). Although the concerns of public health are broader than those of the many distinct and diverse professional disciplines, including those of dentistry and dental hygiene, these disciplines are necessary for the attainment of optimal public health.[1] Public health can accomplish its mission only if partnerships can be fostered and nurtured among governmental and nongovernmental public health agencies, private organizations, and individuals.[5,6]

Definition of Public Health

How *public health* is defined can provide insight into the complexity surrounding the use of the term. Defining the word *health,* for example, is not simple. The traditional dictionary definition of health is being free from pain or disease.[7] This limited definition has proved insufficient to address issues of public health concern. In 1948 the World Health Organization (WHO) created a more encompassing definition of health in its constitution. WHO defines *health* as "a state of complete physical, mental and social well-being and not merely the absence of disease or infirmity."[8] The concept of a close relationship among mind, body, health, and society is not new. Aristotle espoused it in the third century BCE. He wrote that the "health of body and mind is so fundamental to the good life that if we believe men have any personal rights at all as human beings, then they have an absolute moral right to such measure of good health as society alone is able to give them."[9]

Some believe that the WHO concept of health may be unrealistic in that freedom from disease, stress, frustration, and disability is actually incompatible with the process of living and aging. Rene Dubos, for example, wrote, "Complete and lasting freedom from disease is but a dream remembered from imaginings of a Garden of Eden designed for the welfare of man."[10] Pickett and Hanlon[8] suggest considering health as a continuum under which a disease or injury may lead to an impairment, which may lead to a disability, which may lead to a dependency requiring external resources or aids to carry out activities of daily living. Health in this continuum then can be defined as "the absence of a disability."[8]

In 1920 Winslow[11] developed a widely used definition of *public health:*

> The science and art of preventing disease, prolonging life, and promoting physical and mental efficiency through organized community effort for the sanitation of the environment, the control of

communicable infections, the education of the individual in personal hygiene, the organization of medical and nursing services for the early diagnosis and preventive treatment of disease, and the development of the social machinery to insure everyone a standard of living adequate for the maintenance of health, so organizing these benefits as to enable every citizen to realize his birthright of health and longevity.[11]

This definition shows great understanding in that Winslow recognized the impact of social, educational, and economic factors on health. Although he did not include either health care services or mental health within his concept of public health, his definition was advanced for its time. Since then the focus of public health has continued to expand. It has moved from its earliest beginnings dealing with individual hygiene to include sanitary engineering, preventive physical and mental medical science, social behavioral aspects of personal and community medicine, and more recently the promotion and assurance of comprehensive health services for all.[8]

Public health now can be thought of as being concerned with four broad areas: (1) lifestyle and behavior, (2) the environment, (3) human biology, and (4) the organization of health programs and systems. Thus public health is concerned with keeping people as healthy as possible and controlling or limiting factors that impede health; it is the organization and application of public resources to prevent dependency that would otherwise result from disease or injury.

Public health, in essence, determines the health status of the community; identifies populations potentially affected or at risk for a particular problem; analyzes the dimensions of the problem through the use of epidemiologic methodology; and then plans, implements, and evaluates the appropriate interventions.[12]

Another way to view public health practice is to divide it, somewhat arbitrarily, into six categories:

1. *Epidemiology.* Epidemiology is considered the basic science of public health.
2. *Statistics.* Although epidemiology and statistics are two separate disciplines, they combine to form the basis for the assessment functions in public health and for the collection and analysis of information and data.
3. *Biomedical sciences.* Because a major portion of disease is caused by microorganisms and genetic factors, the prevention and control of diseases in populations require an understanding of how these factors affect the body.
4. *Environmental health sciences* has always been a classic part of the public health infrastructure and is concerned with preventing the spread of disease through water, air, and food. Much of the great improvement in the health status of Americans is because of improved environmental health.
5. *Social and behavioral sciences* form the basis for understanding the role of behavior and social status in relation to health status, life expectancy, and utilization of services. Research, and its application in these sciences, is most likely to have a significant impact on solving public health problems.
6. *Health policy and management* or *health administration.* As part of its assurance function, public health seeks to understand the dimensions and operation of the health care delivery system to address problems such as quality of care and disparities in regard to obtaining care.[13]

Public Health and Community Health

The title of this book uses the term *community dental health,* whereas this chapter uses the term *dental public health.* Although both terms often are used interchangeably, a distinct difference exists between them. Both *community* and *public* mean a collection of people, a population, or a group of people having something in common.[7] From that perspective the terms *public health* and *community health* can be considered equivalent. Current usage, however, tends to define *public* to mean a general collection of people without regard to a specific geographic area in which they live. *Community* is used to indicate a collection of people who are located in a defined geographic area such as a city, nation, or state. In this regard, a *community* is more commonly defined as a group or collection of people who live in a specified geographic area that is of a limited size.[7] For example, although one can refer to the community of St. Louis, the home base of the publisher of this book, one would not refer to the public of St. Louis.

Another concept of community is a group or collection of people having similar attributes.[7] For example, although one can refer to a community of dentists, dental hygienists, or dental assistants, one would not refer to a public of those professions. Another meaning of community is that of a particular location in which someone lives. For example, one might ask someone in which community she or he lives, but it would not make sense to ask someone in which public she or he lives.[7]

Oral Health

This book also has in its title the term *dental health.* The term *oral health* has recently come into greater prominence and is replacing in certain instances the term *dental health.* Although the terms *dental* and *oral* in regard to health still are being used interchangeably, use of the term *dental* is still more common. That may not be the case in the future. The use of the term *oral* will most likely continue to increase because the term *dental,* in the eyes of the public, is limited primarily to the teeth. The term *oral,* however, refers to not only the teeth and gingivae and their supporting tissues and bone but also the hard and soft palate, the lining of the mouth, the throat, the tongue, the lips, the salivary glands, the masticator muscles, the lower and upper jaws, and the temporomandibular joints.[14]

The Public's Perspective on Public Health

What much of the public, including many in the clinical health professions, does not realize is that public health has been primarily responsible for the most dramatic and significant improvements in the health of the U.S. population. Since 1900 the average life expectancy of persons in the United States has increased by more than 30 years, with 25 of those years (83%) being attributed to advances in public health. The Centers for Disease Control and Prevention (CDC) selected a public health "top 10 list" for the twentieth century. Fluoridation of drinking water, which was initiated in 1945, is on the list because it has played an important role in the reduction of tooth decay in children (40% to 70%) and of tooth loss in adults (40% to 60%) in the United States. The other nine are vaccinations, motor-vehicle safety, safer workplaces, control of infectious diseases, decline in deaths from coronary heart disease and stroke, safer and healthier foods, healthier mothers and babies, family planning, and recognition of tobacco use as a health hazard.[15]

Thus public health practitioners must

face the reality that the public has a limited understanding of the role and function of public health. A major reason for this is that when public health is functioning optimally, it is invisible. For example, when a person eats at a restaurant in the United States and does not get sick, turns on the tap to get a drink of water and out comes uncontaminated water, walks outside and breathes the air and does not choke, walks into a building and does not become enveloped by secondhand smoke, he or she probably does not think of it, but the reality is that public health has been doing its job. The public takes for granted a safe water supply, that food is not contaminated, that garbage is collected, and that a system safely removes and treats human waste. When we eat at restaurants, we expect that someone has established food safety standards and that the restaurant has been inspected to ensure that those standards have been met. And we expect that a monitoring system is in place to detect outbreaks of disease in case of a breakdown in the established standards of hygiene.

In 1996 a poll conducted by Louis Harris and Associates found that few Americans have any real idea what the term *public health* means. When, however, its meaning was explained to them, "almost everyone believed it to be very important."[16]

Although media coverage of public health issues has continually increased, the stories are rarely labeled as public health stories and most people do not recognize them as such. Even though the stories deal with obvious public health problems such as acquired immunodeficiency syndrome (AIDS), food-borne diseases, lead or mercury poisoning, harmful drug interactions, or polluted air, most people do not recognize them as public health stories because of the multidisciplinary nature of the field and the complex ethical and political issues that are inherently part of each story.[17]

Regardless of the definition of public health, a lack of understanding associated with it will continue. One way to more clearly explain public health and to describe its mission and purpose is by indicating that public health[18]

- Prevents epidemics and the spread of disease
- Protects against environmental hazards
- Prevents injuries
- Promotes and encourages healthy behaviors
- Responds to disasters and assists communities in recovery
- Ensures the quality and accessibility of health services

More specifically, public health is less food poisoning because of food inspection programs, less death and disability from car accidents because of requirements for seat belts and air bags, less lung cancer because of smoking cessation programs, less heart disease because of public education regarding diet and blood pressure screening, less childhood disease because of immunization programs, fewer infant deaths because of prenatal care programs, and fewer dental caries because of water fluoridation.

WHAT IS DENTAL PUBLIC HEALTH?

Dental public health is a field of study within the broader field of public health. Its philosophy and substance reflect public health and its focus on the community rather than on the individual patient. An early dental public health worker, J. W. Knutson, defined public health as follows:

> Public health is people's health. It is concerned with the aggregate health of a group, a community, a state, or a nation. Public health in accordance

with this broad definition is not limited to the health of the poor, or to rendering health services or to the nature of the health problems. Nor is it defined by the method of payment for health services, or by the type of agency responsible for supplying those services. It is simply a concern for and activity directed toward the improvement and protection of the health of a population group in the aggregate.[19]

As applied to dentistry, this definition implies that dental public health is concerned only with the dental health of aggregate populations and not individuals. Now is a good time to reevaluate definitions such as these and amend them to more accurately reflect that individuals, as well as groups, are of concern to the activities and interests of public health. A modification of Knutson's definition to include this concept would be the following: Dental public health is a concern for and activity directed toward the improvement and promotion of the dental health of the population as a whole, as well as of individuals within that population. This expanded concept of public health to include a focus on individuals recently has been gaining increasing acceptance with the emergence of the term the *new public health,* in which the traditional conception of public health is expanded to include "the health of the individual in addition to the health of populations."[9]

As with the more general term *public health,* a better-understood explanation of dental public health may be best achieved by giving specific examples. Dental public health is less tooth decay because of fluoridated water and school fluoride programs, less periodontal disease because of public education programs, greater access to high-quality early diagnosis and treatment of dental disease because of dental care delivery programs and research, less tooth damage among athletes because of mouthguard programs, and less oral cancer because of tobacco cessation and cancer screening programs.

The ADA has recognized dental public health as one of nine specialties of dentistry. The American Board of Dental Public Health (ABDPH), which is the regulatory agency for the specialty, was established in 1954. Dental public health's mission is set forth in the definition adopted by the ABDPH. It is a modification of the previously mentioned Winslow definition of public health.[11] The ABDPH defined *dental public health* as

[T]he science and art of preventing and controlling dental disease and promoting dental health through organized community efforts. It is that form of dental practice that serves the community as a patient rather than the individual. It is concerned with the dental health education of the public, with research and the application of the findings of research, with the administration of programs of dental care for groups, and with the prevention and control of dental disease through a community approach.[19a]

Dental public health, like public health, recently has expanded its focus to include the dental care delivery system and its impact on oral health status. The reason for this is that the development of alternative delivery systems such as dental health maintenance organizations, independent practice associations, point-of-service organizations, and preferred-provider organizations are having an increasing impact on the public's health. Public health's interest in access to comprehensive and quality dental care for the American public requires that attention be paid to the increased role of third-party payers (e.g., insurance companies, managed care plans) and the increasing emphasis on cost control.

In today's complex society, therefore,

dental health issues cannot be the exclusive concern of any one sector of dentistry. In view of current economic, political, and social factors, which are increasingly influencing the health services delivery system in the United States, dental public health, organized dentistry, and dental hygiene will of necessity find it mutually beneficial to work together more closely because the overall mission of these groups is the same: optimal dental health for all Americans and universal access to comprehensive care.

PUBLIC HEALTH PRACTICE

Two themes determine public health practice: the scientific knowledge regarding the causes and control of disease and the belief of the public that the disease can be controlled and that doing so is a public responsibility.[1] An early example in this country of the importance of both of these themes is Lemuel Shattuck's *Report on the Sanitary Conditions of Massachusetts*. This report was published in 1850 and is considered one of the most important documents in the history of public health in the United States.[1,8] The scientific basis in Shattuck's report consisted of vital statistics that demonstrated differences in disease rates in different communities. Although he considered that individual behavior was responsible in part for these differences, he argued that because the larger community could be affected, as well as the individual, public action was necessary. It was not until after the Civil War that increased public acceptance of the government's role developed, and Massachusetts established a state board of public health in 1869.[1] The Great Depression in the 1930s was another event that affected public health by altering the beliefs of people. The great social and economic insecurity during that period led people to look more to government to intervene in the social and economic structure of their lives.

A Report on the Future of Public Health

In 1988 the Institute of Medicine (IOM) published *The Future of Public Health*.[1] The report stated that public health in this country has deteriorated "like a two-lane highway in the shadow of an interstate." The landmark report declared the current system to be fragmented and rudderless to the point of "disarray" and exposed a litany of weaknesses, gaps, and challenges that threatened to overwhelm "this nation that has lost sight of its public health goals."[20] Part of the cause for the decline in public health has been that advances in technology and science over the past decades have led society to focus on diagnosis and cure of disease rather than a public health infrastructure that deals with community efforts aimed at the prevention of disease and promotion of health.

The major problems cited in the report that require public health action include the AIDS epidemic, pollution-related diseases, the surge in chronic diseases characteristic of an aging population, inadequate funding of public health agencies, and the growing health care needs of the indigent.

The IOM report identified three core public health functions: assessment, policy development, and assurance.[1] The American Public Health Association, the national organization that addresses issues of public health concern, delineated these three core functions as follows[21]:

- Assessment can be best understood as a process whereby factors that threaten the health of a population are identified, followed by a determination as to whether resources are available to effectively deal with the identified health problems. Public health agencies must assess personal health, environmental health, community concerns and resources, and data on the quality, range, and use of public and private medical and dental services.

- Policy development is the development of policy by public health agencies in response to specific community and national health needs. Public health agencies must develop comprehensive public health policies to improve health conditions, ensure that policies are politically and organizationally feasible, and respect community values; devise measurable objectives and implementation strategies; and identify resources needed to implement the health policies developed.
- Assurance means that public health agencies are responsible for seeing that conditions contributing to good health, including high-quality services, are available to all. These agencies also must provide essential public health and environmental health services; respond to personal and environmental health emergencies; administer quality assurance programs; and guarantee care for those not served in the current health care marketplace, including recruiting and retaining health care practitioners to provide appropriate services.[21,22]

With the increasing public health focus on chronic diseases and injury prevention, the assurance function has taken on a more prominent role in recent years. As we enter the twenty-first century, heart disease, stroke, and cancer are the leading causes of death in the United States, whereas pneumonia and tuberculosis led the list at the beginning of the twentieth century. Currently, public health efforts seek to reduce cigarette smoking and improve diet. Workplace safety has become an increasing concern for many occupational groups, such as convenience store clerks who are at high risk for violent attacks. The leading cause of death among children under age 14 in industrialized countries is preventable injuries.[23] Because automobile accidents are a major cause of death and injury, public health measures for "assuring conditions in which people can be healthy" include ensuring well-designed highways and cars and the use of seat belts.[1]

Impact of *The Future of Public Health* Report on Public Health Practice

The IOM report, *The Future of Public Health*, served as a catalyst to wake up and bring together the public health community at the federal, state, and local levels, along with other members of society concerned with the health of the public, in the realization that all was not well with the country's public health system. Arguably, the report's most important contribution was the development of the previously mentioned three core public health functions of assessment, policy development, and assurance.

Since publication of the IOM report, a number of agencies and organizations have worked to respond to the problems and recommendations in the report. This section traces some of the responses devised by these groups. Immediately recognizing the value of these core functions, the CDC, a federal agency in the Department of Health and Human Services (DHHS), created the Public Health Practice Program Office (PHPPO) in 1989 for the purpose of further clarifying the role of public health agencies in addressing the core functions.

Soon after its formation, the PHPPO convened a meeting of representatives from the major public health organizations: the Association of State and Territorial Health Officials (ASTHO), American Public Health Association (APHA), National Association of County and City Health Officials (NACCHO), Association of Schools of Public Health (ASPH), U.S. Conference of Local Health Officials (USCLHO), and Health Resources and Services Administration (HRSA). Their task was to clarify and describe the local public health agency activities that are necessary to ensure that the three core functions of public health are implemented. The deliberations of these organizations led to the following set of 10 organizational practices, organized under the three core public health functions[24,25]:

1. Assessment
   a. Assess the health needs of the community
   b. Investigate the occurrence of health effects and hazards in the community
   c. Analyze the determinants of identified health needs
2. Policy development
   a. Advocate for public health, build constituencies, and identify resources in the community
   b. Set priorities among health needs
   c. Develop plans and policies to address priority health needs
3. Assurance
   a. Manage resources and develop organizational structure
   b. Implement programs
   c. Evaluate programs and provide quality assurance
   d. Inform and educate the public

Dental Public Health's Response to Public Health Core Functions

A work group of dental public health leaders was convened by the CDC and the Association of State and Territorial Dental Directors (ASTDD) in 1993 to elaborate on the three core public health functions for dental health. The group developed the following functions[26]:

1. Assessment
   a. Establish and maintain a **state-based oral health surveillance system** for ongoing monitoring, timely communication of findings, and the use of data to initiate and evaluate intervention.
2. Policy development
   a. Provide **leadership** to address oral health problems with a full-time state dental director and an adequately staffed oral health unit with competence to perform public health functions.
   b. Develop and maintain a **state oral health improvement plan** and, through a collaborative process, select appropriate strategies for target populations, establish integrated interventions, and set priorities.
   c. Develop and promote **policies** for better oral health and to improve health systems.
3. Assurance
   a. Provide oral health **communications and education** to policy makers and the public to increase awareness of oral health issues.
   b. Build **linkages** with partners inter-

ested in reducing the burden of oral diseases by establishing a state oral health advisory committee, community coalitions, and governmental work groups.

c. Integrate, coordinate, and implement **population-based intervention** for effective primary and secondary prevention of oral diseases and conditions.
d. Build **community capacity** to implement community-level interventions.
e. Develop **health system interventions** to facilitate quality dental care services for the general and vulnerable populations.
f. Leverage **resources** to adequately fund public health functions.

Public Health Functions Steering Committee

By 1993 public health leaders had realized that although the three core functions of public health were widely accepted in the public health community, they had failed to communicate public health's role to elected officials, policy makers, and the public. To remedy that, public health officials decided that public health needed a list of essential public health services. In 1993 and 1994 the Public Health Service convened the Public Health Functions Steering Committee. The committee included representatives of federal, national, state, and local public health agencies. In 1995 the committee released a document, "Public Health in America," that specified the following 10 essential public health services[2,27]:

1. Monitor health status to identify community health problems.
2. Diagnose and investigate health problems and health hazards in the community.
3. Inform, educate, and empower people about health issues.
4. Mobilize community partnerships to identify and solve health problems.
5. Develop policies and plans that support individual and community health efforts.
6. Enforce laws and regulations that protect health and ensure safety.
7. Link people to needed personal health services and ensure the provision of health care when otherwise unavailable.
8. Ensure a competent public health and personal health care workforce.
9. Evaluate effectiveness, accessibility, and quality of personal and population-based health services.
10. Conduct research toward new insights and innovative solutions to health problems.

In 1997 the ASTDD developed a comparable set of 14 essential state dental public health services to promote oral health in the United States.[28]

The 1995 Institute of Medicine Follow-up Report

In 1995 the IOM formed the Committee on Public Health to determine the progress made since the release of its 1988 report. To assist the committee, the IOM assembled a panel of people from government, academia, industry, and citizen and other private sector groups. After a 9-month period of study, the IOM published a report detailing the committee's analysis of the progress made since the 1988 report was published.[29] This report concluded that since 1988 a significant strengthening of public health practice in governmental public health agencies and in other settings had occurred. In addition, however, the committee "encountered evidence that many of the problems identified in the *Future of Public Health* were still with us."[29]

National Public Health Performance Standards

In 1997 the IOM published *Performance Monitoring to Improve Community Health,* which promoted the use of performance measures, standards, and monitoring to help ensure that needed public health functions are provided.[30,31]

In that same year the Public Health Practice Program Office at the CDC, in partnership with the major national public health organizations, began a new initiative, the National Public Health Performance Standards Program. The purpose of this initiative was to advance the capacity of public health agencies to better address the public health weaknesses highlighted in the *Future of Public Health* report.[32-34] The Standards Program will focus on the following goals: (1) improve quality and performance, (2) increase accountability, and (3) increase the science base for public health practice.[32]

Institute of Medicine Year 2000 Study of Public Health

In March 2001 a report prepared by the CDC for the U.S. Senate was released. The report found that the U.S. public health infrastructure is insufficient to protect Americans from emerging threats. The CDC proposed a major national initiative linking local, state, and federal agencies to address gaps in the public health workforce's capacity and competency, information and data systems, and organizational capacities of local and state health departments and laboratories. The *public health infrastructure* is defined as the underlying foundation that supports the planning, delivery, and evaluation of public health activities.[35]

This report, in asserting that the nation's current public health system could not protect Americans from emerging threats, was proved unfortunately to be prescient. This deterioration, which had been virtually overlooked by much of the country, was suddenly placed in the national spotlight on September 11, 2001. On that day, the United States was suddenly and deliberately attacked by terrorists who flew two airplanes into New York's World Trade Center, resulting in the collapse of its Twin Towers, and another plane into the Pentagon in Washington, D.C.[36]

Unfortunately, it had to take September 11 and the subsequent days of public anxiety caused by the fear of future biological attacks for the state of the nation's public health system to be questioned. It has become apparent that the system is not sound and lacks support. We must acknowledge the need of repair immediately. Only time will tell whether the impact of 9/11 will result in the revitalization of public health.[36a]

Since 1988 several other public health threats have emerged. Among these are the following[20]:

- New and reemerging infectious diseases (e.g., a resurgence of tuberculosis), which have been identified as an urgent public health problem demanding a response that may be beyond the financial means of many public health

agencies. A number of these diseases have become resistant to antibiotics, threatening to reverse hard-won gains.
- The rising tide of violence that has come to be viewed as a major public health problem.
- An antiregulatory movement that has been sweeping through Washington, threatening government's ability to enforce standards and regulations, especially in the areas of environmental and occupational health and safety.
- Food-borne and waterborne microbes going undetected and environmental hazards not addressed.

Dental Public Health Response to *The Future of Public Health*

Leaders in the dental public health community recognized that the important pronouncements contained in the IOM report also applied to dental public health.[1] As a result, an in-depth review of dental public health's origins, scope of responsibilities, and future challenges and roles was included. The findings from this review were published in *The Future of Dental Public Health Report*. In response to the question "Where does dental public health stand today?" the report acknowledged that the current environment in which federal, state, and local dental health programs exist is conflicting, inconsistent, and infused with ambiguous policies. Although the oral health needs are documented with persistent and emerging oral health problems, oral health is given a low priority by health planners. The report states that the contributions of dental public health professionals are not well understood by either the dental profession or the broad field of public health. The report suggests that dental public health leadership "must strive to articulate the public's oral health needs more clearly to dental, public health and health policy makers."[37] The following five interrelated goals are recommended for dental public health as a pathway to improved effectiveness[37]:

1. Earn support from the public.
2. Earn support from policy makers.
3. Earn support from program administrators.
4. Earn support from the dental community.
5. Ensure recruitment and professional development of dental public health personnel.

Elements for Successful Public Health Programs

Public health successes include reductions in lead poisoning, traffic fatalities, smoking, and dental caries. Although much is still to be accomplished in regard to these successes, they are the result not of dental or medical technology but of social, behavioral, and environmental change. Issacs and Schroeder[38] have suggested four elements responsible for successful public health programs:

- The need to have highly credible scientific evidence that can persuade policy makers and withstand attack from those whose interests are threatened.
- The need for passionately dedicated advocates committed to solving a public health problem who can withstand the tremendous pressure applied by those who are not committed to solving the problem.

- The need for a strong partnership with the media because it is only through the media that the public can be reached sufficiently to express its support of solving a public health problem.
- The realization that laws and regulations at the state, local, and especially federal levels of government have been critical elements in addressing and solving public health problems. Despite all the criticism that has been directed at governmental regulation, it is that regulation which has significantly improved people's health. Regulations will continue to be "the underpinning that protects the health of the American public."[38]

PREVENTION IN PUBLIC HEALTH PRACTICE

Prevention has always been the bedrock of public health practice. The essence of public health will continue to remain what it has been for the past 2000 years: prevention rather than cure. The Roman poet Ovid best captured this essence 2000 years ago when he wrote, "Resist beginnings: the prescription comes too late when the disease has gained strength by long delays."[39]

Prevention can be viewed from a three-tiered perspective: (1) primary prevention seeks to avoid the occurrence of an illness or injury by preventing exposure to risk factors; (2) secondary prevention attempts to minimize the severity of the illness or the damage because of an injury-causing event once it has occurred; and (3) tertiary prevention attempts to limit the disability resulting from an injury or disease. Using oral cancer prevention as an example, primary prevention would include efforts to discourage teenagers from smoking or chewing tobacco. Secondary prevention would include screening programs to detect cancer early, so treatment can be initiated to reduce the effect of the disease. Tertiary prevention would involve the rehabilitation of cancer patients.[17]

Another approach to developing intervention programs is to consider a disease or injury as a result of a chain of causal events involving an agent, a host, and the environment. In regard to dental caries, for example, the agent is a disease-causing microorganism, the host is a susceptible person, and the environment includes the means of transmission by which the agent reaches the host. Prevention can be accomplished by breaking the chain of causation at any of these stages.[17]

RECENT DEVELOPMENTS IN DENTAL PUBLIC HEALTH PRACTICE

EVIDENCE-BASED PUBLIC HEALTH PRACTICE

Since the publication of the last edition of this book, the term *evidence-based practice* has been adopted, popularized, and incorporated within both dental and medical practice, as well as within public health practice. The major reason for the increasing popularization of the term is the increasing belief that clinical practice was too often based on opinions and not on demonstrated effectiveness and knowledge that benefits outweigh harms. Evidence-based care is the integration of clinical judgment with the best available research and evidence and the patient's values in making clinical decisions.[40]

The goal of evidence-based practice is to facilitate the timely and appropriate translation into practice of research findings that results in improved practice outcomes. Evidence-based practice incorporates the judicious use of the best evidence available from systematic reviews, when possible, with knowledge of patients' preferences and practitioners' experiences, to make recommendations for the processing of the right care for the right patient at the right time.[41,42]

The current belief that too many procedures and programs have been based on insufficient evidence makes it highly likely that the term will continue to gain increasing acceptance in public health. The expectation is that use of an evidence-based approach will improve the health return on investments, improve the nation's health, and reduce expenditures for interventions that are found to be ineffective.[43]

POPULATION HEALTH

The term *population health* has been increasingly appearing in the literature. Although the dictionary definition of *population* is similar to that of *public,* and one could correctly equate the terms *public health* and *population health,*[7,44] the word *population* often is used in connection with the clinical care setting, such as in the phrase "population-based health services." In this context it describes services in the clinical setting that are focused on improving the health status of the public, rather than on the actual treatment of that population. These services include "health promotion, community health protection, personal prevention and assistance in gaining access to care."[45,46]

The term *population health* is also now being used in the public health setting because of the increasing awareness that, depending on the identified public health problem, the selected intervention should be targeted at the appropriate population, be it at the systems, community, or individual level. For example, the level at which the intervention would be targeted would depend on which level is determined to be the most effective and efficient way to prevent or reduce the problem. At the systems level, a population-based intervention would focus on creating changes in organizations, policies, laws, and structures and would not focus directly on individuals or communities but rather on the systems that serve them. Changing the system often offers a long-lasting and cost-effective way to have the greatest impact on the individuals who collectively form the community. An example of such an intervention is water fluoridation.

A population-based approach at the community level would focus on creating change in communities and would be directed toward groups of persons within the community or, at times, toward all persons in the community. An example of such an intervention is a school dental sealant program.

A population-based approach at the individual level would focus on creating improvements in the health status of individuals, either singly, in families, or in groups. An example of such an intervention is the distribution of fluoride mouth rinses to any child who lacks access to a public fluoridated water supply.[47,48]

FOCUS ON HEALTH CARE AT THE EXPENSE OF PUBLIC HEALTH

In 1977 Dever[49] proposed a model for developing health policy that incorporated a broader concept of health that included, in addition to the system of health care organization, lifestyle (self-created risks), environmental risk, and human biology. Dever was concerned with the apparent mismatch of public resources expended on health care–related activities and factors contributing most prominently to morbidity and mortality. He noted that the United States focused most of its health resources on health care despite the extensive role that these other factors played in the level of health of its population. Although more than two decades have passed since Dever's observations were made, they remain valid.[50]

A 1990 analysis of causes of death in the United States found that the role of lifestyle in mortality rate had changed little since 1977. Half of all deaths could still be attributed to tobacco, diet and activity patterns, alcohol, microbial agents, toxic agents, firearms, sexual behavior, motor vehicles, and illicit drug use. With health resources continuing to be focused on personal health care, the mismatch between resources and health determinants continues. When it is noted that less than 1% of the aggregate amount for all health care in the United States is spent on population-based public health activities, the mismatch is even more extensive than many may realize.[50] Public health receives only 3% of the total health dollar.[51]

DENTAL PUBLIC HEALTH PRACTICE

As previously mentioned, prevention is the bedrock of public health practice, and it is also the foundation for the practice of dental public health. Dental public health practitioners share the belief that the public's dental health "can be improved by altering conditions—behavior, the environment, biological interactions, and the organization of services—that might otherwise, at a future time, have an adverse impact on health."[8] The practice of dental public health requires a set of methods and skills to make that belief a reality. This section describes how those who practice dental public health seek to accomplish their goals. Dental public health practice can be considered as engaging in the processes and activities required to carry out the three previously mentioned IOM core public health functions: assessment, policy development, and assurance. To address and respond to those core functions, three categories of management-related activities have been identified: program planning, implementation, and evaluation.[9,52]

PROGRAM PLANNING (See Chapter 13)

Planning is the process of establishing goals and objectives then determining the optimal course of action to achieve them.[53] Dunning[54] has raised a number of important questions that should be addressed if a program is to be planned effectively:

1. What are the dental needs of the community or population?
2. How extensive is the demand for dental treatment in the population?
3. What dental personnel are available to serve the population, and what is the political climate in regard to the type of staffing that can be used?
4. What is the prevailing philosophy of the people regarding the extent of health care they expect to receive and the manner in which they are willing to receive it?
5. To what extent will the prevention of disease obviate the need for treatment? If preventive measures could accomplish this goal, would they be acceptable for a particular society or segment of society?
6. What scope of service will be offered in a public program, who will receive the service, and in what manner will the service be delivered?
7. How can the service be adjusted to the mores of the population?

A similar approach to planning has been devised by the WHO Expert Committee on Dental Health. The committee identified six phases of planning that should be followed in this sequence: (1) collection of preliminary information, (2) establishment of priorities, (3) selection of targets and objectives, (4) consultation and coordination, (5) drafting of the plan, and (6) periodic assessment and readjustment. Those planning a program should view a perceived dental health problem within the context of the prevailing health problems and the overall situation of the respective country, region, or community.[55,56]

Program Implementation

The implementation phase is comparable to the leading organization and directing aspects of the management process. Implementation essentially involves the design and development of the organizational structure that will be used to carry out the plan.[57]

Program Evaluation

Evaluation is comparable to the monitoring or controlling function in the management process. It attempts to determine whether the problem has been improved by the implementation of the program and whether progress has been made toward the stated goals. Action should be taken to correct any performance that impedes that progress. Program evaluation is required if one is to know what, if anything, the program has accomplished, whether the objectives have been achieved, and to what extent the program has contributed to the improvement of the dental health of the community (see Chapter 14). Without information regarding conditions that existed before a program has begun (baseline information), it is not possible to determine the program's impact.[58]

The main criteria for evaluation of dental health programs include the following:

1. *Effectiveness.* Has the stated objective been attained?
2. *Efficiency.* How much has the attainment of the stated objective cost, and how did that cost compare with the anticipated costs?
3. *Appropriateness.* Has priority been given to the most useful strategy for the attainment of the stated objectives, and is the strategy acceptable?
4. *Adequacy.* Has the program addressed the overall health problem, or was it directed at only part of it? Did the program equitably address the needs of all segments of the population?

From a public health perspective it is important to understand that quality of dental care is not just the quality of individual services. Schonfeld[59] has suggested that four levels be used to evaluate the quality of dental care programs: the first would evaluate the provided individual restoration, procedure, or service; the second would evaluate the impact of that procedure or service on the overall health of the mouth; the third would consider the patient's total oral health and the influence that dental care has had on the attitude toward dentistry and on dental-related behavior; and the fourth would look at the family and the community, evaluate the level of dental care provided for groups and communities, and determine the number and social distribution of persons receiving adequate dental care.[59]

A continuing system of evaluation can indicate the following:

1. Whether the prevalence of dental disease is changing
2. Whether existing disease is being treated at a greater or lesser rate than new disease is occurring
3. If any groups in the community are not receiving the appropriate level of care that is needed
4. If providers of services are performing at acceptable levels
5. Whether the provided preventive or educational measures are effective in reducing needs or promoting demands for treatment[60]

Dental Public Health Practitioners

People who are interested in careers and leadership roles in dental public health should be knowledgeable in both oral health practice and dental public health. Most dental public health practitioners are initially educated as dentists or dental hygienists then pursue graduate-level training in dental public health. Dental public health training programs are offered primarily at schools of public health and schools of dentistry. A committee established by the American Board of Dental Public Health has developed competency objectives for dental public health specialists. The objectives fall within four overall categories: (1) health policy and program management and administration, (2) research methods in dental public health, (3) oral health promotion and disease, and (4) oral health services delivery systems.[61-63]

The specific areas of knowledge and expertise, aside from those in oral health, include planning, implementation, operation, and evaluation of dental public health programs; the policy-making process; regulation; management information systems; human resources management; financial management; marketing; communications; quality assurance; and risk management.[61-63]

Contrast between Clinical and Dental Public Health Practice

The question often is asked, "What are the differences between clinical dental practice and dental public health practice?" Box 1-1 indicates the major conceptual differences. Although differences exist between clinicians treating individual patients and public health workers who deal primarily with populations, the interdependence of these groups cannot be overemphasized.

Public Health Perspective on Dental Disease

To better understand the public health perspective on dental disease, one should keep in mind that a treatment component is an essential element of any dental public health program. This is the case because dental diseases are generally not self-curing. Although preventive procedures are highly successful in reducing the prevalence and incidence of the major dental diseases, prevention has not been able to eliminate them. A comprehensive public health program therefore includes both a preventive and a treatment component.[64]

At least three unique characteristics of the two most common dental diseases of the mouth, dental caries and periodontal disease, are important to consider: (1) they are of almost universal prevalence; (2) after they progress to a certain point they gener-

BOX 1-1

Contrasting Aspects of Dental and Dental Public Health Models of Practice

Dental Model	Dental Public Health Model
Purpose: to maximize the dental interests of individual patients	Purpose: to maximize the dental health status of a population, community, or public
Work content: to provide personal dental health services for patients to improve their dental health	Work content: to develop, implement, and evaluate dental health programs and to create health services for improving the public's oral health
Practitioner is concerned with risk-benefit calculus for individual patients	Practitioner is concerned with relative cost benefits of different community interventions or strategies
Practitioner's primary moral obligation is to individual patients	Practitioner is obliged to think in terms of how best to allocate community resources
The ideal is the provision of state-of-the-art services	The use of appropriate technology, which may not be state-of-the-art
Patient-specific needs are relevant for decision making	Population-based measures of need are of primary importance
Outcomes are measured in terms of changes in individual patients	Outcomes are measured in terms of community change

Modified from Gray BH: *Milbank Q* 70:535, 1992.

ally do not undergo remission or termination if left untreated, but accumulate to result in a backlog of unmet needs; and (3) they usually require technically demanding, expensive, and time-consuming professional treatment. Both clinicians and nondental public health practitioners frequently underestimate the importance of these characteristics.[64]

At a forum held in 1994 on the occasion of World Health Day/The Year of Oral Health, Richard L. Wittenberg, the president and chief executive officer of the American Association for World Health, stated that "for too long oral health has been a topic overlooked or dismissed as a secondary health issue." He called for raising the awareness of critical and oral health issues and motivating change in communities across the United States. He cited the following facts that he said "were staring us in the face":[65]

- More than 20 million U.S. workdays are lost annually because of oral disease or the need for dental care.
- Each year, 8600 people die as a result of oral cancer, much of which should be preventable.
- Early childhood caries is preventable but still affects thousands of young children because of lack of awareness of proper infant feeding.
- The elderly have special oral health needs and are vulnerable to periodontal disease and oral cancers.
- Many populations in the United States do not have access to fluoridated water,

a highly effective means of preventing tooth decay.
- Dental sealants can be nearly 100% effective in preventing dental decay but are woefully underused.

After these comments, Carlyle Guerra de Macedo, then the director of the Pan American Health Organization (PAHO), pointed out that oral health's role as an integral part of general wellness has been long overlooked by the citizens of the world. Because health encompasses more than just the absence of disease, the maintenance of good oral health in relation to the entire healthy self should be stressed. Yet in the case of oral health, preventive measures have not been implemented to their fullest potential, even though relatively small investments would yield lifelong benefits.[65]

Approximately 150 million Americans lack dental insurance, an important factor in seeking care. Although the overall dental health of Americans has improved significantly since the 1960s, low-income populations continue to have high levels of dental disease. Large disparities continue to exist, as evidenced by the following key dental health indicators: untreated tooth decay, restricted activity days because of pain and discomfort from oral health problems, and tooth loss. Low-income children and adults continue to experience higher levels of dental disease and use dental care less frequently than higher-income people do. In 1996, for example, 28% of low-income people reported making a visit to the dentist in the preceding year, compared with 56% of high-income people.[66] Approximately 40% of Americans do not visit the dentist each year, and a much larger percentage do not receive what the readers of this book would call comprehensive care. One of the primary missions of dental public health is addressing these inequities in our society.[65]

PUBLIC HEALTH PERSPECTIVE ON THE USE AND DELIVERY OF DENTAL SERVICES

Several important distinctions, especially concerning dental care, exist in regard to the need for care, the demand for care, and the actual use of services. A dental need is considered to exist when an individual has dental disease, although the individual may not perceive this need. A demand for care exists when an individual perceives a need for and wishes to receive care, even though that person may not actually obtain treatment. Use occurs only when the individual actually receives care. Sheiham's concept of need and demand considers that one may perceive a need, may desire that the need be treated, and then, in an attempt to make a demand on the delivery system, find the system unable or unwilling to provide treatment.[67] For example, the individual may not be able to afford care, an available source of care may not exist, or the provider might not accept the individual for treatment.

As stated, a major concern of public health is the issue of access to care and the fact that access to health services is not equitably distributed among population groups in this country. This has been especially true in regard to the delivery of dental services. Access to basic medical and dental care for all our citizens is still not a reality. The uneven distribution of health services hits the poor and minorities hardest, with substantial numbers of underserved people "who are different ethnically from the controlling group."[14] The United States and

South Africa are the only developed countries with no national policy ensuring that all citizens have access to health care.

The term *rationing* has been used in regard to limiting the distribution and allocation of health services. Aside from the Oregon Health Program, there is currently no official government policy to ration care. The term *de facto rationing,* however, is being used to describe situations in which care is denied or not provided because of economic or social factors that are brought about by the nature of society and its health care system.[68] That term can be applied to the United States to describe the situation in which millions of Americans do not get the care that they need. Although the term *rationing* has to date been applied primarily to medical services, it should not be long before it begins appearing in the dental literature.[69]

Forms of Dental Health Services

Historically, dental health services in the United States have been classified into three groups:

1. Services provided by dental health personnel and financed by the patient or a source other than the government
2. Services provided by nongovernment dental personnel partly or entirely remunerated by the government
3. Services provided by dental personnel employed by the government, such as military personnel

The prevailing philosophy in the United States continues to place the primary responsibility for health and the acquisition of health services on the individual and not on society, even though increased involvement for payment by the federal, state, and local governments has occurred. In the 1940s the ADA established the Council on Dental Health. One of the fundamental principles formulated by a council subcommittee was that the responsibility for the health of the people of the United States is first that of the individual, then the community, then the state, and last the nation.[70] This attitude that the individual has the first responsibility contrasts with an attitude in European countries suggesting that society as a whole is responsible. By the 1970s state-operated social programs were the norm in Europe. Some suggest that the catastrophic events Europe experienced, primarily the effects of two wars in the first half of the twentieth century, hastened the development of social welfare programs in European countries. The United States largely escaped the physical and social devastation of those wars.[71,72]

Impact of Health Care Reform and Managed Care on Public Health

During the past 15 years an evolving revolution has occurred in the financing and delivery of health care services. Although this revolution to date has affected medicine and public health significantly more than it has dentistry and dental public health, this change has increasingly affected dentistry.

The revolution has involved the increasing movement toward a health care system driven by market forces. The initial projection was that the majority of Americans would be enrolled in managed care plans in which one of the emerging integrated health systems would manage the care of their subscribers primarily under a capitated payment system. Under such a payment system, unlike that of a fee-for-service system, a predetermined payment is made to the integrated health system, which essentially agrees to provide all needed health services. Under the fee-for-service system, payment is made only for those services that have been provided. By 1999 approximately 92% of persons with employer-sponsored health insurance coverage were enrolled in managed care plans.[72a]

What had not been projected is that there would later be a diminishing interest in a capitated payment system and an increasing interest in a modified fee-for-service system. It was also not projected that there would be a reversal from more restrictive to less restrictive plans.[72b,72c]

What is ironic about this reversal from the public health policy perspective is that the very mechanisms that were put into place to hold down health care costs are the ones that are now opposed by both consumers and providers.[72d] As health policy analyst Drew Altman suggested, the American people "want to have their cake and eat it too. At the same time, they are demanding forms of managed care that are least able to control health care spending."[72b]

The theory underlying capitated plans was that organizations providing care under a capitated system become accountable for the health and wellness of their subscribers. Theoretically, the healthier their subscribers, the fewer services required and the less it costs the health care plan. If these plans are to be accountable for the health and financial risks associated with the community of the individuals they enroll, the plans will be required to manage the care of their "communities," or population of subscribers.

The concept of health care providers managing the health and health care of a population is a relatively new one for providers but a traditional one for public health. The management of a population's health requires the skills and competencies encompassed within the public health disciplines, such as epidemiology, administration, environmental health, biostatistics, health services research, and health education. In fact, the skills and competencies of the public health disciplines are the basic tools for assessing the health needs of populations, developing programs of intervention, and evaluating their costs, efficacy, and outcomes.[73]

However, at the same time that health care plans are employing public health–trained personnel and focusing more on the health status of their subscribers, concern is developing that this focus will be directed only at those aspects of health that have an impact on the bottom line of the plan's financial statement, rather than on a concern for all aspects of a population's health and environment (the focus of public health).[74]

The question that is most asked in regard to the role of public health in a managed care environment is, "Who will be responsible for maintaining the public's health?" Will it still be public health agencies, will it be integrated health care systems, or will it be a combination of both? It was stated earlier that the capitation system for paying for health care gives managed care organizations (e.g., health maintenance organizations [HMOs], the prototype of prepaid managed care plans) a potential interest in actively improving their enrollees' health status because the plans' expenses should be lower and their profits higher if the enrollees use fewer services. An HMO interested in truly taking responsibility for meeting its enrolled population's health needs could take a public health approach and address these needs as if they occurred in a community of enrollees, and focus on overall prevention.

Although prevention may pay in the longer run, it is an investment in the future; therefore it may be in a plan's interest to expend resources on keeping an enrollee healthy only if that enrollee remains with the plan long enough to allow the plan to realize savings from the reduced use of more expensive services. Prevention measures such as exercising, developing healthful eating habits, and dental health education require up-front investments that may not "pay off" until years later. Efforts to control more general public health problems such as community violence and reducing environmental hazards require complex and expensive programs that would benefit the entire community, as well as the plan's subscribers in a given community. In this type of situation the incentive for cooperative agreements between plans and public health agencies could exist. Although the potential exists for public health agencies and managed care organizations to develop closer working relationships, agencies that operate in the name of public health should be wary of delegating core functions and responsibilities to managed care organizations.[75]

The challenge facing the dental care delivery system will be no different than the one now facing the rest of the health care delivery system. The mandate in health care today is to realign economic incentives to produce fair prices, real value, reasonable profits, and predictable cost growth while improving or maintaining access to care, reducing inappropriate care, improving quality, and promoting optimal health. The challenge from a public health perspective is to ensure that access and quality are not sacrificed in the effort to control costs[76] (see Chapters 3 and 5).

PUBLIC HEALTH PROGRAMS

Achieving the overall mission of public health involves the activities of a broad spectrum of nongovernmental agencies, groups, organizations, and individuals. The governmental public health agency, however, has a unique and crucial role to play in ensuring that the vital elements are in place so that the public health mission can be adequately addressed and achieved.[1] For this reason the governmental role in public health receives the most emphasis in this chapter.

Government can be defined as "the formal institutions and processes through which binding decisions are made for a society."[77] Government is the institutions or processes by which individuals and groups within a society or state are controlled and regulated for various purposes, such as the common defense, general welfare, or internal peace. Virtually all political theorists have regarded government as indispensable for the functioning of society. James Madison, the fourth president of the United States, in his contention that a society could not exist without government, pointed out that the differing opinions, passions, and interests of individuals and groups inevitably create friction, conflict, and strife within society. As a result, government is needed to regulate and resolve these conflicts in an orderly and peaceful fashion.[78] Historical analyses make it clear that a society requires people to make and enforce decisions that affect conduct within that society.

Much has recently been publicly proclaimed about the evils and ineffectiveness of government, such as former President Ronald Reagan's statement that "government is not the solution to our problems, government is the problem." Whether one believes, as did patriot Thomas Paine, that government "is a necessary evil" or as Thomas Jefferson did that "that government is best which governs least," government is a vital part of every society.[78] Without government no effective means would exist of ensuring safe water, food, and products; controlling environmental hazards; licensure of health care providers; or police and fire protection. Without governmental involvement in public health, daily life could revert back to the days when sewage was running down the streets of our major cities. Without government public health anarchy would reign.[79,80]

No constitutionally defined role exists for the federal government in the maintenance of public health, and such activities have traditionally been the province of the states under their police power. Nonetheless, over the years a continuing gradual development of a federal presence in the health field has occurred. This has come about primarily because of (1) the responsibility for special population groups, such as merchant seamen, members of the armed forces, veterans, and Native Americans; (2) constitutional power to regulate interstate commerce, from which most of the regulatory power of the federal government in health is derived; (3) grants-in-aid to states and institutions for a wide variety of activities; and (4) sponsorship and financial participation in the payment for health services (for example, Medicaid and Medicare).[81,82] (See Appendix A for a description of the departments of the federal government.)

FEDERAL GOVERNMENT PROGRAMS

HEALTHY PEOPLE 2010

Beginning in 1979, the U.S Public Health Service adopted a management by objectives (MBO) approach to addressing public health problems. This MBO process requires the development of a set of measurable goals; using these goals as a guide to developing interventions, programs, and actions; and then regularly measuring the progress made during the process of achieving the goals.

The first set of goals to be developed was for the year 1990. These goals were published as *Healthy People: The Surgeon General's Report on Health Promotion and Disease Prevention.* A set of specific objectives directed toward meeting those goals was defined. The *Healthy People* planning process was designed to encourage states and local communities to use these national objectives as a basis for developing objectives of their own. In 1987 the Public Health Service began the process of setting objectives for the year 2000: *Healthy People 2000.* Most states subsequently developed their own 2000 objectives.

In 1995 the Public Health Service published a status report on the progress made toward the year 2000 goals. Of the 17 *Healthy People 2000* oral health objectives, the only one that has been met was the reduction of deaths from oral and pharyngeal cancers. Progress was made in the majority of the objectives, and the decline in dental decay among 15-year-olds nearly met the objective.[17,83]

The federal government has recently published its set of goals for the year 2010. These goals have been set at even higher levels than the year 2000 goals. *Healthy People 2010* for the first time establishes the nation's preventive agenda along with a scoreboard for monitoring health status. The publication has two broad types of objectives—measurable and developmental. The measurable objectives are similar to the majority of the preceding *Healthy People 2000* objectives, but they now have baselines and available data for national measurement purposes. The developmental objectives represent desired outcomes or health status for which current surveillance systems cannot yet provide data.

Healthy People 2010 has two major goals: to increase the quality and years of life and to eliminate health disparities. Unlike *Healthy People 2000, Healthy People 2010* includes a focus on infrastructure with the goal of ensuring the capacity to provide the essential public health services at the federal, state, and local levels so that the year 2010 goals can be accomplished.[24]

ORAL HEALTH OBJECTIVES AND HEALTHY PEOPLE 2010

Goal 21 of *Healthy People 2010* addresses oral health. The overall goal is to "prevent and control oral and cranial facial diseases, conditions, and injuries and improve access to related services." Goal 21 is based on the contentions that "Oral health is an essential of health throughout the life" and that "no one can be truly healthy unless he or she is free from the burden of oral health and craniofacial diseases and conditions."[24] Under Goal 21, 17 specific objectives were developed. Three examples of these objectives are presented here.

Objective 21-5 is to "reduce periodontal disease." Available research showed a baseline of 48% of 35- to 44-year-olds with gingivitis and 22% with destructive periodontal disease in the 1988–1994 baseline period. The target is to reduce these percentages from 48% to 41% for gingivitis and from 22% to 14% for destructive periodontal disease. Although the percentage reductions might appear modest, the effect of just a small percentage change would affect millions of people.

Objective 21-8 is to "increase the proportion of children who have received dental sealants on their molar teeth." The 1988–1994 baseline data indicate that the percentage of 8-year-olds with sealants was 23% and the percentage of 14-year-olds with sealants was only 15%. The target is to increase the percentages for both groups to 50% by 2010.

Objective 21-11 addresses the lack of dental care for the special population of those in long-term care institutions. The objective is to "increase the proportion of long-term care residents who use the oral health care system each year." Baseline data showed that only 19% of all nursing home residents received dental services in 1997. The target is to raise the percentage from 19% to 25%.[83]

FEDERAL AGENCIES

The beginnings of a formalized federal government role in public health began in 1798 in response to the expanding hazardous and unregulated maritime trade. In that year Congress passed a Marine Hospital Service Act for the relief of sick and disabled seamen. The sum of 20 cents per month was required to be paid to the government by ship owners for every seaman employed on their ships. This represented the first prepaid medical and hospital insurance plan in the world. This plan was under the administration of what eventually became a public health agency. In 1878 Congress passed the first port quarantine act. In 1902 Congress renamed the Marine Hospital Service the Public Health and Maritime Service and placed it under the director of the Surgeon General. In 1912 the Public Health and Maritime Service was renamed the Public Health Service. At that time Public Health Service involvement in public health was limited to research at its Hygiene Laboratory (predecessor of the National Institutes of Health), a small number of field epidemiologic studies, and direct care to merchant seamen through a network of hospitals and relief stations.[84] In 1912 the Army Dental Corps was established, and in 1913 the Navy Dental Corps was created. Also in 1913 the Department of the Interior initiated contractual arrangements with itinerant dentists to provide care on Indian reservations.[84]

In March 1919, after the end of World War I, veterans of that war were made a new category of federal beneficiary and were eligible to receive dental services from the Public Health Service. In June 1919 Dr. Ernest E. Buell, who had served as a major in the Army Dental Corps, became the first commissioned dentist in the Public Health Service and later the first Chief of the Dental Section.[84]

The U.S. Public Health Service Commissioned Corps should be distinguished from the current U.S. Public Health Service, an umbrella agency composed of eight constituent agencies. The U.S. Public Health Service Commissioned Corps is one of the seven uniformed services and is primarily composed of commissioned corps officers.[85]

Dentistry is 1 of 11 categories of health professionals in the U.S. Public Health Service Commissioned Corps, and dentists have been commissioned since 1919. Clinical positions available to entry-level dental officers are found in the Federal Bureau of Prisons (FBOP), the Indian Health Service (IHS), the National Health Service Corps (NHSC), and the U.S. Coast Guard (USCG).[86] Research, regulatory, and administrative programs are found in the National Institute of Dental Research (NIDR), the CDC, the Food and Drug Administration (FDA), and the Agency for Healthcare Research and Quality (AHRQ).[86]

A sign of progress made in the past 15 years is that dental hygienists can now be commissioned in the U.S. Public Health Service with a focus either on public health planning and evaluation activities or on the clinical treatment of patients and the implementation of community prevention and promotion programs. Dental hygienists in the U.S. Public Health Service Commissioned Corps come under the category of Health Service Officers, 1 of the 11 Public Health Service professional categories. Although a graduate degree is not required for the commissioning of a dental hygienist (the minimum academic requirement is a bachelor's degree), a master's degree is preferred for hygienists interested in working in a public health position.

FEDERALLY FUNDED HEALTH CENTERS

Dental health care programs that are part of neighborhood, rural, migrant, and homeless health centers—funded largely through federal dollars—have experienced extreme difficulties in recent years. Approximately half of these centers lack a dental program, and no standards have been established for preventive dental care for children. Between 1984 and 1989, the dental personnel at these centers declined by 11%, and approximately 60 centers previously offering dental services no longer provided them.[87]

FEDERALLY FUNDED DENTAL ACTIVITIES

Dental activities undertaken by the federal government can be placed in two categories and are distributed among the several agencies of the Department of Health and Human Services, which has been allocating approximately 1.25% of its budget for these activities.[88]

The first group of dental activities consists of programs that seek to improve the nation's capability to provide better oral health protection. They include biologic research, disease prevention and control, planning and development programs in dental labor, education and services research, and regulation and compliance functions such as quality assessment. These programs account for approximately 40% of the Department of Health and Human Services' dental budget. The remaining 60% is assigned to the second group, which includes those programs concerned with the provision of dental services.[88]

LEADERSHIP MEETING ON ORAL HEALTH

Leaders of both governmental and nongovernmental agencies and associations interested in addressing the nation's dental health problems and the dental health of the public realize that better coordination among the leaders from the communities of interest (including the public, professions, all levels of government, academia, business, and grant makers) is a necessity. Better coordination among federal health agencies is also a necessity.

A good start was made in an attempt to better achieve this goal when, in June 2000, the Deputy Secretary of the Department of Health and Human Services convened the "Leadership Meeting on Oral Health." At this meeting, dental health leaders gathered to discuss issues of mutual concern and to begin to address the need for better and more coordination and cooperative working agreements in order to solve dental public health problems. The attendees expressed agreement on the need for better coordination and in coordinated public-private partnerships. The goals of the meeting were as follows[89]:

- To acknowledge that disparities in oral health and access to care constitute both a personal health and public policy problem
- To explore facets of oral health with communities of interest
- To invite state government and private sector groups to partner with the Department of Health and Human Services in a coordinated campaign to improve the oral health of vulnerable populations, particularly low-income and special-needs children and the elderly

Although the initial meeting results showed promise, it is too soon to tell if this thoughtful and well-intentioned beginning will result in an ongoing and productive process.

ORAL HEALTH INITIATIVE

Recently, an initiative of two agencies in the U.S. Department of Health and Human Services—the Health Care Financing Administration (HCFA), now known as the Centers for Medicare and Medicaid Services (CMS), and the HSRA—has been in discussion. The purpose of the initiative would be to

- Strengthen public and private oral health delivery systems
- Enhance collaboration among Department of Health and Human Services agencies to maximize the effectiveness of dental Medicaid and Children's Health Insurance Programs (CHIP)
- Encourage the application of scientific advances to the practice of dentistry to reduce the burden of disease

Determining whether this initiative will achieve its mission and goals is not yet possible.[90]

U.S. SURGEON GENERAL'S PROPOSED NATIONAL ORAL HEALTH PLAN

In the first year of the new millennium, the U.S. Surgeon General released the first official and comprehensive report on oral, dental, and craniofacial health in the nation's history. The report alerts Americans to the full meaning of oral health and its importance to general health and well-being.[14,90a,90b]

The surgeon general, in his report to the nation, suggested the creation of a National Oral Health Plan "to eliminate oral health disparities and improve the quality of life by facilitating collaborations among individuals, health care providers, communities and policy makers at all levels of society and by taking advantage of existing initiatives."[14] For more information on the proposed plan, see Chapter 2. It is too soon to determine whether the National Oral Health Plan will come to fruition and if so whether it will achieve its goals.

Dental Activities of State and Local Public Health Agencies

Unfortunately, few national data exist on current activities of either the dental or medical activities of state and local health departments. The reason is that funding formerly available from the Public Health Service for collection of this information has been withdrawn.[91] Although all states have public health departments or agencies with responsibilities for state public health functions, not every state health agency has an oral health program. Nor have all state oral health programs sufficient resources to adequately address oral health needs. Only 30 states and 5 territories in the year 2000 had full-time dental directors. In 20 states the state dental director position was part time or vacant. Twenty-one had two or fewer full-time equivalents staffing their dental health programs. In 25 states, fewer than 10% of counties with local health departments had dental health programs.[14] At one time virtually all state health departments had a dentist directing their dental health programs. More recently, in addition to the downsizing of these state dental programs, few dentists have been directed to the programs. The status of dental public health programs at the state level indicates that the status of these programs has been on the decline in regard to staffing, organizational status, and financial and organizational support. Evidence unquestionably suggests that "state dental public health programs have been weakened by ever tightening budgets, poorly articulated oral health needs and priorities, and the failure to modify and integrate traditional dental program activities into more broadly based health programs."[37]

In 1995 the Association of State and Territorial Dental Directors published the *Future of Dental Public Health Report*. The report indicated that "little information had been gathered about local dental public health programs and that local programs varied widely across the nation, but a lack of data about them made generalization about differences, clientele served, population density, organizational structure, and funding difficult."[92] Over the years, however, the number of local dental public health programs has decreased significantly. A study of 150 local dental programs published in 1988 found that 20% reported that their dental program ranked "low" or "lowest" in the organizational structure in which they operated, and only 34% believed that their programs had a high priority in their organizations.[93] The most current data indicate that of the 50 states and the District of Columbia, 71% have full-time dental directors and 17% have part-time dental directors; in 11% the dental director's position is vacant.[94]

NONGOVERNMENTAL DENTAL PUBLIC HEALTH ORGANIZATIONS

Four national-level organizations exist whose primary mission is the advancement of dental public health:

American Association of Public Health Dentistry (AAPHD). This organization includes dental public health practitioners. AAPHD is affiliated with the American Dental Association.

Oral Health Section of the American Public Health Association (APHA). The APHA is the major national association for public health practitioners and is comparable to the American Dental Hygienists' Association and the American Dental Association. The section's membership is composed primarily of dental hygienists and dentists.

Association of State and Territorial Dental Directors (ASTDD). ASTDD's membership is composed of the dental directors of state and U.S. territorial health departments. The Surgeon General's Report acknowledged the important role of ASTDD in assessing the resources needed to achieve the national objectives included in *Healthy People 2010.* Significant gaps were identified by ASTDD in the dental public health infrastructure and the capacity of state and local public health agencies of most states. The report indicated that states had a significant need for oral health surveillance systems and for staff with public health expertise. Similar gaps in regard to many local public health departments without adequate oral health programs or appropriately trained personnel were highlighted in the report.[14,95] In May 2000 the AAPHD joined the ASTDD for their first joint annual meeting. The purpose of the two major dental public health organizations meeting is to more effectively address the population's oral health needs.[96,97]

American Board of Dental Public Health (ABDPH). This organization is responsible for certifying dental specialists in the field of dental public health. It is one of the nine dental specialty boards and is affiliated with the American Dental Association. All members of the ABDPH are dentists. No specialties in the field of dental hygiene currently exist.

In addition to these organizations, both the ADA and the ADHA address issues of public health interest. Both organizations recently have been focusing more on dental public health–related issues in their attempt to increase the strength and effectiveness of the profession and to improve the oral health of the population. The major reason for this increased interest is the perception on the part of organized dentistry that it is facing critical issues, such as the rising cost of dental education, the increased indebtedness of students, the supply and distribution of dental personnel, the increasing number of alternative forms of developing services, deregulation, and a highly competitive marketplace.[98]

In the early 1980s, to address the projected future problems confronting the dental profession, the ADA established the Special Committee on the Future of Dentistry, which produced a report covering a series of issues and their implications.[98] Although this document is almost two decades old, its concern that the future would bring to the dental profession a more complex and more challenging set of problems that will need to be addressed using the knowledge and skills of the dental public health field is still relevant.

In 1999 the ADA established a task force to explore the future of dentistry. Since then, the ADA has been sponsoring the Future of Dentistry Project. The Future of Dentistry Project report has been completed and it suggests that public health has an important role to play in helping dentistry accomplish its twenty-first century mission.[99,100]

PUBLIC HEALTH CHALLENGES FOR THE TWENTY-FIRST CENTURY

The first revolutionary public health achievement of the late nineteenth and early twentieth centuries focused on environmental intervention to reduce the effects of infectious agents. The second revolution, later in the twentieth century, was the progress in methods and interventions to reduce the toll of chronic diseases and related behavioral risk factors. Looking ahead as we enter the twenty-first century, an increasing need will develop for more interorganizational cooperative intervention to counter the human-generated threats to our physical environment.[43]

The American Public Health Association, in addressing the question of what major twenty-first century public health challenges will need to be addressed by the public health field, suggested the following[101,102]:

- Protecting against terrorists and bioterrorist threats
- Global health risks caused by environmental disasters and disease outbreaks
- Racial disparities in health status
- Increasing levels of chronic diseases among the aging
- Properly utilizing available genetic and technical knowledge about human health
- Providing access to high-quality primary and preventive care for all citizens
- Improving quality of health care delivery, including both physical and mental health services
- Changing behaviors and lifestyles to improve quality of life
- Improving the safety of domestic and imported food
- Reducing global death and disease rates resulting from smoking
- Improving the quality of the environment
- Reducing the number of hungry and malnourished children

Dental public health challenges for the twenty-first century include the following:

- To achieve the recognition that dental/oral health means more than healthy teeth—it means the health of the entire craniofacial complex
- To close the gap between levels of medical and dental access to care and between untreated and undiagnosed medical and dental disease
- To better recognize that oral health can have a significant impact on the overall health and well-being of the U.S. population
- To increase the use of public-private partnerships to improve the nation's oral health
- To build an effective dental health infrastructure that meets the oral health needs of all Americans
- To develop a viable, effective National Oral Health Plan to improve the oral

health status of the entire U.S. population
- To more effectively influence lifestyle behaviors that negatively influence oral health
- To increase the use of evidence-based practice in both clinical dental practice and public health practice[14]
- To prevent the potential that the implementation of evidence-based methodology will be used to control costs without sufficient concern for the quality of care

Alfred Sommer, dean of the School of Hygiene and Public Health, Johns Hopkins University, in an address to a group of public health professionals describing the future of public health, stated that its viability lies in "developing a data system for measuring and tracking the health of the public more effectively; integrating curative and preventive services at both individual and societal levels; and evaluating success and modifying the system when needed to achieve it."[103]

In examining its challenges for the twenty-first century, the CDC concluded that the fundamental challenge is "improving the quality of people's lives by preventing disease, injury and disability through collaboration with public and private partners throughout the world." In its 1999 report *An Ounce of Prevention, What Are the Returns?* CDC outlined 19 cost-effective strategies to prevent disease and injury and promote healthy lifestyles. One of these strategies was the promotion of water fluoridation to prevent dental caries.[104]

Health care writer Laurie Garrett[105] perceptively points out that although methodologies discovered in the twentieth century will continue to form the basis of global public health efforts in the twenty-first century, innovations based on biomedical sciences, such as genetics, will be of increasing importance. She indicates, however, that no matter what technologic advancements may unfold in the twenty-first century, the basic factors essential to maintaining and improving the public's health are ancient and nontechnologic: "clear water and waste disposal; correct social and medical control of epidemics; widespread or universal access to maternal and child health care; clean air; knowledge of personal health needs administered to a population sufficiently educated to be able to comprehend and use the information in their daily lives; and, finally, a health care system that follows the primary maxim of dentistry and medicine: do no harm."[105] Public health in the twenty-first century "will rise or fall with the ultimate course of globalization. If the passage of time finds ever-widening wealth gaps, a disappearing middle class, international financial lawlessness, and still rising individualism, the essential elements of public health will be imperiled, perhaps nonexistent, all over the world."[105]

Former Surgeon General C. Everett Koop made the most concise and meaningful statement on the value and importance of public health in the twenty-first century: "Health care is vital to all of us some of the time but public health is vital to all of us all of the time."[106]

In 1977 Harold Hillenbrand, former executive director of the ADA, stated the following:

> The United States is the only industrially developed country in the world without a coherent, identifiable national health program and has only now reached the stage of making a statement of intent. . . . The delivery of dental health care is not now, if it ever was, solely a problem for the dental profession. Real solutions must be found in the unselfish collaboration of dentists, the other health professions, the dental auxiliaries, social and behavioral scientists, epidemiologists, educators,

statisticians, government and public health officials, consumers, and a whole host of others. There are enough problems to challenge and plague us all.[107]

Since then little has changed. Hillenbrand's words are as appropriate in the new millennium as they were in 1977. The dental and dental public health professions still must accomplish much to meet the dental needs of the people in the United States and "enough problems to challenge and plague us all."

REFERENCES

1. Institute of Medicine Committee for the Study of the Future of Public Health, Division of Health Care Services: A vision of public health in America: an attainable ideal. In *The future of public health,* Washington, DC, 1988, National Academy Press.
2. Corso LC et al: Using essential services as a foundation for performance measurement and assessment of local public health systems, *J Public Health Manag Pract* 6(5):1, 2000.
3. American Dental Association History and Mission. Available at www.ada.org/ada/history/strategic.html.
4. American Dental Hygienists Association Profile of ADHA. Available at www.adha.org/aboutadha/profile.htm
5. Crucett JB: Building constituencies to promote health: A case study, *J Public Health Manage Pract* 6(2):62, 2000.
6. Kimberly JD: Coalition, partnership, and constituency building by a state public health agency: a perspective, *J Public Health Manage Pract* 6(2):55, 2000.
7. Urdang L, editor: *The Random House college dictionary, revised,* New York, 1988, Random House.
8. Pickett G, Hanlon JJ: Philosophy and purpose of public health. In *Public health administration and practice,* ed 9, St Louis, 1990, Mosby.
9. Tulchinsky TH, Varavikova EA: *The new public health: an introduction for the 21st century,* San Diego, 2000, Academic Press.
10. Pickett G: Public health. In *Encyclopedia Americana, international edition,* Danbury, CT, 1999, Grolier.
11. Winslow CEA: The untilled field of public health, *Mod Med* 2:183, 1920.
12. Koplan JP: Defining public health, *Curr Issues Public Health* 1:241, 1995.
13. Turnock BJ: *Public health: what it is and how it works,* Gaithersburg, MD, 2001, Aspen.
14. US Department of Health and Human Services: *Oral health in America: a report of the surgeon general,* Rockville, MD, 2000, US Department of Health and Human Services, National Institute of Dental and Craniofacial Research, National Institutes of Health.
15. Centers for Disease Control and Protection: Ten Great Public Health Achievements—United States, 1900-1999, *MMWR Morb Mortal Wkly Rep* 48(12):241, 1999.
16. Taylor H: *Public health: two words few people understand though almost everyone thinks public health functions are very important,* New York, 1997, Louis Harris & Associates, Inc.
17. Schneider MJ: *Introduction to public health,* Gaithersburg, MD, 2000, Aspen.
18. US Department of Health and Human Services: *NPHSP: national public health performance standards: what gets measured gets done,* Atlanta, 1999, Centers for Disease Control and Prevention, Public Health Practice Office, US Department of Health and Human Services.
19. Knutson JW: What is public health? In Pelton WJ, Wisan JM, editors: *Dentistry in public health,* ed 2, Philadelphia, 1955, WB Saunders.

19a. American Board of Dental Public Health: *Guidelines for graduate education in dental public health,* Ann Arbor, MI, 1970, American Board of Dental Public Health.

20. Public health system under siege, *American Medical News* p 2, Jan 8, 1996.
21. American Public Health Association: *Public health in a reformed health care system: a vision for the future,* Washington, DC, 1993, American Public Health Association.
22. Keppel KG, Freedman MA: What is assessment? *J Public Health Manage Pract* 1:1, 1995.
23. Sleet DA, Rosenberg ML: Injury control. In Sutchfield FD, Keck CW, editors: *Principles of public health practice,* Albany, NY, 1997, Delmar.
24. Novick LF: A framework for public health administration and practice. In Novick LF, Mays GP, editors: *Public health administration: principles for population-based management,* Gaithersburg, MD, 2001, Aspen.
25. Dyal W: Ten organizational practices of public health: a historical perspective, *Am J Prev Med* 11(6):6, 1995.
26. Association of State and Territorial Dental Directors: *Building infrastructure and capacity in state and territorial oral health functions,* Jefferson City, MO, 2000, Association of State and Territorial Dental Directors.
27. Kender K, Landrum LB, Bryan, JL: The role of states in ensuring essential public health services: development of state-level performance measures, *J Public Health Manage Pract* 6(5):26, 2000.

28. Burt BA, Eklund SA: *Dentistry, dental practice and the community,* ed 5, Philadelphia, 1999, WB Saunders.
29. Institute of Medicine: *Health communities: new partnerships for the future of public health,* Washington, DC, 1996, National Academy Press.
30. Turnock BJ: Can public health performance standards improve the quality of public health practice? *J Public Health Manage Pract* 6(5):19, 2000.
31. Institute of Medicine: *Performance monitoring to improve community health,* Washington, DC, 1997, National Academy Press.
32. Halverson PK: Performance measurement and performance standards: old wine in new bottles, *J Public Health Manage Pract* 6(5):vi, 2000.
33. Mays GP, Halverson PK: Conceptual and methodological issues in public health performance measurement: results from a computer-assisted expert panel process, *J Public Health Manage Pract* 6(5):59, 2000.
34. Roper WL, Mays GP: Performance measurement in public health: conceptual and methodological issues in building the science base, *J Public Health Manage Pract* 6(5):66, 2000.
35. Centers for Disease Control and Prevention: *Public health's infrastructure: a status report,* Atlanta, 2001, Department of Health and Human Services.
36. Stapleton S: Dispatch from the front lines, *Am Med News* 44(48):24, 2001.

36a. Phalen K: Victim of its own success? *Am Med News* 44(49):22, 2001.

37. Corbin SB, Martin FR: The future of dental public health report—preparing dental public health to meet the challenges: opportunities of the 21st century, *J Public Health Dent* 54:80, 1994.
38. Issacs SL, Schroeder SA: Where the public good prevailed, *American Prospect* p 26, June 4, 2001.
39. Ovid: *Remedia amoris,* Oxford, England, 1961, Oxford University Press.
40. Anderson V: Evidence-based care: is the defense ready? *Dental Economics* p 28, Nov 2000.
41. Ismail A et al: Systematic reviews and the evidence-based dentistry: professional and policy implications, *J Am Coll Dent* 66(1):6, 1999.
42. Mertz E et al: Evidence based dentistry. In *Improving oral health systems in California,* San Francisco, 2000, University of California.
43. Fielding J: Public health in the twentieth century: advances and challenges, *Annu Rev Public Health* 20:xiii, 1999.
44. Nerenz DR: Who has responsibility for a population's health? *Milbank Q* 74:43, 1996.
45. Washington Department of Health: *Core public health functions: a progress report from the Washington State Core Government Public Health Functions Task Force,* Olympia, WA, 1993, Washington Department of Health.
46. Ibrahim MA et al: Population-based health principles in public health practice, *J Public Health Manage Pract* 7(3):75, 2001.
47. *Minnesota Department of Health public health interventions. Examples from public health nursing,* St Paul, 1996, Division of Community Health Services, Section of Public Health Nursing.
48. US Department of Health and Human Services: *For a healthy nation: returns on investment in public health,* Washington, DC, 1994, US Government Printing Office.
49. Dever GEA: Epidemiological model for health policy analysis, *Social Indicators Research* 2(4):451, 1976.
50. Salmon ME: Public health policy: creating a healthy future for the American public, *Fam Commun Health* 18:1, 1995.
51. Gordon L: Public health is more important than health care, *J Public Health Policy* 14(3):261, 1993.
52. Mann ML: Planning for community programs. In Jong A, editor: *Dental public health and community dentistry,* St Louis, 1981, Mosby.
53. Hodgetts BM, Cascio DM: *Modern health care administration,* Madison, WI, 1993, Brown & Benchmark Publishers.
54. Dunning JM: Dental needs, resources, and objectives. In Dunning JM, editor: *Principles of dental public health,* ed 2, Cambridge, MA, 1970, Harvard University Press.
55. World Health Organization Expert Committee on Dental Health: *Organization of dental public health services report, WHO technical report series no 298,* Geneva, 1965, World Health Organization.
56. World Health Organization Expert Committee on Dental Health: *Planning and evaluation of public dental health services report, WHO technical report series no 589,* Geneva, 1976, World Health Organization.
57. Stoner JAF: *Introduction to management,* Englewood Cliffs, NJ, 1978, Prentice-Hall.
58. Dunning JM: A word of warning in incremental dental care, *N Y J Dent* 38:56, 1968.
59. Schonfeld HK: Peer review of quality of dental care, *J Am Dent Assoc* 79:1376, 1969.
60. Burt BA: Administration of public dental treatment programs. In Slack GL, editor: *Dental public health,* Bristol, UK, 1974, John Wright & Sons.
61. American Board of Dental Public Health: Competency objectives for dental public health, *J Public Health Dent* 50:338, 1990.
62. Rozier GR: New opportunities for dental public health, *American Association of Public Health Dentistry's Communique* 9:1, 1990.
63. Rozier GR: Proceedings: workshop to develop competency objectives in dental public health, *J Public Health Dent* 50:330, 1990.

64. Young WO: Dentistry looks toward the twenty-first century. In Brown WE, editor: *Oral health dentistry and the American public,* Norman, OK, 1974, University of Oklahoma Press.
65. American Association for World Health: *Oral health for a happy life,* Washington, DC, 1994, American Association for World Health.
66. US General Accounting Office: *Oral health factors contributing to low use of dental services by low-income populations,* GAO/HEHS-00-149, Washington, DC, 2000, US Government Printing Office.
67. Sheiham A: Planning for manpower requirements in dental public health. In Slack GL, editor: *Dental public health,* Bristol, UK, 1974, John Wright & Sons.
68. Lundberg GD: National health care reform: an aura of inevitability is upon us, *JAMA* 265:2566, 1991.
69. Block LE, Freed JR: A new paradigm for increasing access to care—the Oregon health plan, *J Am Coll Dent* 63:30, 1996.
70. Wilson WA: The future role of government in dental practice and education, *J Am Coll Dent* 40:111, 1973.
71. Burt BA: Financing for dental care services. In Striffler DF, Young WO, Burt BA, editors: *Dentistry, dental practice and the community,* ed 3, Philadelphia, 1983, WB Saunders.
72. Willcocks AJ: Dental health and the changing society. In Slack GL, editor: *Dental public health,* Bristol, UK, 1981, John Wright & Sons.
72a. Dudley RA, Luft HS: Managed care in transition, *N Engl J Med* 344(4):1087, 2001.
72b. Brubaker B: Health costs up 11%, survey finds yearly rise is biggest since '92 some insurors see hike ahead, *Washington Post* Sept 7:E1, 2001.
72c. Bureau of National Affairs: MCOS adopt less restrictive products, seek to smooth provider relationships, *BNA's Health Care Policy Report* 10(3):97, 2002.
72d. Landa AS: Health system pressure is on, and building, *Am Med News* 45(5):10, 2002.
73. Lamm RD: Critical challenge, *Public Health Rep* 111: 224, 1996.
74. Pew Health Professions Commission: *Critical challenges: revitalizing the health professions for the twenty-first century, the third report of the Pew Health Professions Commission,* San Francisco, Dec 1995.
75. Brown RE: With managed care, what role for public health? *Nations Health* 26:2, 1996.
76. Sumaya CV: Oral health for all: the HRSA perspective, *J Public Health Dent* 56:35, 1996.
77. Shafritz JM: *The Harper-Collins dictionary of American government, concise edition,* New York, 1993, Harper Perennial.
78. Carey GW: Government. In *Encyclopedia Americana, international edition,* Danbury, CT, 1999, Grolier.
79. Siege relief, *American Medical News* p 17, Jan 8, 1996 (editorial).
80. Kent C: A long-neglected system strains to respond to a rising threat, *American Medical News* p 7, Jan 8, 1996.
81. Wilson FA, Neuhauser D: *Health services in the United States,* ed 2, Cambridge, MA, 1985, Ballinger.
82. Brandt E: The federal contribution to public health. In Scutchfield FD, Keck CW, editors: *Principles of public health practice,* Albany, NY, 1997, Delmar.
83. US Department of Health and Human Services: *Healthy people 2010: understanding and improving health,* Washington, DC, 2000, US Department of Health and Human Services, US Public Health Service.
84. Snyder LP: Seventy-five years of dentistry in the Public Health Service and the Commissioned Corps: public health through service, research and prevention. In *PHS dental notes special edition,* Bethesda, MD, 1994, US Public Health Service.
85. Missions of US Public Health Service and the Commissioned Corps. Available at www.os.dhhs.gov/phs/corps/history.htm.
86. Furman LJ, Arnold M: *Final draft—US Public Health Service dental programs,* Rockville, MD, 1999, US Public Health Service Dental Category, DEPAC.
87. Corbin SB, Martin FR: The future of dental public health report—preparing dental public health to meet the challenges: opportunities of the 21st century, *J Public Health Dent* 54:80, 1994.
88. Greene JC: Federal programs and the profession, *J Am Dent Assoc* 92:689, 1976.
89. *Leadership meeting summary,* Atlanta, 2000, Division of Oral Health Centers for Disease Control and Prevention.
90. US Department of Health and Human Services, HRSA Oral Health, Oral Health Initiative. Available at www.hrsa.gov/oralhealth/.
90a. Slavkin HC: The Surgeon General's Report and special-needs patients: a framework for action for children and their caregivers, *Special Care Dent* 21(3): 88, 2000.
90b. Anonymous: Oral health in America: a report of the Surgeon General, *J Calif Dent Assoc* 28(9):685, 2000.
91. Public Health Foundation: *Public health agencies 1990: an inventory of programs and block grant expenditures,* Washington DC, 1990, Public Health Foundation.
92. Association of State and Territorial Dental Directors: *State dental directors,* Jefferson City, MO, 1995, The Association.
93. Kuthy R, Odum JG: Local dental programs: a descriptive assessment of funding and activities, *J Public Health Dent* 48:36, 1988.
94. Association of State and Territorial Dental Directors: *Status of state dental programs,* Jefferson City, MO, 2000, The Association.

95. Association of State and Territorial Dental Directors: Home page. Available at www.astdd.org.
96. King R: Coming together for a new millennium: national oral health conference, *J Public Health Dent* 61(1):42, 2001.
97. Edelstein B: On common ground: keynote address at the Joint Annual Meeting of the American Association of Public Health Dentistry and the Association of State and Territorial Dental Directors, *J Public Health Dent* 61(1):3, 2001.
98. American Dental Association: *Strategic plan report of the American Dental Association's Special Committee on the Future of Dentistry: issue papers on dental research, manpower education, practice and public and professional concerns,* Chicago, 1983, American Dental Association.
99. Furlong A: Gazing into the future, *ADA News* 32(6):1, 2000.
100. American Dental Association: *Future of dentistry,* Chicago, 2001, American Dental Association.
101. American Public Health Association: *Public health challenges in the next century,* Washington, DC, 1999, American Public Health Association.
102. Koplan JP, Fleming DW: Current and future public health challenges, *JAMA* 284(13):1696, 2000.
103. Sommer A: Viewpoint on public health's future, *Public Health Rep* 110:657, 1995.
104. Centers for Disease Control and Prevention: *An ounce of prevention . . . What are the returns?* ed 2, Atlanta, 1999, US Department of Health and Human Services.
105. Garrett L: *Betrayal of trust,* New York, 2000, Hyperion.
106. Association of Schools of Public Health: What is public health? Available at www.asph.org/aa_section.cfm/3.
107. Ingle J, Blair P, editors: *International dental care delivery systems,* Cambridge, MA, 1978, Ballinger.

CHAPTER

2

THE SURGEON GENERAL'S REPORT ON ORAL HEALTH IN AMERICA: DEFINING CHALLENGES FOR THE FUTURE

Mark D. Macek

In April 1997 Donna Shalala, then Secretary of the Department of Health and Human Services, commissioned the Surgeon General's Report on Oral Health in America (Surgeon General's Report). The Secretary charged the report to "define, describe and evaluate the interactions between oral health and general health and well-being (quality of life), through the life span, in the context of changes in society."[1] During the next 3 years, under the direction of the Office of the Surgeon General and the National Institute of Dental and Craniofacial Research, Project Director Caswell A. Evans, D.D.S., M.P.H., coordinated the efforts of a highly qualified project team and a cadre of contributing authors and content experts. By early 2000 the project team's dedication and determination paid off, and the first-ever Surgeon General's Report on Oral Health was completed.

The Surgeon General's Report represents a thorough review of the important issues relating to oral and craniofacial health and disease. The report describes the craniofacial complex and its many integral parts. It lists the epidemiology of common oral and craniofacial diseases and disorders. It explains the potential and established links between oral health and general health and portrays the mouth and face as a mirror of general health and disease. It describes how oral health is promoted and maintained and how oral diseases are prevented. The report also shows the oral health needs of the community and lists the many and varied opportunities that exist to enhance oral health in the future. In short, the Surgeon General's Report symbolizes a stepping-off point for the next millennium, bringing important oral health issues into focus, defining challenges for the future, and equipping public health professionals and policy makers with the tools to effect change.

This chapter intends to fulfill a number of objectives. It provides a brief history of the U.S. Public Health Service, presents a chronology of Surgeons General throughout time, and places the current Surgeon General's Report in the context of previous reports. The chapter also summarizes the Surgeon General's Report and its important messages to the American public. Although the chapter provides a thorough synopsis, it does not intend to provide a critical review of the Surgeon General's Report. The breadth of such a critical review would be well beyond the scope of this chapter. Finally, the chapter places the Surgeon General's Report in the broader context of selected oral health initiatives at the national, state, and local levels.

A BRIEF HISTORY OF THE U.S. PUBLIC HEALTH SERVICE

During our nation's early history, port cities found themselves poorly equipped to handle the health care needs of merchant sailors. On July 16, 1798, in an attempt to remedy the situation, President John Adams signed *An Act for the Relief of Sick and Disabled Seamen,* providing for "the temporary relief and maintenance of sick or disabled seamen in the hospitals or other proper institutions now established in the several ports of the United States, or in ports where no such institutions exist, then in such other manner as he (the Secretary of the Treasury) shall direct" (1 Stat. L. 605).[2] The Act called for a tax of 20 cents per month against the wages of all American sailors. Funds were to be used to provide health care to merchant seaman in existing marine hospitals or to construct new hospitals, where necessary. The Act gave the authority for local collection and administration of a Marine Hospital Fund. In 1799 a new law granted that naval personnel would also be beneficiaries of the Marine Hospital Fund, a provision that lasted until 1811, when the U.S. Navy created its own hospital system.[3]

Local administration of the service left administration of the hospitals subject to the whims of politicians and customs collectors. During the next several decades, the Marine Hospital Fund health care system devolved into a disjointed, poorly functioning organization of hospitals.[4] In 1849 the Marine Hospital Fund appointed Drs. George Loring and Thomas Edwards to lead a commission charged with evaluating the Fund hospitals. Their report placed the Fund hospitals and their local administrators in a less than favorable light. Loring and Edwards were also the first to recommend a "chief surgeon" to provide central leadership to the Fund system. During the Civil War, the Marine Hospital Fund fell into further disarray, as some hospitals were overrun by soldiers, and others were abandoned completely. In 1869 the Treasury Secretary, then administrator of the Fund, commissioned Drs. Stewart and Billings to inspect and report on the hospitals. Again, the hospital system was found to be in dismal shape.

During the following year, in response to the unfavorable report, the Secretary initiated some organizational changes.[4] In 1871 Dr. John Maynard Woodworth, General Sherman's chief medical officer during the Civil War, became the first Supervising Surgeon of the Marine Hospital Service (a position later to be renamed Supervising Surgeon General and then simply Surgeon General). Woodworth brought his experiences with disciplined military service to the position and set in motion a series of reforms that would shape the Marine Hospital Service to come. Dr. John B. Hamilton, successor to Woodworth, wanted to make Woodworth's reforms permanent, and his campaign to do so was successful when, on January 4, 1889, President Cleveland signed an *Act to Regulate Appointments in the Marine Hospital Service of the United States* (25 Stat. L. 639). The Act specified that the medical officers would thereafter be appointed by the president, with the advice and consent of the Senate, after passing an examination. These reforms have remained in the Marine Hospital Service to the present.

Over the next three decades, the Surgeons General orchestrated a broader scope for the Marine Hospital Service, which also resulted in two changes in name.[5] During the tenure of Surgeon General Wyman, for example, the budget for the Marine Hospital Service nearly tripled and the number of staff physicians more than doubled. In 1902, in an effort to reflect the new responsibilities of Marine Hospital Service physicians in combating infectious disease, Wyman guided the Congress to change the name of the Marine Hospital Service to the Public Health and Marine Hospital Service and had the term *Supervising* eliminated from the Surgeon General title.

Between 1912 and 1920 the Public Health and Marine Hospital Service gained greater notoriety and responsibility.[6] During the tenure of Surgeon General Rupert Blue, Congress passed legislation that changed the name of the Public Health and Marine Hospital Service to the Public Health Service. The charge of the newly named Service was to investigate diseases and conditions that resulted from sanitation, sewage, and pollution of U.S. streams and lakes. During Blue's period, as a result of demands for health care personnel during World War I, the Public Health Service allowed the commissioning of reserve officers, including pharmacists, sanitary engineers, and dentists.

Changes in the Public Health Service took place at a dramatic rate after World War I. Between 1920 and 1936 the Public Health Service introduced the new fields of epidemiology and biostatistics to various public health problems throughout the country.[7] In 1939 President Roosevelt combined the Public Health Service with a number of other educational, health, and welfare offices into the Federal Security Agency.[8] In 1942 the Public Health Service launched a campaign against malaria in military training camps called Malaria Control in War Areas (MCWA); in 1946 the MCWA program became a permanent agency of the Public Health Service and was renamed the Communicable Disease Center, which later became the Centers for Disease Control, and, finally, the Centers for Disease Control and Prevention (CDC). In 1948 Congress added the National Institutes of Dental Research (NIDR) to the National Institutes of Health, and H. Trendley Dean was named the first director of the new dental institute.[9] In 1953 additional agencies, hospitals, and the Office of Vital Statistics were combined with the Federal Security Agency to create the Department of Health, Education, and Welfare (HEW). In 1955 the Public Health Service took over the medical care of American Indians from the Bureau of Indian Affairs.[10]

During the 1970s, prompted by a sweeping reorganization of HEW by Secretary Gardner (1965–1968), the Public Health Service evolved from a three-agency structure into a six-agency structure.[11] In 1972 the Public Health Service consisted of the newly arrived Federal Drug Administration (FDA), National Institutes of Health, and Health Services and Mental Health Administration (HSMHA). The HSMHA consisted of the Indian Health Service, National Center for Health Statistics, CDC, Regional Medical Program, Public Health Service hospitals and health planning programs, and other agencies. In 1973 the six agencies included the CDC; Health Services Administration (HSA); Health Resources Administration (HRA); Alcohol, Drug Abuse, and Mental Health Administration (ADAMHA); and a combination of the FDA, National Institutes of Health, and four new agencies created by HSMHA.

Today, the Public Health Service is as vital as ever, coordinating research, health care administration and financing, disease prevention and health promotion, and the investigation of infectious disease outbreaks throughout the United States and the world. The Public Health Service has come a long way from its origins as the Marine Hospital Service. Its focus is vastly different today than it was more than 200 years ago, yet the Public Health Service maintains at its core the goal of bringing relief to those who are ill. Much of this continuity in focus should be credited to its long line of leaders—the Surgeons General.

BOX 2-1

Surgeons General of the U.S. Public Health Service

John M. Woodworth	1871–1879 (died)
John B. Hamilton	1879–1891
Walter Wyman	1891–1911 (died)
Rupert Blue	1912–1920
Hugh S. Cumming	1920–1936
Thomas Parran, Jr.	1936–1948
Leonard A. Scheele	1948–1956
Leroy E. Burney	1956–1961
Luther L. Terry	1961–1965
William H. Stewart	1965–1969
Jesse L. Steinfeld	1969–1973
S. Paul Ehrlich (acting)	1973–1977
Julius B. Richmond	1977–1981
C. Everett Koop	1981–1989
Antonia C. Novello	1990–1993
M. Joycelyn Elders	1993–1994
Audrey Manley (acting)	1995–1997
J. Jarrett Clinton (acting)	1997–1998
David Satcher	1998–2002
Kenneth Moritsugu (acting)	2002–

SURGEONS GENERAL OF THE U.S. PUBLIC HEALTH SERVICE: A CHRONOLOGY

Including Surgeon General Satcher, 16 persons have occupied the Office of Surgeon General since John Woodworth assumed the position in 1871 (Box 2-1). Most of the Surgeons General have been men. The first woman to assume the position was Surgeon General Novello, who served from 1990 through 1993. Dr. Novello was also the first Hispanic Surgeon General. In 1993 M. Joycelyn Elders became the second woman and the first African-American to assume the position. Surgeon General Satcher, who was appointed by the Clinton administration in 1998, became the first African-American man to hold the office.

From 1871 until the present, the Surgeons General have taken on a variety of responsibilities and have assumed various roles. Before 1968, for example, the Office of the Surgeon General assumed full responsibility for leading the Marine Hospital Service (and later the Public Health Service), including program development, administration, and financial management. In the position as head of the Marine Hospital Service or Public Health Service, the Surgeon General reported directly to the president or his Cabinet. In 1968 President Johnson reorganized the federal government and took management of the Public Health Service away from the Office of the Surgeon General and placed it in the hands of the Assistant Secretary for Health (ASH). With this reorganization, the Surgeon General was to become a principal deputy to the ASH, losing administrative responsibilities and, instead, offering advice regarding professional medical issues.

Since 1968 the relation between the Surgeon General and the ASH has changed several times. In 1972 the Surgeon General was again asked to report directly to the Secretary, rather than the ASH. In 1977 the positions of Surgeon General and ASH were combined. In 1981 they again became separate positions. In 1987 the Office of the Surgeon General was reestablished as a staff office within the Office of the Assistant Secretary for Health, and the Surgeon General regained administrative authority of the Commissioned Corps of the Public Health Service. Finally, between 1998 and 2001, the positions of Surgeon General and ASH were once again combined.

REPORTS OF THE SURGEONS GENERAL THROUGHOUT HISTORY

Beginning in the mid-1960s the Surgeon General of the U.S. Public Health Service had endeavored to educate the nation about important public health problems by releasing reports on a regular basis. To date, the Office of the Surgeon General has released more than 50 such reports. The vast majority of them have dealt with cigarette smoking and other tobacco-related health issues (Box 2-2); however, beginning in the 1980s, other reports have introduced such diverse topics as disabilities among children, acquired immune deficiency, nutrition and health, child abuse, physical activity, suicide, youth violence, mental health, responsible sexual behavior, and oral health. From the beginning, the reports of the Surgeons General have had a tremendous influence on health and health-related behaviors in the United States.

The first report *(Smoking and Health: Report of the Advisory Committee of the Surgeon General of the U.S. Public Health Service)*, released in 1964 during Surgeon General Terry's tenure, introduced the causal relation between cigarette smoking and lung cancer. The report took the nation by storm. In January 1964, before a standing-room-only press conference, the Surgeon General announced the findings of his Advisory Committee on Smoking and Health. During the conference, Terry stated that "cigarette smoking is causally related to smoking in men," and added, "the magnitude of the effect of cigarette smoking far outweighs all other factors. The data for women, though less extensive, point in the same direction."[12] As a result of this report, the Federal Trade Commission immediately called for warning labels on cigarette packaging and Congress passed legislation requiring their use. The influence of the first Surgeon General's report on smoking and health was far reaching. The report not only effected a dramatic change in the way that the average citizen viewed smoking, but it established prestige for the reports that would follow and secured a special place for the Surgeon General in the public's eye.

In 1979 Surgeon General Richmond released *Healthy People—The Surgeon General's Report on Health Promotion and Disease Prevention.*[13] The document was important because it defined, for the first time, national health objectives against which progress during the following decade could be mea-

BOX 2-2

Reports of the Surgeon General of the U.S. Public Health Service

2001	Surgeon General's Call to Action to Promote Sexual Health and Responsible Sexual Behavior
	National Strategy for Suicide Prevention: Goals and Objectives for Action
	Women and Smoking: A Report of the Surgeon General
	Youth Violence: A Report of the Surgeon General
2000	Reducing Tobacco Use: A Report of the Surgeon General
	Oral Health in America: A Report of the Surgeon General
1999	Mental Health: A Report of the Surgeon General
	The Surgeon General's Call to Action to Prevent Suicide
1998	Tobacco Use among U.S. Racial/Ethnic Minority Groups: A Report of the Surgeon General
1996	Physical Activity and Health: A Report of the Surgeon General
1994	Preventing Tobacco Use Among Young People: A Report of the Surgeon General
	Surgeon General's Report for Kids about Smoking
1992	Surgeon General's Report to the American Public on HIV Infection and AIDS
	Smoking and Health in the Americas: A Report of the Surgeon General
1990	The Health Benefits of Smoking Cessation: A Report of the Surgeon General
1989	Reducing the Health Consequences of Smoking—25 Years of Progress: A Report of the Surgeon General
1988	The Surgeon General's Letter on Child Sexual Abuse
	The Surgeon General's Report on Nutrition and Health
	The Health Consequences of Smoking—Nicotine Addiction: A Report of the Surgeon General
1987	The Surgeon General's Report on Acquired Immune Deficiency Syndrome
1986	Smoking and Health. A National Status Report: A Report to Congress
	The Health Consequences of Involuntary Smoking: A Report of the Surgeon General
	The Health Consequences of Using Smokeless Tobacco
1985	The Health Consequences of Smoking—Cancer and Chronic Lung Disease in the Workplace: A Report of the Surgeon General

sured. This chapter discusses the oral health priority area for these "Healthy People 1990" objectives, as well as the "Healthy People 2000" and "Healthy People 2010" objectives, in a later section.

One of the most influential reports written during the 1980s was *The Surgeon General's Report on Acquired Immune Deficiency Syndrome,* released by Surgeon General Koop.[14] This document, much of which was written by Koop himself, described sex education in elementary schools, addressed the proper use of condoms and other prophylactics, and called for tolerance of those infected with the human immunodeficiency virus (HIV). Although the report used explicit language and, to many, was controversial, it was also immensely popular among public health professionals and the public. The Surgeon General's report on HIV, as well as the document that followed *(Understanding AIDS),* brought useful, accurate, and nonjudgmental information to a nation that was frightened of a serious

BOX 2-2

Reports of the Surgeon General of the U.S. Public Health Service—cont'd

1984	The Health Consequences of Smoking—Chronic Obstructive Lung Disease: A Report of the Surgeon General
	Chronic Obstructive Lung Disease
1983	The Health Consequences of Smoking—Cardiovascular Disease: A Report of the Surgeon General
1982	Report of the Surgeon General's Workshop on Children with Handicaps and Their Families
	The Health Consequences of Smoking—Cancer: A Report of the Surgeon General
1981	The Health Consequences of Smoking—The Changing Cigarette: A Report of the Surgeon General
1980	The Health Consequences of Smoking for Women: A Report of the Surgeon General
1979	Healthy People—The Surgeon General's Report on Health Promotion and Disease Prevention
	Smoking and Health
1977–78	The Health Consequences of Smoking
1976	The Health Consequences of Smoking: Selected Chapters from 1971 through 1975 Reports
1975	The Health Consequences of Smoking
1974	The Health Consequences of Smoking, 1974
1973	The Health Consequences of Smoking, 1973
1972	The Health Consequences of Smoking
1971	The Health Consequences of Smoking: A Report of the Surgeon General
1969	The Health Consequences of Smoking: 1969 Supplement to the 1967 Public Health Service Review
1968	The Health Consequences of Smoking: 1968 Supplement to the 1967 Public Health Service Review
1967	The Health Consequences of Smoking. A Public Health Service Review
1964	Smoking and Health: Report of the Advisory Committee of the Surgeon General of the Public Health Service

public health problem of which they knew little.[15]

On May 25, 2000, at Shepherd Elementary School in Washington, D.C., Assistant Secretary for Health and Surgeon General David Satcher released *Oral Health in America: A Report of the Surgeon General*.[16] The document was the first-ever Surgeon General's report exclusively dedicated to oral health issues and was the fifty-first in a series of Surgeon General's reports since 1964. In his presentation to the American public that day, Surgeon General Satcher summarized key themes of the report and placed the findings in a broader context of general health and well-being. Dr. Satcher stated that oral health meant much more than healthy teeth; that oral health was integral to general health; that safe and effective disease prevention measures existed that everyone could adopt to improve oral health and prevent disease; that profound disparities in oral health existed in the United States; and that general health risk factors, such as tobacco use and poor dietary practices, also affected oral and craniofacial health.

SUMMARY OF THE SURGEON GENERAL'S REPORT ON ORAL HEALTH

The Surgeon General's Report was a comprehensive document, with more than 300 pages of text, tables, figures, illustrations, and references. This section summarizes the landmark report's organization, major findings, and framework for action. To be faithful to the Surgeon General's Report, this section borrows liberally from the original document. Interested persons are encouraged to read the Surgeon General's Report in its entirety if they wish to have access to greater detail.[16]

ORGANIZATION OF THE REPORT

The project team and contributing authors divided the Surgeon General's Report into five parts, each part relating to a particular question. Part One asked, What is oral health? This central question was addressed across two chapters. The first of these chapters affirmed that oral health meant more than healthy teeth, a theme that would recur throughout the report. The chapter stated that oral health meant being free of diseases and conditions that affect the full complement of oral, dental, and craniofacial tissues, collectively known as the craniofacial complex. This distinction is important because the function of the craniofacial tissues is often taken for granted, despite providing for such uniquely human traits as speech and facial expression. The first chapter also followed the lead of the World Health Organization by stating that oral health simultaneously included physical, mental, and social well-being, and this connection between oral health and general health represented a second theme of the report.[17] In spite of the authors' desire to define oral health in broad terms, however, the chapter also stressed the importance of two leading tooth-related problems, dental caries and the periodontal diseases. The second chapter of Part One provided an overview of the craniofacial complex during development. Together, the two chapters of Part One provided the background against which the remainder of the Surgeon General's Report could be more fully appreciated and understood.

Part Two asked, What is the status of oral health in America? This question was addressed across two chapters. The first of these chapters described a variety of oral diseases and conditions, including dental and periodontal infections, selected mucosal infections, oral and pharyngeal cancers and precancerous neoplasms, developmental disorders, injuries, and selected chronic and disabling conditions. The first chapter also stated that research regarding pathology of the craniofacial complex might provide scientists with models of systemic pathology, given that craniofacial tissues had counterparts in other parts of the body. The chapter reached the following conclusions:

- Microbial infections are the primary cause of the most prevalent oral diseases.
- The etiology of diseases and conditions affecting the craniofacial complex are multifactorial, involving a complex interplay between genetic, environmental, and behavioral factors.
- Several inherited and congenital conditions affect the craniofacial complex, and resultant disfigurement and impair-

ment frequently affect other systems throughout the body.
- The oral cavity provides a route for tobacco, alcohol, and inappropriate diets that, in turn, contribute to diseases that affect tissues in the craniofacial complex and elsewhere.
- A number of systemic conditions first appear as primary oral symptoms.
- Conditions related to orofacial pain are common and often have complex etiologies.

The second chapter of Part Two described the distribution of the oral diseases and conditions listed in the first chapter. The authors derived most of their descriptive statistics from large surveys representative of the civilian, noninstitutionalized U.S. population. These data sources included the National Health Interview Survey (NHIS), National Health and Nutrition Examination Survey (NHANES), surveys conducted by the National Institute of Dental Research (currently the National Institute of Dental and Craniofacial Research) during the 1970s and 1980s, and others.[18-25] The second chapter stated, however, that "there is no single measure of oral health or the burden of oral diseases and conditions, just as there is no single measure of overall health or overall disease" (Surgeon General's Report, p. 61).[16] The chapter reached the following conclusions:

- Most Americans have enjoyed major improvements in oral health during the last five decades.
- Despite these general improvements, profound disparities in oral health still exist among specific population subgroups.
- Oral diseases and conditions affect humans throughout their life span, and most Americans have experienced dental caries.
- Conditions that severely affect the face and craniofacial structures are more prevalent among the younger and older age cohorts.
- Orofacial pain can greatly reduce quality of life and restrict major life functions and is a common symptom of diseases and conditions affecting the craniofacial complex.
- National and state data regarding many oral diseases and conditions are limited or nonexistent.
- Research should strive to create better measures of oral disease and illness, explain the determinants of disparities across population subgroups, and develop effective interventions to reduce or eliminate these disparities.

Part Three of the Surgeon General's Report asked, What is the relation between oral health and general health and wellbeing? This question was addressed across two chapters. The first chapter characterized the face and oral cavity as a reflection of health and disease in the body and described numerous established and potential linkages between oral health and general health. It also showed how diagnostic tests of saliva were available to detect antibodies, drugs, hormones, and environmental toxins, as well as to determine the integrity of the mucosal immune system.[26,27] The first chapter reached the following conclusions:

- Several systemic diseases and conditions have oral manifestations, and when these manifestations represent initial clinical signs the craniofacial complex provides a unique means of informing clinicians of the need for further assessments.

- The oral cavity is the portal of entry for microorganisms that affect general health.
- Pharmacologic agents used in the treatment of systemic illness may cause adverse oral signs and symptoms and reduce compliance with treatment.
- Immunocompromised and hospitalized patients are at greater risk of oral infections.
- Diabetics are at greater risk of periodontitis, and diabetics with periodontitis have greater difficulty controlling their blood glucose levels.
- Data suggest an association between periodontal diseases and systemic conditions such as cardiovascular disease, strokes, and adverse pregnancy outcomes; however, the Surgeon General's Report states that additional research is necessary to determine whether these associations are causal.

The second chapter of Part Three focused on the relation between oral health problems and quality of life. The authors set the stage for this relation with a description of the role that oral health value systems have played in society and across cultures. The authors went on to describe the effect that poor oral health had on the functions of daily living, such as communication, social interaction, and intimacy.[28] The chapter reached the following conclusions:

- Oral health is associated with self-reported well-being and quality of life as measured along functional, psychosocial, and economic dimensions.
- Impaired oral health may adversely affect diet, nutrition, sleep patterns, psychologic status, social interactions, and school- and work-related activities among some individuals.
- Cultural values influence oral health and well-being and may play a role in oral health care utilization behaviors and the perpetuation of acceptable oral health and esthetic norms.
- Oral and craniofacial diseases and their treatment place a burden on society in the form of lost productive work time among adults and lost school time among children and adolescents.
- Oral and pharyngeal cancers adversely affect society in terms of premature death and years of life lost.
- Self-reported effects of oral and craniofacial conditions on social functioning include limitations of verbal and nonverbal communication, social interaction, and intimacy.
- Self-reported effects of facial disfigurement include loss of self-image and self-esteem, anxiety, depression, and social stigma that, in turn, may limit educational, career-related, and marital opportunities, as well as other social interactions.
- Reduced oral health–related quality of life is associated with poor oral health status and access to oral health care treatment.

Part Four asked, How is oral health promoted and maintained, and how are oral diseases prevented? These related questions were addressed across three chapters. The first chapter reviewed the evidence regarding current prevention measures, with particular emphasis on the prevention of dental caries (Table 2-1). In addition, the chapter acknowledged a need for the prevention of periodontal diseases, facial injuries, and oral and pharyngeal cancer; however, the authors suggested that current preventive measures were at an early stage. The authors also stated that studies regarding the knowledge, attitudes, and behaviors of

Table 2-1. Quality of Evidence, Strength of Recommendation, and Target Population of Recommendation for Each Modality to Prevent and Control Dental Caries

*Modality**	*Quality of Evidence (Grade)*	*Strength of Recommendation (Code)*	*Target Population†*
Community water fluoridation	II-1	A	All areas
School water fluoridation	II-3	C	Rural, nonfluoridated areas
Fluoridated dentifrices	I	A	All persons
Fluoride mouth rinses	I	A	High risk‡
Fluoride supplements			
Pregnant women	I	E	None
Children age <6 years	II-3	C	High risk
Children age 6 to 16 years	I	A	High risk
Persons age >16 years	N.A.	C	High risk
Fluoride gels	I	A	High risk
Fluoride varnishes	I	A	High risk
Dental sealants	I	A	High risk§

Modified from US Department of Health and Human Services. Public Health Service. Centers for Disease Control and Prevention: Recommendations for using fluoride to prevent and control dental caries in the United States, *MMWR Morb Mortal Wkly Rep* 50:1, 2001; and Association of State and Territorial Dental Directors (ASTDD), New York State Health Department, Ohio Department of Health, and School of Public Health, University of Albany, State University of New York: Workshop on guidelines for sealant use: recommendations, *J Public Health Dent* 55(5 spec no):263, 1995.

NOTE: Criteria for quality of evidence and strength of recommendation designations are adapted from Table 5.3, US Preventive Services Task Force (USPSTF): *Guide to clinical preventive services*, ed 2, Baltimore, 1996, William & Wilkins.

N.A., no published studies of effectiveness of fluoride supplements in controlling dental caries among persons age >16 years.

*Assume that the modalities are used as directed in terms of dosage and age of user.

†The quality of evidence for targeting some modalities to persons at high risk is grade III, representing the opinion of respected experts, and is based on considerations of cost-effectiveness that were not included in the studies establishing efficacy or effectiveness.

‡Groups believed to be at high risk for caries are members of families of low socioeconomic status or with low levels of parental education, those seeking dental care on an irregular basis, and persons without dental insurance or access to dental service. Individual factors contributing to increased risk are currently active dental caries; a history of high caries in older siblings or caregivers; exposed root surfaces; high levels of infection with cariogenic bacteria; impaired ability to maintain oral hygiene; reduced salivary flow caused by medications, radiation treatment, or disease; and the wearing of orthodontic appliances or prostheses.

§Assessment of risk is based on both patient- and tooth-specific factors.

health practitioners and the public showed numerous educational opportunities. The chapter reached the following conclusions:

- Community water fluoridation benefits individuals of all ages and every socio-economic status; however, more than one third of the U.S. population is without this public health benefit.
- Individuals, health care providers, and communities have access to effective disease prevention measures, particularly for dental caries and gingivitis.
- Community-based approaches for the

prevention of oral and pharyngeal cancers and orofacial trauma require further development.
- Community-based prevention measures remain unavailable to substantial segments of the underserved population.
- A gap exists between research and the dissemination of findings for oral disease prevention, health promotion, and knowledge.
- Approaches for disease prevention and health promotion, such as tobacco cessation, appropriate use of fluorides, and dietary supplementation, represent opportunities for partnerships between community-based programs and oral health practitioners, as well as collaborations among various health professionals.
- Community-based health promotion programs require a concerted effort among social service agencies, health care providers, and educational services, at both the state and local levels.

The second chapter of Part Four stated that attaining and maintaining oral health required a commitment to individual care, as well as professional care. The authors argued that, as understanding of oral disease epidemiology and pathology grew, health care providers could incorporate new preventive, diagnostic, and treatment strategies into their practices. The chapter added that practitioners could work closely with their patients to facilitate new, more healthful behaviors, while reinforcing existing practices. The chapter reached the following conclusions:

- Achieving and maintaining oral health require individual action, in combination with professional health care and community efforts.
- Primary prevention of oral and craniofacial diseases and conditions is possible with proper diet and nutrition, oral hygiene, and health-promoting behaviors, including the appropriate utilization of professional services.
- All primary health care providers can contribute to improved oral health, and interdisciplinary care is needed to manage the oral health/general health interface.
- Nonsurgical interventions are available to reverse the progression of certain oral and craniofacial diseases.
- Acquired knowledge and the development of molecular and genetic tests should facilitate risk assessment and treatment.
- Health care providers ought to administer tobacco cessation and other health promotion programs in their practices.
- Biocompatible rehabilitative materials and biologically engineered tissues should greatly enhance the treatment options available to health professionals in the future.

The final chapter of Part Four described the role of health professionals in the oral health care system of the United States. It also listed obstacles that limit the nation's capacity to improve oral health. The chapter reached the following conclusions:

- Dental, medical, and public health delivery systems each provide services that affect oral health; however, private practice dentists provide the majority of clinical oral health care.
- Expenditures for dental services alone made up $53.8 billion (4.7% of total U.S. health expenditures) in 1998; however, this value probably underestimated true expenditures, because ex-

penditure data are unavailable for oral and craniofacial health care provided by other health professionals.

- The public health infrastructure is insufficient to address the oral health care needs of disadvantaged groups, and the integration of oral and general health programs is lacking.
- Expansion of community-based disease prevention programs and removal of barriers to care are necessary to meet the needs of the total population.
- Dental insurance coverage is increasing, but still lags behind medical insurance coverage.
- Dental benefits under Medicaid do not ensure that oral health treatment is provided to low-income groups. Barriers include lack of patient and caregiver understanding of the importance of oral health, low reimbursement rates to providers, and administrative burdens.
- A narrow definition of *medically necessary dental care* limits oral health care services for insured persons, particularly the elderly.
- The dentist-to-population ratio is declining, raising concerns about the ability of the dental workforce to adequately meet the population's needs.
- Approximately 25 million persons live in areas lacking adequate dental care services (Health Professional Shortage Areas).
- Educational debt is increasing for dentists.
- The proportion of minorities in the oral health professions is disproportionate to their distribution in the general population.
- Current and projected demand for dental school faculty and oral health research scientists is not being met.
- Reliable and valid oral health outcome measures do not exist and must be developed.

Part Five asked, What are the needs and opportunities to enhance oral health? This question was addressed across three chapters. The first of these chapters described the determinants of oral health throughout the life stages, although it emphasized America's most vulnerable populations, children and older persons. The authors stated that the most essential of these determinants included biology and lifestyle, the physical and social environment, and organization of the health care system. The authors also stated that these determinants were not independent, but would interact. The chapter reached the following conclusions:

- Major factors affecting oral health and general well-being include biology and genetics, the environment, personal behaviors, access to care, and the organization of health care. These factors interact over the life span and determine the health of individuals, population groups, and communities.
- The burden of oral diseases and conditions is disproportionately borne by individuals with low socioeconomic status and by those with poor general health.
- Access to care is important to oral health, and health insurance increases access.
- Preventive measures such as dental sealants and protective mouth gear exist, but are inconsistently used and reinforced.
- Nursing homes and other long-term care facilities have limited capacity to deliver oral health care services to their residents, and this is of particular

concern given that their residents are at increased risk for oral diseases.

- Anticipatory guidance and risk assessment and management facilitate oral health care for children and the elderly.
- Federal and state assistance programs for selected oral health care services exist; however, their scope is limited and reimbursement rates are unsatisfactory compared with usual fees for care.

The second chapter described innovations in genetics, biotechnology, and biomimetics and explained how these areas might affect oral health care in the future. It also showed how changes in global demographics and technology were related to the oral health of all Americans. The chapter stated that the twenty-first century offers the promise of a new era for health shaped by the union of six cultural movements, any one of which would be sufficient to transform the human condition:

- Biologic and biotechnologic revolutions.
- Redistribution of the world's population by rapid and sizable migrations within countries and across borders.
- Changing demographics in developed, as well as developing, nations.
- Changing patterns of disease, including the emergence and reemergence of infectious diseases, and changes in the organization of health care.
- Real-time, worldwide communication via the Internet, cable, satellite, and wireless technologies.
- Continuing growth of information technology, specifically in computer speed, memory, and complexity.

The chapter also concluded that oral and craniofacial health issues would continue to be diverse and complex, and two major themes would remain: the need and demand for oral and craniofacial health care services and the role, functions, and mix of health care professionals.[29]

The final chapter of Part Five summarized the major findings of the Surgeon General's Report. The primary conclusion of the report was that oral health is essential to general health and well-being. The chapter called for a National Oral Health Plan that would lay the groundwork for improving oral health in the United States. The chapter also proposed five general actions that could be used to that end: increasing understanding of oral health and disease by the public, practitioners, and policy makers; expanding the science and evidence base; enhancing program integration and an oral health infrastructure; reducing barriers to oral health care services; and promoting private-public partnerships to address health disparities. The following section describes the major findings in greater detail.

Major Findings

The project team and contributing authors described eight major findings in the Surgeon General's Report. These findings reflected the conclusions presented at the end of each of the five parts, as well as the two principal themes described in Part One: *oral health means much more than healthy teeth* and *oral health is integral to general health.* The authors also related the eight major findings to two other principal themes. The first of these themes stated that "safe and effective disease prevention measures exist that everyone can adopt to improve oral health and prevent disease" (Surgeon General's Report, p. 18), and the second theme stated that "general health risk factors, such as tobacco use and poor dietary practices, also affect oral and craniofacial health" (Surgeon General's Report, p. 18).[16]

FINDING 1: ORAL DISEASES AND DISORDERS, IN AND OF THEMSELVES, AFFECT HEALTH AND WELL-BEING THROUGHOUT LIFE

According to the Surgeon General's Report, the burden of oral diseases and disorders was extensive, affecting Americans across the life span. A number of developmental disorders affected children from birth, such as congenitally missing teeth, congenital problems involving the tissues of the tooth, and craniofacial birth defects or syndromes. Oral clefts, for example, were among the most common types of congenital malformations in the United States, with incidences in the general population of 1.2 cases of cleft lip (with or without cleft palate) per 1000 live births and 0.6 cases of cleft palate per 1000 live births.[24] In addition, dental caries was one of the most common disorders to affect children ages 5 through 17 years; prevalence of dental caries was higher than that of asthma, hay fever, and chronic bronchitis (Fig. 2-1). More than 39 million Americans (22%) age 18 years or older have reported at least one of five types of orofacial pain during the preceding 6 months.[30] The vast majority of oral and pharyngeal cancers occurred in persons age 35 years or older, and the 30,000 cases of oral and pharyngeal cancer each year accounted for approximately 2.4% of all cancers in the United States.[23,31]

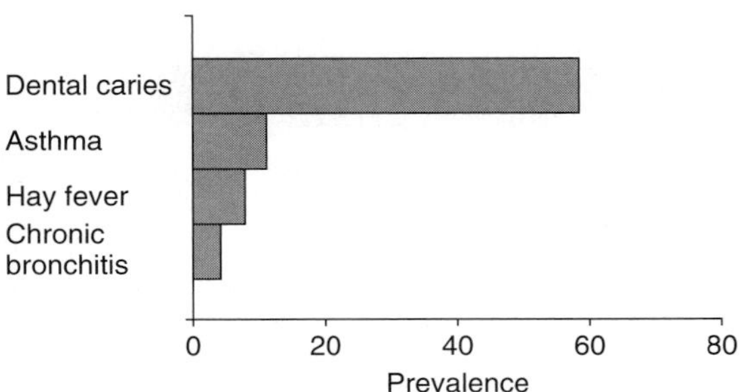

Fig. 2-1. Prevalence of common childhood diseases among children ages 5 through 17 years. (From the CDC/NCHS, 1996. Unpublished data from 1996 NHIS and NHANES III.)

The authors noted that, across the life span, the burden of oral diseases and conditions was particularly severe among vulnerable populations. For example, the prevalence of unrestored dental caries was consistently higher among those below the federal poverty level (FPL) than it was among those at or above the FPL (Fig. 2-2). Age-adjusted incidence rates showed that oral and pharyngeal cancers were the seventh most common cancer among white males, whereas oral and pharyngeal cancers were the fourth most common cancer among African-American males.[23,32] In addition, African-Americans were less likely to be diagnosed with a localized oral or pharyngeal cancer than were whites, and at every stage of diagnosis African-Americans had lower 5-year survival rates than did whites[23] (Fig. 2-3). Prevalence of edentulism was higher among non-Hispanic whites and non-Hispanic blacks than it was among Mexican-Americans, and a poverty status differential also existed among non-Hispanic whites and non-Hispanic blacks (Fig. 2-4).

In addition, the authors noted that many of these oral diseases and conditions undermined self-image and self-esteem, discouraged normal social interactions, led to chronic stress and depression, and incurred great financial burden. The authors also stated that many of these disorders interfered with vital human functions and activities of daily living.

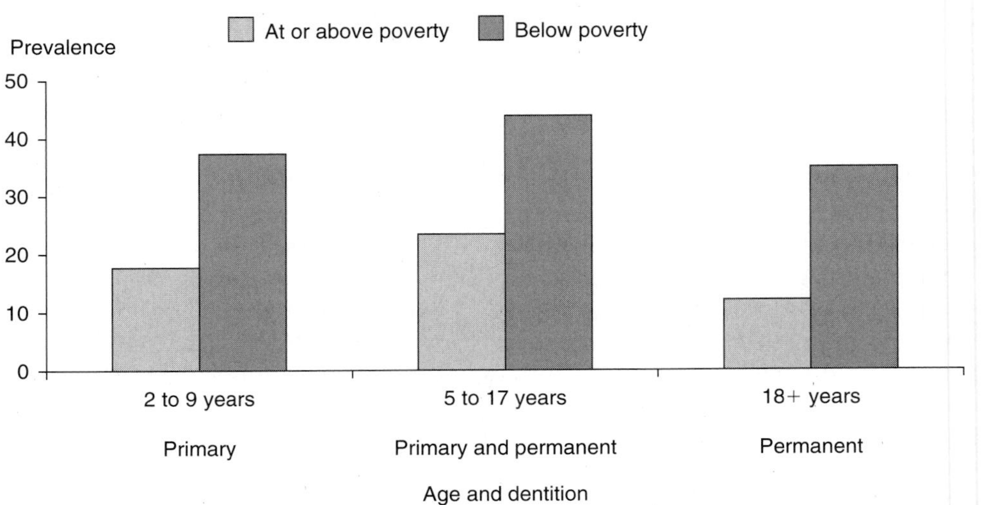

Fig. 2-2. Prevalence of unrestored dental caries among persons age 2 years or older, by poverty status. (From the CDC/NCHS, 1996. Unpublished data from NHANES III.)

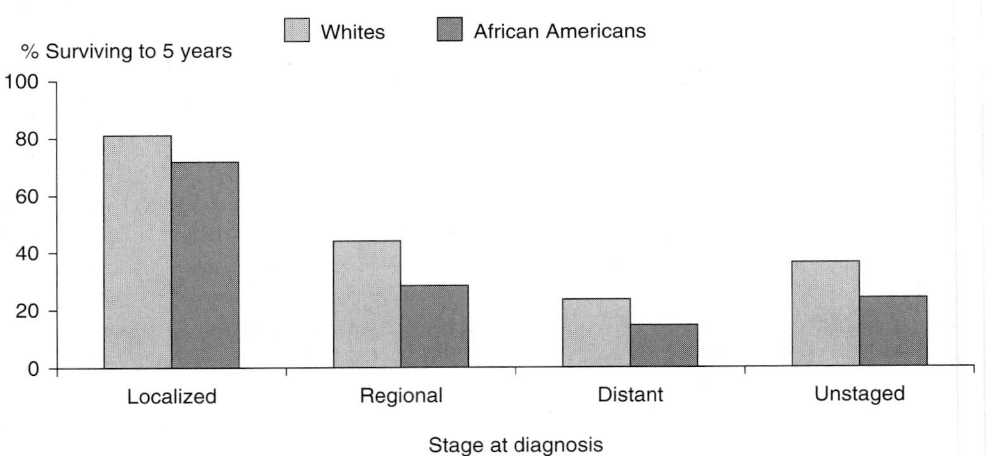

Fig. 2-3. Five-year oral and pharyngeal cancer survival rates among adults, by stage at diagnosis and race. (From Ries LA et al, editors: *SEER cancer statistics review, 1973-1996,* Bethesda, MD, 1999, National Cancer Institute, with permission of Oxford University Press.)

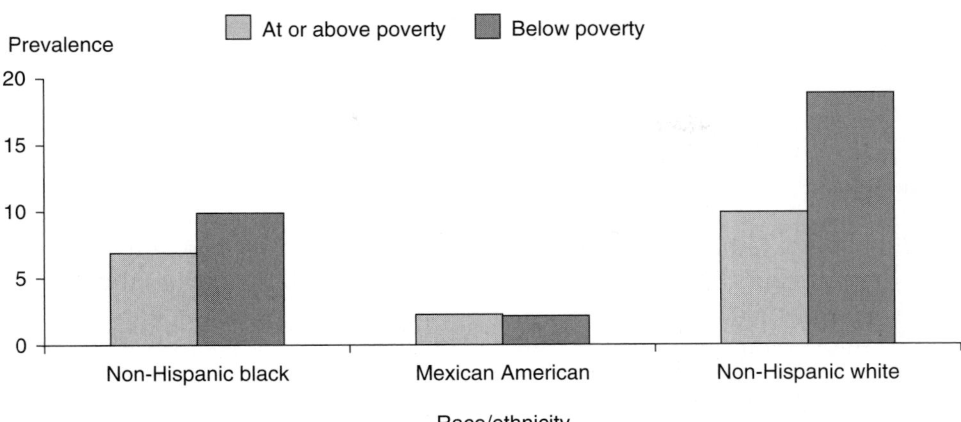

Fig. 2-4. Prevalence of edentulism among adults age 18 years or older, by race/ethnicity and poverty status. (From the CDC/NCHS, 1996. Unpublished data from NHANES III.)

FINDING 2: SAFE AND EFFECTIVE MEASURES EXIST TO PREVENT THE MOST COMMON DENTAL DISEASES—DENTAL CARIES AND PERIODONTAL DISEASES

The authors of the Surgeon General's Report listed the modalities that practitioners and public health officials have used to prevent and control dental caries in the United States, including community water fluoridation, school water fluoridation, dietary fluoride supplements, school-based fluoride mouth rinse programs, fluoride varnishes, dental sealants, fluoridated dentifrices, and fluoride gels.[33-35] The authors summarized the epidemiologic evidence supporting the majority of these modalities and reached some important conclusions.

- *Community water fluoridation.* Strong evidence suggested that this modality was effective in preventing coronal and root caries among children and adults.[36,37] Given the modest cost of fluoridating water systems that serve large populations, this modality was a highly cost-effective measure, as well. Community water fluoridation benefited all populations served by the water system, regardless of demographics or socioeconomic status.
- *School water fluoridation.* This modality had limited application, given the limitations of the evidence for effectiveness and difficulties in implementation and operation.[38] The Surgeon General's Report suggested that public health officials should base their decisions to initiate or continue using this modality on an assessment of current disease risk, availability of alternative modalities, and periodic evaluation of its effectiveness.
- *Dietary fluoride supplements.* The epidemiologic evidence from studies conducted before 1980 supporting the effectiveness of home use of daily dietary fluoride supplements was weak for school-age children residing in areas with less than optimal concentrations of fluoride in the water system.[39-41] By contrast, the evidence supporting the effectiveness of

school-based dietary fluoride supplement programs was strong.[39,40] One requirement for the success of school-based programs, however, was the involvement of highly motivated teachers and students.[42]

- *School-based fluoride mouth rinse programs.* Epidemiologic evidence from studies conducted before 1985 supported the effectiveness of 0.2% sodium fluoride mouth rinses in preventing coronal caries in school populations.[33] The cost-effectiveness of this modality was reduced with declining dental caries prevalence. The report suggested that public health officials should consider this modality for schools and classrooms where children are at high risk for dental caries, but it should not be used among preschool populations.
- *Fluoride varnishes.* The United States has not approved the use of fluoride varnishes with an anticaries indication. Evidence from studies conducted in countries other than the United States indicated that this modality may be efficacious, although the recommendations for the frequency of application were still in question. The results of cost-effectiveness studies were equivocal.[43-50]
- *Dental sealants.* The epidemiologic evidence strongly supported the effectiveness of this modality in preventing dental caries on pit-and-fissured tooth surfaces.[51-53] The authors noted that cost-effectiveness studies showed that this modality should be limited to high-risk children and high-risk teeth.[54,55]

The authors also listed a number of ways to prevent and control periodontal diseases. They noted that personal oral hygiene practices such as tooth brushing and flossing, as well as the use of nonprescription antimicrobial mouth rinses, were effective in preventing and controlling gingivitis.[55,56] They also noted that community-level measures to prevent and control gingivitis by increasing the public's understanding of the role that plaque plays in the condition have received mixed reviews. Although knowledge and attitudes were improved, the educational programs exhibited positive results only over a short time period.[57]

FINDING 3: LIFESTYLE BEHAVIORS THAT AFFECT GENERAL HEALTH, SUCH AS TOBACCO USE, EXCESSIVE ALCOHOL USE, AND POOR DIETARY CHOICES, ALSO AFFECT ORAL AND CRANIOFACIAL HEALTH

The authors cited several epidemiologic studies that identified tobacco and alcohol as major risk factors for oral and pharyngeal neoplasms.[58-60] Blot and colleagues[61] reported that tobacco and alcohol together accounted for 75% to 90% of all oral and pharyngeal cancers in the United States. The authors also stated that tobacco use was associated with periodontitis because the risk of alveolar bone loss was substantially higher among heavy smokers than among those who did not smoke.[62] In addition, the authors wrote of the association between diets high in carbohydrates and dental caries incidence, pointing to studies of the frequency and timing of dietary intake.[63,64]

FINDING 4: PROFOUND AND CONSEQUENTIAL ORAL HEALTH DISPARITIES EXIST WITHIN THE U.S. POPULATION

The discussion in Finding 1 highlighted some of the oral health disparities that existed in the United States across age cohorts, gender, race/ethnicity groups, and socioeconomic status (SES). The Surgeon

General's Report suggested that differential barriers to oral health care and unequal utilization of treatment services explained, in part, some of these disparities. In the United States, for example, gender, race/ethnicity, income, and dental insurance status each influenced utilization of oral health care services.[65,66] Table 2-2 shows that a higher proportion of females reported a dental visit in the last year than did males. The table also shows that a lower proportion of non-Hispanic blacks and Hispanics reported a dental visit than did non-Hispanic whites. These disparities appeared to remain when controlling for level of education. A smaller proportion of persons

Table 2-2. Oral Health Care Utilization among Adults Age 25 Years or Older, by Selected Characteristics and Year

	*1983**	*1989**	*1990*	*1991*	*1993*
Total†‡	53.9	58.9	62.3	58.2	60.8
Age					
25 to 34 years	59.0	60.9	65.1	59.1	60.3
35 to 44 years	60.3	65.9	69.1	64.8	66.9
45 to 64 years	54.1	59.9	62.8	59.2	62.0
65 years and older	39.3	45.8	49.6	47.2	51.7
65 to 74 years	43.8	50.0	53.5	51.1	56.3
75 years and older	31.8	39.0	43.4	41.3	44.9
Gender‡					
Male	51.7	56.2	58.8	55.5	58.2
Female	55.9	61.4	65.6	60.8	63.4
Poverty status‡§					
Below poverty	30.4	33.3	38.2	33.0	35.9
At or above poverty	55.8	62.1	65.4	61.9	64.3
Race and Hispanic origin‡					
White, non-Hispanic	56.6	61.8	64.9	61.5	64.0
Black, non-Hispanic	39.1	43.3	49.1	44.3	47.3
Hispanic‖	42.1	48.9	53.8	43.1	46.2

From Bloom B, Gift HC, Jack SS: Dental services and oral health: United States, 1989, *Vital Health Stat* 10(183):1, 1992.

NOTES: Data are based on household interviews of a sample of the civilian noninstitutionalized population. Denominators exclude persons with unknown dental data. Estimates for 1983 and 1989 are based on data for all members of the sample household. Beginning in 1990, estimates are based on one adult member per household. Estimates for 1993 are based on responses during the last half of the year only.

*Data for 1983 and 1989 are not strictly comparable with data for later years. Data for 1983 and 1989 are based on responses to the question, "About how long has it been since you last went to a dentist?" Starting in 1990, data are based on the question, "During the past 12 months, how many visits did you make to a dentist?"

†Includes all other races not shown separately and unknown poverty status and education level.

‡Age adjusted.

§Poverty status is based on family income and family size using Bureau of the Census poverty thresholds.

‖Persons of Hispanic origin may be of any race.

Continued

Table 2-2. Oral Health Care Utilization among Adults Age 25 Years or Older, by Selected Characteristics and Year—cont'd

	*1983**	*1989**	*1990*	*1991*	*1993*
Education‡					
Fewer than 12 years	35.1	36.9	41.2	35.2	38.0
12 years	54.8	58.2	61.3	56.7	58.7
13 years or higher	70.9	73.9	75.7	72.2	73.8
Education, race, and Hispanic origin‡					
Fewer than 12 years					
White, non-Hispanic	36.1	39.1	41.8	38.1	41.2
Black, non-Hispanic	31.7	32.0	37.9	33.0	33.1
Hispanic‖	33.8	36.5	42.7	28.9	33.0
12 years					
White, non-Hispanic	56.6	59.8	62.8	58.8	60.4
Black, non-Hispanic	40.5	44.8	51.1	43.1	48.2
Hispanic‖	48.7	56.5	59.9	49.5	54.6
13 years or higher					
White, non-Hispanic	72.6	75.8	77.3	74.2	75.8
Black, non-Hispanic	54.4	57.2	64.4	61.7	61.3
Hispanic‖	58.4	66.2	67.9	61.2	61.8

with a low SES reported a dental visit than did those with a high SES.

The authors of the Surgeon General's Report reminded the reader, however, that differences in utilization across these sociodemographic characteristics were not necessarily related to access problems. For example, respondents to the 1989 NHIS reported the reasons why they had not visited a dentist in the previous 12 months[65] (Table 2-3). For all age groups except those age 65 years or older, *no dental problem* was reported as the main reason. In contrast, the main reason among those in the oldest age cohort was *lack of teeth,* and this was also the second most frequently reported reason among persons of all ages.

Cost was the third most frequently reported reason among persons of all ages and the second most frequently reported reason among persons ages 2 through 34 years. As the 1989 NHIS data suggested, the reasons for *no dental visit* varied across gender, race/ethnicity, and SES.[65] In general, a higher proportion of men than women reported *no dental problem,* whereas a higher proportion of women than men reported *lack of teeth* and *cost* as the main reasons for no dental visit in the last year. In addition, a higher proportion of non-Hispanic blacks and Hispanics reported *no dental problem* than did non-Hispanic whites; however, a lower proportion of these minorities reported *lack of teeth* and *cost* as a reason than did non-Hispanic whites. Persons with higher SES, as mea-

Table 2-3. Distribution of the Reasons for No Dental Visit in the Last Year among Those without a Visit

	Total	*Fear*	*Cost*	*Access Problem*	*No Dental Problem*	*No Teeth*	*Not Important*	*Other Reason*
Age								
All ages	100.0	4.3	13.7	1.7	46.8	14.3	2.3	8.7
2 to 17 years	100.0	1.3	15.0	1.5	56.8	0.2	1.9	11.9
18 to 34 years	100.0	5.9	19.1	2.4	52.4	0.7	3.2	9.5
35 to 64 years	100.0	5.8	12.8	1.5	43.3	17.8	2.2	8.4
65 years or older	100.0	2.2	4.1	1.1	31.2	49.7	1.1	3.9
Race								
White	100.0	4.4	14.3	1.8	44.3	15.7	2.4	9.4
Black	100.0	4.0	11.4	1.0	58.5	8.8	1.5	5.1
Hispanic origin								
Hispanic	100.0	4.0	19.1	1.8	56.1	3.5	2.6	5.9
Non-Hispanic	100.0	4.3	13.0	1.7	45.7	15.6	2.2	9.1
Family income*								
<$10,000	100.0	3.8	19.7	1.7	42.8	22.5	1.4	6.4
$10,000-$19,999	100.0	4.0	18.8	1.5	47.0	17.4	1.7	6.5
$20,000-$34,999	100.0	4.8	13.7	1.7	51.3	11.5	2.3	11.1
$35,000 or higher	100.0	5.9	6.8	2.6	52.3	8.1	4.1	14.1

From Bloom B, Gift HC, Jack SS: Dental services and oral health: United States, 1989, *Vital Health Stat* 10(183):1, 1992.
NOTE: Data are based on household interviews of the civilian noninstitutionalized population.
*Persons with unknown income not shown separately.

sured by family income, were more likely to report *no dental problem* as a reason for no visit and less likely to report *lack of teeth* and *cost* as a reason than were persons with lower SES. It is somewhat paradoxical that the racial and ethnic minorities, who were more likely to suffer from dental caries and oral and pharyngeal cancers and less likely to use oral health care services than were their nonminority counterparts, were also less likely to recognize a dental problem. Although the authors concluded that disparities in access to care and utilization of services explained some of the oral health disparities, they also recognized that a number of factors and complex interrelations required further investigation, such as self-perceived need, locus of control, oral health attitudes, and knowledge.

FINDING 5: ADDITIONAL INFORMATION IS NEEDED TO IMPROVE AMERICA'S ORAL HEALTH AND ELIMINATE HEALTH DISPARITIES

The authors concluded that inadequate data existed in the United States regarding oral health, illness, behaviors, and use of services for the population as a whole, as well as for many of the nation's subpopulations. In particular, the authors recognized that few data existed to describe the plight of racial and ethnic minorities, the homeless, persons with disabilities, rural populations, the institutionalized, the very young, and the frail elderly. They also stated that insufficient data exploring oral health issues in relation to gender and sexual orientation existed. Data at the state and local levels were also lacking, and this absence was especially devastating, because the data were essential for program planning and evaluation. Given that program planning also relies on good cost-benefit and cost-effectiveness studies, the authors established that these types of analysis were also in short supply. The authors stated that researchers must generate data regarding the outcomes of dental treatment and continue to define and monitor oral health quality of life and general measures of oral health.

FINDING 6: THE MOUTH REFLECTS GENERAL HEALTH AND WELL-BEING

The Surgeon General's Report stated that the oral cavity was readily accessible and provided health care practitioners and individuals with a window into their general health status. The report also stated that the mouth exhibited signs of a number of systemic conditions, including nutritional deficiencies, HIV infection, and other immune system problems, as well as signs of general infection and stress. As practitioners and researchers gain the ability to accurately assess new substances in saliva, the oral cavity will also enable the diagnosis of specific diseases and the measurement of the concentration of a variety of drugs, hormones, and other molecules of interest. The report added that, in the near future, practitioners might also be able to use cells and fluids in the mouth for genetic analysis to help uncover risks for disease and predict outcomes of medical treatments.

FINDING 7: ORAL DISEASES AND CONDITIONS ARE ASSOCIATED WITH OTHER HEALTH PROBLEMS

The report stated that oral infections might be the source of systemic infections among persons with weakened immune systems. The report also described the link between oral signs and symptoms and other general health conditions.

During the past decade, researchers have described a number of intriguing associations between oral infections—primarily periodontal infections—and diabetes, heart disease, stroke, and adverse pregnancy outcomes. The Surgeon General's Report concluded that there is insufficient epidemiologic evidence to conclude that oral infections lead to the other conditions, however. Chapter 5 of the report described the quality of the evidence supporting the investigations that claimed an association. The chapter included observational, experimental, animal, and population-based studies in its assessment of the evidence. The chapter also offered operative mechanisms proposed to support an association between oral infections and systemic conditions, when they existed. A summary of the evidence is beyond the scope of this section; interested readers are encouraged to consult the Surgeon General's Report for a thorough review of the pertinent literature.

The report described several implications for the linkages between oral infections and systemic conditions. For example, recognition of established oral signs and symptoms might assist in the early diagnosis and prompt treatment of some systemic diseases and conditions. In addition, the report concluded that research into the potential use of oral and nasal vaccination routes could lead to enhanced immunity, and investigations into the host susceptibility factors that contribute to the dissemination of oral infections to other parts of the body could lead to early prevention of disease. The report also placed the potential connection between periodontal infections and heart disease, stroke, and adverse pregnancy outcomes into a broader context. If any of these associations prove to be causal, the report suggested that major changes in health care delivery and the way that health professionals are trained should be expected to follow. To minimize adverse health outcomes and morbidity, the report urged that health professionals, the public, drug manufacturers, and researchers be made aware of the oral complications of pharmaceuticals and other therapies for disease management and health prevention.

FINDING 8: SCIENTIFIC RESEARCH IS KEY TO FURTHER REDUCTION IN THE BURDEN OF DISEASES AND DISORDERS THAT AFFECT THE FACE, MOUTH, AND TEETH

The Surgeon General's Report recognized that the science base for dental diseases was extensive and provided a strong foundation for improvements in prevention. The report also recognized, however, that the science base for craniofacial and other oral health conditions was not as strong and needed greater attention. The authors acknowledged that research has led to a variety of strategies to improve oral health through prevention, early diagnosis, and treatment; however, they also stated that future investigations ought to focus on more targeted and effective interventions and ways to enhance appropriate adoption by the public and health professionals. The report concluded that the application of powerful new diagnostic tools and techniques and advancements in genetics, genomics, neuroscience, and cancer hold great promise for the health of Americans.

A Framework for Action

The Surgeon General's Report suggested that all Americans could benefit from "the development of a National Oral Health Plan to improve quality of life and eliminate health disparities by facilitating collaborations among individuals, health care providers, communities, and policymakers at all levels of society and by taking advantage of existing initiatives" (Surgeon General's Report, p. 284).[16] The report listed the following key components of the national plan.

CHANGE PERCEPTIONS REGARDING ORAL HEALTH AND DISEASE SO THAT ORAL HEALTH BECOMES AN ACCEPTED COMPONENT OF GENERAL HEALTH

As subcategories of this component, the Surgeon General's Report called for changing public perceptions, policy makers' perceptions, and health providers' perceptions. Toward changing public perceptions, the report recognized that many persons fail to recognize the importance of oral and craniofacial symptoms, especially when compared with indications of general health and illness. As a result, the proper treatment of diseases and conditions is often postponed, thus exacerbating problems and complicating care. To address this lack of public recognition, the report recommended that the public be made aware of the meaning of oral health, as well as the relation between oral health and general health. The report also suggested that such messages should be culturally sensitive, to reflect the diversity of American society. Toward changing policy makers' perceptions, the report suggested that policy makers who were well informed would be more likely to include oral health services in health promotion and disease prevention programs, care delivery systems, and reimbursement schedules. Toward informing policy makers, the report stressed that every conceivable approach should be used, both formally and informally. Toward changing health providers' perceptions, the report acknowledged the fact that nondental health professionals infrequently receive training in oral health and disease during their professional education. This lack of training is disheartening, because nondental health professionals are in a position to enhance oral health as part of their practices. To address this shortcoming, the report suggested that physicians include an oral examination as part of a general physical examination, advise their patients about the adverse oral health effects of tobacco and diet, and refer patients to oral health professionals before medical or surgical procedures that could damage oral tissues.

ACCELERATE THE BUILDING OF THE SCIENCE AND EVIDENCE BASE AND APPLY SCIENCE EFFECTIVELY TO IMPROVE ORAL HEALTH

The report pointed to the abundance of behavioral and biomedical research, clinical trials, and population-based investigations that have shaped advances in oral and craniofacial health over the last several decades. In spite of this abundance of research, however, the report highlighted a lack of progress in the study of etiology and distribution of oral diseases and conditions and the scarcity of descriptive data at the state and local levels. The report suggested that for successes to continue into the future, data collection initiatives must focus on differences across subgroups in the population. With these data, policy makers would have sufficient information at their disposal for the introduction of appropriate and effective oral health policy. In addition, researchers must study the interaction of genes with environmental and behavioral variables. The report recommended that the findings from these new studies must be effectively translated into health care practice and healthful lifestyles. The report also called for intensified attention to the complex relations between oral inflammatory diseases and other systemic conditions, such as diabetes and cardiovascular disease.

BUILD AN EFFECTIVE HEALTH INFRASTRUCTURE THAT MEETS THE ORAL HEALTH NEEDS OF ALL AMERICANS AND INTEGRATES ORAL HEALTH EFFECTIVELY INTO OVERALL HEALTH

The report concluded that the public health capacity for addressing oral health was insufficient to meet the demand and was not integrated with other public health programs. The result of these insufficiencies included disparities in oral health among the nation's needy segments. The report acknowledged that resources, such as personnel, equipment, and facilities, were lacking.

REMOVE KNOWN BARRIERS BETWEEN PEOPLE AND ORAL HEALTH SERVICES

The Surgeon General's Report recognized that lack of dental insurance, both public and private, was one of the barriers to oral health care services in the United States, and this lack translated into poorer oral health outcomes among those who lived near or below the federal poverty level. The report also showed that low reimbursement rates to dentists caused lack of participation by oral health professionals in many public dental insurance programs. Although public initiatives such as the Children's Health Insurance Program have helped address the concerns of children and adolescents, the report stated that additional programs should be implemented for those with physical, mental, and emotional disabilities.

USE PUBLIC-PRIVATE PARTNERSHIPS TO IMPROVE THE ORAL HEALTH OF THOSE WHO WILL SUFFER DISPROPORTIONATELY FROM ORAL DISEASES

The report stated that the resources of public health agencies, private industry, social services organizations, educators, health care providers, researchers, the media, community leaders, voluntary health organizations, consumer groups, and concerned citizens must be brought to bear collectively to reduce or eliminate oral health disparities in the nation. The report went on to state that these collaborations would build and strengthen cross-discipline, culturally competent, community-based, and community-wide efforts and demonstration programs to expand initiatives for disease prevention and health promotion. Examples of such initiatives included programs to prevent tobacco use, promote better dietary choices, and encourage the use of protective gear to prevent sporting injuries.

SETTING CHANGE IN MOTION

The Surgeon General's Report provided a solid framework for setting in motion improvements in oral health. This section highlights some of the initiatives that have developed in concert with the report or as a direct result of the attention that the report has brought to oral health issues in the United States. This section discusses federal and state initiatives separately and provides organized dentistry's response. The discussion is not meant to be exhaustive but is meant to provide insight into the kinds of programs that are expected to reduce disparities, set reasonable objectives, encourage research, and improve the dissemination of information to the public and health professionals.

Federal Initiatives

To increase awareness of the Surgeon General's Report among policy makers and public health professionals, the Office of the Surgeon General presented the Face of a Child: Surgeon General's Conference on Children and Oral Health in June 2000. The conference was supported by a variety of federal agencies, including the Agency for Healthcare Research and Quality, CDC, FDA, Indian Health Service, Health Resources and Services Administration, National Institutes of Health, and U.S. Department of Agriculture. The goals of the conference (www.nidcr.nih.gov/sgr/children/children.htm) were to do the following:

- Highlight findings of the Surgeon General's Report on Oral Health
- Increase appreciation of the importance of oral health to overall health and well-being and of the need to integrate oral health into policy, research, professional training, and medical care for children
- Engage the child health and welfare community and the public in a discussion of ethical, legal, historical, and policy issues underlying all areas of children's health
- Promote effective community partnerships and coalitions to eliminate disparities in children's access to oral health care and in their health outcomes

Conference themes were consistent with those of the Surgeon General's Report and included the following:

- Using oral health as an indicator of children's social and health problems

- Ensuring a healthy start for children by including oral health in general health care
- Using ethics, laws, and health policies to improve children's oral health
- Building effective partnerships to eliminate disparities in children's access to oral health care and improve their health

In tackling these goals and themes, the conference addressed several items listed in the "Framework for Action" in the Surgeon General's Report, including changing perceptions about oral health and disease, building an effective health infrastructure, and using public-private partnerships to improve oral health, particularly among those who suffer disproportionately from oral diseases.

In 1979 *Healthy People—The Surgeon General's Report on Health Promotion and Disease Prevention* proposed national goals for reducing premature deaths and preserving independence for older adults.[13] In 1980 *Promoting Health/Preventing Disease: Objectives for the Nation* became the first document to propose specific national health objectives for the United States.[67] The report included a number of oral health objectives (Box 2-3) and charged the nation to meet these targets by 1990. A decade later, the U.S. Department of Health and Human Services released *Healthy People 2000: National Health Promotion and Disease Prevention Objectives,* a list of health objectives for the nation, including 17 oral health objectives (Box 2-4).[68] According to a 1998–1999 review of progress toward meeting the *Healthy People* oral health objectives for 2000, the United States had met only the objective for reduction of oral cancer deaths (13.7).[69] Although the nation showed progress toward meeting eight of the oral health objectives (13.1, 13.4, 13.6, 13.8, 13.9, 13.14, 13.15, and 13.17), it also showed trends that were moving away from meeting three objectives (13.3, 13.5, and 13.12) and mixed trends for objective 13.2. No data beyond baseline were available to assess progress toward four of the oral health objectives (13.10, 13.11, 13.13, and 13.16) during the 1998–1999 review.

In the same year that the Office of the Surgeon General released the Surgeon General's Report, the U.S. Department of Health and Human Services also released the health objectives for 2010 (Box 2-5) in a document entitled *Healthy People 2010: With Understanding and Improving Health and Objectives for Improving Health.*[70] As did its predecessors, the *Healthy People 2010* document contained an oral health priority area. The overall goal for the oral health priority area was to "prevent and control oral and craniofacial diseases, conditions, and injuries and improve access to related services".[70] Unlike the *Healthy People 2000* objectives and in keeping with one of the "Framework for Action" items from the Surgeon General's Report, the *Healthy People 2010* objectives emphasized reduction of health disparities by setting the target for each objective as "better than the best." For example, *Healthy People 2000* objective 13.2 called for a reduction in untreated dental caries in children, but set different targets, depending on race, ethnicity, or SES. The implication of these subgroup-specific targets was that it was acceptable for one population group to have a higher proportion of untreated disease than it was for another group. By contrast, *Healthy People 2010* objectives set a single target for all population subgroups that was better than the target for the population subgroup with the most favorable experience, as defined during the *Healthy People 2000* time period.

BOX 2-3

Healthy People 1990 Objectives for the Oral Health Priority Area

1990 OBJECTIVES, FLUORIDATION AND DENTAL HEALTH

HEALTH STATUS

a. By 1990, the proportion of 9-year-old children who have experienced dental caries in their permanent teeth should be decreased to 60%.
b. By 1990, the prevalence of gingivitis in children ages 6 to 17 years should be decreased to 18%.
c. By 1990, in adults, the prevalence of gingivitis and destructive periodontal disease should be decreased to 20% and 21%, respectively.

RISK REDUCTION

d. By 1990, no public elementary or secondary school (and no medical facility) should offer highly cariogenic foods or snacks in vending machines or in school breakfast or lunch programs.
e. By 1990, virtually all students in secondary schools and colleges who participate in organized contact sports should routinely wear proper mouth guards.

PUBLIC AWARENESS

f. By 1990, at least 95% of schoolchildren and their parents should be able to identify the principal risk factors related to dental diseases and be aware of the importance of fluoridation and other measures in controlling these diseases.
g. By 1990, at least 75% of adults should be aware of the necessity for both thorough personal oral hygiene and regular professional care in the prevention and control of periodontal disease.

SERVICES

h. By 1990, at least 95% of the population on community water systems should be receiving the benefits of optimally fluoridated water.
i. By 1990, at least 50% of schoolchildren living in fluoride-deficient areas that do not have community water systems should be served by an optimally fluoridated school water supply.
j. By 1990, at least 65% of schoolchildren should be proficient in personal oral hygiene practices and should be receiving other needed preventive dental services in addition to fluoridation.

SURVEILLANCE

k. By 1990, a comprehensive and integrated system should be in place for periodic determination of the oral health status, dental treatment needs, and utilization of dental services (including reasons for and costs of dental visits) of the U.S. population.
l. By 1985, systems should be in place for determining coverage of all major dental public health preventive measures and activities to reduce consumption of highly cariogenic foods.

From US Department of Health and Human Services. Public Health Service: *Promoting health/preventing disease: objectives for the nation,* Washington, DC, 1980, US Department of Health and Human Services.

In January 2001 the CDC's Division of Oral Health and the Association of State and Territorial Dental Directors (ASTDD) unveiled the National Oral Health Surveillance System (NOHSS) on the CDC web page (www.cdc.gov/nohss). CDC and ASTDD designed the NOHSS "to help public health programs monitor the burden of oral disease, use of the oral health care delivery system, and the status of community water fluoridation on both a state and national level." The surveillance system in-

BOX 2-4

Healthy People 2000 Objectives for the Oral Health Priority Area

Health Status Objectives

13.1 Reduce dental caries (cavities) so that the proportion of children with one or more caries (in permanent or primary teeth) is no more than 35% among children age 6 through 8 and no more than 60% among adolescents age 15

13.2 Reduce untreated dental caries so that the proportion of children with untreated caries (in permanent and primary teeth) is no more than 20% among children age 6 through 8 and no more than 15% among adolescents age 15

13.3 Increase to at least 45% the proportion of people age 35 through 44 who have never lost a permanent tooth because of dental caries or periodontal diseases

13.4 Reduce to no more than 20% the proportion of people age 65 and older who have lost all of their natural teeth

13.5 Reduce the prevalence of gingivitis among people age 35 through 44 to no more than 30%

13.6 Reduce destructive periodontal diseases to a prevalence of no more than 15% among people age 35 through 44

13.7 Reduce deaths caused by cancer of the oral cavity and pharynx to no more than 10.5 per 100,000 men age 45 through 74 and 4.1 per 100,000 women age 45 through 74

Risk Reduction Objectives

13.8 Increase to at least 50% the proportion of children who have received sealants on the occlusal (chewing) surfaces of permanent teeth

13.9 Increase to at least 75% the proportion of people served by community water systems providing optimal levels of fluoride

13.10 Increase use of professionally or self-administered topical or systemic (dietary) fluorides to at least 85% of people not receiving optimally fluoridated public water

13.11 Increase to at least 75% the proportion of parents and caregivers who use feeding practices that prevent baby bottle tooth decay

Services and Protection Objectives

13.12 Increase to at least 90% the proportion of all children entering school programs for the first time who have received an oral health screening, referral, and follow-up for necessary diagnostic, preventive, and treatment services

13.13 Extend to all long-term institutional facilities the requirement that oral examinations and services be provided no later than 90 days after entry into these facilities

13.14 Increase to at least 70% the proportion of people age 35 and older using the oral health care system during each year

13.15 Increase to at least 40 the number of states that have an effective system for recording and referring infants with cleft lips or palates to craniofacial anomaly teams

13.16 Extend requirement of the use of effective head, face, eye, and mouth protection to all organizations, agencies, and institutions sponsoring sporting and recreation events that pose risk of injury

13.17 Reduce smokeless tobacco use by males age 12 through 24 to a prevalence of no more than 4%

From US Department of Health and Human Services. Public Health Service: *Healthy people: national health promotion and disease prevention objectives,* Washington, DC, 1991, US Department of Health and Human Services.

BOX 2-5

Healthy People 2010 Objectives for the Oral Health Priority Area

21.1	Reduce the proportion of children and adolescents who have dental caries experience in their primary and permanent teeth
21.2	Reduce the proportion of children, adolescents, and adults with untreated dental decay
21.3	Increase the proportion of adults who have never had a permanent tooth extracted because of dental caries or periodontal disease
21.4	Reduce the proportion of older adults who have had all their natural teeth extracted
21.5	Reduce periodontal diseases
21.6	Increase the proportion of oral and pharyngeal cancers detected at the earliest stages
21.7	Increase the proportion of adults who, in the past 12 months, report having had an examination to detect oral and pharyngeal cancers
21.8	Increase the proportion of children who have received dental sealants on their molar teeth
21.9	Increase the proportion of the U.S. population served by community water systems with optimally fluoridated water
21.10	Increase the proportion of children and adults who use the oral health care system each year
21.11	Increase the proportion of long-term care residents who use the oral health care system each year
21.12	Increase the proportion of low-income children and adolescents who receive any preventive dental service during the past year
21.13*	Increase the proportion of school-based health centers with an oral health component
21.14	Increase the proportion of local health departments and community-based health centers, including community, migrant, and homeless health centers, that have an oral health component
21.15	Increase the number of states and the District of Columbia that have a system for recording and referring infants and children with cleft lips, cleft palates, and other craniofacial anomalies to craniofacial anomaly rehabilitative teams
21.16	Increase the number of states and the District of Columbia that have an oral and craniofacial health surveillance system
21.17*	Increase the number of tribal, state (including the District of Columbia), and local health agencies that serve jurisdictions of 250,000 or more persons that have in place an effective public dental health program directed by a dental professional with public health training

From US Department of Health and Human Services. Public Health Service: *Healthy people 2010,* ed 2, 2 vols, Washington, DC, 2000, US Government Printing Office.
*Objective in development or to be reassessed.

cluded a variety of indicators of oral health status, guidelines for oral diseases and health care, information on state dental programs, and links to other sources of oral health information. Each of these indicators was evaluated and approved by the Council of State and Territorial Epidemiologists and the Association of State and Territorial Chronic Disease Program Directors. At its inception, the NOHSS included eight main oral health indicators, including dental visits, teeth cleaning, complete tooth loss, fluoridation status, caries experience, untreated caries, and cancer of the oral cavity and pharynx. The CDC and ASTDD designed the system so that new indicators could be added in the future, based on data sources and surveillance capacity available to most states. Current sources of data include national surveys, such as the National Health and Nutrition Examination Survey, National Health Interview Survey, and the Fluoridation Census, as well as state-based surveys, such as the Behavioral Risk Factor Surveillance System, Youth Risk Behavior Surveillance System, Pregnancy Risk Assessment Monitoring System, ASTDD's Basic Screening Survey, and annual synopses of state dental public health programs. In creating the NOHSS, the CDC and ASTDD helped accelerate the building of the science and evidence base and thus addressed one of the "Framework for Action" items in the Surgeon General's Report.

In April 2000 the U.S. General Accounting Office released *Oral Health: Dental Disease Is a Chronic Problem among Low-Income Populations.*[71] The intent of the report was to determine the dental health status of Medicaid beneficiaries and other vulnerable populations and establish the extent to which these groups have dental coverage and use oral health care services. The authors analyzed currently available national surveys of oral health, as well as Medicaid payment data. In so doing, the U.S. General Accounting Office addressed two of the "Framework for Action" items contained in the Surgeon General's Report (building the science and evidence base and applying science to the improvement of oral health), as well as removing known barriers between people and oral health services.

During the latter half of 2000, in an effort to meet two of the "Framework for Action" items, several collaborating agencies invited applications for research designed to lead to a reduction in health disparities in the United States by focusing on craniofacial and oral diseases, disorders, and health. The request for proposals, entitled *Centers for Research to Reduce Oral Health Disparities,* was sponsored by the National Institute of Dental and Craniofacial Research, HRSA, National Institute of Child Health and Human Development, National Institute of Nursing Research, CDC, Office of Behavioral and Social Science Research, Office of Research on Minority Health, and Office of Research on Women's Health. The research centers were to support science that would lead to an understanding of the factors associated with health disparities and support the development, testing, and evaluation of interventions designed to reduce health disparities, with a particular interest in oral, dental, and craniofacial diseases and disorders. The sponsoring agencies were to provide to highly qualified applicants $1.5 million in support per year over a 7-year period. In providing the funds, the collaborating federal agencies intended that research institutions would discover some of the determinants of oral health disparities in the United States and create initiatives designed to reduce or eliminate the differentials.

State Initiatives

In 2001 the National Institute of Dental and Craniofacial Research and the National Cancer Institute invited applications from eligible institutions for grants to aid in research leading to the development of state models for oral cancer prevention and early detection programs. The request for proposals, entitled *State Models for Oral Cancer Prevention and Early Detection,* was directly related to "Frameworks for Action" items (building an effective science base, building an effective health infrastructure, and using public-private partnerships to improve oral health) in the Surgeon General's Report and several priority areas of *Healthy People 2010.* In addition, the sponsoring agencies viewed this initiative as a first step in the use of oral health assessments as part of an evaluation of overall systemic health. The aims of the request included the following: support an epidemiologic assessment of the level of oral cancer within the state; assess the level of knowledge of oral cancer risk factors among health professionals and the public; document and assess practices in diagnosing oral cancers in the health professions; and assess whether the public is receiving an oral cancer examination annually from a health care provider. The request suggested that a statewide assessment, as opposed to any other strategy, was an important approach, because each state had particular demographics, oral cancer epidemiology, and practice acts governing its health professionals.

Also in 2001, CDC's Division of Oral Health and ASTDD launched a collaborative program intended to provide summaries of dental public health initiatives across the 50 states and the District of Columbia. The project, entitled *Synopses of State Dental Public Health Programs,* exists as a web page (ww2.cdc.gov/nccdphp/doh/synopses/index.asp) and is available to those who require access to current information regarding personnel, resources, and oral health programs at the state and local levels.

Organized Dentistry's Response

Nine months before the release of the Surgeon General's Report, the American Dental Association (ADA) convened a conference that focused on improving the delivery of oral health care services to Medicaid recipients, particularly children and young adults. The Achieving Improvements in Medicaid (AIM) conference evolved from discussions that occurred during the 1998 Building Partnerships to Improve Children's Access to Medicaid Oral Health Services conference, sponsored by the Health Care Financing Administration (currently Centers for Medicare and Medicaid Services), Health Resources and Services Administration, and National Center for Education in Maternal and Child Health.[72] The 1998 conference identified several barriers to oral health care services for Medicaid recipients, including the following:

- Inadequate funding and reimbursement
- Lack of understanding of the importance of oral health to overall health
- Inappropriate utilization practices
- Administrative barriers
- Workforce issues

The goal of the AIM conference was to bring together, in an open forum, state and local policy makers, practitioners, and experts to identify ways to diminish barriers identified during the 1998 conference. Specifically, the participants were to do the following:

- Individually and collectively take responsibility for improvements to the system
- Foster application of successful strategies that improve access through sharing of program innovations and generating new ideas
- Immediately obtain the commitment of every attendee to an action step to affect change

Although AIM preceded the Surgeon General's Report, the conference effectively captured the spirit of the report's "Framework for Action" items. Specifically, the conference both directly and indirectly called for the building of an effective infrastructure that would meet the oral health needs of all Americans, requested the removal of known barriers to oral health care services, and emphasized public-private partnerships and strategies for the improvement of oral health.

SUMMARY

In May 2000 *Oral Health in America,* the first Surgeon General's Report to focus exclusively on oral health issues, was released to the nation. The report carefully divided relevant issues into five parts, each pertaining to a particular question: (1) What is oral health? (2) What is the status of oral health in America? (3) What is the relation between oral health and general health and well-being? (4) How is oral health promoted and maintained, and how are oral diseases prevented? and (5) What are the needs and opportunities to enhance oral health? The report also introduced four themes: (1) Oral health means much more than healthy teeth. (2) Oral health is integral to general health. (3) Safe and effective disease prevention measures exist that everyone can adopt to improve oral health and prevent disease. (4) General health risk factors, such as tobacco and poor dietary practices, have a negative effect on oral and craniofacial health.

The Surgeon General's Report relates a story of dramatic change in focus for oral health issues and improvements in oral health over the last century. The report also reminds the reader that the nation faces some serious challenges for the future. Although oral health has improved in the United States over the last century, disparities in health still exist. Specific population groups, such as infants and young children, the poor, those residing in rural locations, the homeless, persons with disabilities, racial and ethnic minorities, the institutionalized, and the frail elderly, experience a greater burden of oral and craniofacial diseases. There are also great disparities in access to oral health care and utilization of preventive services, each paramount to the establishment and maintenance of optimal health. In addition, the report recognizes that insufficient data exist to describe these population groups. The lack of data will make the development and evaluation of solutions a more difficult task.

In response to the release of the Surgeon General's Report, several federal, state, and local entities introduced initiatives that were intended to address the five questions and four themes of the report. These initiatives, including the Surgeon General's Conference on Children and Oral Health, national health objectives for 2010 *(Healthy People 2010),* a number of joint projects between the CDC and ASTDD, the ADA's AIM program, and other relevant reports and calls for research proposals, sprang forth from a recognition that solving the nation's oral health concerns required a highly coordinated and deliberate approach. These initiatives provide the impetus for change in policy, implementation of effective public health programs, and initiatives to follow. The Surgeon General's Report never claimed to have all of the answers. Rather, it posed meaningful questions that were to be addressed by organizations in the best position to develop solutions. The initiatives serve as an early example of what will continue to be an exciting and challenging time for anyone interested in oral health.

By publishing the Surgeon General's Report, the Office of the Surgeon General has made available important and timely information to health care practitioners, public health professionals, policy makers, and the public. For access to the report, the Office of the Surgeon General provides an electronic version of the document on their web page (http://surgeongeneral.gov/library/oralhealth) and offers a free hard copy of the report to all who request one.

REVIEW QUESTIONS

1. The Surgeon General's Report argues that *oral health means more than healthy teeth.* Why is such an argument necessary? What evidence exists to support such a claim?
2. The Surgeon General's Report acknowledges a lack of epidemiologic research, health services research, and outcomes data at the national, state, and local levels. How has this lack of data affected oral health in the United States? Propose some strategies that could be used in the future to increase the amount of data available to policy makers and public health practitioners. What are some of the barriers to implementing these strategies?
3. Several oral health disparities exist in the United States today. List three of the disparities and discuss how the Surgeon General's Report proposes addressing them.
4. List three ways that the oral cavity may reflect general health and well-being. How might this "reflection" be important to oral health practitioners? How might it be important to medical and other nondental practitioners?
5. This chapter describes a number of ways that changing oral health has been set in motion. Discuss one way at the national level and one at the state level. Propose methods for monitoring the success of these strategies.

REFERENCES

1. Evans CA, Kleinman DV: The Surgeon General's report on oral health in America: opportunities for the dental profession, *J Am Dent Assoc* 131:1721, 2000.
2. Schamel CE et al: *Guide to the records of the United States House of Representatives at the National Archives, 1789-1989: bicentennial edition,* Washington, DC, 1989, National Archives and Records Administration.
3. Straus R: The unorganized marine hospital fund. In *Medical care for seamen: the origin of public medical service in the United States,* New Haven, 1950, Yale University Press.
4. Mullan F: Sailors, sinecures, and reforms. In *Plagues and politics. The story of the United States Public Health Service,* New York, 1989, Basic Books.
5. Mullan F: Science, immigrants, and the public health movement. In *Plagues and politics. The story of the United States Public Health Service,* New York, 1989, Basic Books.
6. Mullan F: Public health warriors. In *Plagues and politics. The story of the United States Public Health Service,* New York, 1989, Basic Books.
7. Mullan F: Public health within limits. In *Plagues and politics. The story of the United States Public Health Service,* New York, 1989, Basic Books.
8. Miles R: *The Department of Health, Education, and Welfare,* New York, 1974, Praeger.
9. Harris RR: *Dental services in a new age: a history of the National Institute of Dental Research,* Rockville, MD, 1989, Montrose Press.
10. Mullan F: The coming of HEW. In *Plagues and politics. The story of the United States Public Health Service,* New York, 1989, Basic Books.
11. Mullan F: Care, cost, and prevention. In *Plagues and politics. The story of the United States Public Health Service,* New York, 1989, Basic Books.
12. US Surgeon General's Advisory Committee on Smoking and Health: *Smoking and health: report of the advisory committee to the Surgeon General,* Washington, DC, 1964, US Government Printing Office.
13. US Department of Health and Human Services. Public Health Service: *Healthy people—the Surgeon General's report on health promotion and disease prevention,* Washington, DC, 1979, US Department of Health and Human Services.
14. US Department of Health and Human Services. Public Health Service: *Surgeon General's report on acquired immune deficiency syndrome,* Washington, DC, 1987, US Government Printing Office.

15. US Department of Health and Human Services. Public Health Service. Centers for Disease Control and Prevention: *Understanding AIDS,* Washington, DC, 1988, US Government Printing Office.
16. US Department of Health and Human Services. Public Health Service. National Institutes of Health. National Institute of Dental and Craniofacial Research: *Oral health in America: a report of the Surgeon General,* Bethesda, MD, 2000, National Institute of Dental and Craniofacial Research.
17. World Health Organization: *Constitution of the World Health Organization,* Geneva, 1948, World Health Organization Basic Documents.
18. Massey JT et al: *Design and estimation for the National Health Interview Survey, 1985-94,* Hyattsville, MD, 1989, National Center for Health Statistics.
19. US Department of Health and Human Services. Public Health Service. Centers for Disease Control and Prevention. National Center for Health Statistics: Design and estimation for the National Health Interview Survey, 1995-2004, *Vital Health Stat* 2(130):1, 2000.
20. US Department of Health and Human Services. Public Health Service. Centers for Disease Control and Prevention. National Center for Health Statistics: Plan and operation of the Third National Health and Nutrition Examination Survey, 1988-94, *Vital Health Stat* 1(32):1, 1994.
21. US Department of Health and Human Services. Public Health Service. National Institutes of Health. National Institute of Dental Research: *Oral health of United States adults. The national survey of oral health in U.S. employed adults and seniors: 1985-86,* Bethesda, MD, 1987, National Institute of Dental Research.
22. US Department of Health and Human Services. Public Health Service. National Institutes of Health. National Institute of Dental Research: *Oral health of United States children. The national survey of dental caries in U.S. school children: 1986-87,* Bethesda, MD, 1989, National Institute of Dental Research.
23. Ries LA et al, editors: *SEER cancer statistics review, 1973-1996,* Bethesda, MD, 1999, National Cancer Institute.
24. Schulman J et al: Surveillance for and comparison of birth defect prevalences in two geographic areas—United States, 1983-88, *MMWR Morb Mortal Wkly Rep* 42:1, 1993.
25. Tomar SL: Total tooth loss among persons aged greater than or equal to 65 years—selected states, 1995-1997, *MMWR Morb Mortal Wkly Rep* 48:206, 1997.
26. Malamud D, Tabak L, editors: Saliva as a diagnostic fluid, *Ann N Y Acad Sci* 694:128, 1993.
27. Mandel ID: The diagnostic uses of saliva, *J Oral Pathol Med* 19:119, 1990.
28. Patrick DL, Bergner M: Measurement of oral health status in the 1990s, *Annu Rev Public Health* 11:165, 1990.
29. Casamassimo P: *Bright futures in practice: oral health,* Arlington, VA, 1996, National Center for Education in Maternal and Child Health.
30. Lipton JA, Ship JA, Larach-Robinson D: Estimated prevalence and distribution of reported orofacial pain in the United States, *J Am Dent Assoc* 124:115, 1993.
31. American Cancer Society: *Cancer facts and figures,* Atlanta, 1999, American Cancer Society.
32. Wingo PA et al: Annual report to the nation on the status of cancer, 1973-1996. With a special section on lung cancer and tobacco smoking, *J Natl Cancer Inst* 91:675, 1999.
33. US Department of Health and Human Services. Public Health Service. Centers for Disease Control and Prevention: Recommendations for using fluoride to prevent and control dental caries in the United States, *MMWR Morb Mortal Wkly Rep* 50:1, 2001.
34. Association of State and Territorial Dental Directors (ASTDD), New York State Health Department, Ohio Department of Health, School of Public Health, University of Albany, State University of New York: Workshop on guidelines for sealant use: recommendations, *J Public Health Dent* 55(5 spec no):263, 1995.
35. US Preventive Services Task Force (USPSTF): *Guide to clinical preventive services,* ed 2, Baltimore, 1996, Williams & Wilkins.
36. Murray JJ, Rugg-Gunn AJ, Jenkins GN: *Fluorides in caries prevention,* ed 3, Boston, 1991, Wright.
37. Newbrun E: The fluoridation war: a scientific dispute or a religious argument? *J Public Health Dent* 56(5 spec no):246, 1996.
38. US Department of Health and Human Services. Public Health Service. Centers for Disease Control and Prevention: Engineering and administrative recommendations for water fluoridation, 1995, *MMWR Morb Mortal Wkly Rep* 44:1, 1995.
39. DePaola PF, Lax M: The caries-inhibiting effect of acidulated phosphate-fluoride chewable tablets: a two-year double-blind study, *J Am Dent Assoc* 76:554, 1968.
40. Driscoll WS, Heifetz SB, Korts DC: Effect of chewable fluoride tablets on dental caries in schoolchildren: results after six years of use, *J Am Dent Assoc* 97:820, 1978.
41. Stephen KW, Campbell D: Caries reduction and cost benefit after 3 years of sucking fluoride tablets daily at school. A double blind trial, *Br Dent J* 144:202, 1978.
42. Ismail AI: Fluoride supplements: current effectiveness, side effects and recommendations, *Community Dent Oral Epidemiol* 22:164, 1994.
43. Clark DC et al: The final results of the Sherbrooke-Lac Megantic fluoride varnish study, *J Can Dent Assoc* 53:919, 1987.
44. de Bruyn H, Arends J: Fluoride varnishes—a review, *J Biol Buccale* 15:71, 1987.

45. Helfenstein U, Steiner M: Fluoride varnishes (Duraphat): a meta-analysis, *Community Dent Oral Epidemiol* 22:1, 1994.
46. Twetman S, Petersson LG, Pakhomov GN: Caries incidence in relation to salivary mutans streptococci and fluoride varnish applications in preschool children from low- and optimal-fluoride areas, *Caries Res* 30:347, 1996.
47. Kirkegaard E et al: Caries-preventive effect of Duraphat varnish application versus fluoride mouthrinses: 5-year data, *Caries Res* 20:548, 1986.
48. Koch G, Petersson LG, Ryden H: Effect of fluoride varnish (Duraphat) treatment every six months compared with weekly mouthrinses with 0.2 percent NaF solution on dental caries, *Swed Dent J* 3:39, 1979.
49. Seppa L, Pollenen L: Caries preventive effect of fluoride varnish applications performed two or four times a year, *Scand J Dent Res* 98:102, 1990.
50. Vehmanen R: An economic evaluation of two caries preventive methods, dissertation, Turku, 1993, University of Turku.
51. Llodra JC et al: Factors influencing the effectiveness of sealants—a meta-analysis, *Community Dent Oral Epidemiol* 21:261, 1993.
52. Ripa LW: Sealants revisited: an update of the effectiveness of pit and fissure sealants, *Caries Res* 27(suppl 1):23, 1993.
53. Weintraub JA: The effectiveness of pit and fissure sealants, *J Public Health Dent* 49(5 spec no):317, 1989.
54. Heller KE et al: Longitudinal evaluation of sealing molars with and without incipient dental caries in a public health program, *J Public Health Dent* 55:148, 1995.
55. Loe H, Thelade E, Jensen SB: Experimental gingivitis in man, *J Periodontol* 36:177, 1965.
56. Ismail AI, Lewis DW: Periodic health examination, 1993 update: 3. Periodontal diseases: classification, diagnosis, risk factors and prevention. Canadian Task Force on the Periodic Health Examination, *Can Med Assoc J* 149:1409, 1993.
57. Horowitz AM et al: Effects of supervised daily dental plaque removal by children aged 3 years, *Community Dent Oral Epidemiol* 8:171, 1980.
58. Rothman K, Keller A: The effect of joint exposure to alcohol and tobacco on risk of cancer of the mouth and pharynx, *J Chronic Dis* 25:711, 1972.
59. Decker J, Goldstein JC: Risk factors in head and neck cancer, *N Engl J Med* 306:1151, 1982.
60. Wight AJ, Ogden GR: Possible mechanisms by which alcohol may influence the development of oral cancer—a review, *Oral Oncol* 34:441, 1998.
61. Blot WJ et al: Smoking and drinking in relation to oral and pharyngeal cancer, *Cancer Res* 48:3282, 1988.
62. Grossi SG et al: Assessment of risk for periodontal disease. II. Risk indicators for alveolar bone loss, *J Periodontol* 66:23, 1995.
63. Gustafsson BE et al: The Vipeholm dental caries study. The effect of different levels of carbohydrate intake on caries activity in 436 individuals observed for five years, *Acta Odontol Scand* 11:232, 1954.
64. Burt BA, Ismail AI: Diet, nutrition and food cariogenicity, *J Dent Res* 65(spec iss):1475, 1986.
65. Bloom B, Gift HC, Jack SS: Dental services and oral health: United States, 1989, *Vital Health Stat* 10(183):1, 1992.
66. US Department of Health and Human Services. Public Health Service. Centers for Disease Control and Prevention. National Center for Health Statistics: Preliminary data from the Centers for Disease Control and Prevention, *Mon Vital Stat Rep* 46(1 suppl 2):1, 1997.
67. US Department of Health and Human Services. Public Health Service: *Promoting health/preventing disease: objectives for the nation,* Washington, DC, 1980, US Department of Health and Human Services.
68. US Department of Health and Human Services. Public Health Service: *Healthy people: national health promotion and disease prevention objectives,* Washington, DC, 1991, US Department of Health and Human Services.
69. US Department of Health and Human Services. Public Health Service. Centers for Disease Control and Prevention. National Center for Health Statistics: *Healthy people 2000 review, 1998-99,* Hyattsville, MD, 1999, National Center for Health Statistics.
70. US Department of Health and Human Services. Public Health Service: *Healthy people 2010: with understanding and improving health and objectives for improving health,* ed 2, 2 vols, Washington, DC, 2000, US Government Printing Office.
71. US General Accounting Office: *Oral health: dental disease is a chronic problem among low-income populations,* Washington, DC, 2000, US General Accounting Office.
72. American Dental Association: Report of AIM for change in Medicaid conference, August 2-3, 1999, Chicago, 1999, American Dental Association.

CHAPTER

3

THE U.S. DENTAL CARE DELIVERY SYSTEM AND MANAGED CARE: AN OVERVIEW

Howard L. Bailit • Tryfon Beazoglou

This chapter provides an overview of the U.S. dental care delivery system. It is not intended to be a thorough review of the system but rather a brief description of its main components.

A dental care delivery system is efficient when its structure, organization, and performance satisfy the dental needs of the population it serves in the best way possible. This requires efficiency in the education and training of its dental manpower, as well as in the production, distribution, consumption, and financing of dental services. To remain efficient over time, a dental care delivery system must adapt to the changing needs of the population it serves.

DENTAL EDUCATION

An important component of a dental care delivery system is the production of dental manpower, which includes dentists and auxiliary personnel.

The typical education and training of dentists in the United States consists of (1) a college degree (4-year predental program) and (2) an undergraduate dental education (4-year program with emphasis in basic sciences during the first 2 years and clinical sciences in the last 2 years).[1] Graduates of such a program, once they pass a state or regional license examination, are permitted to practice dentistry in specific states.

In the past 70 years dental education and training has changed substantially in structure, intensity, and duration. Predental education today has reached, and in many cases has surpassed, the 4-year post–high school education.

Progress in biomedical sciences and the desire to effectively meet the ever-changing dental needs of the American people has led to the division of labor in the dental care delivery system. This division of labor, on the one hand, has led to the creation of allied professions (e.g., dental hygienist, dental assistant, laboratory technician) that require fewer years of education and training and, on the other hand, to postgraduate dental training and specialization. More specifically, today only approximately 42% of dental school graduates practice dentistry immediately (general practitioners); 29% receive postgraduate training in general dentistry (Advanced Education in General Dentistry [AEGD], General Practice Residency [GPR]); and the remaining 29% enter one of the eight recognized dental specialties.[1]

Recent evaluations regarding the effectiveness of dental education and training underline some obvious weaknesses. They include (1) the need for more effective integration between predental and dental education, (2) the need for more effective integration between basic and clinical sciences, (3) the lack of periodic certification of practicing dentists, and (4) the need for more effective utilization of auxiliary personnel.

Proposals to correct these and other shortcomings of the dental education system are contained in the Pew Commission report, the Institute of Medicine report, and more recently in the advocacy of the "oral physician."[2-4] A consequence of these proposals would be an increase of at least 1 year in dental education.

ALLIED DENTAL PERSONNEL

Dental hygiene is a licensed dental profession. The great majority of dental hygienists work in the office of private dental practitioners, but approximately 7% are employed by community health centers, school systems, public health departments, nursing homes, and hospitals. State dental licensing boards determine the scope of hygiene practice. In addition to traditional duties such as screening examinations, the application of topical fluorides, patient education, and prophylaxes, in approximately 30 states hygienists can administer injectable dental anesthetics. Some states require hygienists to work under the direct supervision of a dentist, but others allow them to work under indirect supervision without the dentist being physically present. One state, Arizona, permits hygienists to operate independent practices.

As of 1996 approximately 94,000 professionally active dental hygienists were treating patients. The number of hygienists is increasing as more dentists employ at least one part-time or full-time hygienist. In 1998 approximately 70% of general dental practitioners employed a hygienist. The demand for hygienists appears to be increasing as the oral health of the American people improves. Recent data show a large upsurge in the percentage of patients receiving examinations and prophylaxes—services often provided by hygienists—and a decline in the percentage receiving restorative services. This trend is likely to continue as water fluoridation and other preventive methods reduce the prevalence of caries.

The number of hygienists being trained has increased substantially in the past 10 years in response to greater demand by dentists. In 2000 256 accredited dental hygiene schools graduated more than 6000 students annually. Most students are enrolled in 2-year programs that are located in community colleges and technical schools. Approximately 27% of students graduate from 4-year programs based at universities. Twelve universities have master's degree programs specially designed to train dental hygiene educators.

The other two major allied dental health professions are dental assisting and dental laboratory technologists. These occupations are not state-licensed professions, but graduates of accredited programs are certified. In 1996 201,400 dental assistants and

54,000 dental laboratory technologists were active in practice. Dental assistants work under the direct supervision of dentists, assisting them with the equipment and materials used in patient care. In contrast, most dental laboratory technologists work in independent dental technology laboratories, constructing prostheses based on dentists' prescriptions. Some large dental practices employ their own dental laboratory technologists.

Approximately half of dental assistants and dental laboratory technologists are educated in 1-year accredited programs; the rest receive their education on the job. Currently, the demand for both occupations appears to be greater than the supply.

The broader dental education system produces approximately 3900 dentists, 4500 dental hygienists, 4500 dental assistants, and 600 laboratory technicians per year, though these numbers have fluctuated significantly over the years (Table 3-1).

Table 3-1. Number of Graduates from Dental Schools and Allied Dental Education Programs, 1970–1998

Year	*Dentists*	*Hygienists*	*Dental Assistants*	*Lab Technicians*
1970	3749	2465	2955	359
1975	4959	4568	5972	836
1980	5256	5184	5958	1068
1985	5353	4024	5855	986
1990	4233	3953	3940	596
1994	3875	4553	4490	608
1998	3930	5261	4720	490

Data from Weaver R, Haden NK, Valachovic R: US dental school applicants and enrollees: a ten-year perspective, *J Dent Educ* 64(12):867-874, 2000; and Haden NK, Morr K, Valachovic R: Trends in allied dental education: an analysis of the past and a look to the future, *J Dent Educ* 65(5):480-495, 2001.

STRUCTURE AND ORGANIZATION OF THE DENTAL CARE DELIVERY SYSTEM

Characteristics of Dentists

The trends in dental education and increases in population and income over time have led to an increase in dental manpower. The most recent available data (Table 3-2) indicate that in 1998 the total number of dentists in the United States was 183,000 whereas the number of active private practitioners was 138,449 (less than 76% of the total). Table 3-2 indicates that the number of people per active private practitioner was 1952. It is estimated that the dentist/population ratio was approximately 58 per 100,000 in 2000 and will be 47 per 100,000 by 2020. According to these estimates, the absolute number of active dentists started to decline in 2001.[5]

Table 3-2. Number of Dentists, Population, and Population/Dentists Ratio in the United States 1998

Category of Dentist	*Percent*	*Number*
Total number of dentists	100.00	183,000
Professionally active dentists	81.61	149,350
Active private practitioners	75.66	138,449
Male	86.36	119,565
Female	13.64	18,884
Population		270,299,000
Population/active private practitioners		1,952

From American Dental Association: *Distribution of dentists in the United States by region and state, 1998,* Chicago, 2000, The Association.

Table 3-3. Distribution of Active Private Practitioners by Specialty in the United States, 1991

Dental Specialty	*Percent*	*Number*
General practitioner	81.51	112,564
Specialist	18.49	25,530
Oral and maxillofacial surgeon	3.76	5,188
Endodontist	1.86	2,567
Orthodontist	6.04	8,342
Oral pathologist	0.08	108
Public health dentist	0.18	244
Prosthodontist	1.68	2,323
Periodontist	2.76	3,810
Pediatric dentist	2.13	2,948
TOTAL	100.00	138,094

Data from American Dental Association: *Distribution of dentists in the United States by region and state, 1991,* Chicago, 1993, The Association.

Another important trend is the changing gender of the dentist workforce. The number of female dentists is increasing rapidly and accounted for almost 14% of the total number of active private practitioners in 1998.[6]

Table 3-3 shows the distribution of active dentists in private practice by specialty. General practitioners account for approximately 80% of practitioners. This 80/20 split between general practitioners and specialists is the opposite of that in medicine.

Table 3-4 presents the distribution of active practitioners across the nine regions of the country. Dentists are in every area, but significant variation in the number of people per dentist among regions exists. The primary determinants of the number of dentists in an area are population and per capita income.[7]

Table 3-5 shows the age distribution of active private practitioners. This table carries an important message regarding the future supply of dental manpower. In the

Table 3-4. Distribution of Active Private Practitioners in the United States by Region, 1998

Geographic Region	*Number of Active Private Practitioners*	*Population (Thousands)*	*Population/Dentist Ratio*
New England	8,325	13,430	1613
Middle Atlantic	24,748	38,292	1547
South Atlantic	21,391	48,945	2288
East South Central	6,788	16,471	2426
East North Central	23,012	44,195	1920
West North Central	8,995	18,695	2078
West South Central	11,962	30,014	2509
Mountain	7,865	16,813	2138
Pacific	25,351	43,445	1714
Total	138,449	270,299	1952

From American Dental Association: *Distribution of dentists in the United States by region and state, 1998,* Chicago, 2000, The Association.

next 10 to 20 years the number of retiring dentists will outpace the new entrants into the profession.

Characteristics of Dental Practices

The organization and characteristics of dental practices play an important role in determining the efficiency of the delivery system. First, the size of a dental practice may have significant consequences on access to dental care, as well as the unit cost or fees of dental services. The presence of economies or diseconomies of scale and the extent of dental markets are the main determinants of the dental practice size.

Table 3-6 indicates that dentists are organized in small-size practices. In fact, almost 96% of all dental practices consist of one-dentist (82.6%) or two-dentist (13.3%) practices. Approximately 4% of all dental practices are considered group practices: three or more dentists who share expenses or revenue. Given that this pattern of dental practice size has persisted for many years, it strongly suggests lack of significant economies of scale with larger practice size. This and additional evidence seem to run contrary to conventional wisdom that larger practices are more efficient than smaller practices.[8]

Table 3-7 offers additional evidence of the relatively small size of dental practices. This table shows the square feet of office space, number of operatories, and number of auxiliary staff members in an average dental practice. It also gives the frequency of use of specific units of equipment. Table 3-8 provides further details regarding the frequency and number of specific types of auxiliary staff members employed by dental practices. Although the average dental practice employs four auxiliaries, the number varies from zero to more than seven auxiliary staff members (Table 3-9).

Dentists, auxiliary staff, equipment, and dental office space are contributing factors in the production of dental services. Conventional measures of dental output are number of visits and gross billings in 1 year. When visits are used as an output measure of a dental practice, Table 3-10 shows that the contribution of dentists is approxi-

Table 3-5. Age Distribution of Active Private Practitioners in the United States, 1998

Age of Dentist	*Number of Dentists*	*Percent of Total*
<35	18,274	13.2
35–44	41,946	30.3
45–54	43,054	31.1
55–64	22,703	16.4
65+	12,459	9.0
Total	138,436	100.0

From American Dental Association: *Distribution of dentists in the United States by region and state, 1998,* Chicago, 2000, The Association.

Table 3-6. Distribution of Active Private Practitioners and Dental Practices by Size

Size of Practice	*Percent of All Dentists*	*Percent of All Practices**
One dentist	65.8	82.6
Two dentists	21.1	13.3
Three or more dentists	13.1	4.1

From the 1998 survey of dental practice, ADA, March 2000.

*The total number of practices (110,230) was estimated assuming that the mean number of dentists in the category "three or more dentists" is four.

Table 3-7. Mean Office Space, Number of Operatories, Number of Auxiliaries, and Office Equipment, All Active Private Practitioners, 1998

Square feet of office space	1,755
Number of operatories	4.4
Number of auxiliaries	4.2
Dental office equipment*	% using
1. Composing light curing unit	92.6
2. High speed air handpiece with fiberoptics	71.2
3. Panoramic X-ray unit	54.1
4. Ultrasonic scaling unit	86.8
5. Electrosurgical unit	45.1
6. Nitrous oxide analgesic equipment	57.4
7. Automatic X-ray film processor	78.8
8. Sterilizable handpiece	97.9
9. Intraoral video camera	19.1
10. Surgical laser	1.7
11. Biologic indicator	71.2
12. Silver recovery unit	13.7
13. Amalgam separator	16.8
14. Computer processing services	62.3

From the 1998 survey of dental practice, ADA, March 2000.

*The source for the use of dental office equipment is the 1994 Survey of Dental Practice, ADA, August 1995.

Table 3-8. Auxiliary Personnel in Dental Practices, All Dentists, 1998

Type of Auxiliary Personnel	*% of Practices*	*Mean Number**
Dental hygienists	62.5	1.6
Chairside assistants	92.3	1.6
Secretary/receptionists	89.2	1.3
Dental lab technician	6.6	1.1
Bookkeeper/business personnel	35.8	0.9
Sterilization assistant	14.6	0.9

From the 1998 Survey of Dental Practice, ADA, January 2000.

*For dentists that employ this type of auxiliary personnel.

Table 3-9. Percent of All Independent Dentists Employing Auxiliary Personnel (Part-time or Full-time)

Number of Employees	*Percent*
No employees	1.4
One employee	5.7
Two employees	9.4
Three employees	12.3
Four employees	14.4
Five employees	14.1
Six employees	12.2
Seven or more employees	30.5

From the 1998 Survey of Dental Practice, ADA, January 2000.

Table 3-10. Relative Contribution of Major Inputs in the Production of Dental Services

Production Inputs	Dental Output: Number of Visits (%)	Dental Output: Gross Billings (%)
Dentist(s)	45.63	32.71
Auxiliary staff	36.89	51.40
Equipment	17.48	15.89
Total	100.00	100.00

From Crakes G: An economic estimation of dental practice production process, doctoral dissertation, 1984, University of Connecticut.

Table 3-11. Percentage Distribution of Sources of New Patients, All Dentists, 1998

Sources of New Patients	% of New Patients
Patients	58.7
Other dentists	17.1
Other professionals	3.6
Advertising	5.9
Capitation/close panel contracts	4.6
All other	7.1

From the 1998 Survey of Dental Practice, ADA, January 2000.

mately 46% whereas the contributions of auxiliary staff and equipment are approximately 37% and 17%, respectively. In contrast, when gross billings are used as an output measure, the contribution of dentists decreases to approximately 33% and that of auxiliary staff increases to approximately 51%; equipment contributes approximately 16%. Clearly, the contribution of auxiliary staff in the gross billings of a dental practice is not only significant but exceeds that of the dentist(s).

The preference of most dentists to organize their practices in small units is important, given the fact that production of dental services is characterized by constant returns to scale (i.e., cost per unit involved in the production of dental services does not decline with size of the practice).[8] Thus employers and other group buyers of dental services have little economic incentive to promote larger, more organized dental practices. Likewise, dentists have valid reasons to retain the current practice structure, because it is efficient and meets patient needs. For example, patients select dentists on the bases of proximity and referrals by other patients (Table 3-11). As a result, dental practices tend to draw from a limited geographic area. This in turn imposes several limitations on the number of dentists a viable practice can support. Clearly, the relatively small size of dental practices is a significant advantage in terms of access to dental care. In other words, for a given number of active dentists, the smaller the size of a dental practice the larger the number of dental practices operating in a community. Consequently, more dental practices implies better access, lower indirect costs (travel expenses, travel time), and increased use of dental services, other things being equal.[9]

FINANCING OF DENTAL CARE SERVICES

Health care expenditures in the United States reached $1210.7 billion in 1999, representing more than 13% of the gross national product, the value of all goods and services produced in the United States (Table 3-12). The absolute, relative, and per capita amounts of health care expenditures are the highest in the industrialized world.

Table 3-12. Gross National Product (GNP), National Health Care Expenditures (NHCE), and Their Share of the GNP, 1960–1999

Selected Years	*Gross National Product (Billions $)*	*National Health Aggregate (Billions $)*	*Care Expenditures Per Capita ($)*	*NHCE/GNP (%)*
1960	530.6	26.9	141.50	5.07
1970	1046.1	73.2	340.78	7.00
1975	1648.4	130.7	582.18	7.93
1980	2830.8	247.2	1051.47	8.73
1985	4238.4	428.2	1720.37	10.10
1990	5832.2	697.5	2687.86	11.96
1995	7420.9	993.3	3638.48	13.39
1998	8786.7	1149.1	4089.32	13.08
1999	9288.2	1210.7	4355.04	13.03

Data available on the Center for Medicare and Medicaid Services website (http://www.hcfa.gov).

Table 3-13. National Health Care Expenditures and Sources of Payment, 1960–1999

Selected Years	*National Health Care Expenditures (Billions $)*	*Source of Payments*		
		Private Direct (%)	*Private Insurance (%)*	*Public Funds (%)*
1960	26.9	48.7	21.9	24.5
1970	73.2	34.4	22.4	37.2
1975	130.7	29.0	24.8	41.5
1980	247.2	24.4	28.2	42.4
1985	428.2	21.8	31.9	41.6
1990	697.5	21.3	33.3	40.8
1995	993.3	17.2	32.6	45.9
1998	1149.1	17.4	32.6	45.5
1999	1210.7	15.4	33.1	45.3

Data available on the Center for Medicare and Medicaid Services website (http://www.hcfa.gov).

As a result, much of the impetus for the development of means to control health care expenditures can be attributed to corporate and public concern over both the absolute level of expenditures and the rate of increase in expenditures over time. This push emanates from two major characteristics of the health care system: (1) health care expenditures are paid mostly indirectly (84.6%); and (2) the government (federal, state, and local) is a major payer (45.3% of total expenses). In addition, both of these dimensions are increasing over time (Table 3-13).

Aggregate expenditures for dental care services amounted to almost $56 billion in 1999, yielding an average per capita expense

Table 3-14. Aggregate and Per Capita Expenditures for Dental Services and Their Sources of Payment, 1960–1999

	Expenditures for Dental Services		*Source of Payment*		
Selected Public Years	*Aggregate (Billions $)*	*Per Capita ($)*	*Direct (%)*	*Private Insurance (%)*	*Private Funds (%)*
1960	1.96	10.87	97.2	1.9	1.0
1970	4.67	22.77	90.8	4.5	4.7
1975	7.96	36.84	82.1	11.8	6.1
1980	13.32	58.63	66.3	28.6	5.1
1985	21.65	91.00	56.6	40.1	3.4
1990	31.57	126.54	48.7	48.0	3.3
1995	45.00	171.23	46.8	48.2	4.5
1998	53.83	199.18	47.8	47.5	4.7
1999	56.05	201.62	45.8	49.4	4.6

Data available on the Center for Medicare and Medicaid Services website (http://www.hcfa.gov).

of approximately $202. In contrast to medical care, dental care is almost exclusively financed by private sources (95.4%). The share of the government (local, state, and federal) in financing dental care is less than 5% and is not growing over time (Table 3-14). In comparison, government financing of physician and hospital services amounted to 32% and 59%, respectively, and is growing. Out-of-pocket payments for dental care by consumers amounted to 45.8% of the total dental care expenditures in 1999, and private third-party payments amounted to 49.4%.

Table 3-14 suggests substantial growth in dental benefit plans in the last 30 years. However, several obstacles seem to be developing to prevent further expansion of the proportion of the population covered. Specifically, the bulk of dental insurance, both indemnity and managed care, is employer sponsored. Employers are resisting efforts to expand coverage and are, in fact, actively attempting to reduce or eliminate their contribution. More recently, these efforts have accelerated as the cost of medical and dental care has increased dramatically. In any event, the period of rapid expansion of dental benefit plans seems to be over.

Clearly, dental expenditures grew substantially between 1960 and 1999. This growth reflects the combined effects of changes in dental prices, population, and per capita use. Figure 3-1 shows the trend over time of three price indices: the Consumer Price Index (CPI), the price index for medical care services, and the price index for dental care services. The price index for dental services rose faster than the CPI, but at a rate lower than the price index for medical care services. The price effects on dental expenditures are shown in Fig. 3-2. This figure indicates that aggregate nominal expenditures for dental services are rising at an increasing rate and that aggregate real expenditures (deflated by the price index of dental services) have increased at a decreasing rate since the early 1970s. Figure 3-3 provides the per capita nominal and real dental expenditures (per capita use). Clearly, per capita use of dental services has been remarkably stable in the last 15 years

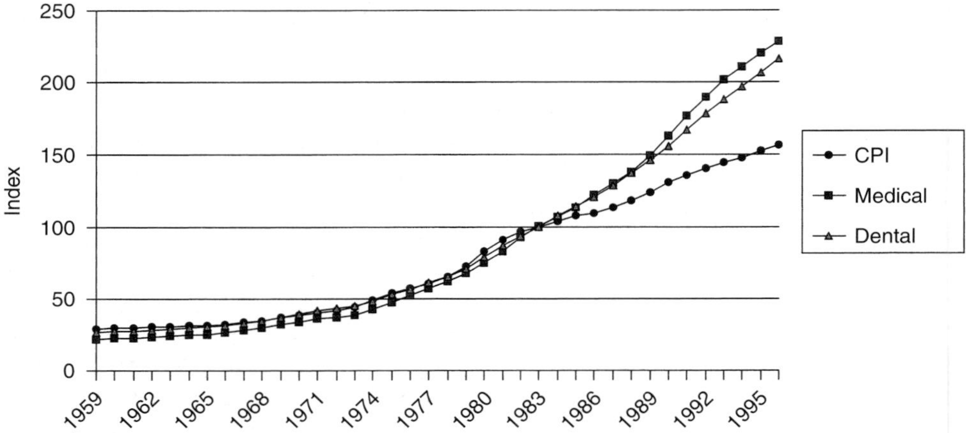

Fig. 3-1. Price indexes for all items (CPI), medical care, and dental care, 1959–1995.

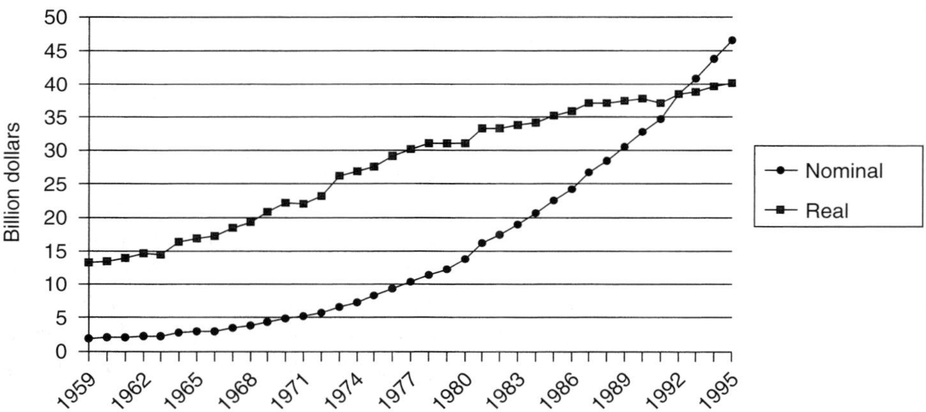

Fig. 3-2. Aggregate nominal and real dental expenditures, 1959–1995.

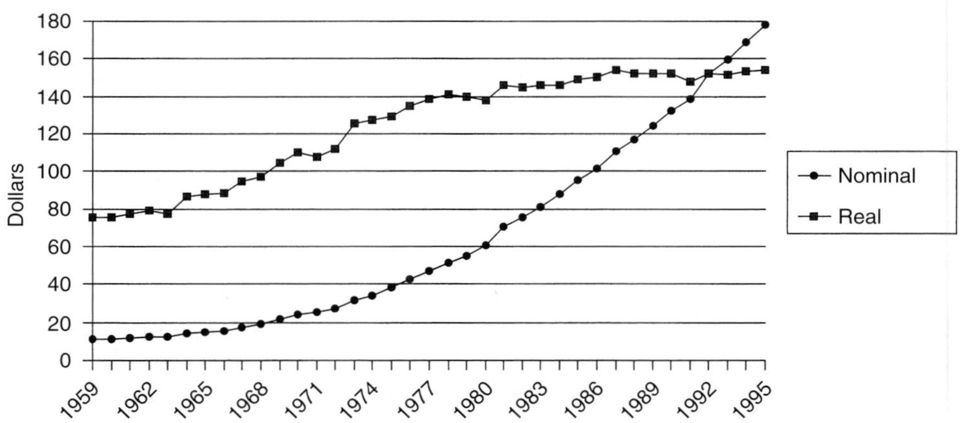

Fig. 3-3. Per capita nominal and real dental expenditures, 1959–1995.

in spite of the significant improvement in the oral health of the U.S. population.

It is worth noting that the share of dental care expenditures in the total health care budget has fallen from 7.55% in 1960 to 4.63% in 1999. This is largely due to the rapid increase in medical expenditures in the 1970s and 1980s.

PERFORMANCE OF THE DENTAL CARE DELIVERY SYSTEM

Dentistry in the United States is considered the finest in the world and has been since World War II.[10] The following discussion is a brief assessment of the performance of dentistry in the United States, with the use of structural (education/training), process (services, access), and outcome (oral health status) measures.

STRUCTURAL MEASURES

The education and training of practicing dentists in the United States is the most extensive in the world. A typical program lasts almost 10 years and consists of predental, dental, and postdental education.

PROCESS MEASURES

The dental sector provides primary care services and increasingly effective diagnostic, preventive, and cosmetic services. Per capita use of dental services has been relatively stable in the last 10 to 15 years, and dental price inflation has been lower than that of hospital and physician services. Approximately 50% to 60% of the U.S. population visits dental practices at least once per year. The average number of visits per person per year is 2.1.[11]

OUTCOME MEASURES

The most important measure of performance of the dental care delivery system is the oral health status of the American population, which is among the best in the world. The oral health of the U.S. population has been characterized by a marked reduction in (1) the prevalence of caries, (2) the amount and severity of periodontal disease, and (3) the percentage of the adult population that is edentulous.[12-15] Similar improvements can be found in a variety of other oral health conditions. Of course, a substantial amount of dental need still exists, particularly in lower socioeconomic class groups.

OVERUTILIZATION OF DENTAL CARE SERVICES

The evidence for the overuse of dental services by patients and overtreatment by dentists is mixed.[16] For example, it has been argued that excessive treatment is relatively rare and that the use of expensive services that may have only a marginal impact on oral health is a much greater problem.[17] The current lack of adequate research on the clinical cost-effectiveness of different dental treatments provides ample room for competent dentists of goodwill to disagree on the need for treatment.

MANAGED DENTAL CARE[18-21]

Managed care developed in the late 1980s in response to rapidly rising health care costs. Public and private employers who pay for a large percentage of health care in the United States supported the development of managed care as a competitive market-based (versus government regulation) approach to controlling health care costs. Now, more than 85% of employed Americans and their dependents receive medical care in some type of managed care plan (e.g., health maintenance organization). Several major differences exist between traditional dental indemnity insurance and managed care. In the latter there is a defined network of providers, a specific population of patients eligible to receive care from those providers, an economic incentive for patients to obtain care in the provider network, and, most importantly, providers assume some financial risk for delivering care to the population for a predetermined amount of money. Contrast this to the usual indemnity insurance system in which an insured person can go to any provider, providers are not organized into formal networks, and they have no financial risk. Generally, without financial risk (indemnity plans) providers tend to deliver more services and with risk (managed care) less care.

Although managed care has had a profound impact on the delivery of medical care, it has had much less effect on dentistry. In part this is because the majority of Americans do not have dental insurance, and without insurance coverage there can be no managed care. Another reason is that under indemnity dental insurance patients still pay a large percentage (40% to 60%) of costs out-of-pocket in the form of deductibles and co-insurance. As a result, dentistry does not have the same problems with rapidly rising costs as medicine has. The medical care system also has a large excess capacity of hospitals and physicians, making it easier for managed care companies to negotiate lower reimbursement rates for the promise of more patients. In contrast, most communities do not have an excess supply of dentists.

Today, of the 105 million people who are covered by employer-based dental insurance, approximately equal numbers are enrolled in managed care and indemnity insurance plans. The percentage enrolled in managed care is growing rapidly. Yet managed care is unlikely to have much impact on the dental delivery system within the next 5 to 10 years. To understand the reasons for this, it is important to know more about how dental managed care is organized.

The two dominant dental managed care products are dental health maintenance organizations (DHMOs) and preferred-provider organizations (PPOs). In DHMOs managed care companies contract with individual dental practices to form a network of practices to provide care to a defined population of patients. Usually, basic services (e.g., examinations, diagnostic tests, and simple restorative care) are provided for a capitation fee. That is, dentists agree to provide these services for a set monthly fee per eligible person regardless of how much care is needed or demanded by patients. Even if members do not seek care, dentists still receive the monthly capitation fee. Likewise, dentists receive the same capitation amount for patients who need and demand large amounts of care. This financial arrangement gives dentists strong incentives to control utilization and expenditures.

DHMOs seldom include expensive tertiary services, such as crowns, bridges, and periodontal surgery, under the capitation fee structure. These services are paid for on a fee-for-service basis much as in an indemnity insurance plan, although the fees are often discounted. For capitated or noncapitated services, members must go to a DHMO-contracted practice to get their care. If they go to a non-DHMO practice, the services are not covered benefits, and patients must pay for them entirely out-of-pocket. In this sense DHMOs limit patients' freedom of choice to select any dentist.

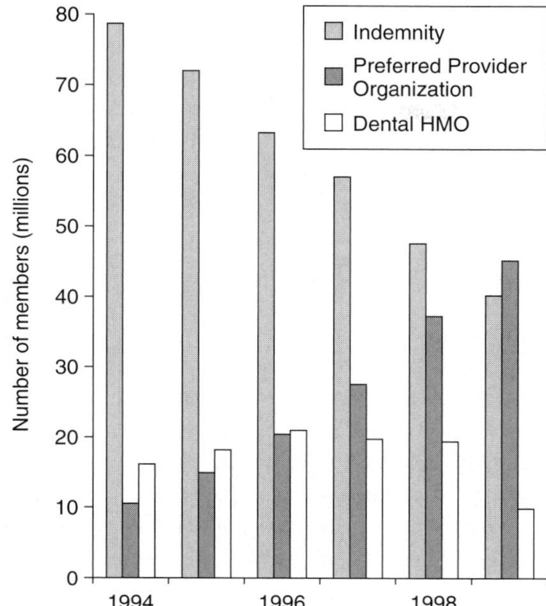

Fig. 3-4. Enrollment in employer-sponsored group dental insurance by product, 1994–1999.[1,2]

Figure 3-4 shows that enrollment in DHMOs grew rapidly in the early 1990s but is now declining. The reason for the decline is that most dentists have reservations about DHMOs and capitation payment and are unwilling to join DHMO networks. In fact, only 20,000 of the 138,000 professionally active dentists in the United States participate in DHMO networks; the majority of these dentists are in three states (California, Florida, and Texas). Another reason for the decline in DHMO enrollment is patient dissatisfaction with access to care. Apparently, some networks do not have adequate numbers of dentists, and some DHMO dentists carefully control patients' access to care. In part, these access problems are the result of DHMO premiums being approximately half of indemnity premiums. Thus a DHMO plan may cost employers $250 per member per year and an indemnity plan $550 per member per year. Although the lower costs per member are attractive to some employers, dentists in DHMO networks have to control access and utilization carefully, and this results in more patient complaints.

In a PPO plan, managed care companies also contract with individual dental offices to form a network of practices to provide care to a defined population of employees and their dependents. The companies negotiate the fees that participating dentists can charge PPO patients. Usually these fees are from 15% to 25% below the usual and customary fee charged by area dentists. Further, patients can elect to go to a PPO practice or to a non-PPO practice to obtain care at any time. Often, to give patients an incentive to obtain care within the PPO network, the co-insurance charges are lower within network practices. Clearly, PPOs are similar to traditional indemnity plans because dentists are paid on a fee-for-service basis and patients can go to any dentist. In this sense PPOs offer patients greater freedom of choice. More than 60,000 dentists participate in PPO networks, and PPOs are the fastest growing managed care product. Figure 3-4 shows that employees are switching from indemnity to PPO plans in large numbers. If current trends continue, the great majority of people who receive dental insurance from their employers will be members of PPO plans within 5 years.

Even though most insured patients will be in a managed care plan (specifically PPOs) within a few years, managed care is unlikely to have a significant impact on the traditional dental delivery system. This is because PPOs do not appear to be very effective in controlling dental care expenditures. Although dentists agree to discounted PPO fees, these discounts do not have much impact on aggregate costs. This is because with lower co-insurance rates within PPO networks, patients demand more services because they pay less for them out-of-pocket. Also, dentists have a great deal of flexibility in changing the mix of services they provide to patients, keeping aggregate expenditures at the same level as indemnity plans without discounted fees. Indeed, annual per member premium costs for PPOs are little different than for indemnity plans.

In addition to employer-based insurance, managed dental care, mainly DHMOs, is the predominant way that most states provide their Medicaid populations dental insurance. Mostly made up of dependent children and single mothers, they can only obtain dental care if they go to a DHMO dentist. States usually contract with a dental managed care company directly or indirectly through a medical managed care company to administer the program. Only 20% to 30% of eligible children participating in dental Medicaid managed care programs visit dentists annually. This is approximately the same rate of utilization seen in nonmanaged care plans.

It is becoming more apparent in both medicine and dentistry that managed care may not be able to meet the primary goal that employers envisioned for this new approach to organizing the delivery system. Managed care is not keeping increases in health care expenditures to the general rate of inflation as demanded by employers. Managed care has also led to considerable backlash among physicians, dentists, and patients. This is the reason for "patient protection act" legislation now seen at both the state and federal levels. How this is all going to turn out is anybody's guess at this time. This is an especially acute problem in medicine, because annual premium increases are in the 8% to 15% range, and this rate of increase is not sustainable. It is likely to lead to millions more people being uninsured. Health care costs and managed care are certain to be contentious political issues for many years to come as this nation tries to come up with a method of providing all Americans with access to high-quality, affordable medical and dental care.

ADAPTING TO CHANGE

The health care environment has changed significantly in recent years in response to a variety of demographic, economic, and professional forces. For example, advances in biomedical technology have increased the ability to diagnose and treat disease, have expanded the potential population likely to benefit from these services, and have increased the demand for facilities, equipment, and personnel consistent with this new knowledge base. Changes have occurred in the racial and ethnic composition of the U.S. population. A growing proportion of the population is over 65 years of age. Additional changes in the environment include the declining significance of manufacturing in the U.S. economy, the emerging dominance of the service sector, and the increasing participation of women in the labor force. These changes, among others, have altered the prevailing patterns of morbidity and mortality, as well as treatment methods.

An even more significant change affecting the health care environment during this period is the growth of third-party payment mechanisms, both public and private. For example, governmental provision of health care coverage for the poor (Medicaid) and the elderly (Medicare) resulted in a tremendous expansion in the demand for medical care services. Other governmental programs supported a significant growth in numbers and types of health manpower, health care facilities, and research in both basic and applied sciences.

These efforts to increase the availability of care, improve access to care, and make medical care more equitable have produced ever-increasing levels of health care utilization, prices, and expenditures. Not surprisingly, this led to other efforts to stem the growth in health care expenditures, particularly given concerns about overutilization and the overall efficiency, effectiveness, and equity of these expenditures.

In short, most individuals, providers, and health care organizations face an increasingly complex and dynamic environment characterized by a scarcity of resources, increased competition, and an increase in the number and variety of regulatory and planning bodies, consumer-interest groups, and business coalitions. All of these people and organizations now have more influence over the quantity and quality of care available and the conditions under which it will be provided. In this environment, managed care (including HMOs and PPOs) has become the dominant system of medical coverage; the share of traditional indemnity medical care insurance coverage has been reduced to 18%.

Dentistry has also experienced and weathered a number of changes. Among them were the growth and decline in the number and size of dental schools, the emergence and proliferation of third-party payment mechanisms (indemnity insurance and managed care), the decline in the incidence of dental caries, the introduction of new technologies, professional advertising, and, more recently, infection control regulations. Perhaps the greatest impact on dentistry comes from the cyclic fluctuation in economic activity at the national, regional, and local levels. The downturn (trough) of these fluctuations seems to coincide with the periodic reemergence of managed care. The latter is a troubling issue for a number of dentists despite the fact that its economic impact is small.

As a result of these changes, a number of opinions and beliefs among dentists, educators, insurers, and policy makers formed during this period lack a factual foundation. Some of these beliefs are related to dentistry and its main features, and others are associated with the various forms of third-party payment mechanisms. The latter, through marketing techniques and rhetoric, have generated much confusion as to what they represent, how big they are (market share), and the nature of their contribution, if any, to improvements in the dental care delivery system. A major part of the misunderstanding arises from the notion that what is effective and applicable in the medical care sector is also effective and applicable in the dental sector.

The notion that managed dental care has become a powerful force and is poised to take over the dental sector is more myth than reality. As previously noted, the dental sector is largely devoid of the features and conditions that have fostered managed care in the medical sector. Performance measures suggest that dental care has been "managed" well by independent fee-for-service providers receiving payments directly from patients and indemnity insurance plans.

It is noteworthy that the mix of dental services has changed and will continue to change. Diagnostic, preventive, and aesthetic services will continue to grow, and an effective recall system is a necessity. As a result, the trend to employ more auxiliary personnel will also continue.

Dentistry faces two major challenges. The first is to learn to adapt to the changing environment. The oral health status of the U.S. population has improved and will continue to improve. Despite this fact, per capita utilization of dental care services has been roughly constant in the last 15 years. The total population is growing and the number of dentists per capita is declining. In addition, the long-term prospects for the state of the economy are good. On the basis of these trends, it is safe to say that use of dental services per dentist will continue to grow in the next 10 to 15 years. Remember, however, that although the long-term trend appears good, there is nothing to protect dentists from fluctuations in the state of the national or regional economy. Every time we are in an economic downturn, utilization will be less, excess capacity will emerge, and the promotion of managed care plans will increase.

The second challenge to dentistry is to find a way to address the lingering problems of substandard oral health and limited access for the poor, medically disabled, and elderly in inner cities and rural areas. The dental care delivery system must find a way to meet this challenge.

SUMMARY

Overall, the U.S. dental care delivery system is relatively effective and efficient and the future looks bright. Given current trends on both the supply and demand sides of dental markets, dentists and dental auxiliary staff will have ample opportunities to practice their professions and will be well compensated for their care.

REVIEW QUESTIONS

1. Discuss the contribution (share) of auxiliary staff and dentists in the production of dental services (gross billings, visits).
2. Discuss the efficiency of dental practices with respect to their size (solo, group).
3. Discuss the financing of dental care, private and public, and contrast it with that of medical care.
4. What are the major reasons for current trends in managed care insurance products?
5. The demand for dental hygienists has increased significantly in the past several years. What is causing this increased demand?

REFERENCES

1. Kennedy JE, Crall JJ: A model for dental education in the year 2005, *Forum* 13:S1, 1992.
2. *Healthy America: practitioners for 2005—an agenda for action for U.S. health professional schools,* Durham, NC, 1991, Pew Health Professions Commission.
3. Institute of Medicine: *Dental education at the crossroads: challenges and change,* Washington, DC, 1995, National Academy Press.
4. Nash DA: The oral physician . . . creating a new oral health professional for a new century, *J Dent Educ* 59:586, 1995.
5. American Association of Dental Schools: *Deans briefing book, academic year, 1993-1994,* Washington, DC, 1995, The Association.
6. American Dental Association: *Distribution of dentists in the United States by region and state, 1998,* Chicago, 2000, The Association.
7. Beazoglou TJ, Crakes GM, Doherty NJ: Determinants of dentists' geographic distribution, *J Dent Educ* 56: 735, 1992.
8. Crakes GM: An economic estimation of the dental practice production process, dissertation, 1984, University of Connecticut.
9. House DR: A full-price approach to the dental market: implications for price determination, *J Health Polit Policy Law* 5:593, 1981.
10. Eggleston FK: Reactor paper, *J Dent Educ* 60:908, 1996.
11. US Department of Health and Human Services: *Vital and health statistics. Dental services and oral health: United States, 1989,* series 10, no 183, Hyattsville, MD, 1992, US Department of Health and Human Services.
12. Brown LJ, Beazoglou T, Heffley D: Estimated savings in U.S. dental expenditures, 1979-89, *Public Health Rep* 109:195, 1994.
13. Brown LJ, Oliver RC, Loe H: Evaluating periodontal status of US employed adults, *J Am Dent Assoc* 121:226, 1990.

14. Graves RC, Stamm JW: Oral health status in the United States, *J Dent Educ* 49:341, 1985.
15. Meskin LH, Brown LJ: Prevalence and patterns of tooth loss in U.S. employed adult and senior populations, 1985-86, *J Dent Educ* 52:686, 1988.
16. Grembowski D, Milgrom P, Fiset L: Variation in dentist service rate in a homogeneous patient population, *J Public Health Dent* 50:235, 1990.
17. Bailit HL: Is overutilization the major reason for increasing dental expenditures? Reflections on a complex issue, *J Dent Pract Admin* 5:112, 1988.
18. Bailit H. Managed medical and dental care: current status and future directions, *J Am Coll Dent* 62:7, 1995.
19. Bailit HL: Dental insurance, managed care and traditional practice, *J Am Dent Assoc* 130:1721, 1999.
20. Beazoglou T, Guay AH, Heffley D: Capitation and fee-for-service dental benefit plans: economic incentives, utilization, and service-mix, *J Am Dent Assoc* 116:483, 1988.
21. Beazoglou TJ, Heffley D, Mark H: Managed care and dentistry: reality and myth, *Conn State Dent Assoc J* 71:49, 1995.

CHAPTER

4

MEDICAID AND THE STATE CHILDREN'S HEALTH INSURANCE PROGRAM

James Crall

Established in 1965 by Title XIX of the Social Security Act (SSA), Medicaid is a jointly funded federal-state entitlement program that provides benefits for medical and health-related services to America's poorest people. Medicaid covers three main groups of low-income Americans: parents and children, the disabled, and the elderly. In fiscal year (FY) 1998, 41.4 million people were enrolled in the Medicaid program and 40.6 million beneficiaries accessed services, including 18.9 million children (47%), 7.9 million adults (19%), 6.6 million individuals who were blind or disabled (16%), and 3.9 million elderly (10%).[1] As such, Medicaid covered more Americans than Medicare or any other health insurer and one fifth of all children in the United States. More recently, Congress created the State Children's Health Insurance Program (SCHIP) as Title XXI of the SSA in 1997 to provide coverage for children in low- to moderate-income families who do not qualify for Medicaid.

Although roughly half of all Medicaid beneficiaries are children, only 17% of expenditures go for children's services. The vast majority of all Medicaid spending is associated with services for the elderly (30%) and disabled (42%). Medicaid spending from federal and state sources totaled $161.2 billion in 1997 (compared with $214.6 billion for Medicare, the primary federal health care program for the elderly and disabled). The federal government pays at least 50% of the cost of Medicaid in every state and up to 78% in some states (national average = 57%).[2]

Although large in scope, Medicaid benefits are subject to specific eligibility regulations set by both state and federal governments. As originally enacted, Medicaid was limited to persons eligible for Aid to Families with Dependent Children (AFDC), now referred to as Temporary Assistance for Needy Families (TANF). Over the last three decades, eligibility rules have been amended and Medicaid coverage has been broadened to include additional populations. As a result, beneficiary regulations have become considerably more complex.

Medicaid rules are further complicated by the fact that states have discretion, within broad national guidelines set by the Centers for Medicare and Medicaid Services (CMS), formerly the Health Care Financing Administration (HCFA). Accordingly, states can establish their own eligibility standards; determine the type, amount, duration, and scope of Medicaid services; set payment rates for services; and administer their individual programs. Given this relative autonomy over key implementation measures, Medicaid programs can vary considerably from state to state.

Considerable attention has been focused on Medicaid dental services in recent years, in part because of greater recognition that individuals covered by Medicaid are disproportionately affected by dental diseases and in part because of widespread concerns about the level of access afforded by Medicaid dental programs. For example, children covered by Medicaid are three to five times as likely to have untreated dental disease than their more affluent counterparts.[3] Growing awareness of these issues has led to a series of federal initiatives and prompted several states to implement policies and operational changes aimed at increasing provider participation, access to services, and overall Medicaid program performance.

ELIGIBILITY AND ENROLLMENT

Three basic groups of low-income people are eligible for Medicaid:

- *Parents and children.* In 1997 Medicaid covered approximately 21 million low-income children and 8.6 million low-income adults in families with children, the vast majority of whom were women.[2]
- *Disabled.* Roughly 6.8 million individuals with disabilities were covered by Medicaid in 1997, largely as a result of receiving cash assistance from the Supplemental Security Income (SSI) program. The remainder generally qualified by incurring large hospital, prescription drug, nursing home, or other medical or long-term care expenses.[2]
- *Elderly.* More than 4 million adults age 65 and over were covered by Medicaid in 1997, slightly less than half because of SSI eligibility and most of the remainder because of extensive health care expenses.[2]

Federally mandated eligibility groups include the following:

- Low-income families with children, who meet certain eligibility requirements in the state's AFDC plan
- Infants, up to 1 year of age, born to Medicaid-eligible pregnant women
- Children under age 6 and pregnant women* whose family income is at or below 133% of the federal poverty level†
- Children under age 19 in families with incomes at or below the federal poverty level
- Recipients of adoption assistance and foster care under Title IV-E of the SSA
- SSI recipients
- Specifically protected groups, including those who lose SSI payments because of earnings from work or increased Social Security benefits

States have the option to extend Medicaid eligibility to "categorically needy" groups.

*Pregnant women remain eligible for Medicaid through the end of the calendar month in which the sixtieth day after the end of the pregnancy falls.

†2001 U.S. Department of Health and Human Services poverty guideline examples: $17,650 for a family of four, $14,630 for a family of three.

Examples of the optional groups that states may cover as categorically needy (and for which they will receive federal matching funds) under the Medicaid program include but are not limited to the following:

- Infants up to age 1 and pregnant women not covered under the mandatory rules whose family incomes are below 185% of the federal poverty level
- Optional targeted low-income children
- Children under age 21 who meet income and resources requirements for TANF, but who otherwise are not eligible for TANF
- Certain aged, blind, or disabled adults who have incomes above those requiring mandatory coverage, but below the federal poverty level

Many states have elected to provide a "medically needy" category of eligibility that allows persons who have too much income to qualify under the mandatory or optional categorically needy groups to receive Medicaid benefits. This option allows them to buy in to Medicaid by incurring medical or remedial care expenses to offset their excess income, thereby reducing it to a level below the maximum allowed by that state's Medicaid plan. States may also allow families to establish eligibility as medically needy by paying monthly premiums to the state in an amount equal to the difference between family income and the income eligibility standard.

MEDICAID TRENDS

Eligibility

As noted earlier, Medicaid has grown significantly from its original eligibility relationship to federal cash assistance programs. Recent congressional legislation provides for expanded coverage to a number of low-income pregnant women, poor children, and some Medicare recipients who are not eligible for any cash assistance program. Legislative changes have focused on both increasing access and improving quality of care, and some have lengthened specific benefits beyond the normal run of Medicaid eligibility and placed restrictions on states' ability to limit specified services.

Since its inception Medicaid has played a prominent role in providing health insurance to low-income children—particularly younger children. Each year more than one third of all births in the United States are covered by Medicaid. In 1998 Medicaid covered 25% of U.S. children under age 3, 22.9% of children between ages 3 and 5, and 15.5% of children between ages 12 and 17.[4] Lower percentages of older children with Medicaid coverage reflect higher income-eligibility criteria for older age groups. Overall, one out of five U.S. children were served by Medicaid in FY 1998.

Mandatory eligibility expansions during the late 1980s contributed to growth in the number of children enrolled in Medicaid. Children (including children with disabilities) represented 54% of the 41.4 million individuals enrolled in Medicaid in FY 1998. The next largest group of enrollees was adults age 21 to 64 (nearly 31%); the elderly, age 65 and over, accounted for the smallest group of enrollees by age.[4]

The proportion of Medicaid beneficiaries with disabilities has increased over time. In 1973 the blind and disabled represented 11% of the total Medicaid population. By 1998 the blind and disabled represented 18% of the total Medicaid population. In contrast, beneficiaries over age 65 decreased from 19% to 11% of the Medicaid population during the past 25 years.[5]

EXPENDITURES

Based on the consistently high ratio of children to adults in Medicaid, it is noteworthy that one of the most pronounced Medicaid service–related trends in recent years has been the exponential increase in spending on behalf of the blind, individuals with disabilities, and the elderly. Expenditures for intensive acute care and for home health and nursing facility services for the aged and disabled have grown sharply during the past two decades. Much of this growth has been attributed to both the increasing size of the Medicaid disabled population and the rising costs associated with institutional long-term care services.

Whereas the aged, the blind, and individuals with disabilities accounted for only 26% of all persons served through Medicaid in 1998, Medicaid payments made on their behalf accounted for 71% of all Medicaid payments. The largest group of persons served through Medicaid, children, accounted for only 16% of all Medicaid program payments.[5]

SERVICES

Most Medicaid beneficiaries are entitled to coverage for the following services, provided they are deemed to be medically necessary:

- Hospital services (inpatient and outpatient)
- Physician services
- Nursing home care
- Nurse-midwife and nurse practitioner services
- Laboratory and x-ray services
- Early and periodic screening, diagnostic, and treatment (EPSDT) services (including dental services) for individuals under age 21
- Federally qualified health center (FQHC) and rural health clinic (RHC) services
- Family planning services

States may also provide home and community-based care waiver services to certain individuals who are eligible for Medicaid. Such services may include case management, personal care services, respite care services, adult day health services, homemaker/home health aide, habilitation, and other services requested by the state and approved by CMS.[4] Dental services per se are not required for Medicaid recipients except as part of EPSDT services, which are described in greater detail later in this chapter.

AMOUNT AND DURATION OF MEDICAID SERVICES

According to federal law, the amount, duration, and scope of each service provided through Medicaid must be "sufficient to reasonably achieve its purpose." States may place appropriate limits on a Medicaid service based on such criteria as medical necessity or utilization control. For example, states may place a reasonable limit on the number of covered physician or dentist visits or may require authorization to be obtained before service delivery.[6]

States have less discretion, however, over medically necessary services provided under EPSDT services. These services must be included in full under each state's program, even if they are not included as part of the covered services in that state's Medicaid plan.

EARLY PERIODIC SCREENING, DIAGNOSTIC, AND TREATMENT SERVICES

The EPSDT service is Medicaid's comprehensive and preventive child health program for individuals under age 21. Enacted in 1967 and amended as part of the Omnibus Budget Reconciliation Act of 1989 (OBRA 89), the legislation provides for periodic screening, vision, dental, hearing, and necessary follow-up services for Medicaid recipients under age 21.

By law, EPSDT services are intended to (1) ensure the availability and accessibility of required health care resources and (2) help Medicaid recipients and their parents or guardians effectively use these resources. This means that states are required to recruit physicians, dentists, and other providers; locate eligible families and inform them about EPSDT services; and ensure that Medicaid-certified physicians, dentists, or other practitioners provide necessary medical and dental examinations, diagnoses, and treatments. Nevertheless, achieving these objectives has been problematic, and obstacles to the delivery of EPSDT services remain.

Screening Services

Each state is required to develop EPSDT periodicity schedules for general health screenings at intervals that meet "reasonable standards of medical practice." Federal law directs states to consult with recognized medical organizations involved in child health care in developing such schedules.

EPSDT screening services must include the following:

- Comprehensive health and developmental history, including assessment of both physical and mental health development.
- Comprehensive unclothed physical examination.*
- Appropriate immunizations according to the schedule established by the Advisory Committee on Immunization Practices (ACIP) for pediatric vaccines.
- Laboratory tests—the minimum laboratory tests or analyses to be performed by medical providers for particular age or population groups.
- Lead toxicity screening—all children are considered at risk and must be screened for lead poisoning.
- Health education—counseling to both parents (or guardians) and children is required to assist them in understanding what to expect in terms of the child's development and to provide information about the benefits of healthful lifestyles and practices, as well as accident and disease prevention.

When screenings indicate the need for further diagnostic or treatment services to evaluate a child's health or correct or ameliorate illnesses and conditions found on screening, children are to be referred to appropriate, qualified health care providers for all necessary services.

*Dental screening services are not required for Medicaid children but generally have been considered to be part of general health screening, at least for very young children. If a dental screening is to be included in a general health screening, the dental screening is to be conducted by qualified providers according to state-specific periodicity schedules. States generally allow a variety of qualified health care and community-based service providers to conduct dental screenings up to an established age threshold, typically set at between 1 and 3 years of age.

Hearing and Vision Services

EPSDT hearing and vision services must include diagnosis and treatment of defects in hearing and vision, including hearing aids and eyeglasses, and are subject to separate periodicity schedules. Where hearing and vision periodicity schedules coincide with (general health) screening schedules, states may include hearing and vision screenings as part of the required minimum screening services.

Dental Services

EPSDT dental services include diagnostic, preventive, and therapeutic or treatment services needed for relief of pain and infection, restoration of teeth, and maintenance of dental health, starting at as early an age as deemed necessary and in accordance with current standards of dental practice. As with hearing and vision services, the law and Medicaid policy require that EPSDT dental services conform to each state's dental periodicity schedule, which must be established after consultation with recognized dental organizations involved in child health care. The periodicity schedule for other EPSDT services (e.g., screening services) may not govern the schedule for dental services.

Parents of children on Medicaid often seek dental services for their children directly (i.e., without a referral). However, when dental care is not initiated by the age specified in each state's dental periodicity schedule (typically between age 1 and 3 years), a "direct dental referral" is required. The dental referral must be for an encounter with a licensed dentist for diagnosis and, if necessary, treatment. Direct referral to a dentist may be met in settings other than a dentist's office. For example, in an area where dentists are scarce or not easily accessible, dental examinations in a clinic or group setting may make the service more appealing to recipients while meeting the state's dental periodicity schedule. Dental periodicity schedules typically also specify recommended intervals for ongoing oral health assessments, health education, and preventive services. Services permitted by the state's practice act also may be obtained from a dental hygienist.

Although an oral screening may be part of a comprehensive physical examination or screening service and may result in a direct dental referral, it does not substitute for examination through direct referral. Referrals to dentists also may occur at times other than those described by the periodicity schedule, as deemed medically necessary (e.g., when oral screening indicates the need for further evaluation, diagnosis, or treatment).

EPSDT Performance Measures

States are required to report annually on Medicaid children's use of various EPSDT services (e.g., number and percent of eligible children receiving recommended general health screenings and dental, hearing, and vision assessments). These reports also serve as measures of states' performance toward meeting EPSDT program goals. The HCFA-416 participation report compiled by CMS for all states for FY 1998 indicated that approximately 14 million, or two thirds of the almost 22 million Medicaid-eligible children, received initial or periodic EPSDT screening services.[7] In contrast, only approximately 4 million, or 18% of all EPSDT-eligible children, received dental assessments during that 12-month period.[7]

Before 2000 states were required to report only the percent of Medicaid-enrolled children who received dental examinations in the preceding 12-month period to document the performance of their dental Medicaid programs. However, recently approved EPSDT reporting revisions now require states to report information annually on (1) the number and percent of Medicaid-eligible children receiving any dental service, (2) the number and percent of eligible children receiving a preventive dental service, and (3) the number and percent of eligible children receiving treatment services (i.e., services beyond diagnostic and preventive dental services). In a related activity, a CMS-supported National Committee on Quality Assurance (NCQA) expert panel has developed recommendations for additional pediatric oral health performance measures.[8]

DENTAL SERVICES IN MEDICAID

Children

EPSDT dental benefits for children include comprehensive diagnostic, preventive, and treatment services. States are required to establish separate dental periodicity schedules that specify the timing and frequency of dental services for Medicaid-eligible children, as well as the timing of initial direct referrals to dentists (generally between 1 and 3 years of age), in consultation with dental organizations involved in child health care.

Medicaid EPSDT coverage includes all dental services deemed "medically necessary," which in this context means services that in the opinion of a qualified provider are required to relieve pain and infections; restore teeth and maintain dental health; or correct or ameliorate defects, illnesses, and conditions discovered by screening services. Orthodontic services are generally limited to cases in which the malocclusion is deemed to be "handicapping" or more severe using various classifying indexes. In the case of children's oral health, the determination of "medically necessary care" must be based on accepted standards of dental and oral health practice, and relevant policies must be developed by recognized dental organizations involved in children's oral health care. "Medically necessary care" also means medical services that directly support the delivery of dental procedures and that, in the judgment of the responsible dentist, are necessary for the provision of optimal-quality therapeutic and preventive oral care to patients with various medical, physical, or behavioral conditions. Such services include but are not limited to sedation, general anesthesia, and use of outpatient and inpatient surgical facilities.

Adults

Federal statutes do not require Medicaid coverage for adult dental services. States that do choose to cover adult dental services as part of their Medicaid programs have the flexibility to determine eligibility criteria and the types of services they will provide. Fifteen states provided adults enrolled in Medicaid with coverage for "basic dental services" (i.e., a limited set of diagnostic, preventive, and therapeutic/restorative services) in 2000; 18 others provided coverage only for services related to dental emergencies (e.g., relief of pain or infection). Still others provided no adult Medicaid dental benefits.[9]

ACCESS TO MEDICAID DENTAL SERVICES

Children

Two recent reports issued by the U.S. General Accounting Office and another issued by the U.S. Department of Health and Human Services Office of Inspector General (OIG) have documented that access to dental services has been a chronic problem for individuals with Medicaid coverage.[9,10] The 1996 OIG report found that less than one in five Medicaid-eligible children received a preventive dental service in 1993.[11] The U.S. Surgeon General's Report on Oral Health, released in 2000, reaffirmed this finding in its statement that "Medicaid has not been able to fill the gap in providing care to poor children."[12]

These low levels of access have been attributed to a variety of factors, including low rates of participation by dentists in Medicaid, issues related to program administration, and enrollee-related issues. Dentists consistently cite inadequate low payment rates as the primary reason for low rates of participation in Medicaid. The General Accounting Office noted that its survey conducted in 2000 found that Medicaid payment rates in most states were well below the prevailing fees charged by more than 90% of practicing dentists in the respective states.[10] Substantial underpayment, combined with cumbersome provider enrollment forms and reimbursement procedures and weak systems linking Medicaid enrollees and dental health providers, has resulted in poor access to dental services for children enrolled in Medicaid. CMS has advised states that actions must be taken to improve Medicaid children's access to dental services and has requested that states develop state plans to address problem areas. Litigation in federal courts is another common approach pursued by Medicaid enrollees and advocacy groups in states with chronic access problems.

Adults

Much less is known about adults' access to dental services in Medicaid because states are not required to report utilization rates as they are for EPSDT services for children. However, in 2000 the General Accounting

Table 4-1. Medicaid and Dental Care Expenditures

Expenditures (in millions)	*1980*	*1985*	*1990*	*1995*	*1998*
Medicaid personal health care	$24,722	$38,922	$71,236	$136,899	$159,212
Total U.S. dental care	$13,323	$21,650	$31,566	$ 45,000	$ 53,829
Medicaid dental care	$ 505	$ 510	$ 756	$ 1,780	$ 1,993
Medicaid dental care expenditures as a percentage of Medicaid personal health care expenditures	2.0%	1.3%	1.1%	1.3%	1.3%
Medicaid dental care expenditures as a percentage of total U.S. dental care expenditures	3.8%	2.4%	2.4%	4.0%	3.7%

Data from Health Care Financing Administration: National health expenditures by type of service and source of funds: calendar years 1960-1999. Available at www.hcfa.gov/stats/nhe-oact/

Office reported a weighted average of 29% of adult Medicaid recipients making a dental visit.[9] CMS has recently directed attention to the issue of the adequacy of oral health care for the elderly in nursing homes, who often are covered by Medicaid.

MEDICAID AND DENTAL CARE EXPENDITURES

Table 4-1 provides data and comparisons for selected years from 1980 to 1998 on expenditures for Medicaid personal health care, total U.S. dental care (including all private/public payers and individuals), and Medicaid dental care services. Note that Medicaid dental expenditures pale in comparison and have declined relative to Medicaid personal health care expenditures since 1980, and they have been a small and somewhat variable portion of total U.S. dental care expenditures.

STATE CHILDREN'S HEALTH INSURANCE PROGRAM (SCHIP)

One of the most significant recent developments related to populations covered by Medicaid is the establishment of the State Children's Health Insurance Program as part of the Balanced Budget Act of 1997. SCHIP, or Title XXI, is the largest effort by Congress since Medicaid to provide health insurance to vulnerable children. The program was created to address the problem of 10 million medically uninsured children. It is distinguished from Medicaid by entitling states (not individual children) to federal allotments to provide "child health assistance." SCHIP provides for a 30% larger federal share of program costs compared with Medicaid and gives states even more latitude in designing eligibility criteria, service benefits, cost sharing, and administration. In its first 3 years, SCHIP reached more than 3 million of the 10 million eligible children. Initial outreach difficulties have been addressed in subsequent legislation to improve enrollment methods.

Under SCHIP, states can extend coverage to children who do not qualify for Medicaid and are not insured through employer coverage. They can cover children up to 200% of the federal poverty level, or 50 percentage points higher than criteria used in their existing Medicaid programs, as long as they cover lower-income children before higher-income children. The overwhelming majority of newly covered children are from "working poor" families—families in which one or both parents are employed full-time but earn too little to afford health insurance.

States may elect to provide SCHIP coverage by expanding Medicaid benefits. If a state elects a Medicaid expansion, it must provide the full range of dental benefits, including whatever orthodontic coverage is provided in its Medicaid program. However, if a state elects a new "state CHIP program," it can base its benefits package on one of three options: (1) "benchmark coverage" (equal to benefits provided to federal employees in their Blue Cross standard option preferred-provider organization plan; equal to benefits offered to state employees in that state; or equal to benefits provided by the health maintenance organization in that state with the largest enrollment); (2) "benchmark-equivalent coverage" (an actuarially determined dollar value of one of the three benchmark coverage plans); or (3) "Secretary-approved coverage" (a set of benefits approved by the Secretary of Health and Human Services).[13]

Dental Services in the State Children's Health Insurance Program

Dental coverage is not a requirement under Title XXI; however, 49 of the 50 states have chosen to offer dental coverage as part of their SCHIP programs and to provide relatively comprehensive benefits. Although not as broad as Medicaid's EPSDT program, coverage under most SCHIP programs includes basic preventive, diagnostic, and restorative services.

States with separate SCHIP programs are delivering dental care through methods not traditionally used under Medicaid. For example, states predominantly deliver dental services under SCHIP through managed care arrangements (even though payments to dentists generally remain on a fee-for-service basis). A recent Urban Institute report acknowledged that whether managed care plans will succeed in improving access to dental care will depend, in large part, on the extent to which states hold the plans accountable for meeting their contractual obligations and the adequacy of the capitation rates paid to plans.[14] The relative success of dental service delivery through SCHIP, supported by higher payment rates and improved provider participation, may provide a model for Medicaid programs to consider in their efforts to improve access.

SUMMARY

Medicaid and the recently established State Children's Health Insurance Program are important programs for facilitating access to dental services for low-income individuals. The design and administration of these programs vary considerably across states, as has their performance. Recent federal and state initiatives have focused on addressing issues identified as contributing to low levels of provider participation and use of dental services. Coverage for dental services under these and other health-related federal programs is restricted according to eligibility criteria, with many states providing little or no dental coverage for low-income adults.

REVIEW QUESTIONS

1. Medicaid provides benefits for what three groups when impoverished?
2. What two groups account for most of Medicaid's funding?
3. What accounts for the complexity of the Medicaid rules?
4. List the federally mandated eligibility groups under Medicaid.
5. What is the early and periodic screening, diagnostic, and treatment (EPSDT) program? What does this program intend to accomplish?
6. What types of dental services are delivered under the EPSDT Medicaid program?
7. How many states provide adult dental services? What are the "basic dental services"?
8. What are the conclusions of the U.S. Surgeon General's Report on Oral Health regarding dental care to poor children?
9. What is the State Children's Health Insurance Program (SCHIP)? How many states have opted to include dental care under this program? What dental services may be provided under this program?

ACKNOWLEDGMENT

The author wishes to acknowledge the contributions of Joanna Parzakonis in the development of this document.

REFERENCES

1. Spisak S, Holt K: Building partnerships to improve children's access to Medicaid oral health services: national conference proceedings, Arlington, VA, 1999, National Center for Education in Maternal and Child Health.
2. Henry J Kaiser Family Foundation: Medicaid: a primer, August 1-3, 1999. Available at www.kff.org/content/1999/2161/pub2161.pdf.
3. Vargas C, Crall J, Schneider D: Sociodemographic distribution of pediatric dental caries: NHANES III, 1988-1994, *J Am Dent Assoc* 129:1229, 1998.
4. Health Care Financing Administration: Medicaid national summary statistics: 1960-99. Available at www.hcfa.gov/medicaid/msis/mnatstat.htm.
5. Health Care Financing Administration: National health expenditures by type of service and source of funds: calendar years 1960-99. Available at www.hcfa.gov/stats/nhe-oact/.
6. Title XIX of the Social Security Act, US Code 42 USC 1396, Public Law #89-97.
7. Center for Medicare and Medicaid services annual EPSDT participation report all states: 1998. Available at www.hcfa.gov/medicaid/ep1998n.pdf.
8. Crall JJ et al: Pediatric oral health performance measurement: current capabilities and future directions, *J Public Health Dent* 59:136, 1999.
9. US General Accounting Office: *Oral health: dental disease is a chronic problem in low-income populations,* GAO/HEHS-00-72, April 12, 2000.
10. US General Accounting Office: *Oral health: factors contributing to low use of dental services by low-income populations,* GAO/HEHS-00-149, September 11, 2000.
11. US Department of Health and Human Services, Office of the Inspector General: *Children's dental services under Medicaid access and utilization,* OEI-09-93-00240, Office of the Inspector General, April 1996.
12. US Department of Health and Human Services: *Oral health in America: a report of the Surgeon General,* Rockville, MD, 2000, US Department of Health and Human Services, National Institute of Dental and Craniofacial Research, National Institutes of Health.
13. Balanced Budget Act of 1997, pub law no 105-33, 1997.
14. Almeida R, Hill I, Genevieve K: Does SCHIP spell better dental care access for children: an early look at initiatives, Urban Institute Occasional Paper no 50, July 2001.

PART

II

DEMOGRAPHIC SHIFTS AND DENTAL HEALTH

CHAPTER

5

DIVERSITY, SOCIOCULTURAL ISSUES, AND COMMUNICATION IN ORAL HEALTH CARE

Hillary L. Broder • Michael Skolnick • Yvette R. Schlussel

We have witnessed extraordinary progress in health care during the last century. Life expectancy has increased dramatically, and a host of medical conditions have been conquered by new biomedical technologies. In the area of oral health, dental caries have been sharply reduced by the introduction of fluoridation, and we no longer expect adults to become edentulous in middle age. As we enter the new millennium, there is a general sentiment that nothing is beyond the scope of science. However, not all Americans have benefited from recent scientific advances. In fact, as the vanguard of health care has advanced, the gaps between the haves and have-nots have become even more pronounced and disturbing. Barriers to oral health care exist. They range from the costs of care and cultural factors related to health beliefs and other psychosocial variables to intrinsic characteristics of the health care system itself. This chapter focuses on the interrelationships between sociocultural factors and health behaviors. It examines the cultural factors themselves, as well as health communication and the importance of cultural competence for the dental professional in achieving the goals of *Healthy People 2010,* namely oral health promotion and the reduction of oral health disparities.[1]

DEMOGRAPHICS

The demographic characteristics of the United States are changing rapidly. In 1990 approximately 24.3% of the population consisted of members of ethnic minority groups; by 2000 that number had grown to 28.7%.[2] Between 1990 and 2000 the black population increased from 11.8% to 12.2% of the total population, Hispanics from 9% to 11.9%, and Asian and Pacific Islanders from 2.8% to 3.8%. Over the same period of time, the white population fell from 75.7% to 71.3% of the total. According to the latest census, 1 of every 10 Americans is foreign born. It is also projected that by 2050 minority-ethnic subpopulations will make up 47.5% of the total population, and that by 2056 whites will be a minority in the United States.[3] In short, the cultural landscape of the United States will undergo seismic changes.

North American culture has been transformed from a melting pot to a mosaic. The American way of life has become a heterogeneous mixture of different cultures, many of which maintain their unique ethnic identities. The growing diversity of the North American population raises serious questions about our health care system. Are the various ethnic subpopulations receiving the quality health care to which they are entitled? How can the health care system address and deal with increasing diversity?

UTILIZATION OF ORAL HEALTH SERVICES

It is commonly accepted that the utilization of professional dental care is essential to achieve and maintain good oral health. The Surgeon General's Report on Oral Health maintains that almost everyone in the United States will experience some form of oral disease over the course of his or her lifetime.[4] To prevent and combat the spread of oral disease, both prophylactic and restorative dental care is administered regularly and proficiently. There is an inverse correlation between unmet dental needs and utilization: that is, people who do not utilize dental care have higher rates of dental problems than those who do.

The most common measure of dental care utilization is the report of *at least one dental visit in the past year.* The proportion of the population over 2 years old with a dental visit in the past year increased from 57.1% in 1986 to 65.1% in 1997.[5,6]

Contrasting data from the Medical Expenditures Panel Survey 1996 (MEPS) indicated that only 44% of the population over 2 years of age visited a dentist in 1996.[7] The Surgeon General's Report on Oral Health notes that there is substantial discrepancy in estimates of dental care utilization because of differences in definitions and sampling methodologies.[3] However, virtually all estimates confirm marked disparities in utilization and unmet needs associated with demographic variables. The factors that affect utilization of dental services are complex. Trends over the past two decades reveal that family income, dental insurance coverage, and education level are positively correlated with the utilization of dental care.[1,4,5] On the other hand, age is inversely correlated with utilization among adults.

Table 5-1 illustrates these trends in oral health utilization and the health disparities by race/ethnicity.[8] Ethnicity is also significantly associated with dental care utilization. Historically, blacks and Hispanics have had lower rates of utilization than whites. The table illustrates that 64% of whites versus 47% of blacks visited the dentist in the past year. The MEPS data indicate comparable disparities between whites and blacks (50% versus 27%, respectively).[7] The consistent disparity is remarkable when one considers other associated variables. For example, although race/ethnicity is correlated with educational level, controlling for the latter does not nullify the disparity in dental care utilization between blacks and Hispanics versus whites.

ACCESS TO ORAL HEALTH CARE

Utilization of and access to care are mediated by a myriad of personal, cultural, and institutional factors. In the Institute of Medi-

Table 5-1. Percentage of Persons 25 Years of Age and Older with a Dental Visit within the Preceding Year, by Selected Patient Characteristics, Selected Years

	1983*	1989*	1990*	1991*	1993*
Total†,‡	53.9	58.9	62.3	58.2	60.3
Age					
25 to 34 years	59.0	60.9	65.1	59.1	60.3
35 to 44 years	60.3	65.9	69.1	64.8	66.9
45 to 64 years	54.1	59.9	62.8	59.2	62.0
65 years and older	39.3	45.8	49.6	47.2	51.7
65 to 74 years	43.8	50.0	53.5	51.1	56.3
75 years and older	31.8	39.0	43.4	41.3	44.9
Gender‡					
Male	51.7	56.2	58.8	55.5	58.2
Female	55.9	61.4	65.6	60.8	63.4
Poverty status‡,§					
Below poverty	30.4	33.3	38.2	33.0	35.9
At or above poverty	55.8	62.1	65.4	61.9	64.3
Race and Hispanic origin‡					
White, non-Hispanic	56.6	61.8	64.9	61.5	64.0
Black, non-Hispanic	39.1	43.3	49.1	44.3	47.3
Hispanic‖	42.1	48.9	53.8	43.1	46.2
Education‡					
Less than 12 years	35.1	36.9	41.2	35.2	38.0
12 years	54.8	58.2	61.3	56.7	58.7
13 years or more	70.9	73.9	75.7	72.2	73.8
Education, race, and Hispanic origin‡					
Fewer than 12 years					
White, non-Hispanic	36.1	39.1	41.8	38.1	41.2
Black, non-Hispanic	31.7	32.0	37.9	33.0	33.1
Hispanic‖	33.8	36.5	42.7	28.9	33.0
12 years					
White, non-Hispanic	56.6	59.8	62.8	58.8	60.4
Black, non-Hispanic	40.5	44.8	51.1	43.1	48.2
Hispanic‖	48.7	56.5	59.9	49.5	54.6
13 years or more					
White, non-Hispanic	72.6	75.8	77.3	74.2	75.8
Black, non-Hispanic	54.4	57.2	64.4	61.7	61.3
Hispanic‖	58.4	66.2	67.9	61.2	61.8

Data from NCHS 1989.

NOTES: Data are based on household interviews of a sample of the civilian noninstitutionalized population. Denominators exclude persons with unknown dental data. Estimates for 1983 and 1989 are based on data for all members of the sample household. Beginning in 1990, estimates are based on one adult member per sample household. Estimates for 1993 are based on response during the last half of the year only.

*Data for 1983 and 1989 are not strictly comparable with data for later years. Data for 1983 and 1989 are based on responses to the question, "About how long has it been since you last went to a dentist?" Starting in 1990, data are based on the question, "During the past 12 months, how many visits did you make to a dentist?"

†Includes all other races not shown separately and unknown poverty status and education level.

‡Age adjusted.

§Poverty status is based on family income and family size using Bureau of the Census poverty thresholds.

‖Persons of Hispanic origin may be of any race.

cine's report entitled *Access to Health Care in America,* access to oral health care is defined as "the timely use of oral health services to achieve the best possible health outcome."[9] Three primary barriers to health care were identified—structural, financial, and personal/cultural.[10] Structural barriers include the shortage of health care providers and lack of facilities in a community. Financial barriers are related to a patient's ability to afford care; lack of insurance or underinsurance is a major obstacle for many patients. Personal barriers include individual characteristics such as sexual orientation, language, and education.

Economics plays a critical role in health care. The cost of dental care and the availability of insurance coverage have a profound impact on the utilization of health care services. Substantial disparities in health insurance coverage exist among different population groups. For adults under age 65 years, 34% of those below the poverty level are uninsured. Among the nonelderly population, approximately 33% of Hispanic persons lacked coverage in 1998, a rate that is more than double the national average.[1] The uninsured use fewer health care services than do insured individuals. Paradoxically, individuals with public insurance (e.g., Medicaid) have higher rates of hospitalization and physician visits than privately insured individuals because of inadequate regular, preventive care.[11,12] Extending the benefits of private insurance to uninsured individuals would significantly increase utilization rates of services by uninsured patients.[13]

Andersen[14] has emphasized that dental care is more discretionary than other types of health services and is therefore more likely to be influenced by social structure, health beliefs, and various enabling factors. "Potential" access to care depends on the presence of enabling resources, such as the availability of health providers and health care facilities, along with income, health insurance, and a regular source of care. More enabling resources increase the likelihood that services will be available and that utilization will take place. "Equitable" access to care is present when the variance in care among different groups is due to differences in age, gender, or the patient's perceived need for services. On the other hand, "inequitable access" to care is present when social structure (e.g., race/ethnicity), health beliefs, and enabling resources (e.g., income and insurance) are responsible for the variance in utilization of health care.

The notion of "inequitable access" and the discretionary nature of dentistry provide valuable information regarding the source of the variance in dental care utilization. Consideration of the impact of culture, ethnicity, income, and health insurance, in determining both need and access to dental care, aids in explaining oral health disparities and targeting interventions. Information about the "usual source of care" may be another critical element of health promotion policy. A recent finding has identified that the existence of a "usual source" of medical care is highly predictive of optimal health status and dental utilization.[15] Additionally, data regarding specific characteristics of such "usual care" may provide insight into improving utilization of dental care by the underserved.

HEALTH PROMOTION AND ADHERENCE TO CARE

Although the terms *compliance* and *adherence* have been used interchangeably in the literature, an important distinction is that adherence is predicated on a mutual agreement by both provider and recipient. This mutuality is deemed essential in effective health communication. Despite medical advancements in reducing disease, adherence is an ongoing, challenging health issue that has received inadequate attention in the education of health professionals.[16,17] What is relevant for successful health behavior change in one group may be irrelevant to another group. What does the patient or community know about the condition or targeted behavior? Who needs to be involved in making the decision to change? Health educators recognize that such questions are linked to the success of a treatment or intervention.[18,19] To implement treatment or create an oral health intervention for an individual or a community, it is crucial to find common ground between the provider and recipient. Successful treatment or intervention depends on the exchange of ideas, attitudes, and behaviors. The process may call for adopting new behaviors or eliminating risk behaviors. To facilitate behavior change and increase adherence with desired goals, mutual understanding and compromise are essential. Surveys, instruments, personal interviews, and focus groups are methods of acquiring salient information. Multiple sources must be tapped to gather data to sensitize us to the needs of the community. The community represents the stakeholders and partners, the target audience, community health providers, and opinion leaders such as newspaper reporters or editors, politicians or teachers, as well as lay advocates for patients.

MODELS OF HEALTH PROMOTION

In our efforts to improve health status and reduce health disparities, an understanding of established theoretic frameworks that incorporate psychologic and social variables is warranted. Across these theoretic frameworks, it is generally recognized that people do not change health behaviors unless there is a perceived payoff and their behavior can lead to this payoff. The Readiness to Change Model identifies four distinct stages of change associated with acquiring or sustaining health promotion/disease prevention behaviors.[20] Although this model is the foundation for numerous health programs, it has not been applied to oral health programs. The stages are (1) *precontemplation,* in which there has been no thought about performing or changing a target behavior; (2) *contemplation,* which represents the phase when consideration of performing or changing behaviors takes place; (3) *action,* in which the target behavior is adopted; and (4) *maintenance,* in which the behaviors continue to prevail. *Relapse,* a regression to any earlier stage, is a recognized part of the model.

As with many intervention programs, baseline assessment of the community or individual is critical to knowing how to best create the program and maintain the targeted behavior. Although the Readiness to Change framework has not been applied to dental behaviors, it offers a promising model for oral health promotion. In the case of the parent or caregiver who has low oral health knowledge about the implications of using a baby bottle with milk at night, the initial program might include an informational exchange before contemplation of behavior change is sought. Fostering behavior through motivational techniques is appropriate during the action and maintenance stages. For example, a scale was recently developed to assess Readiness to Change parenting behaviors associated with risk behaviors of early childhood caries.[21]

The Health Belief Model emphasizes that behaviors such as visiting the dentist or toothbrushing and flossing are dependent on the individual's cognitions.[22,23] Perceived susceptibility to and the severity of a particular condition are integral to the model. Further, the individual's perception of the benefits of and barriers to (e.g., costs) following a particular health-related action are also part of the model. In short, those health behaviors that are believed to have many benefits and few barriers are more likely to be followed.[24,25] After the completion of considerable research, this model has failed to conclusively explain or predict behaviors based merely on oral health beliefs.[26,27] However, this model has formed a foundation for subsequent models and is associated with specific health behaviors.

The Extended Parallel Process Model is a fear appeal theory that is linked to the Health Belief Model.[28] This model proposes that when people perceive a health threat they either control the actual health threat (danger) or control their fear about the danger. They weigh their risk of the health threat (e.g., oral cancer) against actions that they can take that would reduce their risk (e.g., stop smoking). Thus the important variables in this model are the perceived threat, perceived susceptibility, and perceived self-efficacy. A variation of this model has been, in part, adapted in dentistry by examining both motivational variables and a vulnerability dimension.[29]

Social Cognitive Theory postulates the belief that the extent to which one can exert control over one's behavior and health constitutes the driving force of whether persons are willing to engage in behavior change.[30] This theory of behavior change incorporates self-efficacy (cognitive factors) and the social environment (e.g., social support). For example, asking parents whether they believe they can control whether their infants' teeth will decay is viewed as critical in predicting whether parents will engage in health promotion efforts to reduce early childhood caries. This model has been used in health programs aimed at reducing periodontal disease and increasing oral health maintenance in adults.[31,32]

Behavioral analytic theories rely on learning theory approaches—using rewards and reinforcements.[33] The ABC approach examines antecedents, behaviors, and consequences. The antecedents (A) include enabling factors such as the knowledge and skills needed to carry out the targeted behavioral outcome; behaviors (B) represent the sequential steps needed to achieve the outcome and are the natural consequences (C) of learning. This model has not been implemented much in the Western world but has been demonstrably useful in creating behavior adherence in developing areas. In essence, it is a learning theory approach in which barriers are identified and facilitators are implemented—with particular emphasis on skill acquisition and self-efficacy.

Another approach to understanding the delivery of health care services, as previously alluded to, is Andersen's revised Behavioral Model of Health Services Use.[14] In it, he posits that people's use of health services is a function of their predisposition to use services, their need for care, and factors that enable or impede use. Predisposing characteristics or need include demographic factors such as age and gender. Personal variables such as education level, occupation, and ethnicity; coping style and command of resources to deal with problems; and the health of the physical environment are all factors that ultimately affect the utilization of health services. These features, in addition to beliefs about health and health services, are proposed to influence perceptions of need and use of such services. This model of health services includes two important additions: (1) the health care system, which incorporates the relevance of health policy and the organization of the health care system as a factor of utilization; and (2) health outcomes, which include perceived health status and consumer satisfaction. These additions allow for a more complex dynamic model containing feedback loops revealing that health outcomes influence predisposing factors, perceived need, and therefore future health behaviors.

FACILITATORS AND BARRIERS TO CARE

The health delivery system influences oral health attitudes and behaviors.[34,35] The implementation of facilitators in the system may be as important as the elimination or reduction of barriers to care in changing attitudes and behaviors and improving adherence to treatment regimens. If people feel that dentistry is painful and costly, a campaign to alter these perceptions is important. If the dental clinic is viewed as an unwelcoming facility (e.g., child-unfriendly, rude staff, crowded waiting area, unclean), the system will need to understand the expectations and the cultural and health needs and concerns of the community. Efforts to unravel barriers and increase facilitators are laudable, can be costly, and also require the recognition that system change is needed. Noteworthy facilitators for underserved populations in cross-cultural settings include translators or bilingual staff, flexible appointment times, transportation service, reminder phone calls, and child care services.[36-39] Additionally, reducing costs, using sliding pay scales, or affiliating with or enrolling patients into subsidized programs can facilitate access to care. For example, Ryan White funds compensate clinics providing dental care, and funds from social services departments for transportation facilitate access to care for people with limited financial or physical resources. Such funds have increased attendance at clinics and the routine provision of dental care, including anticipatory guidance.[37] It is important to note that health status assessments are deemed necessary to evaluate health interventions, as well as to address policy-relevant issues such as effectiveness.

Recognizing the World Health Organization's definition of health (1958) as "more than the absence of disease" and the identification of sociodental indicators, the development of assessments measuring variations in oral health that can supplement biologically based measures has received increasing attention.[38] Over the past two decades, the development of such assessments for older adults has been accomplished, and currently oral health–related quality-of-life assessments for children are being developed.[39,40] Data from such assessments are valid health indicators or outcomes only if they are sensitive to multicultural populations.

CULTURAL INFLUENCES ON ORAL HEALTH BELIEFS AND PRACTICES

The significance of culture for health is well recognized in that conceptions and expressions of health are culturally determined and vary both between and within cultural groups.[34,41-44] Although measures of disease seemingly have no cultural content, measures of health and quality of life address inherently cultural phenomena. Culture is a complex matrix of interacting elements that is ubiquitous, multidimensional, and complex. It represents knowledge, experience, beliefs, values, meanings, and attitudes, as well as concepts of religion and notions of time, roles, and the universe. In essence, culture is the lens through which we view the world. Johnson[42] defines culture as "learned and shared ways of interpreting the world" that thereby provide individuals with ideas about what is relevant or irrelevant, valued or devalued in life. Thus health is "culture bound," and those interacting cross-culturally can easily become prey to ethnocentrism, in which a health provider or investigator assumes that the values important to the culture in which she or he has been socialized are necessarily shared by all. In health care, communication is complex, requiring careful consideration of cultural concepts of health, illness, and health values and behaviors. Table 5-2 provides examples of specific health-related factors that affect the delivery of dental and health care by ethnicity.[45] It should be noted that the group descriptions are generalizations about ethnic groups with the understanding that there is much diversity within groups. Although the groups in the table are not exhaustive, they are representative of those ethnic groups that are most prevalent in the United States.

Understanding Cultural Backgrounds

If a public health practitioner is to understand why a patient engages in risk behaviors associated with his or her oral health status, the practitioner needs to understand the patient's cultural background. Without this understanding, miscommunication occurs and can lead to adverse health outcomes. Barker[46] has identified distinct categories where miscommunication occurs in health-related issues as a result of differences in definitions of verbal and nonverbal messages. The first area, ethnomedical systems, deals with unique cultural beliefs and knowledge about health and disease held by the cultural group. Specific groups believe in personalistic medical systems in which spirits or sorcerers cause disease (e.g., indigenous people of Central and South America); while others believe in the naturalistic medical system wherein health is associated with a balance or equilibrium in the body (e.g., traditional Chinese medicine). For this reason, an individual adhering to a "hot-cold" balance thinks of some conditions, such as a tooth inflammation, as a hot condition brought on by consumption of too many hot foods. Treatment for conditions such as a jaw or joint problem (cold condition) involves consuming hot foods or medicine. An oral cleft may be perceived as the result of "bad" acts by the mother (e.g., infidelity), the evil eye, or the happenstance whereby a pregnant mother looked at a rabbit during pregnancy.[47-49] In any case, Western medicine generally treats the health condition based on the physical and medical data (radiographs, laboratory tests, and physical examination) with little consideration of the patient's perceptions and beliefs. We tend to consider the mind and body as though they are separate entities. The mind-body connection is intrinsically linked to some cultural health values and the connection of the mind-body and the universe. These linkages can be observed in variations among Native American, African, and Chinese health systems.

Ethnocultural Identity

Vast intragroup diversity is associated with ethnocultural identity. *Ethnocultural identity* refers to the extent to which an individual endorses and practices a way of life associated with a particular cultural tradition.[50] It includes multiple behaviors and values. Ethnocultural identity refers only to one's identity with one's chosen group(s), whereas *acculturation* typically refers to the degree to which an individual identifies with or adjusts to mainstream cultures.[51] Ethnocultural identity is dynamic and is affected by the acculturation process. The individual's identity, values, attitudes, and degree of acculturation influence the health encounter. Four levels of acculturation have been identified: (1) *bicultural*—one who functions equally well in the dominant culture and his or her own culture; (2) *traditional*—one who holds most of the characteristics of his or her culture of origin; (3) *marginal*—one who does not have contact with the dominant culture or culture of origin; and (4) *acculturated*—one who has given up the traits of the culture of origin and has adopted the traits of the dominant culture. The process, termed *assimilation,* involves social, economic, and political integration into a mainstream society to which one has emigrated. Assimilation is closely linked to acculturation, which requires an understanding or assessment by the health practitioner to better understand the person for whom an intervention or program is designed. Such assessments have been investigated.[52,53] One scale, the Brief Acculturation Scale by Burnam and colleagues,[54] identifies three variables: generation in the United States, preferred language, and preferences for persons with whom the individual most often socializes.

CROSS-CULTURAL COMMUNICATION

In working toward the elimination of oral health disparities, it is critical to acknowledge that cross-cultural encounters often result in miscommunication. Barna[55] identifies commonly observed factors accounting for interpersonal misunderstanding:

1. *Assumption of similarities.* Despite varying health beliefs and attitudes between those involved in the interaction, assuming similarities (e.g., projection) can be problematic. A poignant example may be that we assume that because there are universal facial expressions associated with anger, fear, and happiness, body language and visual expressiveness connote emotion in ways that are familiar to us and similar to how we would display such emotions. However, it is important to note that the expressive display or suppression of emotion such as fear or pain can vary within and across cultural groups. If we perceive everything from only our own frame of reference, we will undoubtedly be misinterpreting meaning. Nonverbal communication, such as spatial relations and gestures, is discussed in a later section.
2. *Disclosing health information* is highly variable across cultures. When a provider inquires about bodily function or potential areas of health concern, it should be understood that such information may be private and not readily disclosed—even in a health setting with a familiar provider, and even when treatment is being sought. Thus data from health questionnaires and interviews may underestimate patient symptomatology.
3. *Language differences* are obvious blocks. In addition to simply not un-

Text continued on p. 118

Table 5-2. Communication Issues across Ethnicity

Ethnic Group	*Verbal Communication*	*Nonverbal Communication*	*Self-Care*	*Spirit/Healers, Amulets/Cloth*
Native Americans	Most speak English. Humor is important. Use metaphors. Long pauses are typical. Time flexible, and 56% are high school grads vs. 69% of all groups—1990 census.	Avoid eye contact. Listening is valued cultural skill. Greeting—light touch, handshake. Keep respectful distance.	Traditional medicine may be used first or with Western medicine.	Variable. If medicine bag is worn, do not remove it (whenever possible) or examine it.
Brazilians	Portuguese is major language; varying levels of fluency in English. Do not assume that Brazilians or Portuguese speak Spanish.	Lower-class people may avoid direct eye contact with health professionals to show respect. Personal space is quite close; interpersonally warm; touch to reassure; thumbs up is an appropriate nonverbal sign for "all is well." Avoid North American OK (with thumb and forefinger). Time of little import.	Reluctance to undergo screening may be rooted in fear of uncovering disease and not wanting to deal with bad news.	Strong religious/ spiritual healing. Catholic priests; spiritists; curanderas.
Arab Americans	Arabic. Many speak English. More past and present than future orientation— "on time" is kept for official business.	Respect elders and professionals. Traditional women may avoid eye contact with non-acquaintances and men. Polite—may try to please. Modesty is valued. Very polite—may not disagree outwardly.	Believe in complete rest. Alcohol prohibited among Moslems. Do not eat hot and cold together.	Scarves for women are important—depends on country of origin. Koran or Bible—other amulets to ward off evil eye.

From Lipson JG, Dibble SL, Minarik PA, Broder HL: Personal communication, 1996.

Pain	*Cause of Illness*	*Home/Folk Remedies*	*Informed Consent*	*Concept of Health*
Generally undertreated in this population. Patient may complain of pain to trusted family member.	Illness may be caused by breaking taboos or violation of social proscription or loss of harmony with environment.	Roots/herbs; sweat lodges.	Ask if patient needs to consult anyone before consenting. Some are unwilling to sign written consent.	Health beliefs are holistic and wellness oriented. Do not recognize "silent disease." Religious ceremonies promote health of self and family.
Generally low threshold for pain; men thought to be less tolerant than women.	Divine intervention or fate.	Vast array of teas and special prayers.	Family members should be consulted—decision making should include parents, spouse, or those with more education; less educated patients may be reluctant to ask questions.	Usually considered as absence of pain, suffering, or disease. Health is considered a divine blessing—fatalistic attitude. Weight gain is considered a healthy sign. Health promotion or health screening appointments are uncommon.
Very expressive. Generally low pain tolerance—injections are more effective than pills.	Physical illness is caused by evil eye, stress in family, germs, imbalance of hot and dry and cold and moist.	Prefer Western medicine for treatment. Decision making is collective. Home remedies include religious prayer, herbal teas. Women are the nurturers.	Written consent may be somewhat problematic because verbal consent based on trust is more acceptable. Collective decisions—may be the spokesperson.	Health is a gift from God manifesting in eating, good mood, and no pain. Avoid hot-cold shifts in temperature and wind. Self-help and rehabilitative efforts must be understood and reinforced.

Continued

Table 5-2. Communication Issues across Ethnicity—cont'd

Ethnic Group	*Verbal Communication*	*Nonverbal Communication*	*Self-Care*	*Spirit/Healers, Amulets/ Cloth*
Black/ African Americans	English. Flexible time frame. Older persons are more punctual.	Expressive, affectionate. Handshake is appropriate; use titles on first meeting.	Prefer independence.	Prayer; church is an important African-American institution. Faith and root healers may be used in conjunction with biomedical resources. Women are often the nurturers.
Chinese-Americans	Cantonese and Mandarin are common; English. Elderly women may be unable to read or write.	Eye contact may be avoided. Asking questions may be disrespectful. Keep respectful distance, often shy. Being on time is not valued by traditional Chinese. Elders are highly respected.	Modesty, in particular among women.	Treat with food remedies—use herbal preparations. May be fearful of blood and avoid surgery—leave body intact so soul will have a place to live in future visits to Earth.
South Asians, East Indians	Major languages: Hindu, Urdu, Punjabi; >400 languages; men most educated; older first generation may not speak English.	Touching is not common. Love and caring are expressed thru eyes and facial expressions—not touching. Silence usually means acceptance, approval, or tolerance. At difficult times, people may pray in silence. Modesty, shyness (sharm), and silence are admired from childhood. Direct eye contact may be seen as rude.	Sick individuals expect caregiver or family members to help relieve patient from family responsibilities to ensure recovery.	Hindus worship many gods and goddesses. Caste system. Karma. Muslims: one god. Religious practices include prayer 5 times daily. Sikhs: one god. Western medicine generally well accepted; Hindus believe that rituals will eliminate diseases, sins. Yoga; offerings. May seek spiritual assistance by a pir or advice by homeopathic or Ayurvedic physician.

From Lipson JG, Dibble SL, Minarik PA, Broder HL: Personal communication, 1996.

Pain	*Cause of Illness*	*Home/Folk Remedies*	*Informed Consent*	*Concept of Health*
Generally open. Pain scales helpful to rate discomfort.	Natural causes; improper diet and eating habits; God's punishment; work of evil; spell.	Teas, herbs, warm compresses. Rural areas use folk healers or voodoo in specific locations. Also varies by education.	Avoid medical jargon (long history of abuse as experimental subjects). Clear explanations are important.	Feelings of well-being, able to fulfill role expectations. Free of pain and distress.
May not complain of pain; may use acupressure, acupuncture, or herbs. Use Western doctors for more serious illnesses.	Imbalance of yin (cold) (e.g., fruits, cold liquids, vegetables) and yang (hot) (meats, eggs, hot soup, fried foods).	Soups, herbs, and food (yin/yang balance). Ginseng root is a common home remedy for common ailments.	Involve oldest man of the family with consent explanations.	Health is balance of yin and yang and environment. Harmony important to maintain with body, mind, and spirit.
Would understand a numeric scale to quantify pain. Medication for pain secondary to surgery will usually be taken.	Hindus: karma (actions in past lives) determines person's body constitution in this life and susceptibility to illnesses Muslims: illness can result from bad actions, not necessarily in past life. South Asians may believe that illnessess result from imbalance in bodily humors.	Reciting charms and performing certain rituals will eliminate disease and sins. Yoga is thought to eliminate specific bodily ailments, including mental distress. Common and variable.	Male family member, usually eldest son, has decision-making power in family. Women assume caretaking role.	Health considered a gift—balance of body, mind, and consciousness. Negative emotions are believed bad for health. Respectful of biomedical advancements. Exercise, eat, and sleep are important.

Continued

Table 5-2. Communication Issues across Ethnicity—cont'd

Ethnic Group	*Verbal Communication*	*Nonverbal Communication*	*Self-Care*	*Spirit/Healers, Amulets/ Cloth*
Puerto Ricans	Spanish and English. Elderly are highly respected. Time is not very important. Quality of the interaction is important.	May nod affirmatively but not necessarily agree. Loving and affectionate; interpersonal relations are important. Homemade cooking is an expression of gratitude (*do not refuse*). Elder respect. Rural may not make eye contact out of respect.	Rural and urban differences. Woman is nurturer. Health history must be discussed privately and quietly.	Priests or traditional healers (Espiritistas) use topical herbs, aromatic ointments, or oils. Highly expressionistic.

derstanding a language other than our own, colloquialism, syntax, idioms, and vocabulary are among potential language barriers. For example, the use of a word such as "handicapped" is considered less appropriate in North America than "disabled." Further, we first refer to the person, not the condition: people with disabilities rather than disabled people. In addition, many languages may be spoken within one country—more than 300 dialects are spoken in India, for example, with 16 recognized languages.[56]

4. *Preconceptions and stereotypes.* The expectation that events, observations, or behaviors mean something specific and fit our stereotype causes miscommunication. It has long been contended that stereotypes help one reduce the threat of the unknown by making the world predictable.[57] Such stereotyping may enable the already fearful dental patient to avoid future encounters with dentists because of the preconceived idea that dental professionals are greedy or insensitive. A patient who associates the doctor with discomfort and uncaring behaviors will easily rationalize why she or he should continue to avoid going to the dentist. Thus the stereotype may fulfill the patient's need to avoid dental care.
5. *High anxiety and stress* are often reported in cross-cultural experiences, which are believed to be associated with the presence of uncertainty. Fear of the unknown is a well-known stressor in interpersonal communication.

Pain	Cause of Illness	Home/Folk Remedies	Informed Consent	Concept of Health
"Si Dios quiere" (if God wants) or spiritual forces control life situations and health. Highly outspoken.	Outcome of punishment, sin, or lack of personal attention to health—result of evil forces in the individual.	Often used first. Herbal teas, heat, prayer. Great difference between urban and rural dwellers; urban are more westernized.	Take time—may want verbal approval from other family members. May nod affirmatively but not necessarily mean agreement or understanding of dialogue. Allow time to consider and possibly share with family members, especially elders.	Not being too thin and being clean—llenitos y limpios. "If you are happy, oversized, and have red cheeks, you are healthy." Use of fruit juices.

6. *Tendency to evaluate* augments misperceptions. For example, the mother who comes to her dental appointment late is seen as "irresponsible" based on the health provider's philosophy or value. However, she may prioritize family responsibilities regardless of the scheduled appointment time. In short, the tendency not to appreciate the worldview or family view can lead to counterproductive communication and conflict. When stressed, some of us become frightened, angry, or withdrawn, whereas others transcend and excel. The etiology of human differences is multifactorial—some learned and some innate. Understanding differences and celebrating diversity can only be learned over time and are contingent on our willingness to become aware, become mindful, understand, and communicate effectively.

SOCIOCULTURAL BARRIERS TO CARE

Given that communication facilitates or impedes the effectiveness of a clinical encounter, bridging the gap between clinicians or health educators and patients of different backgrounds, with socioeconomic and cultural differences, is important. An ethnic group is considered a socially and culturally constructed group to which a common set of characteristics (language, customs, physical appearance) is attributed. Within this context, the health provider must walk a tightrope—be sensitive to the characteristics of the ethnic group but not stereotype people. In other words, one must determine the degree to which the individual from one culture has given up the traits of his or her culture of origin and adopted the traits of the dominant culture in which he or she resides. Assessing enabling resources such as socioeconomic status is critical because it may be a stronger influence on health practices and access to care than ethnicity. Income, education, and occupation determine socioeconomic status. Documentation reveals that the cultural distance between doctors and patients affects the quantity and quality of information exchanged.[58,59] Doctors are reported to exchange more information with patients of higher socioeconomic status.[60] Evidence from *Healthy People 2010* articulates that oral health disparities are associated with these sociocultural variables.[7] Because of the greater mobility of North American society, social class has less influence historically on behavior and values here than in other countries. However, social class should be considered, because approximately 40% of the U.S. population now consists of immigrants or first-generation Americans.[61] Many of these individuals emanate from environments where social class has a distinct influence on how people interact in health care encounters. Additionally, disabilities and sexual orientation are sociocultural factors that can affect the health care process whereby patients can be offended even before the instigation of treatment. For example, during intake interviews health providers often assume heterosexuality in the patient when asking the adult about sexual risk behaviors and marital status. These behaviors are potentially inhibiting or alienating to the gay or transgender patient. Physical barriers to care include accessibility issues such as no railings or Braille in the elevators, steep steps, and narrow passageways. Further, specific words that are offensive can inadvertently estrange the individual or family living with disabilities. For example, the term *handicapped clinic* is not only politically incorrect but also offensive. Other behaviors counterproductive to positive, effective health communication include the following: avoiding eye contact with patients having facial differences (e.g., craniofacial anomalies) or those with wheelchairs; spending less time with people who have little education than more highly educated patients or explaining less to those who are of a different ethnicity than the provider; speaking loudly to patients with visual impairment; or infantilizing adults with disabilities.

COMMUNICATION STYLES

One of the most significant differences within and between groups relates to communication styles. *Communication* is defined as "that which happens whenever someone responds to the behaviors or the residue of the behavior of another person."[62] The behavior may be intentional, unintentional, conscious, or unconscious—yet messages are received and understood. Therefore it is important to remember that we are always communicating (exchanging messages), but we may not be communicating what we *want* to communicate. Misunderstandings occur even between friends who have similar values and are known to one another; therefore much attention in cross-cultural interactions is required to transmit the desired message.

Numerous identifiable, relevant facets of the health interaction exist. To begin, the pacing of the verbal exchange during a health interview is significant and should blend with or complement the receiver to increase his or her comfort level during the interview. The appropriate pace can vary across groups. During the initial encounter, discussing the weather, food, and the family may be more appropriate than direct questions. During the encounter, silence may mean that the patient heard or is expressing "no"—although that word is not uttered because it is considered rude.

In many Western dental practices, it may be expected for the clinician or health provider to relate his or her expertise, education, and wealth of experience to the patient. Such a presentation of range of experience or credential sharing can be thought to give the patient and family a sense of security regarding the professional's competence; however, among some cultural groups it is considered arrogant to flaunt one's credentials. Indirect, modest behaviors are expected in high-context cultural groups (e.g., Japanese and Arab) in which the physical context or setting and nonverbal messages are most relevant in the interaction; in low-context cultures (e.g., German and Scandinavian), direct, verbal messages are typically emphasized, expected, and valued.

Personal space differs between people of various groups and can affect the interaction. Feeling too close or too distant may engender a distinct negative effect on the doctor-patient relationship. Latinos or Middle Easterners, who generally prefer a distance of approximately 2 feet during conversation, may perceive the North American health professional as aloof or cold because North Americans generally prefer a distance of approximately 4 to 5 feet during conversation. Observing others within the culture can be enlightening, as well as actually consulting with others who work in the community. Nurses, social workers, or educators can be excellent informational sources regarding the appropriateness of space.

Nonverbal messages are salient but can be difficult to interpret because of diverse meanings across cultures. Smiling during an appointment can be misleading. If the male dentist is speaking with a Vietnamese female patient about her oral health behaviors or attractive smile, she is likely to look away because of modesty. An East Indian woman may perceive the smile of a health professional as inappropriate because the health setting is not a social situation among equals. Thus smiling from the patient or the provider may connote information that is confusing to the culture of the receiver.

Touching is another issue of concern potentially affecting the health encounter. For example, among some Southeast Asians touching the head, a sacred area, may be seen as a violation unless forewarning and an explanation is made. Touching at the initial greeting can vary among groups. In the United States a professional greeting often includes an introduction and handshake. The latter may not always be expected and may actually be offensive or misinterpreted. The strength of the handshake is considered a sign of confidence in the West; however, among people from other regions, a bow or gentle handshake is expected and polite. In Arab cultures, touching patients, especially of the opposite gender, can be considered inappropriate.

Time orientation is another possible source of miscommunication. Punctuality holds importance in most health practices in North America because appointment times typically are scheduled.[63] However, in most Latino groups, the concept of time holds less importance. As previously discussed, personal family activities such as taking care of children is more valued than being punctual for an appointment. Consider the following scenario: when a mother was queried regarding her tardiness, she responded proudly with a smile: "I am a mother." The dental staff believed that she was noncompliant with treatment and did not value dental services. This example does not imply that a dental clinical facility should not have rules for what is "right" or "wrong," but should not presume or attach values to behavior—rather should look, listen, empathize, and communicate if expectations (e.g., adhering to clinical guidelines) are not being met. Thus to bypass negative residue between the patient and clinic staff that can taint subsequent encounters, the need to find common ground is emphasized and reiterated. If family issues arise, it may be helpful to reinforce the office or clinic rules and schedule appointment times early with the knowledge that the patient is typically late and does not hold the same time orientation values as Westerners. Scheduling afternoon appointments when punctuality may be less important to the clinic can be useful. Compromise and adaptation from both sides is critical.

TOWARD CULTURAL COMPETENCE IN THE DENTAL PROFESSIONAL

"What we see as science, the Indians (Native Americans) see as magic. What we see as magic, they see as science. If we can appreciate each other's views, we can see the whole picture more clearly. . . . To heal ourselves or to help others, we need to reconnect magic and science, our right and left brains."[64] As practitioners and public health officials, we need to understand more than the physical symptoms and pathology of disease to help diagnose, prevent disease, and promote health and well-being. Given the mosaic of ethnicities in North America, we are required to be open and sensitive to difference, because we will undoubtedly experience cross-cultural interactions. Despite the fact that the majority of dental school graduates have had little or no formal training in cross-cultural communication, the Institute of Medicine requires the health professional to be culturally competent. Considering the globalization of communications, and increasing waves of immigration to the United States (much of which consists of traditional minority groups), the relevance of addressing issues related to cultural competence in health care is underscored.

Cultural competence is defined as a set of cultural behaviors and attitudes integrated into the practice methods of a system, or its professionals, that enables them to work effectively in cross-cultural situations.[65]

These multicultural behaviors and attitudes are gained through good interpersonal communication skills, knowledge of cultural values and norms, situational factors, and empathic understanding. The culturally competent clinician becomes increasingly sensitive to those issues inherent in health attitudes and behaviors and relearns regularly that there is at least as much diversity within one cultural group as across groups. Socioeconomic status and education, length of time in this country, age, and gender are among the most recognized and important variables contributing to intragroup variability. Manifestations or expressions of the impact of these variables are also diverse. Given the sociocultural differences between dentists and other health providers and patients, understanding of and respect for differences are critical.

Cultural values contribute to decision making, goal setting, and expectations for treatment. Knowledge of cultural values is crucial to understanding those with whom we interact, as is sensitivity to the values that we have accepted from our own cultural group. Several concepts indigenous to successful cross-cultural encounters are worth highlighting. As readily recognized and reiterated throughout this chapter, language and communication patterns can facilitate or impede the health context. If English is not the primary language, or among specific cultural groups, querying individuals about discomfort or pain may be perceived as inappropriate, and more global, vague descriptors may be used. It may be discouraged or viewed as unacceptable to talk about feelings, especially if there is a sense of fatalism associated with a health condition such as bleeding gums or oral cancer. Further, if one asks about quality of life or the concept of well-being, self-expression may be blunted. Such responses have more to do with culture than with perceived symptoms or health status. If there is a language barrier, using translators who are familiar with the culture, as well as with health practices, is essential. In the United States it is more common to find children speaking English than their parents; however, it is inappropriate to use friends or family members, in particular children, as interpreters. Imagine the emotional strain on the child having to deliver bad news, such as a diagnosis of oral cancer. The discussion of risk factors in front of children is a violation of confidentiality and is potentially disruptive to the family system. For example, the middle-aged Latino woman may be reluctant to discuss personal social history items that her adolescent son should interpret. Thus the use of professional interpreters may be ideal. In North America, a telephone service exists in which health translators are available in more than 100 languages. In working with interpreters, the culturally competent clinician or health educator must demonstrate patience. The length of the interview with an interpreter is typically twice the time of that with patients of the same language and background. Explaining the purpose of the meeting to both the patient and interpreter is key. Using short sentences without jargon facilitates understanding. As in most health encounters, having the patient repeat what was heard (e.g., instructions, diagnosis, treatment) helps ensure effective communication. This technique is frequently overlooked in many health encounters and is especially vital in cross-cultural interactions. During the entire session with the interpreter, it is important to observe the patient and not face the interpreter. Observations, including voice intonations and facial expressions, can be highly informative but could be overlooked if the health practitioner is focused on the translator. In short, using a professional interpreter and eliminating a family member or friend in that role respects patient confidentiality and ensures that the patient's needs are being expressed and not confused with those of the patient's significant other (e.g., family member).

Individualism versus collectivism is another potentially important concept requiring consideration in cross-cultural encounters. In the collectivistic orientation, each person is less important than the group and individualism is discouraged. Therefore health decisions often include family members, and excluding an elder or a male figure from the discussion with the patient regarding diagnosis and treatment planning may be viewed as insensitive and unacceptable. In fact, in some cultures, the family or group makes the decision, not the individual. Thus the configuration of effective health communication can be dependent on understanding the role of the family and gender. In the case of an unmarried woman, deference to the parents or older brothers may be indicated among some Middle Eastern families.[66] In North American culture, gender-based stereotypes have led to underdiagnosis and undertreatment of women's cardiovascular symptoms, which were reportedly dismissed by clinicians as minor.[67]

Understanding Nonverbal Gestures

Through our health promotion efforts, many public health providers have experienced frustration in a lack of follow-through by the recipients despite the "agreement" reached. For example, the East Asian man may shake his head in a horizontal direction, which means "no" to the North American but "yes" to the East Asian. Thus what is gestured is agreement, yet according to North American standards is disagreement. Further, in many cultures it is considered disrespectful to disagree with the authority figure. Therefore the Latina may nod seemingly in agreement, when she has no intention of following the prescribed regimen. This misreading is frustrating and underscores the relevance of having a health team comprised of individuals of the same cultural group as the patients or dictates that the health provider must understand the people who are being served and ask the appropriate background questions.

Expectations for Care

Non-Westerners may emphasize the importance of receiving either medication or an injection if there is a problem. Thus the Latino or Chinese patient who arrives for an appointment and has a checkup and radiographs without getting something (e.g., shot, prescription) often feels that the visit was without meaning. Urban African Americans also echo this response. In one study, African-American caregivers of human immunodeficiency virus–positive children who were told that their children needed dental care brought their children in for treatment, and then complained that no treatment was rendered. The expectations were that treatment involved drilling a tooth, not radiographs or treatment planning.[68] Use of alternative or complementary treatments and medical pluralism is increasing in the United States. Acupuncture, therapeutic massage, and meditation are now incorporated into health practices. Herbs are used in conjunction with other Western medicines. It is not uncommon for Latinos or Chinese to use herbal remedies in addition to other health practices. An individual with trigeminal neuralgia explained that after dental care, he must seek relief from an acupuncturist. It is noteworthy that given the thrust of evidence-based care and cost-effectiveness considerations, some health researchers and insurance providers are now supporting complementary treatment regimens. Currently, National Institutes of Health–supported clinical trials using alternative or multiple health interventions to examine treatment outcomes and establish efficacious practice guidelines are underway.[69] In summary, acknowledging peoples' beliefs and health practices is both respectful and imperative in establishing rapport and implementing effective health programs. Such efforts reflect cultural awareness and competence.

The role of religion in health practices can be significant. For example, the use of prayer or other rituals in treatment should be acknowledged, and mutual consensus of accepting a balance of "God's will" in coordination with other interventions should be established between the provider and recipient. Belief in karma and past lives can affect an East Indian patient's readiness to accept and adhere to treatment. Further, if a Moslem patient believes that God's will is dominant, the provider must acknowledge the patient's background and the influence of Allah and prayer.[68] This issue may be critical when expeditious treatment is needed to treat a malignant tumor. Additionally, those who have fatalistic tendencies may be reluctant to undertake immediate treatment or initiate preventive treatment. Using religious or spiritual leaders for advice or guidance and counseling can be both enlightening and imperative when working with patients and their families who are suspicious of or reluctant to accept Western medicine.

TEACHING CROSS-CULTURAL COMMUNICATION SKILLS

Over the past decade, medical school educators have developed curricula in the area of cross-cultural communication that emphasize empathic communication. Factors such as interpersonal communication skills, cultural values and norms, situational factors, and empathic understanding are intrinsic to cultural competence.[70] Empathic communication includes reception to the feelings or experience of the other person, verbal and nonverbal communication of this awareness to the other person, and awareness from the other person that the message is understood. For decades, medical anthropologists have observed that the health or illness belief systems between providers and receivers are often disparate. These differences have been highlighted in the pioneering works of Arthur Kleinman, chair of the Departments of Psychiatry and Medical Anthropology at Harvard Medical School.[71,72] He espouses that the following basic questions facilitate empathic understanding that is from the patient's perspective:

1. What do you call this problem?
2. What do you think caused this problem?
3. Why do you think it started when it did?
4. What do you think this condition does? How does it work?
5. How severe is the condition? What do you think will happen? Will it have a short or long course?
6. What kind of treatment do you think you should receive? What results do you want from treatment?
7. What problems has the condition caused?
8. What do you fear most about the condition?

In developing a teaching framework for culturally competent clinical practice, an adaptation of Kleinman's work called ETHNIC is presented.[73] ETHNIC is an acronym for explanation, treatment, healers, negotiate, intervention, collaborate:

Explanation. Ask the patient to explain his or her condition. (Why do you think you have these symptoms? What do others say or what have you seen or heard or read?)

Treatment. Ask about treatments, medicines, and home remedies. (What kind of treatment do you want?)

Healers. Ask about the use of alternative folk healers or other practitioners.

Negotiate. Negotiate mutually acceptable options that incorporate the patient's beliefs, and ask about expectations.

Intervention. Determine an intervention that is mutually acceptable; this may include healers or cultural practices (e.g., foods eaten/avoided).

Collaborate with the patient, family, healers, staff, and community resources that might influence the acceptance and outcome of care.

Within the context of understanding the patient's life situation, BATHE, a framework for the health interview, is outlined.[74] BATHE is an acronym for background, affect, trouble, handling, empathy:

Background. What is going on in your life? Has anything changed recently?

Affect. How do you feel about your health concern?

Trouble. What about this situation troubles you most? What concerns you?

Handling. How are you coping with or handling this situation?

Empathy. That must be very difficult (or another appropriate term). I can understand that you feel that way.

Cultural Competency

The long-range goal of teaching cross-cultural communication to the health professional is for the clinician to become culturally competent and proficient—that is, understand the patient from his or her point of view and from that group's point of view, be mindful of the factors that influence a health encounter, and understand the varying magnitude of the factors. In general, topics addressed in coursework on cultural competence must address global issues of health and disease, as well as introspection into our own attitudes. Health sensitizers and case reports are used to highlight specific interpersonal behaviors, and to illustrate cultural competence.[75] Trigger tapes may serve to demonstrate positive (desirable) and negative (undesirable) behaviors that are used to underscore relevant topics, as well as modeling. Discussion among students is encouraged using the clinical encounters viewed on the tapes. Use of videotapes, case studies, and role-playing situations, in addition to didactic material related to communication and epidemiology, is helpful. The recent creation of the National Center for Cultural Competence in Washington, D.C., serves as a dissemination center for cross-cultural teaching, health research, and advocacy. The center exemplifies the importance attached to the issue of cultural competence in the health care setting.

FACILITATING CULTURAL COMPETENCE IN THE DENTAL SCHOOL CURRICULUM

One successfully implemented and published teaching model for primary care physicians has been applied to the New Jersey Dental School (NJDS) curriculum for junior students.[76] The LEARN model emphasizes the following behaviors: listen, explain, acknowledge, recommend, and negotiate. It is based on the notion that doctors must effectively communicate to bridge the distance between them and their patients. Further, panel discussions have provided interactive forums to discuss important topics for the study of cultural competence in health care. At NJDS, panel discussions among clinicians of different ethnocultural identities are used for them to share the lessons learned from cross-cultural encounters in oral health care. These discussions allow students to appreciate the power of what the clinician brings to the encounter. Additionally, the students learn about their own cultural values and their potential for bias in working with others who are outside of their cultural group. In essence, dentists serve as role models discussing their experiences with basic "do's and don'ts" in cross-cultural dental health interactions. In another panel forum, people with specific disabilities (e.g., cerebral palsy, blindness) and others are queried about their perceptions and experiences with dental care providers. The testimonials of these individuals highlight the unique characteristics of each individual, as well as the across-group similarities and expectations from the dental professional.

Consonant with the Institute of Medicine's recommendation to use standardized patients, the NJDS program now incorporates a patient instructor program in the curriculum.[77] In the context of its clinical communications program, students interview different patient instructors who are trained to act (portray) specific patient scenarios and then provide instructive feedback to the students.[78] These exercises simulate cross-cultural encounters. The feedback from the patient instructors includes information about extracting the salient content from the "patient" and the student's interpersonal interviewing skills. Issues inherent in the patients' histories include culture-specific health beliefs, treatment expectations, sexual preference, religion, and the role of families and gender in developing appropriate treatment plans. After the sessions, the students have a seminar with the instructor to discuss their learning experience. Students consistently report that this information is enlightening and useful.

Another effective exercise requires students to interview patients, caregivers, or employees (e.g., sheltered workshop) with a target population having a disability (acquired immunodeficiency syndrome, autism) or clinicians (e.g., special care clinic) or individuals from a cultural group other than their own. They tape-record their interview regarding health beliefs, concerns, utilization, health behaviors, and dental/medical history; transcribe the tape; and then reflect on the interview for content, affect, knowledge acquired, and so on. The information and introspection gained from this assignment empowers the students to understand the significance of empathy and to experience the intensity of a cross-cultural interview.

Acknowledging that empathy is easier to achieve when the person with whom we are interacting shares our values, cross-cultural communication in health care sessions underscores that values are relative, not absolute; this reinforces the idea that understanding and accepting others within the framework of the patient's own value system is a prerequisite for effective communication within and across cultural groups. The process from cultural awareness to competency to proficiency is an ongoing professional responsibility. The golden rule of "doing unto others as we would want them to do unto us" applies only if everyone moves to the same music in the same way. Given the mosaic of cultural groups and influences in the United States, it is more mindful to understand and respect that "people walk differently to the rhythm of circumstance." As we learn to accept that culture is dynamic, so too can we learn that attaining cultural proficiency is a lifelong process requiring commitment.

The oral health setting presents a unique opportunity for individuals from different cultures to meet on common ground. Dentists may be among the first health professionals that many young members of ethnic or racial subcultures encounter. This contact within the context of the Western health care system can influence one's oral health attitudes and behaviors. Primary or initial experiences in the dental care setting hold the potential to be interpreted as experiences to be avoided, because of fear of pain or unfamiliar interactions in uncomfortable settings, or ones that are rewarding and worthy of incorporating into one's health behavioral repertoire. To the extent that the oral health care provider or educator has sufficient multicultural knowledge to provide empathic health messages, these encounters may be positively viewed—and thereby are likely to increase dental utilization among the culturally diverse groups in our society.

REVIEW QUESTIONS

1. What demographic characteristics are related to oral health care?
2. What are the primary barriers to oral health care?
3. Identify facilitators to care.
4. What factors account for interpersonal misunderstanding in cross-cultural encounters?
5. What is cultural competence, and why is it important?

REFERENCES

1. US Department of Health and Human Services: *Healthy people 2010: understanding and improving health,* Washington, DC, 2000, US Department of Health and Human Services.
2. US Bureau of the Census: National population estimates. Summary files, Jan 2000. Available at www.census.gov/population/www/estimates/uspop.html.
3. Lavizzo-Mourey R, Mackenzie ER: Cultural competence: essential measurements of quality for managed care organizations, *Ann Intern Med* 124(10):919, 1996.
4. Department of Health and Human Services, US Public Health Service: *Oral health in America: a report of the Surgeon General,* Bethesda, MD, 2000, National Institutes of Health.
5. Bloom B, Gift HC, Jack SS: Dental services and oral health: United States, 1989, *Vital Health Stat* 183:1, 1992.
6. National Center for Health Statistics: *Prevalence of selected chronic conditions: United States, 1990-92. Series 10: data from the National Health Survey no. 194,* Hyattsville, MD, 1997, US Department of Health and Human Services, Centers for Disease Control and Prevention.
7. *Medical Expenditures Panel Survey 1996. Analysis by Center for Cost and Financing Studies,* Rockville, MD, 2000, Agency for Healthcare Research and Quality.
8. National Center for Health Statistics: Design and estimation for the National Health Interview Survey, 1985-94, *Vital Health Stat* 2:110, 1989.
9. Millman M, editor: *Access to health care in America,* Washington, DC, 1993, National Academy Press.
10. Bolden AJ, Henry JL, Allukian M: Implications of access, utilization and need for oral health care by low income groups and minorities on the dental delivery system, *J Dent Educ* 57(12):888, 1993.
11. Bindman AB et al: Preventable hospitalizations and access to health care, *JAMA* 274(4):305, 1995.
12. Billings J et al: Impact of socioeconomic status on hospital use in New York City, *Health Aff (Millwood)* 12(1):162, 1993.
13. Hahn B: Health care utilization: the effect of extending insurance to adults on Medicaid or uninsured, *Med Care* 32(3):227, 1994.
14. Andersen RM: Revisiting the behavioral model and access to medical care: does it matter? *J Health Soc Behav* 36(1):1, 1995.
15. Davidson PL et al: Evaluating the effect of usual source of dental care on access to dental services: comparisons among diverse populations, *Med Care* 56(1):74, 1999.
16. Levanthal H: Theories of compliance and turning necessities into preferences: application to adolescent health action. In Krasnegor NA et al, editors: *Developmental aspects of health compliance behavior,* Hillside, NJ, 1993, Erlbaum.
17. Liptak GS: Enhancing patient compliance in pediatrics, *Pediatr Rev* 17(4):128, 1996.
18. Israel B et al: Review of community-based research: assessing partnership approaches to improve public health, *Annu Rev Public Health* 19:173, 1998.
19. Hatch J et al: Community research: partnership in black communities, *Am J Prev Med* 9:27, 1993.
20. Prochaska JO, DiClemente CC: Stages and processes of self-change of smoking: toward an integrated model of change, *J Consult Clin Psychol* 51:390, 1983.
21. Broder HL, Riesine S, Johnson RL: Role of African American fathers in child-rearing and oral health practices in an inner city environment, Manuscript submitted for publication, 2001.

22. Rosenstock IM, Strecher VJ, Becker MH: Social learning theory and the health belief model, *Health Educ Q* 15:175, 1988.
23. Maiman L, Becker M, Liptak G: Improving pediatrician's compliance enhancing practices, *American Journal of Disorders in Childhood* 142:773, 1988.
24. Becker MH: *The health belief model and personal health behavior,* Thorofare, NJ, 1974, Slack.
25. Smith RA et al: Measuring desire for control of health care processes, *J Pers Soc Psychol* 47(2):415, 1984.
26. Norman P, Conner M: The role of social cognition models in predicting attendance at health checks, *Psychol Health* 8:447, 1993.
27. Kegeles SS, Lund AK: Adolescents' health belief and acceptance of a novel preventive dental activity: a further note, *Soc Sci Med* 19(9):979, 1984.
28. Witte K: Putting the fear back into fear appeals: the extended parallel process model, *Communication Monographs* 59:329, 1992.
29. Maizels J, Maizels A, Sheiham A: Dental disease and health behavior: the development of an interactional model, *Community Dent Health* 8(4):311, 1991.
30. Bandura A: *Social foundations of thought and action: a social cognitive theory,* Englewood Cliffs, NJ, 1986, Prentice Hall.
31. Tedesco LA et al: Self-efficacy and reasoned action: predicting oral health status and behavior at one, three, and six month intervals, *Psychol Health* 8:105, 1993.
32. Tedesco LA et al: Effect of a social cognitive intervention on oral health status, behavior reports, and cognitions, *J Periodontol* 63:467, 1992.
33. Graeff J, Elder J, Booth E: *Communication for health and behaviour change: a developing country perspective,* San Francisco, 1993, Jossey-Bass.
34. Davidson PL et al: Indicators of oral health in diverse ethnic and age groups: findings from the International Collaborative Study of Oral Health Outcomes, *J Med Syst* 20(5):295, 1996.
35. Kiyak HA: Age and culture: influences on oral health behavior, *Int Dent J* 43(1):9, 1993.
36. Broder HL et al: Oral perceptions and adherence with dental treatment referrals among caregivers of children with HIV, *AIDS Educ Prev* 11(6):541, 1999.
37. Broder HL et al: Barriers and facilitators to dental care, Manuscript submitted for publication, 2001.
38. Cohen L, Jago J: Toward the formulation of sociodental indicators, *Int J Health Serv* 6:681, 1976.
39. Slade G: *Measuring oral health and quality of life,* Chapel Hill, NC, 1997, University of North Carolina.
40. Broder HL et al: Development of the child oral health quality of life questionnaire, *J Dent Res* 80:73, 2001 (abstract).
41. Pal DK: Quality of life assessment in children: a review of conceptual and methodological issues in multidimensional health status measure, *J Epidemiol Community Health* 50:391, 1996.
42. Johnson M: Cultural considerations. In B Spiker, editor: *Quality of life and pharmacoeconomics in clinical trials,* Philadelphia, 1996, Lippincott Raven.
43. Hunt S, McEwen J, McKenna S: *Measuring health status,* London, 1986, Croom Helm.
44. Patrick DL, Sittampalam Y, Somerville S: A cross-cultural comparison of health status values, *Am J Public Health* 75(12):1402, 1985.
45. Lipson JG, Dibble SL, Minarik PA, editors: *Culture and nursing care: a pocket guide,* San Francisco, 1996, UCSF Nursing Press.
46. Barker J: Cultural diversity—changing the context of medical practice, *West J Med* 157:248, 1992.
47. Toliver-Weddington G: Cultural considerations in the treatment of craniofacial malformations in African Americans, *Cleft Palate J* 27(3):289, 1990.
48. Meyerson MD: Cultural considerations in the treatment of Latinos with craniofacial malformations, *Cleft Palate J* 27(3):279, 1990.
49. Shaw WC: Folklore surrounding facial deformity and the origins of facial prejudice, *Br J Plast Surg* 34(3):237, 1981.
50. Marsella AJ: Migration, ethnocultural diversity and future worklife: challenges and opportunities, *Scand J Work Environ Health* 4:28, 1997.
51. Sodowsky G, Lai EWM, Plake BS: Moderating effects of sociocultural variables on acculturation attitudes of Hispanics and Asian Americans, *Journal of Counseling and Development* 70:194, 1991.
52. Paniagua FA: *Assessing and treating culturally diverse clients: a practical guide,* Thousand Oaks, CA, 1994, Sage.
53. Suinn RM et al: The Suinn-Lew Asian Self-Identity Acculturation Scale: an initial report, *Education and Psychological Measurement* 47:401, 1987.
54. Burnam MA et al: Acculturation and lifetime prevalence of psychiatric disorders among Mexican Americans in Los Angeles, *J Health Soc Behav* 28(1):89, 1987.
55. Barna LM: Stumbling blocks in intercultural communication. In Samovar LA, Porter RE, editors: *Intercultural communication,* Belmont, CA, 1997, Wadsworth.
56. Rajwani R: South Asians. In Lipson JG, Dibble SL, Minarik PA, editors: *Culture and nursing care,* San Francisco, 1996, UCSF Nursing Press.
57. Becker MH, Maiman LA: Sociobehavioral determinants of compliance with health and medical care, recommendations, *Med Care* 13(1):10, 1975.

58. Cooper-Patrick L et al: Race, gender, and partnership in the patient-physician relationship, *JAMA* 282(6): 583, 1999.
59. Moy E, Bartman BA: Physician race and care of minority and medically indigent patients, *JAMA* 273(19):1515, 1995.
60. McKinlay JB, Potter DA, Feldman HA: Non-medical influences on medical decision-making, *Soc Sci Med* 42(5):769, 1996.
61. Welch M: Required curricula in diversity and cross-cultural medicine: the time is now, *JAMA* 53:121, 1998.
62. Samovar LA, Porter RE, editors: *Intercultural communication,* ed 8, Belmont, CA, 1997, Wadsworth.
63. Zerubavel E: *Patterns of time in hospital life: a sociological perspective,* Chicago, 1979, University of Chicago Press.
64. Hammerschlag CA: *The dancing healers: a doctor's journey of healing with Native Americans,* San Francisco, 1988, Harper.
65. Administration on Aging: Achieving cultural competence: a guidebook for providers of services to older Americans and their families, 2001. Available at www.aoa.gov/minorityaccess/guidbook2001/default.htm.
66. Meleis AI, Hattar-Pollara M: Arab Middle Eastern American women: stereotyped invisible but powerful. In Adams E, editor: *Women of color: a cultural diversity health perspective,* Thousand Oaks, CA, 1994, Sage.
67. Weintraub WS, Kosinski AS, Wenger NK: Is there a bias against performing coronary revascularization in women? *Am J Cardiol* 78(10):1154, 1996.
68. Broder HL et al: Oral health perceptions and adherence with dental treatment referrals among caregivers of children with HIV, *AIDS Educ Prev* 11(6):541, 1999.
69. NIH consensus statement, *Acupuncture* 15(5):1, 1997.
70. Mullavey-O'Byrne C: Empathy in cross-cultural communication. In Cushner K, Brislin RW, editors: *Improving intercultural interactions: modules for cross-cultural training programs,* vol 2, Thousand Oaks, CA, 1997, Sage.
71. Kleinman A, Eisenberg L, Good B: Culture, illness, and care: clinical lessons from anthropologic and cross-cultural research, *Ann Intern Med* 88:251, 1978.
72. Kleinman A: *The illness narratives: suffering, healing, and the human condition,* New York, 1988, Basic Books.
73. Levin S, Like R, Gottlief J: Personal communication. Department of Family Medicine, University of Medicine and Dentistry New Jersey–Robert Wood Johnson Medical School, 1997.
74. Stuart MR, Lieberman JA III: *The 15 minute hour: applied psychotherapy for the primary care physician,* ed 2, Westport, CT, 1993, Praeger.
75. Gropper RC: *Culture and the clinical encounter,* Yarmouth, ME, 1996, Intercultural Press.
76. Berlin EA, Fowkes WC Jr: A teaching framework for cross-cultural health care, *West J Med* 139:934, 1983.
77. Fields MJ, editor: *Dental education at the crossroads: challenges and change,* Washington, DC, 1995, National Academy Press.
78. Broder HL, Feldman CA, Saporito RA: Implementing and evaluating a patient instructor program, *J Dent Educ* 60:755, 1996.

CHAPTER

6

ORAL HEALTH AND THE AGING POPULATION (GERIATRIC ORAL HEALTH)

Rima Bachiman Sehl

The aging phenomenon emerges as the most significant health issue of the twenty-first century. In the coming years, the nation's social and health institutions will continue to be challenged by changing demands for social and health services because of the anticipated growth in the elderly American population. This demographic imperative is expected to have a major impact on the dental profession and the delivery of oral health services to the older adult population, whose oral health needs differ from those of younger adults. The oral and general health status and needs of the older adult reflect a complex interaction of age-related physiologic changes, their psychosocial concomitants, and the various pathologic processes that occur with increasing frequency in aging. This chapter reviews some of the social and economic issues, as well as the biologic and psychologic considerations, that affect the oral health of the elderly. It considers what is currently known about the oral health of older adults and what the profession might expect in the future. Emphasizing the concept of the interdisciplinary team approach to care, the chapter also provides a framework for managing the oral health needs of older adults in various settings.

DEMOGRAPHIC AND SOCIOECONOMIC TRENDS[1-3]

Significant changes in the demographic characteristics of the older population have occurred in the past century. The size of the geriatric population, persons 65 years of age and older, increased dramatically during the twentieth century and is expected to continue to increase at a rapid pace well into the first half of the twenty-first century. The percentage of Americans age 65 and older has more than tripled, from 4% in 1900 to 13% in the year 2000; the number has increased nearly 11 times, from 3 million to 35 million individuals. As Fig. 6-1 demonstrates, the older population will continue to

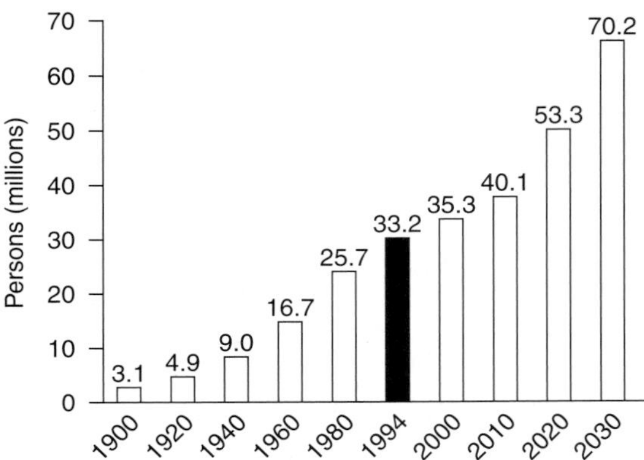

Fig. 6-1. Number of persons age 65 and older (in millions): United States 1900–2030. (Data from U.S. Bureau of the Census.)

grow in the future. The most rapid increase is expected between 2010 and 2030 when the "baby boom" generation, persons born between 1946 and 1964, reaches age 65. By 2030 approximately 70 million older persons will represent 20% of the population.

Another important trend is the change in the racial and ethnic composition of the elderly population. In 2000 approximately 16% of persons age 65 and older were minorities: 8% were non-Hispanic black, 2% were Asian or Pacific Islander, and less than 1% were Native American or Alaskan Native. Persons of Hispanic origin represented 6% of the older population. Minority populations are projected to represent 35% of the elderly population by 2050. Hispanic persons are projected to account for 16% of the older population; 12% of the population is projected to be non-Hispanic black; and 7% of the population is projected to be Asian and Pacific Islander, with the Native American and Alaskan Native populations remaining at less than 1%. Although the older population will increase among all racial and ethnic groups, the Hispanic older population is projected to grow the fastest, from approximately 2 million in 2000 to more than 13 million by 2050. The burgeoning elderly minority population will have major implications for the dental profession. It will necessitate an increased sensitivity to, and a heightened awareness of, the unique cultural issues affecting the planning and provision of oral health care in the various ethnic subgroups.

Of particular interest and concern with respect to the provision of health care and other social services is the increase in the number of very old people. The older population itself is getting older. The population age 85 and older is currently the fastest growing segment of the older population. In 2000 approximately 2% of the population was age 85 and older. By 2050 the percentage in this age group is projected to increase to almost 5% of the U.S. population. The size of this group is especially important for the future of the nation's health care system, because these individuals tend to be in poorer health and require more services than the younger old. Projections by the U.S. Census Bureau suggest that the population age 85 and older could grow from approximately 4 million in 2000 to 19 million by 2050.

Longevity varies considerably with the gender of the person and is greater for American women than men. As the population ages, the distribution by sex also changes. The elderly population is composed of many more women than men. In 2000 women accounted for 58% of the population age 65 and older and 70% of the population age 85 and older. At age 65 there are 122 women for every 100 men. The sex ratio increases with age; at 85 there are 257 women for every 100 men. Of the women over age 65, 47% are widows, and 43% are married. Of the older men, only 10% are widowers, and 77% are married. In 1998 approximately 7% of the older population was divorced, and only a small percentage, less than 5%, had never married. Marital status is a major variable that strongly affects a person's emotional and economic well-being. It influences living arrangements and availability of caregivers among older adults with declining health and function.

Like marital status, the living arrangements of older Americans are important because they are closely linked to income, health status, and the availability of caregivers. Older persons who live alone are more likely to be in poverty than older persons who live with their spouses. In 1998 73% of older men and 41% of older women lived with their spouses, and 17% of older men and 41% of older women lived alone. The majority (68%) of older noninstitutionalized persons live in a family setting, and approximately 30% live alone. Although a small segment (5%) of the over-65 population lives in nursing homes, the percentage increases dramatically with age, ranging from 1% for persons age 65 to 74 years to 5% for persons age 75 to 84 years and 15% for persons age 85 and older.

Social Security is the major source of income for older individuals (40%), followed by income from assets (21%), public and private pensions (19%), earnings (17%), and all other sources (3%). The poverty rate for persons age 65 and older is 11%, approximately the same as the rate for the younger adult population; it is, however, higher for older women and minorities. Although most elderly are retired, approximately 12% are still in the labor force, either working or actively seeking work.

As a group, older adults have significantly less formal education and a higher illiteracy rate than younger adults. Still, the educational level of older Americans has increased in recent years. The percentage of older Americans who had completed high school rose from 28% in 1970 to 67% in 1998. The percentage of older Americans with at least a bachelor's degree also increased to almost 15% during the same period. The percentages are substantially lower for blacks and Hispanics.

If the demographic trends visible in successive cohorts of the elderly persist, the elderly people for whom the dental profession of today will have to care in the future will be significantly different. They will certainly be older, and more of them will be women. There will be more minorities, and most will be better educated.

The increase in the number and proportion of the elderly in the population has been attributed to three basic phenomena: (1) the decline in the birth rate, (2) the aging of the "baby boomers," and (3) the substantial increase in life expectancy during the twentieth century. As Table 6-1 demonstrates, the overall decline in age-specific death rates has led to increases in life expec-

Table 6-1. Life Expectancy at Birth and at 65, 75, and 85 Years of Age, by Gender: United States

	1900			*1997*		
Age	*Both Genders*	*Men*	*Women*	*Both Genders*	*Men*	*Women*
Birth	47.3	46.3	48.3	76.5	73.6	79.4
65	11.9	11.5	12.2	17.7	15.9	19.2
75	7.1	6.8	7.3	11.2	9.9	12.1
85	4.0	3.8	4.1	6.7	6.0	7.0

From *National Vital Statistics Reports*, 47(28):6, 1999.

tancy at birth and also at 65, 75, and 85 years of age. The decline in mortality rate among the very old has been greater than that for any other age group. An important issue for health care professionals is the relationship between changes in the mortality experience of the elderly population and coincident changes in the underlying morbidity and disability experiences. Will future increases in longevity be associated with prolongation of dependency? Or will active life expectancy increase as health promotion and disease prevention strategies for the elderly become increasingly more effective?[4] Currently, an argument can be presented for either view.

AGING, FUNCTION, AND DEPENDENCY

Aging can best be viewed as a biopsychosocial process in which changes occur at various levels in all three components of the biopsychosocial system.[5] From the biologic perspective, gradual declines in the physiologic reserves of most major organ systems begin during the fourth decade.[6] An increasing probability of specific age-related diseases also contributes to the loss of physiologic reserves. Within the psychologic component, age-associated alterations in perceptual and cognitive capabilities also occur.[7,8] From the social perspective, the elderly are faced with different societal attitudes and are confronted by a higher likelihood of losses within their support network because of retirement or the deaths of family and friends.[9] From a clinical standpoint these changes become most significant when they break through the clinical threshold and begin to impair the functional status of the individual.[5] Because of the great variability in functional status among people age 65 and older, addressing the health needs of older adults according to their level of function is more appropriate.

Functioning is a critical indicator of health and well-being in the older person. It is more important than the presence of specific diseases. Impairments in physical and cognitive functioning predict mortality rate and institutionalization among the elderly and the amount of services they receive.

The most common way of assessing functional capacity is evaluating limitation in activities of daily living (ADLs) and instrumental activities of daily living (IADLs), which generally indicate an inability to live independently.[10] ADLs include bathing, dressing, eating, transferring from bed or chair, walking, getting outside, and toileting. IADLs include preparing meals, shopping, managing money, using a telephone, and doing housework. It is apparent that ADL and IADL levels affect the older adult's ability to access and maintain oral health care.

Several scales are used to determine the level of orientation, memory, and cognitive ability.[11] The most commonly used scales are the Short Portable Mental Status Questionnaire (SPMSQ) by Pfeiffer, the Mini-Mental State by Folstein, and the Mental Status Questionnaire by Kahn.[12-14] These brief mental status screening tests can be administered in a dental setting as part of the mental assessment of potentially impaired patients. Poor scores usually indicate an increased probability that a cognitive or dementing disorder is present. Although screening test scores alone do not measure presence of a disorder, they will alert the dental practitioner to request a comprehensive medical evaluation.

The conditions that most frequently cause disability among the elderly are of

Table 6-2. Prevalence of Selected Major Chronic Conditions among Older Adults—United States, 1995

Condition	*% Older Adults*
Arthritis	48.9
Hypertension	40.3
Hearing impairment	33.2
Heart disease	30.8
Visual impairment	18.1
Cancers	17.9
Selected respiratory diseases (chronic bronchitis, asthma, emphysema)	13.8
Diabetes	12.6
Cerebrovascular diseases	7.1

From CDC/National Center for Health Statistics, 1995 National Health Interview Survey.

two kinds: those that are also the leading causes of death, such as heart disease, cancer, and cerebrovascular disease; and chronic conditions that are generally nonfatal, such as dementia, arthritis, orthopedic impairment, visual impairment, and hearing impairment.[15]

Although more than four out of five people age 65 or older have at least one chronic health condition, their disability ranges from minimal problems to total dependence.[10] Table 6-2 lists the prevalence of selected major chronic conditions among older adults. Based on their functional status and level of dependence, older adults have been described as being either independent, frail, or functionally dependent.[16] Independent older adults are those who reside in the community and require no assistance in their necessary ADLs. These individuals make up 80% of the elderly population and are able to access dental care as would younger individuals. The frail elderly have chronic debilitating physical, medical, and emotional problems and are able to maintain some independence in the community only with assistance. Approximately 10% to 15% of the elderly are frail and dependent on various support services. Most of these individuals reside in the community; a small percentage are institutionalized. The functionally dependent are those who are seriously impaired and unable to maintain themselves. Approximately 5% to 10% of the elderly are unable to function independently and are either homebound or institutionalized. Based on the functional status and level of dependence, oral health status, dental needs, utilization of services, and mode of delivery vary from group to group. The present dental care delivery system is least effective in caring for the homebound and institutionalized segment of the elderly population, and they remain the least served.

The elderly can also be characterized according to the historical, cultural, and social events in their lives, as well as their past experiences with the dental care system.[17] Accordingly, the "young old," individuals between 65 and 79 years of age, are better educated, more politically aware, and more demanding of health services. Having somewhat benefited from the availability of fluoride and prevention, they have retained more of their teeth and have been using dental care services at a higher rate than their older cohorts. Characteristically, the "old old," individuals age 80 and older, have experienced dentistry in an era of mass extractions. Consequently the majority of this cohort is edentulous and still believes that losing one's teeth is an inevitable consequence of aging. They are more likely to suffer from medical conditions and to be on medications that affect their oral health. They have grown up with the notion that dentistry is a luxury and therefore tend to be infrequent users of dental services. In addition, the second decade of the twenty-first century will witness the emergence of a yet more vigorous young old cohort—the aging baby boomers of today. Being better educated, having benefited from the availability of fluoride and prevention throughout their entire lives, and having experienced less tooth loss than their parents, they are expected to be more frequent users of oral health care services and more aggressive and demanding of sophisticated care.

USE OF DENTAL SERVICES

Table 6-3 demonstrates the steady increase in the use of dental services by the general population over the past two decades. The percentage of the general adult population reporting use of dental care during the previous year increased from approximately 53.9% in 1983 to 60.8% in 1993.[3,18] Similarly, in 1993 approximately 51.7% of persons 65 years of age and older reported using dental care compared with 39.3% in 1983. However, this proportion is still below the *Healthy People 2000* target of 60%. The mean numbers of visits per person per year for all individuals age 65 years and older have also increased, from 0.8 to 2.1 visits between 1957 and 1989.[19,20] The increase in the utilization of dental services by the older population has not been attributed to changes in the dental delivery system, but is more indicative of changes in the socioeconomic status and dental profile of the younger cohort of older adults.

However, with the possible exception of children under age 6, the elderly, as a group, still have the lowest utilization rate of dental services.[21] Studies also indicate that reported dental care use among minority elders has not increased parallel with elders of all races and ethnic origins.[22] Given the expected future growth in minority elders, attempts should be made by the profession to identify and alleviate barriers to care and to improve access to necessary dental services.

The low utilization of dental services

Table 6-3. Persons (%) with a Dental Visit within the Past Year among Persons 25 Years of Age and Over, according to Selected Age Groups: United States

Characteristic	*1983*	*1989*	*1990*	*1991*	*1993*
Age					
25–34 years	59.0	60.9	65.1	59.1	60.3
35–44 years	60.3	65.9	69.1	64.8	66.9
45–64 years	54.1	59.9	62.8	59.2	62.0
65 years and over	39.3	45.8	49.6	47.2	51.7
65–74 years	43.8	50.0	53.5	51.1	56.3
75+ years	31.8	39.0	43.4	41.3	44.9
Total	53.9	58.9	62.3	58.2	60.8

From Centers for Disease Control and Prevention, National Center for Health Statistics, Division of Health Interview Statistics. Data from the National Health Interview Survey (1995). (Data are based on household interviews of the civilian noninstitutionalized population.)

cannot be explained solely by conventional sociodemographic variables such as age, gender, ethnicity, residence, education, and income. They tend to interact in a complex pattern with other factors, particularly attitudinal factors.[23] Schou[23] divided the factors reported to directly and indirectly influence older persons' utilization of dental services into four main categories: (1) factors related to ill health, (2) sociodemographic factors, (3) service-related factors, and (4) attitudinal or subjective factors. The variables most frequently found within these four categories are listed in Box 6-1.

Studies comparing users and nonusers of dental services often report the dentate status of the elderly as one of the most significant factors related to utilization of dental care.[24-28] The 1985–1986 National Institute for Dental Research (NIDR) survey discovered that among 5000 well elderly, approximately 55% of the dentate elderly had visited a dentist within the past 12 months. Only 13% of the edentate elderly had seen a dentist over the same period. The well dentate elderly used the services of a dentist at approximately the same rate as working adults and the population as a whole.[29] Use of dental services seems to be highly related to presence of teeth. When dentate status is controlled, visit rates are similar between older and younger persons.

Poor general health and functional limitation have been reported as barriers to seeking oral health care by institutionalized and frail homebound elderly.[30,31] Other studies, however, have shown that variables such as functional impairment and the presence of health problems are not as conclusive in predicting or explaining utilization behavior in the elderly; presence or absence of teeth remains the key factor in utilization of dental care.[32,33]

The traditional barrier, cost for services,

BOX 6-1

Factors Influencing Older Persons' Demand for and Utilization of Dental Services

ILL-HEALTH FACTORS

Dental health status
- Edentulousness
- Number of teeth

Experiencing discomfort
General ill health
Mobility, functional limitations

SOCIODEMOGRAPHIC FACTORS

Place of residence
Education
Income
Age
Gender
Cultural
Ethnicity

SERVICE-RELATED FACTORS

Accessibility
- Financial
- Spatiotemporal
- Psychosocial

Dentist behavior
Dentist attitude
Price of service (cost)
Insurance coverage
Satisfaction with service
Transport
Lack of regulations, policies

ATTITUDINAL FACTORS

Personal beliefs
Feeling no need, perceived need
Perceived importance
Fear and anxiety
Resistance to change
Perceived economic strain
Satisfaction with dental visits

From Schou L: Oral health, oral health care, and oral health promotion among older adults: social and behavioral dimensions. In Cohen LK, Gift HC, editors: *Disease prevention—sociodental sciences in action,* Copenhagen, 1995, Munksgaard.

was found by Kiyak[34] to have only a slight influence on the utilization rate of care in the elderly. The same investigator suggested that lack of perceived need is the primary reason for not seeking dental care.[35] This was confirmed in a study by Tennstedt and colleagues,[28] who reported that one fourth of nonrecent dentate users and only 5% of all dentate subjects cited treatment cost or lack of dental insurance as a problem. Although these elders, consistent with other findings, cited a lack of need as the most frequent reason for nonuse of dental care, clinical examinations provided objective evidence of the need for treatment in the dentate subjects. These investigators concluded that lack of importance attributed to oral health and perceived need for oral health care are significant barriers to utilization. This finding underscores the importance of oral health promotion and education in the older adult population.

Because perception of treatment needs affects utilization of services, the discrepancy between actual and perceived need for treatment is a major concern. Treatment needs are generally described in terms of professionally established clinical criteria. The elderly, however, have different standards in evaluating their oral health status and tend to have different expectations for the outcomes of therapy. Because oral health status is influenced by clinical, socioeconomic, and behavioral factors, need assessment cannot be based solely on clinical measures. To improve assessment of needs in older persons, a better understanding of the role of social and behavioral factors is needed.[23]

The use of dental services by the elderly is also partly determined by the education and attitudes of dental professionals. Surveys of dental professionals indicate that many have little or no training in geriatrics and most accept popularly held aging myths.[36,37] Surveys on dental education reveal continuing efforts at both the predoctoral and postdoctoral levels to remedy this situation. The lack of geriatric sophistication by dental professionals often results in dental offices that are poorly located or poorly designed for the purpose of accommodating the needs of the elderly. Adequate nearby parking is often missing. Ramps to assist those who are physically disabled or hallways of sufficient width for the passage of wheelchairs may not be provided.[38,39] Many professionals believe that the elderly or the chronically ill cause discomfort for other patients. Treatment of the elderly is perceived as being more difficult and more time-consuming than treatment of other groups. The enactment of the Americans with Disabilities Act is expected to lessen some of these barriers to care encountered by the functionally disabled elderly.[40] The law requires that private dental offices serve persons with disabilities and that dentists make reasonable modifications to facilitate access to dental offices.

The utilization of dental services by older adults is closely related to oral health status. The decision to access the dentist appears to be based on a variety of sociodemographic and perception-of-need variables. The most regularly cited factors associated with dental utilization include age, income, education, ethnicity, the presence of one or more teeth, and a perceived need for dental care.

DENTAL DISEASE AND ORAL HEALTH STATUS

The pattern of dental disease in the older population has changed over the past 40 years. However, the epidemiologic literature describing the oral health status of older Americans is limited, especially regarding the oldest old (age 85 and older). Although older adults were sampled in national surveys such as the 1960–1962 National Health Examination Survey (NHES) and the 1971–1974 National Health and Nutrition Examination Survey (NHANES), individuals over age 79 were not included in NHES, and NHANES III was the first NHANES to include persons age 75 years and older.[41-43] The 1985–1986 NIDR survey included a sample of adults between 65 and 99 years of age who attended senior centers, but the sample was not representative of the entire older adult population.[29] Regional studies among rural elderly Iowans, elderly in North Carolina, and the New England Elders Dental Study have contributed to knowledge of the epidemiology of dental disease in the elderly and further documented the change in oral disease pattern.[44-48]

Tooth Loss

Despite the general decline in edentulism over the last four decades, 10.5% in the total adult population, the prevalence of edentulism is still high in the older population.[43] Approximately 30% of noninstitutionalized persons age 65 and older are edentulous.[3] Table 6-4 demonstrates the consistent decline in edentulism in this age group; however, rates of total tooth loss still exceed the *Healthy People 2000* target that no more than 20% of the population age 65 and older will be edentulous. Edentulism tends to increase with age and is associated with low income, less education, and minority group status. A substantial decline in edentulism is projected by 2024 for the age 65 to 74 cohort, which is the age 15 to 24 cohort in the 1974 survey, a group that has benefited from preventive activities and advances in dental treatment.[49]

Although the elderly continue to share a disproportionate burden of the problems associated with tooth loss, substantial evidence exists that older adults are maintaining a greater number of teeth into later years. Among dentate older adults, the 1960–1962 NHES survey reported a mean number of 10.6 teeth present for the age 65 to 74 cohort; the NHANES III number was almost 19 for the same age cohort.[41,43] For the age 75 and older cohort, the mean number of teeth retained was 7.1 in 1960–1962 and 16 in the 1988–1991 survey.[41,43]

Dental Caries

The prevalence of coronal caries is decreasing in children and young adults. However, it is difficult to draw conclusions about the prevalence of coronal caries in older adults. Although the mean number of decayed and filled teeth among the age 65 to 74 cohort increased between 1960–1962 and 1985–1986, as shown in Table 6-5, the increase is probably the result of greater retention of

Table 6-4. Percent of Edentulous Older Adults in the United States by Age and Year of Survey

Age (yr)	*NHES[41] 1960–1962*	*NHANES[42] 1971–1974*	*NIDR[29] 1985–1986*	*NHANES III[43] 1988–1991*
65–74	49	46	37	28
75+	61	NA	47	44

NA, data not available.

Table 6-5. Mean Number of Decayed and Filled Teeth among Dentate Adults in the United States by Age, Sex, and Year of Survey

	NHES[41] 1960–1962		NHANES[42] 1971–1974		NIDR[29] 1985–1986	
Age (yr)	Men	Women	Men	Women	Men	Women
45–54	7.1	8.1	9.3	9.4	11.0	11.4
55–64	5.7	7.1	8.3	8.9	9.7	10.6
65–74	4.3	6.0	6.2	7.7	7.4	8.4
75–79	2.7	5.0	NA	NA	6.4	7.6
80+	NA	NA	NA	NA	6.0	6.5

NA, data not available.

teeth within this cohort and may not represent a true increase.[29,41]

In addition to continued coronal caries activity in adults, root surface caries, in their primary and secondary forms, account for a significant amount of dental decay experienced by the elderly.[50] The 1985–1986 survey found that the average percentage of adults ages 18 to 64 with at least one decayed or filled root surface was 21.2%.[29] Among seniors age 65 and older, the average percentage of individuals with at least one decayed or filled root surface was 62.6%. The NHANES III–phase 1 survey demonstrates that the prevalence of root caries and the number of decayed and filled root surfaces are strongly age dependent.[51] Gender differences suggest that men have more treated or untreated root caries than women.[52] In 1988–1994 nearly one third of persons age 65 and older with natural teeth had untreated dental caries in the crown or root of their teeth. A higher percentage of older men (35%) than older women (27%) had at least one untreated dental caries.[3]

Large studies of the incidence of new coronal and root caries have not been performed. Among a sample of 451 dentate Iowans over age 65, a mean of 0.87 new surfaces of coronal decay per person per year and a mean of 0.57 new surfaces of root decay per person per year were noted.[44] Coronal and root caries therefore were still active in this group. Beck[53] estimated that the annual incidence of root caries among older Americans is approximately 1.6 surfaces per 100 surfaces at risk. Tooth survival results in continued exposure to environmental factors and therefore continued risk of disease. Root caries is found only where loss of periodontal attachment has led to exposure of the roots to the oral environment.

Periodontal Disease

The preponderance of current evidence indicates that periodontal disease is age associated, rather than being a consequence of aging. The greater prevalence and greater severity of the disease seen in older people in cross-sectional surveys do not reflect greater susceptibility, but rather the cumulative progression of lesions over time.[54-58] In the NIDR survey 7.6% of employed adults had at least one site with 6 mm or greater loss of periodontal attachment (LPA), compared with 34% of the population age 65 and older.[29] The NIDR data show that with increasing age, there is a gradual decrease in the proportion of sites with 2 to 3 mm LPA and a gradual increase in the proportion of moderately affected sites (4 to 6 mm LPA). The extent of severe disease (6 mm or greater LPA), however, remains relatively low even in the oldest groups. Analysis of the data from NHANES III supports the conclusions reached in other studies that severe periodontal destruction, loss of attachment (LA) of 5 mm or greater, increased steadily in older ages, affecting more than one third of persons in the age 55 to 64 cohort and 40% of those age 65 or older. The extent of LA greater than or equal to 5 mm was not large in any age group. Even among the oldest age group, less than 10% of the sites had LA greater than or equal to 5 mm.[57] In a review of the literature on the epidemiology of periodontal disease among older adults, the authors concluded that although moderate levels of attachment loss are to be found in a high percentage of middle-aged and elderly persons, severe loss is confined to a minority, is evident in only a few sites, and affects only a small proportion of sites examined.[58]

Few longitudinal data exist that describe the progression of periodontal disease with age. Data from a study of a group of tea workers in Sri Lanka who received virtually no dental treatment for 15 years showed that the condition worsened with age for the most susceptible individuals, but among the nonsusceptible, age did not seem to be a factor.[59]

Analysis of the data from the New England Elders Dental Study indicated that of the examined variables, gender, number of dentate arches, and socioeconomic status emerged as the important predictors of periodontal destruction in older adults. Age was not significantly associated with periodontal destruction in this elder population. The investigators further stated that what previously was thought of as an age effect may be due to cohort differences. The great increase in number of teeth in the elderly is the primary difference among cohorts of older persons. With greater tooth retention comes a higher risk of moderate periodontal disease. Longitudinal studies must be conducted to best document this relationship.[60]

ORAL CANCER

Cancers of the oral cavity and pharynx account for 2% to 4% of all cancers diagnosed in the United States. Oral pharyngeal cancer remains the sixth most common type among U.S. white males and the fourth most common among African-American males. Approximately 30,000 new cases and more than 8000 deaths occur annually.[61] Oral cancer, like most cancers, is a disease related to older age. Approximately 95% of all oral cancers occur in persons over 40 years of age, and the average age at the time of diagnosis is approximately 60. Approximately one half of all oral and pharyngeal cancers and the majority of deaths related to oral and pharyngeal cancers occur in people 65 years of age or older.[62] Oral cancer occurs more frequently in males, but the male-female ratio, which in 1950 was approximately 6:1, is now approximately 2:1 and declining. The increase in smoking among women and the greater number of women in the 65-and-older age group are offered as explanations for the reduced ratio.[63] The highest incidence rate is reported for African-American males.[61]

The tongue is the most common site for oral cancer in both men and women. Approximately 85% of all oral cancers occur in the tongue, oropharynx, floor of the mouth, and lips; 8% occur in the gingiva; 3% occur in the buccal mucosa; and less than 2% occur in the hard palate. The remainder occurs in unspecified areas in the mouth.[63]

Tobacco smoking, particularly when combined with heavy alcohol consumption, has been identified as the primary risk factor for developing oral and pharyngeal cancers in the United States. Other risk factors include lifestyle and environmental factors such as a diet lacking in fruits and vegetables and exposure to sunlight without the protection of lip sunscreen or hats.

Despite advances in treatment of cancerous lesions, 5-year survival rates remain poor. Therefore improvement in prevention and control of oral cancer is of critical importance. Both public and professional awareness of the disease is fundamental for minimizing the time from onset of appearance of signs or symptoms to diagnosis. Oral health care providers have a professional obligation to assess their patients' risk factors for oral cancer and to provide tobacco cessation counseling. Because most oral cancers are amenable to early treatment and the mouth is readily accessible, regular oral cancer examinations are imperative for early diagnosis, especially for individuals in their forties and fifties and those who are at high risk.[62]

MANAGEMENT OF THE OLDER ADULT PATIENT

The elderly differ from other age groups in important respects, and these differences demand a multidisciplinary approach by the dental practitioner that is geared to the special needs of the individual patient. The proper management of the older adult patient depends on an understanding of the aging process, the diseases from which the elderly suffer, the treatment and sequelae of these diseases, and the elderly themselves.

THE AGING PROCESS

The process of aging is a multifactorial one in which tissues, organs, and cells age at different rates, with much individual variation. The major results of the aging process are (1) a reduced physiologic reserve of many bodily functions (e.g., cardiac, respiratory, and renal); (2) an impaired homeostatic mechanism by which bodily activities are kept adjusted (e.g., fluid balance, temperature control, and blood pressure control); and (3) an impaired immunologic system and a related increased incidence of neoplastic and age-related autoimmune conditions.[64] The reduction in physiologic reserve and the impairment of the homeostatic and immunologic systems contribute to the increased vulnerability of the elderly to disease during acute illness, trauma as a result of burns, major surgery, and administration of medications. Visits to the dentist or dental hygienist, of course, are potential sessions of increased stress, and the practitioner must modify the management of the patient accordingly.

Many common geriatric diseases, disorders, and impairments, and their management, necessitate alterations in the provision of dental treatment. It is beyond the scope of this chapter to review all geriatric medical conditions, their treatment and sequelae, and their influence on dental treatment. Instead, an attempt is made to provide key principles and a general framework for the management of the older patient.

PATIENT ASSESSMENT

Assessment is the key to developing a comprehensive, appropriate treatment plan. The assessment is a comprehensive multidisciplinary evaluation in which several domains of the elderly patient—physical, mental, social, economic, and functional—are reviewed and integrated into a coordinated plan of care.

The general goals of the assessment are to (1) determine the patient's current general and oral health status and diagnosis; (2) establish a database against which future developments and changes can be compared; (3) establish a good relationship with the patient and the patient's family and caregivers; and (4) determine the priorities for management and intervention in order to prevent or alleviate disease and improve the quality of the patient's life.

The practitioner performing the assessment needs to adopt the following two principles:

1. *Oral health is an integral part of total health,* and therefore oral health care is an integral part of comprehensive care. Oral health is linked to the overall health of the older patient because oral diseases and conditions have consequences that extend beyond the confines of the oral cavity.
2. The *interdisciplinary team approach to care* is the safest and most effective way of providing appropriate dental care to older adult patients. Communication among the patient's multidisciplinary care providers is key to the development of an appropriate treatment plan and the proper coordination of care. In addition, regular communication among providers tends to educate and sensitize nondental providers to the dental aspects of the patient's overall health care and treatment needs, thus optimizing treatment outcomes.

The following elements are incorporated into the assessment process: (1) review of the patient's biopsychosocial systems, (2) determination of the patient's functional status or capacity (both physical and mental), and (3) assessment of the patient's oral health status.

Cognitive Functioning

Because of the multiplicity and complexity of factors that relate to the treatment of the elderly, it is important to evaluate the ability of the patient to communicate and to understand, consent to, and participate in the treatment. The practitioner must determine, either through a psychologic evaluation or through an interview, the capacity of the individual to respond to treatment. Although instances of dementia are not common, they do increase in frequency as the individual ages. Prevalence starts at approximately 1% at age 60 and then doubles approximately every 5 years, reaching approximately 40% at age 85.[65] Data from the National Nursing Home Survey suggest that among inhabitants of nursing homes approximately 47% have some sort of dementing disorder.[66]

The most common type of dementia in the elderly is Alzheimer's disease.[67] It accounts for 50% of all cases of dementia.[65] This disease is characterized by a gradual deterioration of almost every function of the brain. The patient progresses through a series of behavioral changes and losses. Cognitive skills and competency in the life skills decline. Loss of intellectual prowess occurs, and the patient experiences language difficulties, memory loss, concentration difficulties, aberrant emotionality, and altered spatial-motor performance. Verbal and nonverbal communication is affected.[68]

The other types of dementia in the elderly—diffuse Lewy body dementia, frontotemporal dementia, and vascular dementia—account for 15%, 15%, and 10%, respectively, of all cases.[65]

Treatment Planning

Treatment planning decisions for older patients are more complex. The dental practitioner has to take into consideration the normal and pathologic aging changes and their great individual variability, the impact of the presence and interaction of multiple disorders, medications, and psychosocial issues, and the effects of years of accumulated oral changes. The appropriate level and type of dental care the older patient receives is based on the individual's capacity to understand, withstand, and maintain the care planned. For the dentist to provide the most appropriate and effective care with successful outcomes, the treatment plan must be based on the patient's functional capacity and must have maintenance or enhancement of function and quality of life as its primary goal. Given future functional decline and uncertainties in some outcomes of the older person's life, the treatment plan should also have great flexibility and great emphasis on prevention.

Prevention and Oral Health Promotion

Prevention of oral disease, through frequent recalls, regular updating of vital information, and ongoing assessment of the patient's functional status, is the cornerstone of geriatric care. In addition to promoting and monitoring the basic oral hygiene practices (brushing with a fluoride dentifrice, flossing, and maintaining a nutritious well-balanced diet, low in refined carbohydrates), the clinician should be vigilant of the changing physical, psychologic, socioeconomic, and medication status of the older patient and be ready to intervene and make the necessary modifications in the prevention protocol. The most effective strategy for prevention of caries has been increasing tooth resistance through the use of systemic and topical fluorides. Systemic and topical fluoride application has been deemed by many researchers to be the single most important preventive and treatment modality older adults can employ to prevent dental caries.[69] The concentration and the method and frequency of application depend on the level of risk and the ability of the individual to manage the regimen.

Older adults and their caregivers need to be educated to enhance their knowledge and modify their attitudes regarding prevention, regular professional care, use of appropriate oral hygiene devices and chemotherapeutic agents, and the important relationship of oral health to general health. In addition, dental health professionals, as part of the health care team, have a responsibility to evaluate the health status and health risks of their older patients and make the proper referrals.

ORAL HEALTH IN LONG-TERM CARE SETTINGS

Long-term care refers to health, social, and residential services provided to chronically disabled persons over an extended period of time.[70] These services may be provided in a variety of settings, including nursing homes, chronic disease hospitals, mental health facilities, rehabilitation centers, residential facilities, and the individual's own home. With the projected growth of the older population, particularly the 85 and older cohort, the demand for long-term care is expected to increase in the future. In 1990 approximately 7 million older people needed long-term care. By 2005 the number will increase to almost 9 million. By 2020 approximately 12 million older people will need long-term care at home, in the community, or in a nursing home.[71]

The provision of dental care to the nursing home and the homebound elderly presents a special challenge to the oral health care delivery system, in which the mode of care usually requires that the patient travel to the dentist's private office. The nursing home and homebound elderly are characterized as being frail or functionally dependent because of at least one chronic longstanding physical, mental, or emotional disability. Therefore they have dental treatment needs somewhat different from those of the functionally independent cohort. As a group, they experience many barriers to dental care and are currently underserved.

Cognitive decline, lack of motivation, physical impairment, and other chronic medical problems all contribute to a decrease in self-care ability and subsequent increased risk of oral diseases. In addition, difficulties with transportation to the dentist, accessing the dental office, lack of perceived need, preexisting attitudes and expectations, and financing the care are some of the barriers to accessing dental services in this population.

The homebound and nursing home elderly have been characterized as having high rates of edentulism, coronal and root caries, poor oral hygiene, gingivitis and periodontal disease, and soft tissue lesions.[72,73] Table 6-6 depicts the type and prevalence of oral conditions in a sample of dentate nursing home residents.

Poor oral hygiene has been identified as the most significant problem among nursing home residents.[74-77] This is not surprising given the functional impairment affecting most nursing home residents. It does, however, underscore the importance of the regular involvement of caregivers in the residents' oral hygiene maintenance and the need for in-service training of the nursing staff.

Homebound and nursing home elderly also have other characteristics in common that affect the delivery of dental services. As a group, they are older (mean age 80), predominantly female (approximately two thirds), and physically disabled with respect to basic ADLs (more than 90%). Approximately 63% have some disorientation or memory impairment, and 47% have been diagnosed with dementia.[78] Although it is important to recognize the general characteristics shared by nursing home residents, the dentist, as a member of the professional team, needs to be cognizant of the individual needs of each resident. Decisions regarding treatment planning, level of care, and modality of care are usually based on the condition of the resident, other treatment

Table 6-6. Number and Percentage of Nursing Home Residents with Natural Teeth Who Have Oral Problems

Rank Order of Problems	*n = 445*	*%*
1. Poor oral hygiene	321	72.1
2. Sore or bleeding gums	191	42.9
3. Root caries	160	36.0
4. Coronal caries	117	26.3
5. Retained root tips	105	23.6
6. Significant tooth mobility	80	18.0
7. Dry mouth	44	9.0
8. Toothache	34	7.6
9. Intraoral swelling or suppuration	27	6.1
10. Soft tissue lesions	20	4.5

From Kiyak AH, Grayston MN, Crinean CL: Oral health problems and needs of nursing home residents, *Community Dent Oral Epidemiol* 21:49, 1993.

goals, and the anticipated length of stay in the facility.[78]

Delivering dental care to the homebound population presents a different practice environment, and a different set of challenges, than the nursing home setting. The type and the range of dental services provided are limited by the type of equipment and delivery system used. It is important to remember that a dentist in a homebound setting has no backup support available. Complicated and invasive procedures are therefore not appropriate in a homebound setting.[78] This mode of dental service delivery is still in its infancy with respect to regulations and funding mechanisms.

Federal Nursing Home Regulations

As a result of the nursing home reform law of the Omnibus Budget and Reconciliation Act (OBRA) of 1987, all nursing homes that accept Medicaid and Medicare payments are held to providing a new, higher standard of care focusing on the residents' "highest practicable physical, mental and psychosocial well-being."[79] The new law imposed some additional dental care requirements on nursing facilities. In addition to the annual comprehensive assessment, which must include the resident's present dental condition, the final regulation requires that facilities (1) assist residents in obtaining routine and 24-hour emergency dental care; (2) provide or obtain from an outside resource routine and emergency dental services to meet the needs of each resident; (3) may charge a Medicare resident (but not a Medicaid resident) an additional amount for routine and emergency dental services; (4) provide to Medicaid residents emergency dental services and routine dental services (to the extent covered under the state plan); (5) assist the resident in making appointments and by arranging for transportation to and from the dentist's office; and (6) promptly refer residents with lost or damaged dentures to a dentist. Also, a nursing home must ensure that a resident who is unable to carry out activities of daily living receives the necessary services to maintain good nutrition, grooming, and personal and oral hygiene.[79] Analysis of data from the 1995 National Nursing Home Survey suggests that the requirements of the federal law are being met by most facilities. Nursing homes probably provide initial examinations and some oral health services. However, dental professional services are available on an infrequent basis, and there is little evidence for the provision of routine or systematic follow-up services.[80]

Dental Delivery Systems

Four types of dental care delivery systems are available for the homebound and institutionalized elderly.[81]

THE PRIVATE DENTAL OFFICE

The private dental office that has been appropriately designed to receive frail and functionally dependent older adults is the ideal delivery system for those elderly individuals who can be easily transported. This is the most ideal and cost-effective modality for the dentist because no travel or setup and breakdown time is involved. It also allows the dentist to treat the patient in the comfort of an equipped office, with the help of auxiliary personnel. This type of delivery system is, however, expensive and time-consuming for the nursing home, which often must have a staff member accompany the resident. Nursing facilities therefore do not favor such an arrangement.

ON-SITE DENTAL PROGRAMS

On-site dental facilities are appropriate options in large nursing homes where the economy of scale renders them cost effective. They are less disruptive to the functioning of the facility. The disadvantage of on-site facilities is that they cannot be moved to treat bedridden residents. They must be supplemented with a portable dental unit.

PORTABLE DENTAL PROGRAMS

These are self-contained dental units and instrument kits that can be transported by the provider into the facility or the person's home. This type of delivery system is ideal for homebound and bedridden individuals. The current oral health system, however, lacks an effective reimbursement mechanism for this type of delivery system to be attractive to practitioners. It is usually available, in a limited fashion, only to those elderly who can afford it.

MOBILE VAN PROGRAMS

These are vans that are modified to accommodate built-in dental equipment, supplies, a dental team, and patients. A mobile dental office has all the advantages of the private office, in addition to the ability to visit nursing facilities and private homes. Transporting patients to the vehicle may still be a problem, however, especially those who are bedridden.

The American Dental Association (ADA) encourages the appropriate use of portable dental equipment and mobile setups, and dentists have been providing dental services to homebound or institutionalized patients for several years.[82] However, the majority of dentists, like other health professionals, are not attracted to working in institutions such as nursing homes. The apparent reluctance of dentists to treat elderly patients outside the conventional practice has been attributed primarily to low reimbursement levels, inadequate treatment facilities in the nursing home, and inadequate training in gerontology and geriatric dentistry.[83]

FINANCING GERIATRIC ORAL HEALTH

Financing of oral health services for the older population differs from financing in younger groups and from financing for general health services. Dental care, unlike medical care, is heavily financed through the private sector. In 1990 out-of-pocket spending and insurance plans' share combined accounted for approximately 97% of the total dental care expenditure for the elderly and the general population alike; government programs paid less than 3%.[83,84] In contrast, government programs covered 63% of the health expenditures for older persons, compared with only 26% for the population under 65.[1]

Out-of-pocket payment remains the dominant method of paying for dental services. However, the proportion of persons insured for dental services has increased dramatically since the mid-1960s. Currently, approximately 45% of Americans have some form of dental insurance.[85] Unfortunately, few of these programs offer prepaid coverage after the insured reaches retirement age. A descending rate of dental insurance coverage by age has been reported among the elderly, that is, 36% in the age 60 to 64 cohort and only 7% in the 80 and older age cohort are covered by dental insurance.[86] The 1985–1986 NIDR survey found that approximately 52% of all employed adults age 60 or older had dental care coverage, but only 34.5% of nonemployed seniors had similar coverage.[29] The differential in coverage between employed adults and the elderly has occurred as the elderly have retired and left the workforce.

As a group, older adults account for only 10% of the national dental expenditures.[87] However, when they used dental services, the average amount expended was found to be higher than that expended for all age groups. In 1987 an average of $311 was expended by those older adults making one or more visits, compared with $295 of mean annual dental expenditure for all ages. The elderly, however, had the lowest proportion of dental expenses reimbursed by private dental insurance (10% compared with 35% for all ages) and the highest percentage of out-of-pocket dental expenses (79% compared with 56% for all ages).[88] A 1990 survey showed that 44% of persons age 66 and older used dental services, and, among users, 88% of the average total expenditure of $378 was paid out-of-pocket.[84]

Public programs are not a major source of payment for dental services. In 1987 only 3% of the elderly dental expenditures were paid by Medicaid and Medicare.[87]

Medicaid, or Title 19 of the Social Security Act, enacted in 1965, provides federal funds to be distributed among the state public assistance programs. The intent of the program is to provide health benefits to indigent and medically indigent persons. Some services are required under the program; dentistry is not. Medicaid is a joint federal-state program in which the states are allowed to determine eligibility requirements and coverage. In states where dentistry is included, it is usually underfunded and limited in benefits, especially for adults. In addition, Medicaid expenditures for dental care as a percentage of total Medicaid expenditures has been declining steadily since 1977.[89] Except for programs that serve the elderly of a specific group, such as the Dental Services Branch of the Indian Health Service and the Department of Veterans Affairs, Medicaid remains the only source of public financing of dental care for the indigent elderly.

Medicare, or Title 18 of the Social Security Act, also enacted in 1965, is a program intended to provide health insurance for those over age 65. The program pays for hospital and physician services. Dental services, unless provided under special circumstances, are not included. Medicare does not pay for dental services except for limited, medically necessary oral health care. *Medically necessary oral health care* is defined as oral and maxillofacial care that is a direct result of, or has a direct impact on, an underlying medical condition or its resulting therapy. Presently, Medicare guidelines allow for reimbursing hospitals for surgical cases related to oral and pharyngeal cancers and jaw fractures and the fabrication of maxillofacial prostheses.

Until 1977 the ADA had opposed inclusion of dental benefits under Medicare, fearing a fixed-fee schedule and government control of the profession.[90] The ADA's stance today is supportive of the inclusion of more comprehensive dental benefits within Medicare, but only with the proviso that it includes a fee-for-service payment mechanism to dentists, that dentists in private practice have the choice to participate, and that the patients have the freedom to choose their provider.[91]

There have been few successful initiatives to expand dental coverage for the elderly through Medicare and private insurance. The only effective oral health care benefit plan for the older adult population is one that is part of a comprehensive benefits package developed with the understanding that oral health is an integral part of general health and that the two cannot be separated. An infection in the mouth must be considered in the same manner as an infection in any other part of the body.

The unlikely expansion of dental coverage under current health care reform initiatives, coupled with the potential loss of insurance benefits by retirees, may lead to a decrease in the number of elderly persons in the future that will have dental insurance. Thus expenditures for dental services are likely to remain a large source of out-of-pocket expenditures for elderly persons.

GERIATRIC TRAINING AND PERSONNEL NEEDS

Currently, the majority of dental care for the older adult population is provided in the community by general practitioners. According to the ADA, approximately 20% of dentists also provide some care in long-term care settings. With the projected increases in tooth retention and utilization rate, demand for a wider range of dental services by older individuals is also anticipated.

Although the majority of older individuals are relatively healthy and have oral needs similar to those of the rest of the adult population, many experience complex conditions and problems requiring intensive and sophisticated care. These individuals may be living at home or in long-term care facilities. The two cohorts of elderly require different types of dental services, delivered by appropriately trained practitioners.

In 1987 the Department of Health and Human Services recognized the need for three levels of professional training in geriatric dentistry.[92] Because the dental profession will be serving an increasing number and proportion of older patients, all dentists, dental hygienists, and dental assistants should receive basic training in gerontology and geriatric dentistry. To prepare dentists capable of serving functionally dependent older individuals, advanced postdoctoral training (e.g., residency programs with a dental geriatric emphasis) will be required. A small cadre of dental professionals, responsible for educational and research activities as well as specialized consultation, will also be needed. To develop competencies for this leadership group, formal programs of at least 2 years' duration in the form of fellowships or Ph.D. degrees are necessary.[92]

Projections by the American Dental Education Association and the American Society for Geriatric Dentistry indicate a need for approximately 7500 dental practitioners with advanced training in geriatric dentistry as of 2000 and 10,000 practitioners by 2020. It is estimated that the leadership cadre may be approximately 20% of the group with advanced education in geriatric dentistry. They may number approximately 1500 as of 2000 and 2000 by 2020. The leadership cadre will usually be located at dental schools and teaching hospitals. On the basis of these projections, dentists with such advanced preparation will make up approximately 5% of all practicing dentists.[92]

Recognizing the deficiency in the supply of health care personnel adequately prepared to serve the elderly, in 1988 the federal government awarded funding to 23 medical schools to support 2-year fellowship training and 1-year faculty retraining programs for dentists and physicians who are interested in career preparations and professional advancement in geriatrics.[93] The programs offer interdisciplinary training in clinical care, research, teaching skills, and program administration.

Other learning opportunities in geriatric dentistry have evolved over the last 15 years.[94] Short-term intensive experiences offered by regional geriatric education centers have also emerged. These are federally initiated, university-based programs that offer and coordinate geriatric training for several different professions. Forty-one centers were in existence in 1993, and the majority had dental components. In addition, other continuing education experiences of shorter duration are available, offering mixed clinical and didactic training opportunities. Currently, four such programs exist, in Illinois, Kentucky, Minnesota, and Washington.

Important progress has also been made in recent years in expanding geriatric educational efforts as part of the predoctoral and postdoctoral dental programs. Changes in the curricula were initiated by the Geriatric Dentistry Academic Awards Program between 1980 and 1984. The National Institute on Aging funded this program. The purpose of the awards was to assist the preparation of researchers and leaders in academic dentistry and to help develop and strengthen curricula in geriatrics. With a grant from the Bureau of Health Professions of the Health Resources and Services Administration in 1979, the American Hygienists' Association developed the Geriatric Curriculum for Dental Hygiene Education to expand geriatric training in the dental hygiene programs.

SUMMARY AND FUTURE TRENDS

The aging of the nation's population and the apparent decrease in the prevalence of dental caries in children have shifted attention to the oral health needs of older adults. The oral health care professional of today and tomorrow will undoubtedly be called on to treat an ever-increasing number of older adult patients who differ from older cohorts of the past. The majority of the new cohorts of elderly will have more of their own teeth, visit the dentist more often, and demand more sophisticated care. It is important, however, to recognize that the elderly are not a monolithic group. They are a heterogeneous mix of individuals with various levels of functional, socioeconomic, and oral health status. The challenge for the dental profession will be to develop oral health promotion and disease prevention programs and treatment and financing strategies that will meet the unique needs of individuals in each subgroup, especially those in long-term care settings.

With the shift of population toward an older composition with more chronic diseases and medications, a need will arise for expanded courses in internal medicine, pharmacology, gerontology, and geriatrics in the dental curriculum. In addition, the complex nature of the aging process will demand an increase in the interdisciplinary communication among dental health and allied health personnel to optimize treatment outcomes.

Finally, oral health care should be recognized as a primary health care service that is essential to the general health and well-being of older adults. Supported by the major message in the Surgeon General's Report on Oral Health, it is imperative for oral health care professionals to seize the moment and act as agents to facilitate and ensure this change.[95]

REVIEW QUESTIONS

1. List the major factors that have contributed to the increase in the number of elderly in the population.

2. Describe the biologic, psychologic, and social components of aging, and briefly discuss their impact on the functional capacity and dental management of the older individual.
3. Discuss how the increase in the number of "very old" in a population affects the provision of oral health care.
4. List and briefly discuss barriers to access to oral health care for institutionalized and homebound older individuals.
5. List and briefly describe the dental public health challenges generated by the increase in the number of elderly in the population.

REFERENCES

1. American Association of Retired Persons: *A profile of older Americans,* 1997.
2. Federal Interagency Forum on Aging-Related Statistics: *Older American 2000: key indicators of well-being,* 2000.
3. US Department of Health and Human Services, National Center for Health Statistics: *Health, United States, 1999, health and aging,* DHHS pub no 99-1232, September 1999.
4. National Research Council: *The aging population in the twenty-first century: statistics for health policy,* Washington, DC, 1988, National Academy Press.
5. Becker PM, Cohen HJ: The functional approach to the care of the elderly: a conceptual framework, *J Am Geriatr Soc* 32(12):923, 1984.
6. Rossman I: Bodily changes with aging. In Busse EW, Blazer DG, editors: *Handbook of geriatric psychology,* New York, 1980, Van Nostrand-Reinhold.
7. Marsh GR: Perceptual changes with aging. In Busse EW, Blazer DG, editors: *Handbook of geriatric psychology,* New York, 1980, Van Nostrand-Reinhold.
8. Seigler IC: The psychology of adult development and aging. In Busse EW, Blazer DG, editors: *Handbook of geriatric psychology,* New York, 1980, Van Nostrand-Reinhold.
9. Palmore E: The social factors of aging. In Busse EW, Blazer DG, editors: *Handbook of geriatric psychology,* New York, 1980, Van Nostrand-Reinhold.
10. US Senate Special Committee on Aging: *Aging America: trends and projections,* DHHS pub no (FCoA) 91-28001, Washington, DC, 1991, US Department of Health and Human Services, US Government Printing Office.
11. Medalie JH, Pasem HR, Calkins E: Confusion (delirium). In Calkins E et al, editors: *The practice of geriatrics,* Philadelphia, 1986, WB Saunders.
12. Pfeiffer E: A short portable mental status questionnaire for assessment of organic brain deficit in elderly patients, *J Am Geriatr Soc* 23:433, 1975.
13. Folstein MF, Folstein EE, McHugh PR: Mini-Mental State: a practical method for grading the cognitive state of patients for the clinician, *J Psychiatr Res* 12:189, 1975.
14. Kahn RL et al: Brief objective measures for the determination of mental status in the aged, *Am J Psychiatr* 117:326, 1960.
15. Katz P, Dube D, Calkins E: Aging and disease. In Calkins E et al, editors: *The practice of geriatrics,* Philadelphia, 1986, WB Saunders.
16. Ettinger RL, Beck JD: Geriatric dental curriculum and the needs of the elderly, *Special Care Dent* 4(5):207, 1984.
17. Ettinger RL, Beck JD: The new elderly: what can the dental profession expect? *Special Care Dent* 2(2):62, 1982.
18. National Center for Health Statistics: *Health promotion and disease prevention, United States, 1990,* Hyattsville, MD, 1993, National Center for Health Statistics.
19. National Center for Health Statistics: *Dental care: interval and frequency of visits, United States, July 1957-June 1959,* Public Health Service pub no 584-B14, Washington, DC, 1960, National Center for Health Statistics.
20. Bloom B, Gift HC, Jack SS: *Dental services and oral health, United States, 1989,* DHHS pub no (PHS) 93-1151, Hyattsville, MD, 1992, Centers for Disease Control and Prevention, National Center for Health Statistics.
21. Jack SS: *Use of dental services: United States, 1983. Advance data from vital and health statistics, no. 122,* DHHS pub no (PHS) 86-1250, Washington, DC, 1986, US Government Printing Office, National Center for Health Statistics.
22. Jones JA et al: Gains in dental care use not shared by minority elders, *J Public Health Dent* 54(1):39, 1994.
23. Schou L: Oral health, oral health care, and oral health promotion among older adults: social and behavioral dimensions. In Cohen LK, Gift HC, editors: *Disease prevention and oral health promotion,* Copenhagen, 1995, Munksgaard.
24. Holtzman JM, Berkey AB, Mann J: Predicting utilization of dental services by the aged, *J Public Health Dent* 50(3):164, 1990.
25. Grytten J: How age influences expenditure for dental services in Norway, *Community Dent Oral Epidemiol* 18:225, 1990.

26. Ter Horst G, de Wit CA: Review of behavioral research in dentistry 1987-1992: dental anxiety, dentist-patient relationship, compliance and dental attendance, *Int Dent J* 43(3 suppl):265, 1993.
27. MacEntee MI, Stolar E, Glick N: Influence of age and gender on oral health and related behavior in an independent elderly population, *Community Dent Oral Epidemiol* 21:234, 1993.
28. Tennstedt SL et al: Understanding dental services use by older adults: sociobehavioral factors vs need, *J Public Health Dent* 54(4):211, 1994.
29. NIDR, US Department of Health and Human Services, Public Health Service, National Institutes of Health: *Oral health of United States adults, the national survey of oral health in US employed adults and seniors: 1985-86, national findings,* NIH pub no 87,2868, Washington, DC, 1987, US Government Printing Office.
30. Merelie DL, Heyman B: Dental needs of the elderly in residential care in Newcastle-upon-Tyne and the role of formal carers, *Community Dent Oral Epidemiol* 20: 106, 1992.
31. Jones JA et al: Issues in financing dental care for the elderly, *J Public Health Dent* 50(4):268, 1990.
32. Branch LG, Antczak AA, Stason WB: Toward understanding the use of dental services by the elderly, *Spec Care Dent* 6(1):38, 1986.
33. *FDI Technical Report no. 43: delivery of oral health care to the elderly patient. Commission on Dental Education and Practice. Working Group 10,* London, 1992, Federation Dentaire Internationale.
34. Kiyak HA: Recent advances in behavioral research in geriatric dentistry, *Gerodontology* 7:27, 1988.
35. Kiyak HA, Miller RR: Age differences in oral health attitudes and dental service utilization, *J Public Health Dent* 42:29, 1982.
36. Ettinger RL, Beck JD, Glenn RE: Some considerations in teaching geriatric dentistry, *J Am Soc Geriatr Dent* 13:7, 1978.
37. Gluck GM, Lakin LB: Determination of common myths among dental students and dental school faculty. Unpublished data, 1985.
38. Epstein CF: Enhancing the dental office environment for the elderly, *Dent Clin North Am* 33:43, 1989.
39. Ettinger RL, Beck JD, Glenn RE: Eliminating office architectural barriers to dental care of the elderly and handicapped, *J Am Dent Assoc* 98:398, 1979.
40. Americans With Disabilities Act, PL 101-336: Americans with Disabilities Act Title III regulations, 28 CFR Part 36, Nondiscrimination on the basis of disability by public accommodations and in commercial facilities, Washington, DC, 1992, US Department of Justice, Office of the Attorney General.
41. Johnson ES, Kelly JE, Van Kirk LE: *Selected dental findings in adults by age, race, and sex: United States 1960-1962,* PHS pub no 1000, series 11, no 7, Washington, DC, 1965, US Department of Health, Education, and Welfare, Public Health Service, US Government Printing Office.
42. Harvey C, Kelly JE: *Decayed, missing, and filled teeth among persons 1-74 years, United States,* DHHS pub no (PHS) 81-1673, series 11, no 223, Washington, DC, 1981, National Center for Health Statistics, US Government Printing Office.
43. National Center for Health Statistics: National Health and Nutrition Examination Survey (NHANES III), *J Dent Res* 75(spec iss), Feb 1996.
44. Hand JS, Hunt RJ, Beck, JD: Coronal and root caries in older Iowans: 36-month incidence, *Gerodontics* 4(3): 136, 1988.
45. Hunt RJ et al: Incidence of tooth loss among elderly Iowans, *Am J Pub Health* 78:1330, 1988.
46. Warren JJ et al: Dental caries and dental care utilization among the very old, *J Am Dent Assoc* (131): 1571, 2000.
47. Drake CW et al: Eighteen-month coronal caries incidence in North Carolina older adults, *J Public Health Dent* 54(1):24, 1994.
48. Douglass CW et al: Oral health status of the elderly in New England, *J Gerontol* 48(2):M39, 1993.
49. Weintraub JA, Burt BA: Tooth loss in the United States, *J Dent Educ* 49:368, 1985.
50. Hand JS, Hunt RJ, Beck JD: Incidence of coronal and root caries in an older population, *J Public Health Dent* 48:14, 1988.
51. Papas A, Joshi A, Giunta J: Prevalence and intraoral distribution of coronal and root caries in middle-aged and older adults, *Caries Res* 26:459, 1992.
52. Winn DM et al: Coronal and root caries in the dentition of adults in the United States, 1988-1991, *J Dent Res* 75(spec iss):642, Feb 1996.
53. Beck JD: The epidemiology of root surface caries, *J Dent Res* 69:1216, 1990.
54. Page RC: Periodontal diseases in the elderly: a critical evaluation of current information, *Gerodontology* 3:63, 1984.
55. Abdellatif HM, Burt BA: An epidemiological investigation into the relative importance of age and oral hygiene status as determinants of periodontitis, *J Dent Res* 66:13, 1987.
56. Burt BA: Periodontitis and aging: reviewing recent evidence, *J Am Dent Assoc* 125:273, 1994.

57. Brown LJ, Brunelle JA, Kingman A: Periodontal status in the United States, 1988-91: prevalence, extent, and demographic variation, *J Dent Res* 75(spec iss):672, Feb 1996.
58. Locker D, Slade GD, Murray H: Epidemiology of periodontal disease among older adults: a review, *Periodontology 2000* 16:16, 1998.
59. Loe H et al: Natural history of periodontal disease in man; rapid, moderate, and no loss of attachment in Sri Lankan laborers 14 to 46 years of age, *J Clin Periodontol* 13:431, 1986.
60. Fox CH et al: Periodontal disease among New England elders, *J Periodontol* 65(7):676, 1994.
61. Greenle RT et al: Cancer statistics, *CA Cancer J Clin* 50:7, 2000.
62. Horowitz AM et al: Oral pharyngeal cancer prevention and early detection, *J Am Dent Assoc* 131:453, 2000.
63. Silverman S, American Cancer Society: *Oral cancer,* ed 4, St Louis, 1998, Mosby.
64. Medalie JH: An approach to common problems in the elderly. In Calkins E et al, editors: *The practice of geriatrics,* Philadelphia, 1986, WB Saunders.
65. Bolla LR, Filley CM, Palmer RM: Dementia Ddx. Office diagnosis of the four major types of dementia, *Geriatrics* 55(1):34, 2000.
66. *Use of nursing homes by the elderly: preliminary data from the 1985 National Nursing Home Survey, Advance Data 135,* Washington, DC, 1987, National Center for Health Statistics, US Government Printing Office.
67. Katzman R: Alzheimer's disease, *N Engl J Med* 314: 964, 1986.
68. White L et al: Geriatric epidemiology, *Annu Rev Gerontol Geriatr* 6:215, 1986.
69. Stamm JW, Banting DW, Imrey PB: Adult root caries survey of two similar communities with contrasting natural fluoride levels, *J Am Dent Assoc* 120:143, 1990.
70. Doty P, Liu K, Weiner J: Special report: an overview of long-term care, *Health Care Financing Review* 6(3):69, 1985.
71. Department of Health and Human Services: *Healthy people 2000,* Public Health Service DHHS pub no (PHS) 91-50212, Washington, DC, 1990, US Government Printing Office.
72. Berkey D et al: Research review of oral health status and service use among institutionalized older adults in the United States and Canada, *Spec Care Dent* 11:131, 1991.
73. Strayer M, Ibrahim M: Dental treatment needs of homebound and nursing home patients, *Community Dent Oral Epidemiol* 19:176, 1991.
74. Kiyak HA, Grayston MN, Crinean CL: Oral health problems and needs of nursing home residents, *Community Dent Oral Epidemiol* 12:49, 1993.
75. Weyant RJ et al: Oral health status of a long-term care veteran population, *Community Dent Oral Epidemiol* 21:227, 1993.
76. California Dental Association: *California skilled facilities' residents: a survey of dental needs,* Sacramento, CA, 1986, California Dental Association.
77. Empy G, Kiyak HA, Milgrom P: Oral health in nursing homes, *Spec Care Dent* 3(2):65, 1983.
78. Henry RG, Ceridan B: Delivering dental care to nursing home and homebound patients, *Dent Clin North Am* 38(3):537, 1994.
79. National Citizens' Coalition for Nursing Home Reform: *Nursing home reform law: the basics,* Washington, DC, 1991, NCCNHR.
80. Gift HC, Cherry-Peppers G, Oldakowski RJ: Oral health care in US nursing homes, 1995, *Spec Care Dent* 18(6):226, 1998.
81. Ettinger RL: Oral care for the homebound and institutionalized, *Clin Geriatr Med* 8(3):659, 1992.
82. Council on Access, Prevention and Interprofessional Relations: *Portable and mobile dentistry information,* Washington, DC, 1995, American Dental Association.
83. Olsen ED: Dental insurance and senior Americans, *J Am Coll Dent* 58:22, 1991.
84. US Health Care Financing Administration: *Health care financing review,* Winter 1992.
85. Health Insurance Association of America: *Source book of health insurance data,* Washington, DC, 1985, Health Insurance Association of America.
86. Meskin LH et al: Economic impact of dental service utilization by older adults, *J Am Dent Assoc* 120:665, 1990.
87. Center for General Health Services Extramural Research: *Expenditures and sources of payment for medical care, National Medical Expenditure Survey,* Washington, DC, 1987, Agency for Health Care Policy and Research.
88. Kington R, Rogowski J, Lillard L: Dental expenditures and insurance coverage among older adults, *Gerontologist* 35(4):436, 1995.
89. US Department of Health and Human Services, Office of National Cost Estimates: National health expenditures, 1988, *Health Care Financing Review* 11(4):1, 1990.
90. Durante SJ: Medicare: what it did for medicine it can do for dentistry, *J Dental Practice Administration* 5(3): 92, 1988.
91. American Dental Association, Council on Dental Care Programs: *Policies on dental care programs,* Chicago, 1991, The Association.
92. National Institute on Aging: *Personnel for health needs of the elderly through the year 2020,* Bethesda, MD, 1987, Public Health Service, Department of Health and Human Services.

93. Shay K, Berkey DB, Saxe SR: New programs for advanced training in dental geriatrics, *J Am Dent Assoc* 120:661, 1990.
94. American Society for Geriatric Dentistry: *Resource directory of postgraduate educational opportunities in geriatric dentistry,* Chicago, 1993, American Society for Geriatric Dentistry.
95. US Department of Health and Human Services: *Oral health in America: a report of the Surgeon General—executive summary,* Rockville, MD, 2000, US Department of Health and Human Services, National Institute of Dental and Craniofacial Research, National Institutes of Health.

CHAPTER

7

NEW INSIGHTS INTO EARLY CHILDHOOD CARIES AND STRATEGIES FOR PREVENTION

Benjamin Peretz • Eliezer Eidelman

The previous century was marked by the development of the scientific method with the consequent explosion of information and an understanding of the underlying biologic processes. The new millennium has harnessed the information through new technology; new understanding has led to new clinical insights. Every dental school attempts to link the basic biologic sciences with the diagnosis and treatment of dental disease. This chapter traces the embryologic development of dental enamel, speculates about the relationship of embryologic development and dental caries, describes the public health impact of early childhood caries, and suggests strategies for prevention.

ENAMEL FORMATION

Enamel formation of the primary teeth begins with the incisors at approximately 11 to 14 weeks of fetal life.[1,2] The initial phase consists of matrix formation followed by calcification. These two processes begin in utero and are completed by the third postnatal month. Because enamel is a relatively stable structure, defects of the enamel of the primary teeth involving its matrix secretion or maturation, or both, can act as a permanent record of insults occurring during the prenatal or early postnatal periods. Birth itself leaves its mark on the developing teeth. The change from intrauterine life to extrauterine life causes the formation of the neonatal line.[3] This is a narrow line of hypoplasia, seen in the crowns of the primary incisors near the gingiva and in the primary molars in the middle portion of the crown. In a child born through a normal delivery, the neonatal line is seen only microscopically; however, after complicated deliveries the neonatal line is likely to be macroscopic and visible to the naked eye. A wide range of conditions may contribute to these hypoplastic or hypocalcified defects. Systemic maternal disorders associated with enamel hypoplasia of the dentition of the fetus or neonate include diabetes, kidney disease, and viral or bacterial infections. Systemic disorders of the neonate may include premature birth, Rh incompatibility, allergies, tetany, gastroenteritis, malnutrition, infectious diseases, and chronic diarrhea.[4-8] Some researchers have suggested that a common factor in all these conditions—both maternal and fetal or neonatal—is transient hypocalcemia, which may be a predisposing factor for dental caries. Others maintain that linear enamel hypoplasia is a predisposing factor to dental caries.[9] A possible correlation between hypoplastic defects and dental caries was proposed as early as four decades ago.[10,11] However, hypoplastic dental defects may be difficult to distinguish from caries caused by excessive bottle nursing, especially when the caries is subsequent to the defect.[12]

DENTAL CARIES

Dental caries is the most prevalent childhood dental disease. In the 1980s studies of children up to age 12 in Western countries showed a dramatic decline in the prevalence of dental caries and an increasing number of children with caries-free dentitions.[13,14] However, a more recent study warned that the 50% caries-free characterization of U.S. schoolchildren was mythical because it failed to consider decayed primary teeth and it inappropriately averaged in children who were too young to have experienced decay.[15] When decay in primary teeth is also considered, roughly half of children have already experienced decay before first grade. It has been observed that the prevalence of dental caries continues to increase steadily with age until five of every six high school graduates are affected. In light of such opposing opinions, a review of some basic aspects of dental caries is in order.

Dental caries is caused by the demineralization of the dental enamel by organic acids that are the outcome of the metabolism of carbohydrates by microorganisms in the mouth. It is a multifactorial disease, involving four main factors:

1. *Microorganisms. Streptococcus mutans (S. mutans)* is the principal microorganism involved in the carious process.[16] *S. mutans* is present in the mouth only after tooth eruption. Infants whose teeth have not erupted yet do not have this microorganism in their oral cavities.[17,18] Some researchers suggest that there is a continuous transmission of *S. mutans* from the parent's oral cavity to the infant's oral cavity through kissing, sharing of food, and other contact.[19-21] In caries-free children the *S. mutans* count was found to be negligible.[22]
2. *Substrate.* Carbohydrates in the diet provide the microorganisms with the substrate for organic acid production, which leads to enamel demineralization.[16,23] Sucrose has long been considered the "archcriminal" of dental caries.[24,25] *S. mutans* accumulation strongly depends on the amount of sucrose.[26]
3. *Host—tooth enamel.* For caries to occur, a susceptible host is required so that microorganisms can adhere, colonize, and metabolize available carbohydrates. The tooth's morphologic condition and enamel structure are important in this respect; both food debris and microorganisms readily impact in the pit and fissure areas of molar teeth, making them highly susceptible to caries. Although smooth enamel tooth surfaces

are not prone to caries development, bacteria accumulate on and adhere to irregular enamel surfaces, thus accelerating the carious process. In general, the surface of the tooth is more acid resistant than its subsurface. Furthermore, the increase in fluoride content and the decrease in permeability of the enamel of the mature teeth make them more acid resistant than is the immature enamel surface of young teeth. Thus, as a host, the enamel of a young tooth is more prone to dental caries than is the enamel of the mature tooth. In addition, as the tooth enamel matures, the tooth surface may be considered a reservoir of fluoride, thus increasing tooth resistance to caries.[27,28]

4. *Time.* Elapsed time determines the three previous factors. The longer the teeth are exposed to fermentable carbohydrates, the more acid will be produced. This phenomenon increases the probability that caries will occur.

Saliva is a major factor influencing the development or inhibition of dental caries. Saliva is to the tooth enamel what blood is to body cells. Just as body cells depend on the bloodstream to supply nutrients, remove waste, and protect the cells, enamel depends on saliva to perform similar functions. The beneficial actions of saliva include the following:

1. Speeding oral clearance of food particles and dissolving sugars
2. Facilitating the removal of insoluble carbohydrates from the mouth by salivary enzymes
3. Neutralizing organic acids produced by plaque bacteria by salivary buffers
4. Inhibiting demineralization and enhancing remineralization by the action of salivary minerals on tooth structure
5. Recycling ingested fluoride into the mouth
6. Discouraging the growth of bacteria
7. Inhibiting both mineral loss and the adhesion of bacteria by adsorption of salivary proteins to tooth surfaces[29,30]

Children as young as 6 months to 3 years old are already at risk for a distinctive pattern of dental caries known as early childhood caries (ECC), baby-bottle tooth decay (BBTD), or nursing bottle caries. ECC is seen in epidemic proportions in developing countries and among disadvantaged children in Western countries.[31] Because it is so prevalent, ECC requires special attention from both clinical and public health perspectives.

EARLY CHILDHOOD CARIES

Early childhood caries is the term now recommended by the Centers for Disease Control and Prevention to describe a unique pattern of carious lesions in infants, toddlers, and preschool children. This term now covers the previously used terms *baby-bottle tooth decay* and *nursing caries* that describe a form of rampant caries of the primary dentition caused by prolonged use of a bottle of milk or other liquid including carbohydrates.[12,31] Clinically, the decay is first found in the maxillary primary incisors; later it spreads to the maxillary molars, mandibular molars, and rarely the mandibular incisors. It has been postulated that this pattern of caries is related to the following factors:

1. *The chronology of primary tooth eruption.* With the exception of the mandibu-

lar incisors, teeth that erupt early are most affected. Therefore the maxillary incisors are affected most in younger infants and toddlers.[32]

2. *The duration of the harmful habit.* The longer sweet liquid remains around the teeth, the more likely it is that it will be metabolized by oral microorganisms into organic acids that demineralize the tooth enamel.
3. *The pattern of the muscular activity of the sucking infant.* Because the teeth cannot be protected by the tongue, weak muscular activity results in the teeth being bathed in an increasingly large pool of liquid that cannot be effectively washed out by the available saliva.

Thus the occurrence of dental caries in cases of ECC depends on all four factors: microorganisms, substrate, host, and time.

The contents of the feeding bottles must be considered in cases of ECC. Most studies have reported that these bottles all contain some form of sugar.[33-36] How, for example, does milk affect the occurrence of ECC? Cow's milk and mother's milk contain lactose, composed of glucose and fructose, both of which enhance cariogenic bacteria colonization and acid production.[37-39] Some studies report on ECC in children who were fed with cow's milk only and some on ECC in children who were only breast-fed.[40-42] It has also been found that the high concentrations of calcium and phosphate in milk are caries protective.[33,43-46] Apparently, under normal diet conditions milk is not cariogenic and may even provide some protection against caries. However, the diets of most children with ECC are not normal; prolonged exposure to milk leads to its stagnation around the necks of the teeth, especially the maxillary incisors, leading to high acidity (low pH) and subsequent enamel demineralization.[47] In addition to having sweet liquids from bottles, affected children are often given pacifiers dipped in sweets; an association has been established between the use of these comforters and ECC.[48-50]

PREVALENCE

It is difficult to determine the exact prevalence of ECC because every survey is seriously limited. Preschool-age children with ECC are less available for dental examination than are older children. In addition, those children who are examined may not necessarily represent the general population of this age. Instead, the population of children seen at a given dental clinic may be biased because their parents believed that their children had a dental problem.[40] Selection of survey samples from mother-child centers or from child health centers could skew the sample into a particular socioeconomic class.[51] In addition, because the patterns of infant feeding habits are largely culturally and ethnically influenced, survey samples of children from such cultural or ethnic backgrounds will be similarly skewed.[52] For all these reasons it is difficult to make an analogy from the prevalence of ECC in one country with its prevalence in another country.[53-55]

The reported prevalence of ECC may also be influenced by the fact that infants are difficult to examine. Not every pediatric dentist knows that a thorough dental examination of an infant requires that the infant lie with his or her head on the dentist's lap with the legs on the mother. Furthermore, the infant's distress and crying may trouble an inexperienced examiner so much that the examination may be superficial at best.

The diagnosing criteria of ECC are somewhat controversial; some researchers claim that a minimum of one infected incisor is a sufficient criterion for diagnosing the condition.[53] Others maintain that a minimum of two teeth is required, whereas some believe that at least three infected maxillary incisors are required.[48,52,56]

It is generally accepted that the prevalence of ECC in predominantly Western-type cultures is about 5%.[35,40,48,51-56] In certain populations a higher prevalence has been found. In the United States, Hardwick and colleagues[57] reported a 21% prevalence of ECC for urban Hispanic children younger than 5 years. Barnes and colleagues[58] reported a 16% prevalence for urban children and a 37% prevalence for rural Hispanic children. In a preliminary study of children of Mexican-American migrant workers, Weinstein and colleagues[59] found a 29.2% prevalence of ECC among infants age 27.6 months on the average. In a subsequent study the same research group found that in a sample of children with an average age of 17.1 months, 7% had at least one maxillary incisor with decay and more than 30% had at least one incisor with a white spot lesion.[60] A study among Arizona infants and toddlers reported a more complex pattern of prevalence, associated with age: among 13- to 24-month-olds, caries was most prevalent on the buccal and lingual surfaces of the maxillary central incisors (approximately 4% in the 19- to 24-month-olds). In children age 25 to 27 months, caries of the maxillary central incisors was most prevalent on the mesial and distal surfaces (nearly 6%), and among 31- to 33-month-olds, prevalence on these surfaces was nearly 10%. Caries of the lateral incisors showed a similar pattern of change with age, except that the distal surface was consistently the least prevalent.[32]

Disease Progression

ECC has a predictable progression. Initially the teeth are seen to have white spots that are usually decalcification lesions, which may become frank lesions or caries within 6 months to 1 year. Such decalcification lesions do not necessarily progress to cavities because the process may be reversed and the teeth may become remineralized.[61] Undetected, and thus unchecked, early ECC causes severe problems for the child, who may be in considerable pain and may have difficulty eating and talking. The disease is also a serious threat to the health of other primary teeth and subsequently to the health of the permanent dentition. An association between ECC and failure to thrive (FTT) has been found.[62] However, the results of this study do not distinguish clearly whether ECC had caused the FTT or whether the FTT, caused by various general systemic conditions, was itself a predisposing factor in the development of ECC.

The results of a pilot study indicate a strong correlation between BBTD and maternal diseases or complications during pregnancy or delivery.[63] This study compared the pregnancies of the mothers of two groups of age-matched children with similar eating and feeding habits—they all were fed from bottles containing sweet liquids. Compared with the pregnancies of mothers of children with healthy teeth, the pregnancies of the mothers of children with ECC involved more cases of vaginal bleeding, premature uterine contractions, episodes of viral or bacterial infections, and other indications of high-risk pregnancies. There were also more instrumental deliveries (vacuum or forceps) and cesarean sections. Therefore it seems clear that children born of high-risk pregnancies are more likely to have ECC than are children of normal pregnancies.

The biology of ECC may be modified by factors unique to young children: the implantation of cariogenic bacteria associated with feeding and oral hygiene in early childhood.[64] ECC is known to be characterized microbiologically by dense oral populations of mutans streptococci (MS).[65] It is suggested that the development of ECC occurs in three stages. The first stage is characterized by the primary infection of the oral cavity with MS. The second stage is characterized by the accumulation of these organisms to pathologic levels as a consequence of frequent and prolonged exposure to cariogenic substrate. The third stage is characterized by a rapid demineralization and cavitation of enamel, resulting in rampant caries.[66] It has been demonstrated that colonization by MS is stable over time. Over a 2-year period, levels of MS were fairly stable; high levels of infection tended to stay high and were associated with subsequent development of caries.[67]

Furthermore, none of the teeth with undetectable levels of MS developed caries. This indicates that children with ECC are highly susceptible to the development of caries in later years when compared with caries-free children.

The traditional perception of blaming the bottle containing sweetened liquid as responsible per se for ECC must be reconsidered. Most studies have only asked the question, "Did your child ever go to bed with the bottle?" Few studies have investigated related behaviors, such as whether the child quickly finishes the bottle or whether the child uses the bottle ad lib. during the day. The method of bedtime bottle use also has been found to influence caries risk. If the bottle is removed after feeding, no increased caries risk is noted. However, if the bottle remains in the bed, the child is at greater risk of developing ECC compared with those children who had no nighttime bottle.[68] These questions touch the time factor mentioned previously and must be considered whenever disease progression is discussed. Nevertheless, the bottle still must be considered as a risk factor, and to eliminate the baby bottle as a cause of or at least a risk factor for ECC would be premature.[69]

A recent study on caries among Arizona infants and toddlers has revealed some interesting findings: Use of an infant feeding bottle was common; nearly 45% of 13- to 36-month-olds reported still using a bottle. Those children currently using a bottle were more likely to have a prior history of sleeping with a bottle than those who were no longer using the bottle.[32]

Among children age 25 to 38 months, a significant relationship between nighttime bottle use and maxillary anterior caries was found. Of those children with maxillary anterior caries, 46% slept with a bottle. However, the predictive value of these findings is limited because only 19% of those children who reportedly slept with a bottle were found to have maxillary anterior caries. No relationship between nighttime bottle use and maxillary anterior caries was found among 13- to 24-month-olds. Furthermore, no relationship between nighttime bottle use and posterior caries patterns was found in either age group.

Treatment

Treating frank lesions in very young children is invasive and most frequently requires crown preparation for the affected teeth and often pulp treatments. These treatments are most often carried out with the child under general anesthesia (GA) or some form of sedation and thus are risky for the child. Often the indications for either general anesthesia or sedation as the treatment modality are similar, with no clear criteria as to exactly when one mode is superior to the other.

Sedation is generally indicated for children who are uncooperative, fearful of the dental environment, or unable to cope because of other reasons. The ideal goal of sedation is to relax the patient, allowing completion of the dental treatment while maintaining communication and responsiveness. GA may be preferred in treating young uncooperative children with extensive caries, rather than subjecting them to numerous sedation visits, because of an increased sensitization of children to repeated stressful procedures with accompanying decreased cooperative behavior. It is commonly accepted that GA is more radical and relatively more risky than sedation. GA also provokes more stress among parents during treatment.

A study that compared restorations for children with ECC treated under GA or conscious sedation showed that 59% of children treated under GA and 74% of children treated under sedation required further dental treatment. The majority of the required treatment was due to new caries. As for the quality of restorations, general anesthesia yielded better restorations compared with sedation.[70] Furthermore, in the sedation group, success of restorations was more prevalent in patients who exhibited "positive" behavior, that is, were cooperative.

All such treatments are expensive, both from the point of view of the parent and as a general public health expense. In any case, before any invasive treatment is undertaken, the first necessary step in treating ECC, as recommended by most practitioners and educators, is to stop the deleterious habit of unrestrained bottle nursing. It is important to note that not only would stopping the habit cause a decrease in the exposure to the cariogenic liquid, but it would also arrest the carious process and allow the pulp to produce reparative dentin. The formation of this dentin prevents the pulp from being exposed after caries removal. Protecting the pulp reduces the likelihood that the child will require pulp treatments such as pulpotomy or pulpectomy; it also conditions the tooth material so that new adhesive will be more likely to bond to it.[71]

PREVENTION

Most researchers agree that the only rational approach to the treatment of ECC is prevention, which begins with education about oral self-care. Teaching oral self-care is extremely frustrating for health educators; thus it is not surprising that Weinstein and colleagues[72] call one of the chapters in their book "Why Most Plaque Control Programs Do Not Work." Most traditional stand-alone health educational approaches provide general information about ECC, focus on the bottle as the risk factor, and recommend immediate substitution of the cup for the bottle at all feedings by 12 months. Unfortunately, this approach has not been very successful. Considering the seriousness of this disease and how unsuccessful most preventive programs have been, it is surprising how few alternative programs have been suggested. In fact, some authors have suggested that changing oral hygiene measures may be a more effective prevention strategy for ECC than attempting to modify diet.[73]

Future Preventive Behavior of Children and Their Parents

Future preventive behavior of children who had been treated for ECC under GA or under sedation is not encouraging. It was hypothesized that because GA is a more radical and dramatic mode of treatment, parents of those children would change their families' dental health behaviors to avoid future dental disease and the subsequent treatment. However, no difference in plaque levels of both groups was found, as well as in frequency of brushing of both children and parents, and in continuous sleeping with a bottle. However, some preventive behaviors regarding children's dental health, such as decreasing sweet consumption and brushing of children's teeth by parents, were more frequently adopted among the families of children treated using GA.[74]

A recent study that evaluated the susceptibility of children to the future development of caries following comprehensive treatment for ECC showed that despite increased preventive measures for children who experienced ECC, this group of children is still highly predisposed to greater risk of caries incidence in later years. These findings strongly suggest that more aggressive preventive therapies may be required to prevent the future development of carious lesions in children who experienced ECC.[75]

Children who were treated under GA or under sedation behave similarly in the operatory in future dental appointments. Most children sat alone on the dental chair, without the assistance of their parents.[76]

Brushing and dental caries among infants and toddlers are not directly correlated: no significant association was found between frequency of brushing and caries prevalence among 13- to 24-month-olds, but an inverse relationship was found in 25- to 36-month-olds.[32] However, children who reportedly had an adult participating in brushing were more likely to be caries free than children who brushed their own teeth.

The child's risk for ECC should be assessed. As described here, a risk for ECC could be caused by complications or diseases during the pregnancy or by instrumental delivery. Teeth that develop while these complications occur, especially the incisors, are especially at risk for ECC.[63] When risks are high or when the results of the dental examination indicate the presence of ECC, culturally appropriate interventions should be undertaken. Different implantation of MS by various individuals may be the reason for vulnerability to dental caries.

Although weaning to a cup at 1 year is recommended, it may prove difficult for parents who have a sick or temperamentally difficult child and who have little social support. It may also be culturally unacceptable.[77] In many societies, until they are several years old, infants are carried everywhere by their mothers and nursed by them. In other societies in which there are many children per family, it is difficult to encourage weaning from the bottle at an early age. In an attempt to overcome the problem of parents' noncompliance, Weinstein and colleagues[77] tried an original approach: they applied fluoride-containing varnish to the teeth of ECC high-risk populations, a simple and effective method that requires only minimal parental cooperation. The varnish is brushed on dried teeth, and the procedure takes less than 2 minutes. Although the only compliance required from the parents is to bring the children for semiannual treatment, parents in the study demonstrated only approximately

50% compliance after 6 months. The rationale for this approach was to allow the fluoride to arrest the carious process and to enhance the formation of reparative dentin, thus keeping the tooth condition stable even though not restored. This approach is close to the idea that stopping the habit would allow new reparative dentin to be formed. Attempts to enhance follow-up are needed, especially in migrant families living on subsistence wages and in families with more than one child because bringing in one child for a follow-up would entail providing care for the other children and is thus logistically complicated.

The question of who will transmit the preventive information to parents remains to be answered. Currently, dental professionals are not in a position to provide this information. Most children do not see a dentist until age 3 years, if at all.[78] By that age, cariogenic diets are well established and difficult to change, and the carious process already may be under way. Therefore nondental professionals need to have this responsibility. In particular, prenatal educators, pediatricians, family physicians, nurse practitioners, and Women, Infants, and Children (WIC) nutritionists are well placed to have frequent contact with parents and their children at this critical time of dietary development.[69] Also, access to dental care through dental and nondental health professionals must be substantially improved to enable any preventive strategy to be implemented.[32]

The Fetus Is Also a Patient!

With the aim of improving the health education of the general public, health professionals are constantly searching for target populations at high risk for preventable diseases.[60,61,72,79-81] Within this framework, and considering the association between ECC and maternal diseases or complications during pregnancy or delivery, we propose that the dental profession adopt the concept that the fetus is also a patient.[63] Because the quality of intrauterine life affects the quality of the infant's teeth, dental health educators should educate women who may experience complications during pregnancy or delivery about the dangers of ECC and how to avoid it. For example, they could teach appropriate methods for infant bottle-feeding.

The rapid progress in medicine and the increasing ability of modern medicine to maintain high-risk pregnancies, as well as to keep newborns alive after complicated or instrumental deliveries, have resulted in many more infants whose teeth may be affected and could be more vulnerable to dental caries. Thus it is only natural that the dental profession will encounter more young patients at risk for ECC. It is important to warn parents and prospective parents that maternal diseases and complications during pregnancy and delivery may predispose their fetus's/infant's teeth to ECC. These parents in particular should be taught to avoid prolonged bottle-feeding of sweetened liquids to their infants.

GENERAL RECOMMENDATIONS: CARIES PREVENTION IN INFANTS AND CHILDREN

In this chapter we have chosen not to deal with the issue of water fluoridation, which has been discussed at length in the literature. However, we believe that the following recommendations should always be mentioned. It is recommended that an infant be examined soon after eruption of the first primary tooth.[81] This examination should include the soft tissues of the oral cavity, as well as the teeth, to detect defects in the enamel or early carious lesions. At this time the dentist can teach the parents proper maintenance of oral and dental health. Tremendous success has been reported in educating parents about preventive dental treatment for children younger than 4 years of age.[82] A protocol for preventive procedures beginning early in infancy should include the use of fluoride and instruction in proper home dental care.[83,84]

Preventive measures can be divided into two categories: home care and professional dental care.

Home Care

Home care includes the following elements:

1. *Consistent visits to the dentist.* Preferably the first visit should occur before the eruption of the first tooth. Dental visits provide the dentist with the opportunity to teach the parents to wipe their infant's teeth clean with a small piece of gauze held between their fingers. Because it has been found that bacteria are transferred from the parents to the child, parents should be encouraged to keep their own teeth very clean during the time that their infant's teeth are erupting.[20]
2. *Effective oral hygiene.* The infant's teeth should be brushed twice daily, with the whole dentition being brushed both after breakfast and before bedtime.[85]
3. *Use of home-fluoride modalities.* These treatments include fluoridated dentifrices, fluoride supplements (tablets or drops), and fluoride rinse solutions. The most common topical application of fluoride is obtained during brushing with a fluoride dentifrice. Fluoride toothpastes have contributed considerably to the recent decline in the incidence of caries in industrialized countries. Their effect is related more to the frequency of use than to the fluoride concentration.[86] Brushing with a fluoride dentifrice after breakfast and just before bedtime is recommended to maintain an intraoral reservoir of salivary fluoride ions for as long as possible. Such brushing and the use of fluoride tablets or drops require the establishment of a regular daily routine, in which the main responsibility is taken by the parents. Because this demands a high degree of health consciousness and concern by at least one parent, compliance for this regimen has been low.[87] When the fluoride tablets have been given at school, the coverage has been better, but such cases require a time commitment from the teachers, who are not always cooperative. Fluoride supplements should be considered for all children drinking fluoride-deficient water (less than 0.6 ppm).[81] Before supplements are prescribed, however, it is essential to know the fluoride concentration of the patient's drinking water to avoid dental fluorosis. Other sources of fluoride or its removal through the use of in-house filtration systems must be taken into account.

Fluoride rinse solutions are used to provide the tooth enamel surface with a constant supply of fluoride ions, which help remineralize initial carious lesions. This method is recommended only for children 6 years of age or older because younger children may swallow the solution. For this reason fluoride rinse solutions are not appropriate for the treatment of infants with ECC.

All home care methods depend on patient compliance. The child's socialization process and developmental framework must be considered, especially in the design of home care programs for children.

Professional Dental Care

Professional dental care includes the following:

1. *Oral hygiene instructions.* In accordance with the child's developmental framework and socialization process, oral hygiene education should be integrated with general health education dealing with body cleanliness, grooming, and self-esteem.[88] It is also beneficial to involve the parents in health promotion programs for children.[89] Oral health for children should be supportive and cannot be achieved without parallel efforts for a healthy environment, which would support healthy choices and healthy behavior of the individual.
2. *Fluoride gel or varnish applications.* The application of topical fluoride to the teeth increases tooth resistance to caries. Constant and repeated applications of fluoride varnish have been highly successful in preventing BBTD.[77] Nevertheless, now that fluoride action is better understood, dentists must ask themselves if they should give fluoride treatments to all their patients. For example, is it possible that applying topical fluoride to the teeth of patients who have been caries free for 1 or 2 years may be considered as overtreatment?
3. *Pit and fissure sealants.* The issue of pit and fissure sealants has become one of the most important and controversial topics in pediatric dentistry. Some researchers have recommended that sealants be placed over initial caries.[90,91] However, other clinicians and researchers have raised serious objections to this recommendation.[92-94] In any case, because the issue of pit and fissure sealants has enormous implications for public and community dentistry as a means of preventing dental caries in children and young adolescents, elaboration on the subject from some practical viewpoints is necessary.

   Occlusal surface pits and fissures increase the risk of primary and permanent teeth to the ravages of caries attack. Because these areas are least benefited by fluoride, treating them with pit and fissure sealants can be particularly effective for newly erupted noncarious primary or permanent molar and premolar teeth with deep pits or fissures and for the cingulum area of maxillary incisors with deep lingual pits or fissures.[81]

   The issue of sealant retention is of utmost importance. Among the various factors affecting sealant retention, the most important is the ability to keep the tooth surface dry. Contamination of the tooth surface by saliva or gingival fluid may prevent the adhesion of the sealant. Therefore as soon as possible after the tooth erupts, sealants should be placed under conditions permitting sufficient isolation so that contamination of the tooth surface by moisture is prevented. Because gingival fluid can be spread and may interfere even more with the adhesion process, it is necessary that the eruption status of the tooth be such that no operculum covers the distal portion of the occlusal surface. Sealant retention is further affected by the position of teeth in the mouth (the sealants on the more anterior teeth are better retained), the skill of the operator, and the age of the patient (the behavior of younger children may make it difficult to maintain a dry field).[95] Sealants may be applied to the teeth of individual children, with the use of criteria such as caries history, patient's age, length of time the tooth has been exposed in the oral cavity, and tooth surface anatomy. Alternatively, sealants may be used as a public health preventive measure, with members of the dental team applying the sealant under the dentist's supervision. The results of research on sealant retention rates indicate much higher retention when sealants are placed after mechanical preparation; that is, the fissures are widened with a bur before sealant placement.[96] Evidence suggests that the use of an intermediate bonding layer before sealant application may improve sealant retention rates.[97] Because auxiliary workers are not permitted to cut tooth structure, the dentist must perform the mechanical preparation.

4. *Diet counseling.* In addition to reducing the incidence of dental caries by adequate oral hygiene immediately after the ingestion of cariogenic foods, reducing the consumption of cariogenic food can also be helpful.[98,99] However, because controlling dental caries through diet modification is complex, it has been only moderately successful. Furthermore, the precise cariogenicity of any food is not easily predicted. It should be noted that when there is a general decline in the incidence of caries, there is a weaker association between sugar consumption and the incidence of caries, especially when there is an optimal concentration of fluoride in the drinking water.[100] It seems that although most children realize that eating sugar may cause tooth decay, this realization does not cause them to modify their behavior. Community- or school-based programs directed at dietary changes have met with only short-term success, leading to attempts to replace sugar with sugar substitutes in snack foods, beverages, and chewing gums at the population level.[100,101] As clinicians and educators, we have found that teenagers worried about their body image are more motivated than younger children to use sugar substitutes. Of course, it is important to consider the general health of the child and to modulate accordingly our recommendations for decreasing sugar in the diet or using sugar substitutes. The complexity of these individual behavior modifications or social changes suggests that population-wide oral health promotion based on diet modification is less practical than other caries prevention strategies.[100,101] All foods containing even small quantities of sugars or cooked starches can potentially lead to organic acid production by plaque bacteria.[102] This is one of the reasons why is it difficult to judge the relative cariogenicity of various foods. In general, it is more important to control the frequency of sugar consumption and whether it is consumed during daytime activity or im-

mediately before bedtime and the length of time that residual food material remains in the mouth after eating.

SUMMARY

This chapter has shown that ECC is a serious and all too common disease. It has emphasized that the traditional cause of ECC—inappropriate use of the baby bottle—can no longer be considered the sole etiology. The risks for ECC may involve different implantation of MS by different individuals or maternal diseases and complications during pregnancy or delivery. By identifying populations at risk and using existing treatment modalities and appropriate educational approaches, dental caries in general and ECC in particular may be controllable and even preventable. Other treatment strategies that are useful in the prevention of dental disease in children have also been discussed.

REVIEW QUESTIONS

1. How does the understanding of tooth development contribute to an understanding of the development of tooth decay?
2. Explain the prevalence of ECC in developing countries and among minority populations in the United States.
3. How might diet counseling contribute to the prevention of ECC?
4. Why should the prevention of ECC begin during the intrauterine development of the fetus?

REFERENCES

1. Kraus BS, Jordan RW: *The human dentition before birth,* Philadelphia, 1965, Lea & Febiger.
2. Lunt RC, Law DB: A review of the chronology of calcification of deciduous teeth, *J Am Dent Assoc* 89:599, 1974.
3. Shour I, Massler M: Development of the teeth. In Brauer JC et al, editors: *Dentistry for children,* ed 4, New York, 1958, McGraw-Hill.
4. Infante PF, Gillespie GM: An epidemiologic study of linear hypoplasia in anterior teeth in Guatemalan children, *Arch Oral Biol* 19:1055, 1974.
5. Noreen J, Grahnen H, Magnusson BO: Maternal diabetes and changes in hard tissue of primary teeth, *Acta Odontol Scand* 36:127, 1978.
6. Smith DM, Miller J: Gastro-enteritis, coeliac disease and enamel hypoplasia, *Br Dent J* 147:91, 1979.
7. Suckling GW, Pearce EI: Development defects of enamel in a group of New Zealand children: their prevalence and some associated aetiological factors, *Community Dent Oral Epidemiol* 12:177, 1984.
8. Needelman HL et al: Antecedents and correlates of hypoplastic enamel defects of primary incisors, *Pediatr Dent* 14:158, 1992.
9. Nikiforuk G, Fraser D: The etiology of enamel hypoplasia: a unifying concept, *J Pediatr* 98:888, 1981.
10. Grahnen H, Larsson PG: Enamel defects in the deciduous dentition of prematurely born children, *Odont Revy* 9:193, 1958.
11. Rosenzweig KA, Sahar M: Enamel hypoplasia and dental caries in the primary dentition of prematurity, *Br Dent J* 113:279, 1962.
12. Johnsen DC: Characteristics and background of children with "nursing caries," *Pediatr Dent* 4:218, 1982.
13. Brunelle JA, Carlos JP: Changes in the prevalence of dental caries in U.S. school children, 1961-1980, *J Dent Res* 61(spec iss):1346, 1982.
14. Hargreaves JA, Thompson GW, Wagg BJ: Changes in caries prevalence of Isle of Lewis children between 1971 and 1981, *Caries Res* 17:554, 1983.
15. Eidelstein BL, Douglas CW: Dispelling the myth that 50 percent of U.S. schoolchildren have never had a cavity, *Public Health Rep* 110:522, 1995.
16. Loesche WJ: Role of *Streptococcus mutans* in human dental decay, *Microbiol Rev* 50:353, 1980.
17. Berkowitz RJ, Jordan HV, White G: The early establishment of *Streptococcus mutans* in the mouth of infants, *Arch Oral Biol* 20:171, 1975.
18. Catalanoto FA, Shklair IL, Keene HJ: Prevalence and localization of *Streptococcus mutans* in infants and children, *J Am Dent Assoc* 91:606, 1975.
19. Berkowitz RT, Turner J, Green P: Maternal salivary levels of *Streptococcus mutans* and primary oral infection of infants, *Arch Oral Biol* 26:147, 1981.

20. Kohler B, Andreen I, Jonsson B: The effect of caries preventive measures in mothers on dental caries and the oral presence of the bacteria *Streptococcus mutans* and lactobacilli in their children, *Arch Oral Biol* 29:879, 1984.
21. Dasanayake AP et al: Transmission of mutans streptococci to infants following short term application of an iodine-NaF solution to mothers' dentition, *Commun Dent Oral Epidemiol* 21:136, 1993.
22. van Houte J, Gibbs G, Butera C: Oral flora of children with "nursing bottle caries," *J Dent Res* 61:382, 1982.
23. Kleinberg I: The role of dental plaque in caries and inflammatory periodontal disease, *J Can Dent Assoc* 40:56, 1974.
24. Newbrun E: Sucrose, the archcriminal of dental caries, *J Dent Child* 36:239, 1969.
25. Makinen KK: The role of sucrose and other sugars in the development of dental caries: a review, *Int Dent J* 22:363, 1972.
26. Loesche WJ: Nutrition and dental decay in infants, *Am J Clin Nutr* 41:423, 1985.
27. Nyvad B, Fejerskov O: Formation, composition and ultrastructure of microbial deposits on the tooth surface. In Thylstrup A, Fejerskov O, editors: *Textbook of cariology,* Copenhagen, 1986, Munksgaard.
28. Newbrun E: *Cariology,* ed 3, Chicago, 1989, Quintessence.
29. Peretz B, Sarnat H, Moss SJ: Caries protective aspects of saliva and enamel, *N Y State Dent J* 56:25, 1990.
30. Moss SF et al: *Insights into saliva action: a program for the International Association of Dentistry for Children,* New York, 1994, Colgate Palmolive Co.
31. Ripa LW: Nursing caries: a comprehensive review, *Pediatr Dent* 10:268, 1988.
32. Douglass JM et al: Dental caries patterns and oral health behaviors in Arizona infants and toddlers, *Community Dent Oral Epidemiol* 29:14, 2001.
33. Picton DCA, Wiltshear PJ: A comparison of the effects of early feeding habits on the caries prevalence of deciduous teeth, *Dent Pract* 20:170, 1970.
34. Dilley GJ, Dilley DH, Machen JB: Prolonged nursing habit: a profile of patients and their families, *J Dent Child* 47:102, 1980.
35. Goose DH, Gittus E: Infant feeding methods and dental caries, *Public Health* 82:72, 1968.
36. Curzon MEJ, Curzon JA: Dental caries in Eskimo children of the Keewatin District in the Northern Territories, *J Can Dent Assoc* 36:342, 1970.
37. Koulourides T et al: Cariogenicity of nine sugars tested with an intraoral device in man, *Caries Res* 10:427, 1976.
38. Brown CR et al: Effect of milk and fluoridated milk on bacterial enamel demineralization, *J Dent Res* 56:210, 1977 (abstract).
39. Birkhed D et al: Milk and lactose-acid production in human dental plaque, *J Dent Res* 60:1245, 1981 (abstract).
40. Gardiner DE, Norwood JR, Eisenson JE: At-will breast feeding and dental caries: four case reports, *J Dent Child* 44:187, 1977.
41. Kotlow LA: Breast feeding: a cause of dental caries in children, *J Dent Child* 44:192, 1977.
42. Curzon MEJ, Drommond BK: Case report—rampant caries in an infant related to prolonged on-demand breast feeding and a lactovegetarian diet, *Int J Paediatr Dent* 3:25, 1987.
43. Powell D: Milk . . . Is it related to rampant caries of the early primary dentition? *J Calif Dent Assoc* 4:58, 1976.
44. Bibby BG et al: Protective effect of milk against in vitro caries, *J Dent Res* 59:1565, 1980.
45. McDugall WA: Effect of milk on demineralization and remineralization in vitro, *Caries Res* 11:166, 1977.
46. Mor BM, McDugall WA: Effects of milk on pH of plaque and salivary sediment and the oral clearance of milk, *Caries Res* 11:223, 1977.
47. Rugg-Gunn AJ, Roberts GT, Wright WG: Effect of human milk on plaque pH in situ and enamel dissolution in vitro compared with bovine milk, lactose, and sucrose, *Caries Res* 19:327, 1985.
48. Winter GB, Hamilton MC, James PMC: Role of the comforter as an etiological factor in rampant caries of the deciduous dentition, *Arch Dis Child* 41:207, 1966.
49. Holt RD, Joles D, Winter GB: Caries in preschool children: the Camden study, *Br Dent J* 153:107, 1982.
50. Shannon IL, Edmonds EJ, Madsen KO: Honey: sugar content and cariogenicity, *J Dent Child* 46:29, 1979.
51. Currier GF, Glinka MP: The prevalence of nursing bottle caries or baby bottle syndrome in an inner city fluoridated community, *Va Dent J* 54:9, 1977.
52. Kelly M, Bruerd B: The prevalence of baby bottle tooth decay among two Native American populations, *J Public Health Dent* 47:94, 1987.
53. Cleaton-Jones P, Richardson B, Rantsho JM: Dental caries in rural and urban black preschool children, *Commun Dent Oral Epidemiol* 6:135, 1978.
54. Aldy D et al: A comparative study of caries formation in breast-fed and bottle-fed children, *Paediatrica Indonesiana* 19:308, 1979.
55. Richardson BD et al: Infant feeding practices and nursing bottle caries, *J Dent Child* 48:423, 1981.
56. Winter GB et al: The prevalence of dental caries in preschool children aged 1 to 4 years, *Br Dent J* 130:271, 1971.
57. Hardwick FK, McIlveen LM, Forrester DJ: A comparison of nursing caries prevalence in black and Hispanic children, *American Academy of Pediatric Dentistry,* 1991 (abstract).

58. Barnes GP et al: Ethnicity, location, age, and fluoridation factors in baby bottle tooth decay: pilot study at a migrant farmworkers clinic, *J Dent Child* 59:376, 1992.
59. Weinstein P et al: Mexican-American parents with children at risk for baby-bottle tooth decay: pilot study at a migrant farmworkers clinic, *J Dent Child* 59:376, 1992.
60. Domoto P et al: White spot caries in Mexican-American toddlers and parental preferences for various strategies, *J Dent Child* 61:342, 1994.
61. Lee C et al: Teaching parents at WIC clinics to examine their high caries–risk babies, *J Dent Child* 61:347, 1994.
62. Acs G et al: Effect of nursing caries on body weight in a pediatric population, *Pediatr Dent* 14:302, 1992.
63. Peretz B, Kafka I: Biologic factors influencing BBTD, *J Dent Res* 75:34, 1996 (abstract).
64. Seow WK: Biological mechanisms of early childhood caries, *Community Dent Oral Epidemiol* 26(suppl 1):8, 1998.
65. Berkowitz RJ, Turner J, Hughes C: Microbial characteristics of the human dental caries associated with prolonged bottle feeding, *Arch Oral Biol* 29:949, 1984.
66. Berkowitz RJ: Etiology of nursing caries: a microbiologic perspective, *J Public Health* 56:51, 1996.
67. Burt BA et al: Stability of *Streptococcus mutans* and its relationship to caries in a child population over two years, *Caries Res* 17:532, 1983.
68. Johnsen DC: Characteristics and background of children with "nursing caries," *Pediatr Dent* 4:218, 1982.
69. Douglass JM: Response to Tinanoff and Palmer: dietary determinants of dental caries and dietary recommendations for preschool children, *J Public Health Dent* 60:207, 2000.
70. Eidelman E, Faibis S, Peretz B: A comparison of restorations for children with early childhood caries treated under general anesthesia or conscious sedation, *Pediatr Dent* 22(1):33, 2000.
71. Eidelman E, Ulmansky M, Michaeli Y: Histopathology of the pulp in primary incisors with deep dentinal caries, *Pediatr Dent* 14:1372, 1992.
72. Weinstein P, Getz T, Milgrom P: *Oral self care,* ed 3, Seattle, 1991, University of Washington.
73. Gibson S, Williams S: Dental caries in preschool children: associations with social class, toothbrushing habit, and consumption of sugar and sugar-containing foods, *Caries Res* 33:101, 1999.
74. Peretz B et al: Dental health behavior of children with BBTD treated under GA or sedation, and their parents in a recall examination, *J Dent Child* 67(1):50, 2000.
75. Galganny Almeida A et al: Future caries susceptibility in children with early childhood caries following treatment under general anesthesia, *Pediatr Dent* 22:302, 2000.
76. Peretz B et al: Children with BBTD treated under general anesthesia or sedation: behaviour in a follow up visit, *J Clin Pediatr Dent* 24(2):97, 2000.
77. Weinstein P et al: Results of a promising open trial to prevent baby bottle tooth decay: a fluoride varnish study, *J Dent Child* 61:338, 1994.
78. Tang JM et al: Dental caries prevalence and treatment levels in Arizona preschool children, *Public Health Rep* 112:319, 1997.
79. Dunning JM: *Principles of dental public health practice,* Cambridge, MA, 1970, Harvard University Press.
80. Mushlin AI, Appel FA: Diagnosing patient noncompliance, *Arch Intern Med* 137:318, 1977.
81. American Academy of Pediatric Dentistry: Reference manual, *Pediatr Dent* 17(spec iss):2, 1995-1996.
82. Schneider HS: Parental education leads to preventive dental treatment for patients under the age of four, *J Dent Child* 60:33, 1993.
83. Goepfred SJ: Infant oral health: a protocol, *J Dent Child* 53:261, 1986.
84. Goepfred SJ: Infant oral health program: the first 18 months, *Pediatr Dent* 9:8, 1987.
85. Frandsen A: Mechanical oral hygiene practices: state-of-the-science review. In Loe H, Kleinman DV, editors: *Dental plaque control measures and oral hygiene practices,* Oxford, 1986, IRL Press.
86. Naylor MN, Murray JJ: Fluorides and dental caries. In Murray JJ, editor: *The prevention of dental disease,* Oxford, 1983, Oxford University Press.
87. Honkala E et al: Dental health habits in Austria, England, Finland and Norway, *Int Dent J* 38:131, 1988.
88. Blinkhorn AS, Hastings GB, Leather DS: Attitudes towards dental care among young people in Scotland: implications for dental health education, *Br Dent J* 155:311, 1983.
89. Blinkhorn AS, Taylor I, Willcox GF: Report of a dental health education program in Bedfordshire, *Br Dent J* 150:319, 1981.
90. Mertz-Fairhurst EJ, Schuster GS, Fairhust CW: Arresting caries by sealants: results of a clinical study, *J Am Dent Assoc* 112:194, 1986.
91. Frencken JE et al: An atraumatic restorative treatment (ART) technique: evaluation after one year, *Int Dent J* 44:460, 1994.
92. Eidelman E: Intentional sealing of occlusal dentin caries: a controversial issue, *Pediatr Dent* 15:312, 1993.
93. Brannstrom M: Infection beneath composite resin restorations: can it be avoided? *Oper Dent* 12:158, 1987.
94. Liebenberg WH: The fissure sealant impasse, *Quint Int* 25:741, 1994.
95. Ripa LW: Occlusal sealants: rationale and review of clinical trials, *Int Dent J* 30:127, 1980.

96. Shapira J, Eidelman E: Six-year clinical evaluation of fissure sealants placed after mechanical preparation: a matched pair study, *Pediatr Dent* 8:204, 1986.
97. Feigal RJ: Sealants and preventive restorations: review of effectiveness and clinical changes for improvement, *Pediatr Dent* 20:85, 1998.
98. Newbrun E: Sugar and dental caries: a review of human studies, *Science* 217:418, 1982.
99. Schou L: Social factors and dental caries. In Johnson NW, editor: *Dental caries, markers of high and low risk groups and individuals,* Cambridge, 1991, Cambridge University Press.
100. Schou L, Currie C, McQueen D: Using a "lifestyle" perspective to understand toothbrushing behavior in Scottish schoolchildren, *Commun Dent Oral Epidemiol* 18:230, 1990.
101. Corbin SB: Oral disease prevention technologies for community use, *Int J Technol Assess Health Care* 7:327, 1991.
102. Firestone AR, Schmid R, Muehlemann HR: Cariogenic effects of cooked wheat starch alone or with sucrose, and frequency-controlled feeding in rats, *Arch Oral Biol* 27:759, 1982.

PART

III

DISTRIBUTION OF DENTAL DISEASE AND PREVENTION

CHAPTER

8

EPIDEMIOLOGY OF ORAL DISEASES

David G. Pendrys

IMPORTANCE OF ORAL EPIDEMIOLOGY

A fundamental understanding of general epidemiologic principles, as well as knowledge of the epidemiology of oral diseases, can help practitioners, their patients, and society in several ways. A key component of the ethical, rational management of dental patients is an *assessment of risk* for future oral diseases. This assessment of risk is the rational foundation for the development and implementation of individualized preventive strategies for the patient. An understanding of the epidemiology of oral diseases is an essential step in this risk assessment process. Knowledge of how a patient's past and current disease status compares with others of the same age and gender is a valuable first step in the process of assessing the patient's future risk of disease. Knowledge of the underlying determinants of oral diseases (both risk and preventive factors), when compared with the patient's individual history, can meaningfully contribute to the development of an individualized preventive treatment plan for the patient.

A basic understanding of general epidemiologic principles provides the foundation for the important skill of critically interpreting new information as it becomes available in the literature and via presentations. An understanding of the strengths and limitations of epidemiologic research and the relative potential of a particular study design to contribute to a judgment of causation is fundamental to this process. When combined with a basic knowledge of oral disease epidemiology, knowledge of epidemiologic principles allows the practitioner to assess how consistent and coherent the new information is with past information and to judge what its impact will be.

Awareness by the practitioner of the epidemiology of oral diseases can be of broader benefit to society. The practitioner may be called on to be a source of expert guidance to the community on public health matters related to oral health. Only by having an understanding of the distribution and determinants of oral disease within populations and subgroups of the population, along with knowledge of risk and preventive factors, will the oral health practitioner be able to provide that expertise. In addition, the alert practitioner with an understanding of the epidemiology of oral diseases may be the first to identify the presence in the population of an unusual pattern of disease. The result of this can be profound. A classic example is Frederick McKay, who shortly after graduation from dental school called attention to the presence of an unusually high prevalence of enamel staining among his patients in Colorado Springs.[1] His further observation that these same patients had a lower caries prevalence led ultimately to the discovery that optimally fluoridated drinking water could dramatically reduce the incidence of caries, arguably the most important discovery made in the history of dental public health.

INTRODUCTION TO EPIDEMIOLOGY

Epidemiology is a discipline that strives to understand the occurrence of disease among groups of people. One of the more widely cited definitions defines epidemiology as "the study of the distribution and determinants of disease frequency in man."[2] Oral epidemiology is the application of epidemiologic principles to the study of oral diseases.

Epidemiologic investigations usually measure and report findings in terms of either the prevalence or incidence of disease. The *prevalence* of disease is the proportion of existing cases of a disease in a population at one point in time or during a specified period of time.[3] For example, one might report a caries prevalence of 20% in a population of adults, meaning that 20% of the population had existing caries at a particular point or period in time (e.g., spring 2001). The *incidence* of disease is the number of new cases of a disease that occur in a population at risk for the disease during a specific time period (e.g., 1 year or a period of years).[3] For example, one might report the incidence of caries in a population to be 20% per year, meaning that 20% of the population at risk for caries developed new caries during a 1-year period. Edentulous people in the population would not be part of this incidence calculation because these individuals, lacking any teeth, would not be at risk for caries. Sometimes the population at risk and time period are combined into a single measure of person-time (e.g., person-years).[3]

THE DESCRIPTIVE EPIDEMIOLOGIC STUDY

Much of the oral epidemiologic research done in the past has been descriptive in nature. Descriptive epidemiologic studies help define the extent of disease in a population. This type of study asks several basic questions. The first and perhaps most fundamental question is, "What is the disease or health outcome under study?" That is, what exactly defines one person as having the disease and another person as not having it? The formal terminology for this is to *state a case definition.* This is a critical and sometimes challenging first step in the understanding of a disease. Descriptive epidemiology attempts to determine who is getting the disease (e.g., the young, the elderly, males, females) and where the disease is occurring (e.g., across the United States, a particular geographic region, urban versus rural setting). Descriptive epidemiology also seeks to determine the specific timing of disease occurrence, or when it occurs (e.g., all the time, during tooth formation, following gingival recession). The findings of these studies often provide the basis for the generation of hypotheses concerning disease causation and prevention, which can be further investigated epidemiologically.

EPIDEMIOLOGIC STUDIES THAT TEST HYPOTHESES

Epidemiologic investigations that test hypotheses about disease causation and prevention can be broadly grouped into two categories: observational studies and experimental studies.

Observational studies attempt to assess the relationship between exposures and disease by observing exposure-disease associations as they naturally occur in the population under study. This exposure-disease relationship is usually reported in terms of an estimate of the relative risk of disease associated with a particular exposure. The relative risk can be defined as follows:[3]

$$\text{Relative risk} = \frac{\text{Incidence of disease in exposed group}}{\text{Incidence of disease in unexposed group}}$$

Because the relative risk is a ratio, a relative risk of 1.0 (i.e., a 1:1 ratio) represents no difference in risk of disease associated with an exposure. Relative risk estimates above 1.0 suggest increased risk of disease associated with the exposure, whereas relative risk estimates between 0 and 1.0 suggest a protective effect associated with the exposure. Because of the potential for bias and general noise in the data that inherently exists in epidemiologic studies (as contrasted with many laboratory studies), generally relative risk estimates that lie in the ranges of 0.7–1.0 and 1.0–1.5 are considered to be weak evidence of an association.[4] Generally speaking, relative risk estimates of greater than 3.0 or less than 0.3 are considered estimates of a strong association (in the direction of increased risk or protective effect, respectively).[4] Because many diseases may be associated with multiple exposures or other factors (e.g., age), some of which may be related to one another, it is important for risk factor studies to use study designs and statistical techniques that allow for a simultaneous assessment of the relationship between the disease of interest and these multiple exposures or factors.

Three main types of observational, hypothesis-testing epidemiologic studies exist: the cross-sectional study, the case-control study, and the cohort study. The cross-sectional study looks at both the exposure of interest and the disease outcome at the same point in time. A case-control study identifies subjects based on whether the disease of interest is present and then looks backwards in time, often via a history, for associations between the disease and one or more past exposures. The cohort study identifies subjects based on whether they have a particular exposure of interest and then follows them over time to see if an association exists between having the exposure and developing one or more diseases.

THE CROSS-SECTIONAL STUDY

Consider the hypothesis that the presence of a restoration near the gingival margin increases the risk of developing gingival inflammation (gingivitis) among adolescents. If researchers chose to conduct a cross-sectional study to explore this hypothesis, they might examine a group of adolescents for restorations at the gingival margin and then compare the occurrence of gingivitis among adolescents with and without these restorations. The researchers could then determine if there was an association between the presence of restorations and the presence of gingivitis. Although the cross-sectional study is relatively quick and inexpensive to do, its potential to contribute to a judgment of causation is limited because it cannot determine whether the exposure of interest (in this example, a restoration at the gingival margin) occurred before the disease of interest (gingivitis). For example, the argument could be made that adolescents with gingivitis might be less likely to brush because of gingival bleeding and sensitivity and therefore are at greater risk of developing caries requiring restoration near the gingival margin, subsequent to the presence of the gingivitis.

The Case-Control Study

If the researchers had instead chosen to conduct a case-control study to explore this same hypothesis, subjects would have been split into two groups, those with gingivitis and those without, based on an examination. To search for an association with restorations at the gingival margin, a history of restoration placement at the gingival margin before the occurrence of gingivitis would be sought, for example, through past dental records. Thus the case-control study could establish a temporal relationship between the exposure and disease of interest, in this case a history of restoration placement before the occurrence of gingivitis. This type of study is only as good as the techniques it uses to gain a good history of exposure. Also, because a case-control design ordinarily does not allow direct measurement of incidence rates, it must estimate the relative risk using a measure called the *odds ratio,* a valid, but indirect, estimator of the relative risk.[5]

The Prospective Cohort Study

If the researchers had chosen to conduct a prospective (forward-looking) cohort study, adolescents would have been divided into groups based on the presence or absence of restorations at the gingival margin and then followed over time to see who developed gingivitis and who did not. As with the case-control study, the prospective cohort study can establish a temporal relationship between the exposure and disease of interest. However, the prospective cohort design does not rely on a history to determine past exposure. Importantly, because the cohort study allows direct measurement of incidence rates, the relative risk of disease can be directly estimated using the formula given earlier in this chapter. However, this study design requires that subjects be followed for a potentially long period of time, during which they might move away or decide to quit the study. Further, as in this example, subjects initially in the "no restoration" group could develop caries and the need for restorations and thus have a mixed exposure history. Also, if the outcome of interest is rare, the prospective cohort design may not be practical because of the large number of subjects necessary to enroll at the outset to allow for sufficient occurrence of the disease.

The Retrospective (Historical) Cohort Study

The retrospective, or historical, cohort study is a variation of the prospective cohort study that eliminates the need for a prospective follow-up period. It is similar to the prospective cohort in design except that the exposure is determined by past exposure records, so that the follow-up period has already occurred at the time the study is begun. The feasibility of conducting a study of this design depends on the availability of suitable records of past exposure. In the restoration-gingivitis example, it would be reasonable to expect that past dental records would exist on which to historically establish exposure (i.e., the presence of restorations at the gingival margin), so this design might be highly useful.

THE CLINICAL TRIAL

The second broad category of hypothesis-testing epidemiologic studies is the experimental study. Experimental epidemiologic studies can be divided into two main types: the clinical trial and the community trial. Clinical trials are conducted to test new preventive or therapeutic agents, with subjects assigned by the investigator to different treatment groups, usually using some form of random assignment. A new treatment will generally be compared with either the current conventional therapy, if one exists, or a placebo (a nontherapeutic intervention). For example, a clinical trial might be constructed to test the gingivitis-reducing benefit of using a new restorative material for use at the gingival margin. In this example, a recruited sample of subjects who are in need of gingival margin restorations would be randomly (by chance) placed either into the group that will receive the new restorative material or into the group that will receive a currently used (conventional) restorative material. Well-designed clinical trials use a double-blind design, in which neither the subjects nor the investigator knows to which group a subject belongs. This design helps prevent the potential for a biased interpretation of treatment effect (better or worse) that might occur if either the subject or investigator knew to which treatment group (e.g., placebo or experimental agent) a subject belonged. Clinical trials compare the incidence of disease and side effects between the groups in the study to draw inferences about the safety and efficacy of the treatment(s) under investigation.

THE COMMUNITY TRIAL

Community trials are conducted in situations where an intervention can be practically evaluated only at the community level. In these studies, treatment is assigned on the basis of the community rather than the individual. The more that the comparison communities are similar in all aspects except the intervention under study, the more valid this type of study will be. The Newburgh-Kingston water fluoridation trial is a classic example of a community trial.[6]

CAUSATION

Although an epidemiologic study might identify an association between an exposure and a disease, that is not the same thing as "proving" that the exposure caused the disease. Demonstration of an association only indicates that there is some relationship between the exposure and the disease, of which one possibility is a causal relationship. In fact, no epidemiologic study can ever "prove" causation. Causation is a judgment that can only be arrived at following a consideration of all available evidence.[3] Over the years, criteria have been developed to aid in the process of arriving at a judgment of causation. The first criterion is the demonstration of a temporal relationship (i.e., it is established that the exposure of interest has preceded the disease in time). The second criterion when arriving at a judgment of causation is the strength of association (measured as relative risk); the stronger the association, the less likely the association is due to some other biasing factor. However, this criterion does not mean that a weak association cannot be causal. The third criterion is consistency of findings reported from different investigations on different populations. The greater the number of different studies showing a particular association, the less likely the association is due to some bias or deficiency in study design, because it becomes increasingly less likely that all of the studies would share the same particular bias or deficiency. A judgment of causation is further supported if the finding is coherent with existing knowledge, although it should be realized that "existing knowledge" is continuously changing. There is no rule as to when it is appropriate for a judgment of causation to be made. Consideration of the consequences of accepting a judgment of causation balanced against the consequences of delaying acceptance is often part of the process.

EPIDEMIOLOGY OF DENTAL CARIES

THE MEASUREMENT OF CARIES

Caries is the pathologic process of localized destruction of tooth tissues by microorganisms.[7] Dental caries can be described epidemiologically in several useful ways, each of which helps our understanding of caries activity within groups of people. The conventional method of defining dental caries in a population is to measure either the number of teeth or the number of tooth surfaces that are decayed, missing, or filled as a result of caries. When this measure is applied to the permanent dentition, the acronyms DMFT and DMFS are used, indicating the number of decayed, missing, or filled teeth (DMFT) or decayed, missing, or filled surfaces (DMFS).[8] When this measure is applied to the primary dentition, the acronyms deft and defs are used, with e indicating a carious primary tooth that is indicated for extraction.[9] Because of confusion over how this "e" term should be interpreted and applied, recent surveys often simply report decayed or filled teeth (dft) or decayed or filled surfaces (dfs). Measuring caries by surfaces affected (i.e., the DMFS or DFS) is more precise than measuring caries by affected teeth because, for example, a tooth with five surfaces affected by caries would make the same contribution to the DMFT score as a tooth with only one affected surface. At the same time, however, the DMFT can be a useful public health measure because it is an indicator of the number of teeth that have had or require treatment. The missing teeth component of the DMFT and DMFS assumes that missing teeth have been lost because of caries. Although this assumption is reasonable for children, among adults, the older the population, the more likely it becomes that teeth may be lost as a result of other causes, for example, periodontal disease. For this reason a DFS is often used to measure caries in adult populations. Although this measure may underestimate total caries experience (because teeth missing as a result of caries are not included), it avoids a biased overestimate that would result from including missing teeth that were not lost because of caries.

Although the DMFS is a useful measure, it is often important to be more specific in the measurement of the presentation of caries in a population. One important measure with public health implications is the proportion of the overall DMFS that is untreated caries, or the decayed teeth component of the DMFS or DFS. The D/DMFS (D/DFS) ratio is often presented as a percent and is a measure of the level of treatment need in a population: the higher the value of this ratio, the higher the unmet need in the population under study.

A second important way to specify caries activity is on the basis of the type of tooth surface that has been affected by decay. Thus the presence of caries in a population can be described in terms of coronal pit and fissure caries, coronal smooth surface caries, and root surface caries. Describing caries in this surface-specific way can provide greater insights into potential risk factors and allow for more effective planning of preventive strategies.

A third important way to specify caries is to draw the distinction between primary caries, caries that occurs on unrestored tooth surfaces, and recurrent or secondary caries, caries that occurs adjacent to an existing restoration. The presence of these distinct types of caries can have different implications for the management of caries in the individual patient or in the population at large.

Caries in Children

Several demographic factors have been consistently shown to be related to the occurrence of caries. These factors are associated with either the person or the environment in which that person has lived. As with many diseases, age is directly and strongly associated with the prevalence of dental caries. The relationship between age and caries is illustrated in Fig. 8-1, drawn from two National Institute of Dental and Craniofacial Research (NIDCR) surveys of the oral health of U.S. children and adults.[10,11] One can see that with increasing age the number of

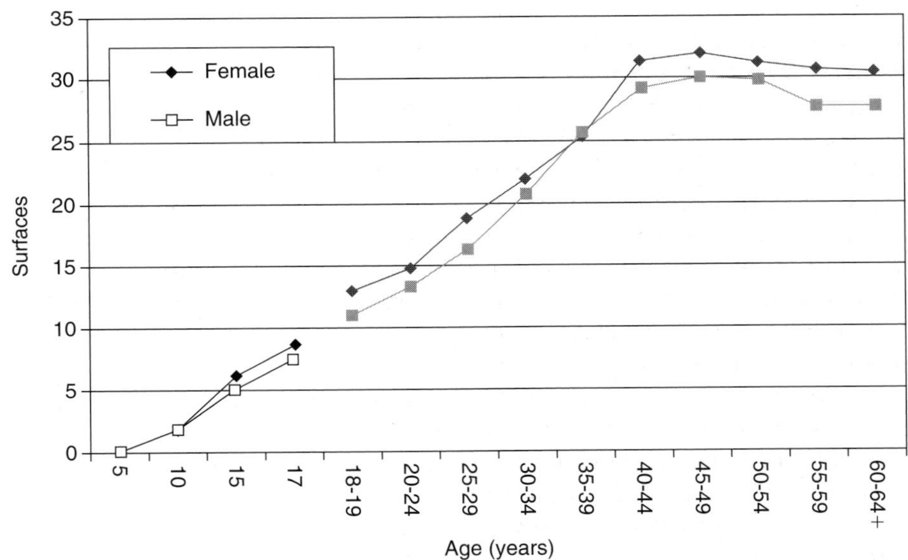

Fig 8-1. Relationship between age, gender, and mean DMFS among U.S. children and mean DFS among U.S. adults. (Modified from US Department of Health and Human Services: *Oral health of United States children: the National Survey of Dental Caries in U.S. School Children: 1986-1987,* National Institutes of Health pub no 89-2247, Washington, DC, 1989, US Government Printing Office; US Department of Health and Human Services: *Oral health of United States adults: the National Survey of Oral Health in U.S. Employed Adults and Seniors: 1985-1986,* National Institutes of Health pub no 87-2868, Washington, DC, 1987, US Government Printing Office.)

surfaces affected by caries increases, plateauing at around 50 years of age. This figure also illustrates the relationship between caries and gender. One can see that the mean DMFS for males tends to lag behind that of females. For example, 14-year-old boys have approximately the same mean DMFS as 13-year-old girls (i.e., 4.2 mean DMF surfaces). One explanation for this finding is the parallel finding that the dentition appears to erupt earlier in girls.[12,13] Thus at any given age the dentition in males has been at risk for a shorter period of time as compared with females.

The relationship between race and caries is more equivocal. Although in the past, some studies had reported a lower caries prevalence among African-American children as compared with Caucasian children, others had reported either a higher caries prevalence among African-Americans or no difference.[14] Two recent national surveys in the United States indicate little difference in caries prevalence between Caucasian and African-American children.[10,13] However, consistent differences in the extent to which caries has been treated were found. For example, the NHANES III survey reported that although the mean DMFS for Caucasian and African-American children was virtually identical, untreated decay was more than twice as high among African-American children.[13]

Historically, the prevalence of caries in the United States has varied by geographic region of the country. This finding can be traced back to the time of the Civil War and continues today.[14] The advent of artificial water fluoridation has had a profound effect on the distribution of caries. Historically, the prevalence of caries would be as much as 60% lower in fluoridated areas as compared with nonfluoridated areas.[15] Today, this type of comparison is less meaningful, because children living in areas not served by a fluoridated water supply may be indirectly benefiting from it by drinking beverages manufactured in a fluoridated community and thus prepared with fluoridated water.[16,17] National survey data show that the greater the number of fluoridated communities in a region, the less the difference in caries prevalence between children living in fluoridated and nonfluoridated communities.[18]

Important secular changes have occurred in the prevalence of dental caries in the United States and elsewhere. Figure 8-2 shows findings drawn from four national surveys.[13,19] Two important trends can be seen in this figure. The first is that the

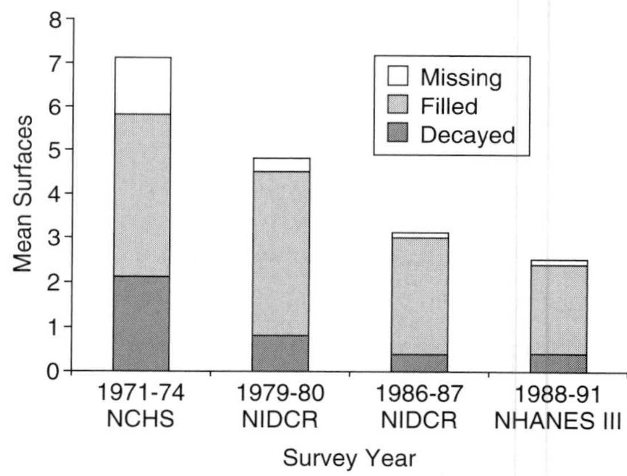

Fig. 8-2. Changes in DMFS prevalence among U.S. children, 1971–1991. (Data from Brunelle JA, Carlos JP: Changes in the prevalence of dental caries in U.S. schoolchildren, 1961-1980, *J Dent Res* 61:1346, 1982; US Department of Health and Human Services: *Oral health of United States children: the National Survey of Dental Caries in U.S. School Children: 1986-1987,* National Institutes of Health pub no 89-2247, Washington, DC, 1989, US Government Printing Office; Kaste LM et al: Coronal caries in the primary and permanent dentition of children and adolescents 1-17 years of age: United States, 1988-1991, *J Dent Res* 75(spec iss):631, 1996.)

prevalence of caries in the United States declined substantially between the early 1970s and late 1980s. Whereas the mean DMFS for U.S. children ages 5 through 17 was 7.1 during the early 1970s, this value had dropped to 2.5 by the late 1980s, a 65% reduction. At the same time, it can be seen from the figure that the proportion of DMFS that is either untreated caries or missing surfaces has also dramatically fallen during this period. As mean DMFS has fallen, the proportion of caries-free children has increased. For example, the percentage of 12- to 17-year-old children in the United States who are caries free had increased threefold from 10.4% in the early 1970s to 32.7% in the late 1980s.[13,19] A similar decline in the prevalence of caries in the permanent dentition of children has occurred throughout other Western countries as well,[20-23] with this decline in Western countries being widely attributed to the use of fluorides.[22]

Although these findings represent significant success on the part of efforts to reduce the prevalence of caries, it is important to remember that these values represent averages over a large (5 to 17 years) age span. For example, although the mean DMFS for 10-year-old children in the 1986–1987 NIDCR national survey was 1.7, the mean DMFS was four times as high (i.e., 8.0 DMF surfaces) among 17-year-olds.[10] Similarly, whereas 97% of 5-year-olds were caries free, only 16% of 17-year-olds were caries free.[10] There has also been a change in the contribution of specific surface types to the total DMFS. Although the proportion of DMF surfaces that were proximal smooth surfaces has decreased by half from 24% to 12% during the past 20 years, the portion of the DMFS that is occlusal and buccal lingual surfaces has proportionally increased.[10] Thus the greatest relative reductions in caries have occurred on the smooth surfaces, again strongly suggesting the role of fluoride in the decline in caries prevalence.[22,24]

A decline in caries prevalence has also occurred in the primary dentition.[10,13,19] A comparison of the 1979–1980 and 1986–1987 NIDCR national surveys showed that mean dfs among 5- to 9-year-old children declined from 5.3 surfaces to 3.9 surfaces, a 26% decline.[10] The NHANES III 1988–1991 survey reported that 50% of 5- to 9-year-old children and 83% of 2- to 4-year-old children were caries free in the primary dentition.[13] A similar decline in the prevalence of caries in the primary dentition has occurred in other Western countries.[20,22,23]

Early Childhood Caries

A distinct form of caries in the primary dentition is early childhood caries (ECC), known formerly in the literature as "nursing caries."[25] A recent, thorough review of ECC illustrates the difficulty in describing this condition epidemiologically because of differences in clinical diagnostic criteria and case definition, study designs, and populations studied.[26] For example, the review reported that the prevalence of ECC ranged from 0.8% to 64% across the 71 population studies they reviewed.[26] Nevertheless, the current best estimate of ECC prevalence in the United States is approximately 5% nationwide.[25,27] However, the literature further indicates important ECC prevalence difference across children of different race, ethnic, and socioeconomic background, with ethnic minority and lower socioeconomic status children being at greatest risk.[28] For example, a recent report of a statewide study of Arizona preschool children who participated in federal assistance programs reported a caries prevalence of

25% by age 3 years.[29] The exact etiologic mechanism(s) responsible for the development of ECC remain to be clearly defined.[30,31] A recent national workshop recommended that ECC be defined as the presence of one or more primary tooth surfaces affected by caries (i.e., decayed, missing, or filled).[32] This workshop further recommended that the term *severe early childhood caries* (S-ECC) be applied to the occurrence of caries that was either atypical, progressive, acute, or rampant in nature, using specific suggested criteria.[32] The development and acceptance of consistent ECC case definitions will be an important step in clarifying both the prevalence and etiologic mechanism(s) of this disease. Despite these current limitations, preventive strategies have been proposed, based on an understanding of the set of risk and preventive factors that may play a role, including early mutans streptococci colonization and poor oral hygiene, frequent ingestion of fermentable carbohydrates, enamel hypoplasia, and limited exposure to fluorides.[26,30,31,33,34] These strategies include community interventions, such as water fluoridation; professional interventions, such as early detection and sealants; and home care, including proper diet and oral hygiene habits.[26]

Coronal Caries in Adults

Nearly all dentate U.S. adults have at least one decayed or filled tooth.[11,35] Mean DFS continues to rise with age until around 50, after which it plateaus at approximately 30 DF surfaces, as illustrated in Fig. 8-1.[11,35] Data from U.S. national surveys of adults indicate that Caucasians have a significantly higher coronal DFS as compared with non-Caucasians. For example, the NHANES III survey reported that Caucasians had a mean coronal DFS twice as high as African-Americans (i.e., 24 surfaces and 12 surfaces, respectively).[35] However, although surveys have estimated that the proportion of untreated coronal caries for the entire U.S. population is less than 15%, this proportion is approximately three times higher in African-American adults than in Caucasians.[11,35]

The prevalence of coronal caries has declined in recent decades among U.S. adults under age 45 years.[36] Actual prevalence estimates vary widely, but a decrease in the prevalence of coronal caries among adults has also been observed in other Western countries.[20,21,37,38]

Root Surface Caries

Wide variation in the methods used to diagnose and report root surface caries, in particular in the case definition used, has made the comparison of findings from different investigations challenging.[39-42] This has led to estimates of root caries prevalence that vary widely.[41] The two most recent U.S. national adult surveys suggest that between 20% and 25% of U.S. adults have at least one root surface that has been affected by caries.[11,35] This prevalence is virtually identical between Caucasians and African-Americans, as is the average root surface DFS, which is approximately equal to one surface.[11,23] The prevalence of root caries increases with age.[11,35,41,43] For example, the findings of the most recent national survey show the prevalence of root surface caries rising steadily from 7% among 18- to 24-year-olds to 56% among those 75 years and older.[35] In contrast to coronal caries, the proportion of untreated root surface caries can be high (50% in the most recent

U.S. national survey).[35] As is the case with coronal caries, minorities have a much higher proportion of untreated root surfaces as compared with Caucasians.[35] Importantly, as with coronal caries, the prevalence and incidence of root caries are lower in areas served by fluoridated drinking water.[41]

In the absence of pathology, root surfaces are not exposed to the oral environment and are therefore not at risk of carious attack. Thus, although root surface DFS is a useful prevalence measure, root caries incidence is best measured in terms of root surfaces at risk.[42,44-46] The Root Caries Index, which counts only exposed root surfaces as being at risk for root surface caries, was developed to address this important issue.[44,45]

Caries "Polarization" and Risk Assessment

Descriptive caries data indicate that in addition to there having been a marked decrease in the prevalence of caries, there has also been a change in the pattern of dental caries in the United States and other countries, with most of the caries occurring among 20% to 30% of the population.[13,23,47,48] For example, the NHANES III survey found that 80% of the total DMFT for children ages 5 through 17 years occurred among 25% of the children.[13] These findings have led to attempts in recent years to develop methods and models by which people at high risk for future caries attack can be identified out of a population generally at low risk.[49-58]

The concept that caries is a multifactorial disease has long been understood and accepted, and individual factors affecting the risk for caries have been identified for many years.[59] These factors include the presence of specific microorganisms, such as *Streptococcus mutans;* dietary factors, such as the proportion and frequency of dietary carbohydrate; salivary factors, such as salivary flow rate; and host factors, such as age and health behaviors.[49,60] A series of analytic epidemiologic investigations has been conducted in an effort to identify comprehensive models of future coronal caries risk; however, the complex, multifactorial nature of the caries process makes this a challenging task.[49-58] To date, past caries experience (i.e., DFS) and salivary *S. mutans* and *Lactobacillus* levels have been found to be the best predictors of future coronal caries risk.[50-58,61] Studies have also identified sugar consumption as an indicator of future caries risk.[62,63] Studies indicate that factors such as fluoridation status, past root caries experience, age, number of teeth, gingival recession, number of decayed coronal surfaces, and use of sugared foods are predictors of root surface caries.[41,63,64]

EPIDEMIOLOGY OF PERIODONTAL DISEASE

Periodontal disease has been defined by Loe[65] as "a group of lesions affecting the tissues surrounding and supporting the teeth in their sockets." The vast majority of periodontal disease cases can be classified as either gingivitis or periodontitis.

Gingivitis is a disease characterized by inflammation restricted to the gingival soft tissues, with no loss of alveolar bone or apical migration of the periodontal ligament along the root surface.[66] Clinically, the signs of gingivitis are erythema, edema, and gingival bleeding.[66] Gingival diseases can be divided into two main categories: those that are associated with the presence of dental plaque and those that are not.[67] Plaque-induced gingival disease can be further categorized as to whether it is related to the presence of plaque only, or whether it is also associated with systemic conditions, such as the presence of blood dyscrasias; use of medications, such as oral contraceptives; or malnutrition, especially ascorbic acid (vitamin C) deficiency.[68] Periodontitis is characterized by inflammation that extends beyond the gingiva to the periodontal structures, causing destruction of the periodontal ligament attachment and alveolar bony support and leading to migration of the junctional epithelium apical to the cementoenamel junction.[69,70] The two major categories of periodontitis are chronic periodontitis (formerly classified as adult periodontitis) and aggressive periodontitis (formerly characterized as early-onset or juvenile periodontitis).[67] These changes in terminology reflect the consensus of a recent workshop organized by the Academy of Periodontology.[71,72] The decision to abandon the terms *adult periodontitis* and *early-onset* or *juvenile periodontitis* was based on the observation that these forms of periodontitis can each occur across a wide age range, affecting children, adolescents, and adults.[72] In addition to these two major categories, other categories of periodontitis include periodontitis as a manifestation of systemic disease, such as hematologic or genetic disorders; necrotizing periodontal diseases, a condition usually seen in the presence of underlying systemic conditions such as human immunodeficiency virus (HIV) infection; abscesses of the periodontium, a condition that, although associated with other forms of periodontitis, is considered a distinct condition in terms of diagnosis and treatment; periodontitis associated with endodontic lesions; and periodontitis associated with developmental or acquired conditions such as tooth anatomy or the presence of dental restorations.[67] Clinically, the signs of periodontitis can include loss of soft tissue attachment, gingival recession, tooth migration, mobility, and tooth loss.[66,73,74] Most cases of gingivitis and periodontitis occur as a result of the presence of bacterial plaque on the gingiva and subgingival tooth surfaces and calculus.[69] It is generally accepted that periodontal disease begins as gingivitis, which progresses, only in some individuals, to periodontitis, with severe periodontitis affecting only a small percentage of the population.[66,75]

Measurement of Periodontal Disease

Historically, several indices were developed in an attempt to provide a standardized method of measuring periodontal disease among groups of people in epidemiologic studies, most notably the Periodontal Index and the Periodontal Disease Index.[76,77] Both of these indices have been criticized on methodologic grounds, especially because they combine gingivitis and periodontitis measures into a common score.[78,79] For this reason, neither of these indices is considered the best method to measure periodontal disease. Another index, which gained considerable international popularity, is the Community Periodontal Index of Treatment Needs (CPITN), developed by the World Health Organization (WHO) to provide a means to summarize treatment needs.[80,81] To do this, the CPITN combines an assessment of gingival health, pocket depth, and the presence of supragingival and subgingival calculus.[80,81] Proponents of the CPITN state that the CPITN allows for a rapid, simple, uniform method by which the average periodontal status and treatment needs of international populations can be determined using minimal equipment. It has been further argued that the use of a widely understood index facilitates the formulation of international goals for periodontal health and that this index has been used in more than 100 countries to generate data for the WHO Global Oral Data Bank.[82] However, critics of the CPITN argue that the combination of gingival health, pocket depth, and presence of calculus into a combined score is not consistent with current approaches to describing periodontal disease and that failure of the CPITN to measure gingival recession leads to an inaccurate estimate of attachment loss.[78] A consensus report of the American Academy of Periodontology concluded that it is an inappropriate measure with which to assess the prevalence and severity of periodontal disease.[83,84]

The Gingival Index (GI) was introduced to provide an index that measured only inflammation of the gingiva and that would allow a clear distinction to be made between the location or quantity of gingivitis and the severity or quality of the gingivitis.[85,86] The GI accomplishes this by applying a four-category qualitative assessment (normal, mild, moderate, or severe inflammation) to four sites on each examined tooth. These values can then be averaged to yield a score for the individual.[85,86] The GI has become a mainstay index of gingivitis.[87] At the same time, it has become generally accepted that periodontitis should be measured and reported separately from gingivitis, characterized in terms of extent, or number of affected sites, and severity in terms of loss of periodontal attachment measured in millimeters.[72] For example, U.S. national surveys have reported the prevalence and extent of periodontitis in terms of loss of periodontal attachment, measured in millimeters.[11,88]

The varied use of different indices in past surveys of periodontal disease has made direct comparison of the findings from one survey to another difficult. This situation illustrates the importance in epidemiology of how disease is measured and how a case of the disease is defined. Nevertheless, some broad conclusions can be drawn from these data. The two most recent U.S. national surveys (the NIDCR U.S. Employed Adult Survey[11] and the NHANES III survey[88]) used similar methodologies, allowing a comparison to be made. Although the NHANES III survey included a broader age range of individuals (younger as well as older) as compared with the U.S. Employed Adult Survey, the findings of the two surveys are generally similar.

Gingivitis

Both of the most recent U.S. national surveys suggest that the prevalence of gingivitis declines from its highest during the second and third decades and remains relatively constant after age 30 years.[11,88] The surveys differ in their estimates of the prevalence of gingivitis, the Employed Adults Survey reporting an average gingivitis prevalence of 44% compared with the NHANES III estimated gingivitis prevalence of 63%.[11,88] These surveys also reported that from one half to two thirds of U.S. adults have subgingival calculus, affecting between 22% and 34% of available sites per person.[11,88]

Chronic Periodontitis

Chronic periodontitis is the most common form of periodontitis.[89] The prevalence, extent, and severity of chronic periodontitis increase with age.[90] The two most recent national surveys both suggest that the loss of some attachment is virtually ubiquitous among U.S. adults. The prevalence estimate for having at least one site with 1 mm or more of attachment loss was between 92.5% (NHANES III) and 99.7% (U.S. Employed Adult Survey).[11,88] Importantly, however, the two surveys are consistent in suggesting that both the prevalence and the extent of more severe attachment loss are markedly lower.[11,88] Whereas the prevalence of attachment loss of 3 mm or greater among U.S. adults is approximately 40% to 45%, the prevalence of attachment loss of 5 mm or greater is less than 15%.[11,88] Similarly, whereas between 7% and 10% of available sites had lost at least 3 mm of attachment, fewer than 3% had lost as much as 5 mm or more.[11,88]

Periodontal disease is recognized as an important cause of gingival recession.[74] The U.S. Employed Adult Survey reported 51% of individuals to have at least one site with 1 mm or more of recession, affecting on average 10% of available sites.[11] Similarly, the NHANES III survey reported this prevalence to be 42%, affecting 11% of available sites.[88]

In both surveys males were found to be more likely to suffer attachment loss and gingival recession.[11,88] The Employed Adult Survey reported African-Americans to have a higher prevalence of attachment loss and gingival recession as compared with Caucasians.[11] The NHANES III data suggested that African-Americans were more likely to have more severe attachment loss (i.e., 3 mm or greater) and more severe gingival recession (i.e., 3 mm or greater) compared with Caucasians.[88] Factors related to socioeconomic status (SES) appear to play an important role in these observed racial differences.[91] An analysis of NHANES III data suggests that the prevalence of both gingivitis and loss of attachment is higher among lower-SES groups.[92]

Aggressive Periodontitis

Aggressive periodontitis is characterized by rapid loss of periodontal attachment and bone destruction in otherwise healthy individuals.[71] There also appears to be a tendency for this condition to cluster within families.[71] Often the severity of periodontal destruction is beyond what would be expected given the amount of plaque present, but it may be self-arresting.[71] Other common features of this disease are the presence of elevated proportions of *Actinobacillus actinomycetemcomitans* and *Porphyromonas gingivalis* in the plaque, phagocyte abnormalities, and the presence of hyperresponsive macrophages.[71] Aggressive periodontitis is classified as either localized or generalized.[71] Localized aggressive periodontitis is characterized by having an onset around the time of puberty with a localized attachment loss on the proximal surfaces of the first molars and incisor teeth and, by definition, no more than two other teeth involved.[71] This form of aggressive periodontitis is also marked by a strong serum antibody response to the infection.[71] Generalized aggressive periodontitis is characterized by an onset that usually (but not always) occurs before age 30 and a generalized loss of interproximal attachment that affects at least three permanent teeth other than the first molars and incisors, with the loss of attachment and alveolar bone occurring in discrete episodes.[71] In further contrast to localized aggressive periodontitis, generalized aggressive periodontitis is marked by a weak serum antibody response to the infection.[71] Aggressive periodontitis is a rare disease, with most reports indicating a prevalence of 1 to 8 cases per 1000.[79,93-96] A U.S. national survey estimated that the prevalence of all forms of aggressive periodontitis was 6.6

cases per 1000, 80% of which were the localized form.[79] The incidence rate for all forms of aggressive periodontitis among 14- and 15-year-olds in the United States was 1.5 cases per 1000 person-years at risk.[97] Familial aggregation of aggressive periodontitis cases has been established.[98,99] Some studies have suggested that the prevalence is higher in females than in males,[93,95] but other studies have not found this relationship,[94,96] most notably the 1986–1987 U.S. national survey.[79] Some studies have reported important racial differences in prevalence.[79,94] The 1986–1987 U.S. survey found African-Americans to be 15 to 22 times more likely than Caucasians to have aggressive periodontitis, depending on whether it was localized or generalized.[79]

Risk Assessment Investigations

Although there has long been a consensus that bacteria are essential for gingivitis and periodontitis to occur,[65,100,101] there is also a consensus that most gingivitis does not become periodontitis.[66] Considerable attention has been given in recent years to attempting to develop models that will predict which individuals and which sites within individuals will progress to periodontitis. In this regard, periodontitis is considered to have multiple risk factors. These factors can be divided into three groups: host factors, specific bacteria, and environmental factors.[101] Host factors include genetic factors, increasing age, and the presence of systemic disease (e.g., diabetes mellitus).[101, 102] Specific gram-negative anaerobic bacteria are associated with periodontitis.[103] These include, for example, *P. gingivalis, Bacteroides forsythus,* and *A. actinomycetemcomitans.*[100,104] Environmental risk factors for periodontitis include such factors as poor oral hygiene, the presence of subgingival calculus, and tobacco smoking, a habit that has been shown to be an important environmental risk factor for periodontitis.[105-109] Although specific factors associated with periodontitis have been identified, important questions remain. For example, it has been observed that although specific bacteria may be isolated from individuals with severe periodontitis, these same bacteria can also be found in individuals free of disease.[100,101] Models that have been developed to date are not yet able to satisfactorily separate persons and individual sites within persons that are at high risk of future periodontitis from those that are at low risk.[110] Currently, the best indicator of future disease at a specific periodontal site is evidence of past disease.[111,112] One complicating aspect of this search for a comprehensive model by which risk for periodontitis can be assessed has been the realization that multiple diseases probably exist under the term *chronic periodontitis.*[112] Thus an important step in the process of risk assessment for periodontitis may be a continued refinement of case definitions for periodontitis.

EPIDEMIOLOGY OF TOOTH LOSS

Prevalence of Tooth Loss

Tooth loss among children and adults in the United States has been declining for many years.[113,114] Edentulism affects 11% of all adults or less, depending on the survey.[11,114] A steady decline in tooth loss has been observed in other countries as well.[38] More than 30% of U.S. adults retain all of their teeth (excluding third molars).[11,115] Tooth loss is higher elsewhere in the world.[116-119]

The loss of teeth is age related, with the average number of retained teeth decreasing and the prevalence of edentulism increasing as age increases.[11,114,115,120-124] Even so, U.S. adults retain more than 75% of their teeth as late as the seventh decade of life, and even the most elderly retain more than half of their teeth.[11,115] Studies suggest that tooth loss is not associated with gender.[11,115,120-122,124]

Causes of Tooth Loss

The principal reported cause of tooth loss across all ages in the United States is caries,[125,126] which has been generally found to be the most common cause of tooth loss in other countries throughout the world.[127-138] However, studies suggest that above age 45 periodontal disease also becomes an important cause of tooth loss,[126-129,133-138] with some studies suggesting that it becomes the most common cause of tooth loss in this age group,[128,129,135,136] whereas others indicate that caries remains the principal cause.[137,138] Studies further suggest that tooth loss is associated with lower SES.[113,114,124,125,139-141]

EPIDEMIOLOGY OF ORAL CANCER

Descriptive Findings

Approximately 30,000 new cases of oral and pharyngeal cancer are diagnosed annually in the United States,[142] the great majority of which are squamous cell carcinomas, as is also true in other parts of the world.[143-145] Recent Surveillance, Epidemiology, and End Results (SEER) data indicate that the annual age-adjusted incidence of oral and pharyngeal cancer in the United States is 9.7 new cases per 100,000.[146] However, these rates vary substantially by gender, with males showing an annual age-adjusted incidence rate of 14.5 per 100,000 compared with 5.6 per 100,000 for females.[146] In the United States, oral and pharyngeal cancer accounts for 3% of new cancers among males and 1.6% of new cancers among females.[142] Oral and pharyngeal cancer rates vary widely across the globe.[147] For example, from 1988 to 1992, standardized oral cancer incidence rates in India were estimated to be as high as approximately 13 per 100,000, compared with incidence estimates of approximately 5 per 100,000 in Scotland and 2 per 100,000 in Finland.[147]

The incidence of oral and pharyngeal cancers increases with age and is relatively uncommon before age 40.[148] Table 8-1 illustrates the variation in incidence rates for oral and pharyngeal cancer in the United States associated with anatomic site, race, and gender. Cancers of the lip and oral cavity account for approximately two thirds of all incident (new) oral and pharyngeal cancers, with the tongue being the most common site of incident cancers of the oral cavity.[148] The overall incidence rate of oral and pharyngeal cancer is higher among men than among women. Although Caucasians have a markedly higher incidence rate for lip cancer, overall, male African-Americans show the highest oral and pharyngeal cancer incidence rates, with these rates being markedly higher for pharyngeal sites.[148]

Recent SEER data indicate that the incidence of oral and pharyngeal cancer decreased in the United States by approximately 1.1% per year from 1981 to 1997, with the decline in incidence rates being relatively similar for Caucasians and African-Americans.[146] This decline contrasts with an overall annual increase of 0.8% during the previous 8-year period.[146]

Table 8-1 Age-Adjusted Oral and Pharyngeal Cancer Incidence Rates (per 100,000) in the United States Stratified by Gender, Race, and Selected Anatomic Sites, 1983–1987

Site	*Caucasian Men*	*African-American Men*	*All Men*	*Caucasian Women*	*African-American Women*	*All Women*	*All Persons*
Lip	3.0	0.1	2.7	0.3	0.1	0.3	1.4
Tongue	3.2	4.9	3.3	1.4	1.5	1.4	2.3
Floor of mouth	1.9	3.2	1.9	0.7	0.6	0.7	1.3
Total oral cavity	11.8	12.8	11.6	4.7	4.3	4.6	7.7
Total pharynx	5.0	11.8	5.7	1.8	2.7	1.9	3.6
Total oral cavity and pharynx	16.8	24.5	17.3	6.5	7.0	6.5	11.3

Modified from US Department of Health and Human Services: *Cancers of the oral cavity and pharynx: a statistics review monograph 1973-1987,* Atlanta, 1991, Centers for Disease Control and Prevention.

A recent analysis of Connecticut Tumor Registry data suggests that there was a long-term decline in age-adjusted lip cancer incidence rates during the 60-year period from 1935 to 1994 (93% decrease for males, 75% decrease for females).[149] Among males there was a relatively steady 60-year decline of 24% in age-adjusted incidence rates for all oral and pharyngeal cancers combined.[149] By contrast, among females there was a relatively steady 50-year, twofold increase in these incidence rates through the early 1980s, with these rates beginning to show a decline only after that period.[149] The effect of this is that although age-adjusted incidence rates among males were approximately ninefold those of females for the 1935–1939 period (17.7 per 100,000 and 2.0 per 100,000, respectively), this fell to an approximately threefold difference (13.5 per 100,000 and 5.2 per 100,000, respectively) for the 1990–1994 period.[149]

Another recent analysis of SEER data suggests that in contrast to the generally declining trends in overall oral cancer incidence rates, incidence rate trends for in situ carcinoma have been increasing, perhaps as a result of increased surveillance.[150] This analysis reported that overall, in situ head and neck cancer incidence rates increased from approximately 6.3 per 1,000,000 person-years in 1976 to 8.0 per 1,000,000 person-years in 1995.[150] Incidence rates for in situ oral cancer alone (exclusive of lip) increased from 1.9 per 1,000,000 person-years to 2.67 per 1,000,000 person-years during that period.[150]

Approximately 8000 deaths occur each year in the United States as the result of oral and pharyngeal cancer, representing 1.7% of all cancer deaths among men and 1% of all cancer deaths among women.[142] Internationally, oral and pharyngeal cancer mortality rates vary markedly. For example, from 1990 to 1993 the age-adjusted oral cancer mortality rate among men in the Netherlands was 2.8 per 100,000, compared with 12.9 per 100,000 in France.[151]

Overall, the 5-year survival rate for oral and pharyngeal cancers is approximately 50%.[148] However, survival rates for oral and pharyngeal cancer vary considerably depending on cancer site, gender, and race. This is illustrated in Table 8-2, which shows that whereas 5-year survival rates for cancer of the lip are approximately 90%, the sur-

Table 8-2 Oral Cancer 5-Year Survival Rates (Percent) in the United States Stratified by Gender, Race, and Selected Anatomic Sites, 1981–1986

Site	Caucasian Men	African-American Men	All Men	Caucasian Women	African-American Women	All Women	All Persons
Lip	91.1	*	91.1	84.5	*	83.7	90.2
Tongue	45.8	19.8	42.8	49.7	43.7	49.1	45.0
Floor of mouth	52.9	31.0	49.8	60.7	44.9	59.2	52.9
Pharynx	31.0	22.3	30.9	38.4	26.4	37.5	32.9
Total oral cavity and pharynx	52.0	26.8	49.0	56.3	42.5	54.8	50.9

Modified from US Department of Health and Human Services: *Cancers of the oral cavity and pharynx: a statistics review monograph 1973-1987*, Atlanta, 1991, Centers for Disease Control and Prevention.

*Valid survival rates could not be calculated because of the small number of cases.

vival rate for cancers of the tongue is approximately half that when all persons are considered together and is only approximately 20% among African-American males, who have the overall poorest oral cancer survival rates. Women tend to have higher survival rates, with the exception of cancer of the lip. Although pharyngeal cancers account for only approximately one third of all incident oral and pharyngeal cancers, they have a relatively poor survival rate, accounting for nearly 50% of all deaths attributed to oral and pharyngeal cancer.[148] From 1979 to 1997 the mortality rate of oral and pharyngeal cancer declined by approximately 1.9% per year.[146] Until 1993 African-Americans showed a somewhat smaller annual percent decline in mortality rate from oral cancer (1.3%) compared with the annual decline for Caucasians between 1977 and 1997 (1.9%).[146] However, more recently (1993 to 1997) the annual percent decline in mortality rate for African-Americans grew to 4.5%.[146] Cancer stage is also an important predictor of survival.[152] Overall, localized oral cancer has an 81% 5-year survival rate, compared with 42% for cancers that have spread regionally and 17% for those with distant metastases.[152] Overall, individuals with a history of oral cancer are more likely to develop additional new aerodigestive tract cancerous lesions, with 25% of all oral cancer deaths caused by these so-called second primary cancerous lesions.[152]

Risk and Protective Factors

Smoking tobacco and drinking alcoholic beverages have both been shown to increase the risk of oral and pharyngeal cancer, based on consistent evidence from many studies, conducted by different researchers, across many different populations.[153-162] A dose-response relationship has also been demonstrated between both smoking and drinking and oral cancer, with a history of heavy smoking or heavy drinking over many years having been shown to convey a strong risk for developing oral cancer.[153-162] Importantly, many studies have demonstrated that a history of both smoking and drinking conveys an increased risk of oral cancer that is greater than the sum of the increased risks associated with either smoking or drinking alone.[153,155-158,160] This same relationship has been observed between smoking and drinking combined and the risk of oral epithelial dysplasia, a histopathologic condition associated with increased risk of oral cancer.[163] At the same time, studies have reported that high fruit consumption is associated with a decreased risk of oral cancer.[164-166]

Smoking and drinking account for 75% of the oral cancers in the United States and the world.[153,167] It is important therefore that studies have also demonstrated that when smoking is discontinued, the risk for oral cancer, adjusted for drinking, falls over time to levels similar to those of people who have never smoked.[153,155,158,159,161] This evidence suggests that many cases of oral cancer are preventable.

Use of smokeless tobacco has been shown to be a risk factor for oral cancer.[162,168,169] An estimated 5.3 million adults use smokeless tobacco in the United States, the vast majority of whom are men (4.8 million).[170] An additional 7.9 million adults are estimated to have been former smokeless tobacco users.[170] The Centers for Disease Control and Prevention estimates that approximately 18% of high school students and 7% of middle school students are current or past users of smokeless tobacco.[171] Among boys, approximately 29% of high school students and 11% of middle school students are estimated to be past or current users of smokeless tobacco (compared with approximately 8% and 3% for high school and middle school girls, respectively).[171] An analysis of national survey data indicated that adolescents who were current snuff users were 18 times more likely to develop white or red soft tissue lesions than nonusers.[172] A study of U.S. female snuff dippers reported a strong risk of cancer of the gingiva and buccal mucosa associated with this habit.[162]

Local intraoral factors such as oral hygiene, inadequate dentition, mouthwash use, and the wearing of dentures have been suspected as being risk factors for oral cancer. Past studies that have investigated this question have produced inconclusive findings.[154,157,158] A more recent study of a Brazilian population reported that although there was no association with denture use per se, a history of oral sores caused by ill-fitting dentures conveyed a twofold increase in the risk of oral cancers.[173] This study reported a similar increased risk associated with a history of less than daily toothbrushing.[173]

EPIDEMIOLOGY OF THE ORAL MANIFESTATIONS OF HUMAN IMMUNODEFICIENCY VIRUS INFECTION

The Human Immunodeficiency Virus/Acquired Immunodeficiency Syndrome Epidemic

As of the year 2000, approximately 53 million people had been infected with HIV worldwide since the beginning of the epidemic in the early 1980s, with the overwhelming majority of cases occurring in developing countries.[174] Of these, nearly 22 million had died, including more than 4 million children.[174] In 2000 more than 5 million new HIV cases and 3 million deaths related to acquired immunodeficiency syndrome (AIDS) occurred, with approximately 36 million people infected with HIV worldwide.[174] In the United States, approximately 754,000 cases of HIV/AIDS had been diagnosed through June 2000, including approximately 8800 children under age 13 years.[175] As of that same date, nearly 439,000 deaths had occurred in the United States attributable to AIDS, including approximately 5000 children.[175] Sexual contact and injected drug use continue to account for the majority of AIDS cases in U.S. adults.[174,176] More than 90% of the pediatric AIDS cases in the United States have been children born to HIV-infected mothers.[177]

Oral Lesions Associated with HIV/AIDS

Oral lesions are among the earliest signs of HIV infection.[178] Oral lesions associated with HIV infection include those of fungal, bacterial, and viral origin, as well as neoplastic lesions.[179] Oral candidiasis, a fungal infection most often associated with *Candida albicans,* is highly prevalent among those infected with HIV.[178-180] Estimates of the prevalence of oral candidiasis among HIV-infected adults range between 30% and 50%, and it is the first sign of infection in approximately 10% of HIV-infected adults. Estimates for the prevalence of oral candidiasis in HIV-infected children have ranged widely, from 20% to 72%.[181]

Oral hairy leukoplakia (OHL) is a white, irregular lesion found predominantly on the lateral borders of the tongue.[178,182] The Epstein-Barr virus has been found to be associated with the occurrence of OHL.[178,179] OHL occurs most often in HIV-infected adults and occurs only rarely in noninfected individuals.[178] Past estimates put the prevalence of OHL in HIV-infected adults at approximately 25%; however, more recent estimates suggest that the use of protease inhibitor therapy has resulted in a substantially lower prevalence of approximately 11%.[183] OHL is rare in HIV-infected children, with an estimated prevalence of 2%.[180,184]

Herpes simplex virus (HSV) infections are common in HIV-infected patients, with an estimated prevalence of 10% to 20%.[179] Chronic recurrent herpetic lesions are the most common viral infection in HIV-infected children, with prevalence estimates ranging as high as 24%.[181] HSV infections can appear as gingivostomatitis or as vesicles that rupture to form ulcers.[180,185]

The most common oral malignancy associated with AIDS is Kaposi's sarcoma (KS), an endothelial cell multicentric neoplasm that appears as a red, blue, or purple nodule or nodules.[179] The oral cavity may be the sole site of KS in the AIDS patient.[179] However, the prevalence of KS among AIDS patients appears to be steadily declining, with a prevalence of 14% among adult male AIDS patients.[186] KS is rarely observed in HIV-infected women and children.[186]

Non-Hodgkin's lymphoma (NHL) is the second most common AIDS-associated malignancy.[179,186] NHL is found in approximately 3% of AIDS patients; however, the prevalence has been increasing as survival times have increased.[178,186] The Epstein-Barr virus has been identified in the majority of these lesions, which appear clinically as a solitary mass or ulcer.[178,186] To date, NHL has not been reported in children.[185]

Current evidence suggests that HIV infection is a risk factor for periodontal attachment loss.[187] Two specific periodontal conditions have been reported to be associated with HIV infection: linear gingival erythema (LGE) (formerly HIV-associated gingivitis) and necrotizing ulcerative periodontitis (NUP) (formerly HIV-associated periodontitis).[187,188] LGE is characterized by a linear band of erythema affecting the gingival margin.[189] An association between candidal infection and the occurrence of LGE has been suggested.[187] NUP is characterized by necrosis involving the gingival tissues, the periodontal ligament, and alveolar bone.[190] Studies of LGE in adults have estimated the prevalence at 5% to 30%.[191-193] Recent estimates suggest that with the use of protease inhibitors, the prevalence of ulcerative periodontal disease in HIV patients has decreased to less than 2%.[183] LGE has also been reported in HIV-infected children, although estimates of its prevalence vary widely, from 0% to 48%.[194]

Recent evidence suggests that the occurrence of HIV-related salivary gland disease has increased in recent years, with an estimated prevalence of approximately 5%.[183] Enlargement of the parotid gland occurs in HIV-infected children, although prevalence estimates vary widely, from 11% to 47%.[181] (See Chapter 9 for additional information about HIV and other transmissible diseases.)

EPIDEMIOLOGY OF OROFACIAL CLEFTING

DESCRIPTIVE FINDINGS

Clefting of the lip can result from any disturbance in the normal timing and positioning of the facial prominences during development of the embryo.[195] Clefting of the palate is caused by the improper growth, elevation, or fusion of the palatine shelves or a rupture of these shelves subsequent to fusion.[195] Cleft lip, either with or without the presence of a cleft palate, occurs with an incidence of approximately 1 per 1000 births and is the second most common congenital defect.[195,196] However, there appear to be important differences in incidence related to race/ethnicity and gender.[195,197,198] For example, the incidence rate in Sweden (approximately 1.3 per 1000 births) is approximately twice the rate of 0.6 per 1000 births in France,[197] and the rate in Japan has been estimated at 2.1 per 1000 births.[195] The rate for California Caucasians (approximately 1 per 1000 births) is higher than the rate for California African-Americans (approximately 0.7 per 1000 births). Cleft lip, with or without cleft palate, is seen approximately twice as often in males as compared with females.[197] The incidence of cleft palate in the absence of cleft lip is lower, with a rate of approximately 0.4 per 1000 births.[195] Again, there are differences related to race/ethnicity and gender.[195,198] For example, the incidence rate of cleft palate alone in France (approximately 0.3 per 1000 births) contrasts with a rate of approximately 0.6 per 1000 births in Sweden.[197] In contrast to cleft lip, the prevalence of cleft palate in the absence of cleft lip is markedly higher in females.[195,197,198]

ETIOLOGY

More than 300 identifiable syndromes associated with oral clefting have been identified, but approximately two thirds of oral clefts are so-called nonsyndromic (i.e., not associated with a specific syndrome).[195,196] Nevertheless, considerable evidence suggests that genetic factors play an important role in the etiology of both cleft lip with and without cleft palate and cleft palate alone.[195,196,198] For example, the identical twin of a child with cleft lip has been estimated to be 400 times as likely to have a cleft lip as someone in the general population.[196,199] The sibling of someone with cleft lip is more than 30 times as likely to have a cleft lip as someone in the general population.[196,199] Other factors for which an association with oral clefts has been suggested include certain environmental exposures, such as cigarette smoking and alcohol ingestion, and increased parental age.[195,198]

EPIDEMIOLOGY OF TEMPOROMANDIBULAR DISORDERS

The term *temporomandibular disorders* (TMD) refers to a set of signs and symptoms associated with a broad group of underlying disorders.[200] Historically, the signs and symptoms most often related to TMD are pain, either in the temporomandibular joint (TMJ) area or muscles of mastication; limitation or deviations in the range of mandibular motion; or noises in the TMJ during mandibular function.[200,201] This definition is manifestational, based on signs and symptoms only, as contrasted with etiologic, based on an underlying cause or causes. In fact, these TMD signs and symptoms have been shown to be related to a host of underlying etiologies.[202] Therefore, although the epidemiology of these disorders has been extensively investigated, the absence of a consensus on case definitions and methodology has made interpretation of findings difficult, if not impossible.[200,203,204] As recently as 1992, Dworkin and LeResche[205] commented that diagnostic methodologies of demonstrated reliability and validity did not exist for TMD. In their meta-analysis of 51 TMD studies, De Kanter and colleagues[206] reported that 25% of the studies gave no case definition for TMD at all, approximately half of the studies failed to identify the population being studied, and only 12% reported assessing the reliability of their methods. Not surprisingly, these 51 studies report a range for TMD prevalence of 6% to 93%.[206] The limited value of these findings to elucidate the true prevalence of these disorders is self-evident and suggests that these studies may have been investigating disorders of differing etiologies, all under the same manifestational label of TMD.[204] A National Institutes of Health Technology Assessment Conference Statement, discussing this lack of consensus in the definition of TMD disease, noted that even the term *temporomandibular disorders* itself is not universally accepted.[207]

These important methodologic concerns notwithstanding, it has been estimated that more than 10 million people in the United States have TMD symptoms of one sort or another and that one in three adults will develop pain in the temporomandibular region for some period of time during their lifetime.[208,209] A report of findings from a U.S. national survey estimated that 6% of the population had reported having had TMJ pain.[209] However, most TMD cases are self-limiting and resolve without treatment.[210] A serious concern associated with this confusion over case definitions is that some patients may undergo care that is ineffective and perhaps harmful.[208] This is especially true because most papers pertaining to TMD therapy are not reports of controlled clinical trials, the standard for evaluating new therapy, nor have these papers reported findings on the outcomes from the treatments they describe.[211] A new set of diagnostic criteria for research studies was introduced entitled Research Diagnostic Criteria for Temporomandibular Disorders (RDC/TMD).[212] The RDC/TMD was developed in an attempt to rectify the lack of standardized diagnostic criteria by which the different etiologic disorders, previously all labeled simply TMD, could be defined.[212] The RDC/TMD lists criteria by which three main groups, as well as subgroups, of TMD disorders can be identified. In brief, the groups identified are as follows: (1) myofacial pain, either with or without limited opening; (2) disc displacements often with associated TMJ clicking and limitation of mandibular movement; and (3) pain and tenderness in the joint capsule or the synovial lining of the TMJ, osteoarthritis of the TMJ, or degenerative disorder of the TMJ.[212] Ultimately, practical standardized diagnostic methods will need to be available for use by the clinician.[203]

In the absence of a set of accepted, etiologically clear case definitions for TMD, the identification of risk and preventive factors for most cases has been extremely challenging. The literature to date has failed to establish malocclusion or routine dental/medical procedures as underlying causes of TMD.[210] By contrast, considerable evidence suggests a link between biopsychosocial factors, such as emotional status and psychosocial adaptation, and the development of TMD.[210,213,214]

EPIDEMIOLOGY OF ENAMEL FLUOROSIS

Enamel fluorosis is a subsurface enamel hypomineralization or porosity that occurs when a child ingests above-optimum amounts of fluoride while enamel formation is occurring.[215] Clinically, the appearance of enamel fluorosis can vary from faint white flecks in its mildest presentation, to more noticeable snow flaking or mottling of the enamel, sometimes with accompanying brown staining of the enamel. Enamel fluorosis is an aesthetic concern, except in the most severe cases, in which pitting of the enamel or loss of enamel integrity can occur. A number of indices have been developed to measure enamel fluorosis. Each of these indices has particular strengths, thus the choice of the "best" index will depend on the specific use to which it will be placed.[216]

ENAMEL FLUOROSIS PREVALENCE

The contribution of fluoride to the observed secular decline in caries prevalence has been broadly accepted.[24,217] Paralleling this decline in caries prevalence has been an observed increase in the prevalence of enamel fluorosis.[218,219] Circa 1940 the prevalence of enamel fluorosis in optimally fluoridated areas was approximately 16%, being mostly of the very mildest forms.[218] During the same period the prevalence of enamel fluorosis in nonfluoridated areas was on average less than 1%.[218] By conservative estimate, since that time the prevalence of fluorosis has increased on average 43% (7 percentage points) in fluoridated areas and tenfold in nonfluoridated areas.[218] At the same time, some studies have reported an increase in the severity of fluorosis that is being observed.[219-222]

RISK FACTORS FOR ENAMEL FLUOROSIS

Because the goal of fluoride use in dentistry has always been to achieve the maximum benefit with minimum side effects, a series of investigations, using analytic epidemiologic techniques, has sought to identify the specific causes or risk factors for this increase in enamel fluorosis prevalence. Enamel is at risk of developing fluorosis only during its formation. Therefore only the ingestion of fluoride during the first 6 to 8 years of life can be a risk factor for enamel fluorosis. The use of multifactorial analyses has been important because there are numerous potential sources of ingested fluoride during early childhood.[218] Because of the inherent long follow-up required in fluorosis investigations (i.e., exposure can occur during the first year of life, but the permanent teeth do not begin to erupt until approximately age 6), most of these studies have used a case-control design.

Although the studies have been of variable quality, some consistent patterns have emerged. A growing body of studies has demonstrated an association between the use of fluoride toothpaste by preschool children and enamel fluorosis.[220,222-228] These findings are coherent with previous research, which indicated that preschool children tend to swallow much of the dentifrice they put into their mouths and that the majority of the fluoride thus ingested is absorbed into the gastrointestinal tract.[229,230] These findings have led to recommendations that parents supervise their preschool children's toothbrushing to ensure that no more than a pea-size amount of fluoride toothpaste is used and to encourage the child to spit out the toothpaste, not swallow it.[226,227] The findings have also led to a call for a reduced-fluoride toothpaste, specifically for use by preschool children.[231,232]

The use of fluoride supplements during the first 6 to 8 years by children living in nonfluoridated areas has been shown to be strongly associated with enamel fluorosis.[220,221,227,228,233] The findings of these studies led to a joint decision in 1994 by the American Dental Association and the American Academy of Pediatrics to reduce the fluoride supplement dosage schedule.[234,235] The use of fluoride supplements by children living in fluoridated areas, an inappropriate practice, not surprisingly has been shown to be very strongly associated with enamel fluorosis.[223]

Studies have further demonstrated that the use of infant formula before 1979 was an important enamel fluorosis risk factor.[223-225] In 1979, based on early evidence, the manufacturers of infant formula in the United States voluntarily agreed to regulate the fluoride concentration of their products at a low level, an action which subsequent studies indicate occurred.[236-238] Findings suggest that this action may have been sufficient to eliminate infant formula use as an enamel fluorosis risk factor in nonfluoridated areas.[220] However, the hypothesis has been put forward that the addition of even relatively low concentrations of fluoride from concentrated infant formula to optimally fluoridated water may produce a beverage containing an above-optimal concentration of fluoride.[238,239] The findings from a recent investigation support this hypothesis, suggesting that the use of formula prepared from concentrate, especially powdered concentrate, may remain a potentially important source of fluoride when mixed with already optimally fluoridated water.[222] However, further studies will be needed to confirm whether this is indeed the case.

REVIEW QUESTIONS

1. Discuss two examples from the chapter that illustrate the importance of case definition as it relates to understanding the underlying etiology of a disease, as well as its prevention and treatment.
2. Discuss an example from the chapter that illustrates how an understanding of epidemiologic principles, as well as knowledge of the specific epidemiology of an oral disease, can aid in its prevention and treatment.
3. Discuss an example from the chapter that illustrates the importance of risk assessment for targeting preventive strategies.
4. Discuss an example from the chapter that illustrates the importance of studies that look simultaneously at several risk factors when trying to understand the causes of a disease.
5. Discuss an example from the chapter that illustrates how an understanding of

epidemiologic principles can help the health professional critically review and make judgments about scientific papers in the literature.

6. Discuss an example from the chapter that illustrates the importance of understanding the concept of judgment of causation when interpreting the role of potential risk or preventive factors for disease.

REFERENCES

1. Black G, McKay F: Mottled teeth: an endemic developmental imperfection of the enamel of the teeth heretofore unknown in the literature of dentistry, *Dental Cosmos* 58:129, 1916.
2. MacMahon B, Pugh T: *Epidemiology: principals and methods,* Boston, 1970, Little, Brown.
3. Henekins C, Buring J: *Epidemiology in medicine,* Boston, 1987, Little, Brown.
4. Monson R: *Occupational epidemiology,* Boca Raton, 1990, CRC Press.
5. Schlesselman J: *Case-control studies,* New York, 1982, Oxford University Press.
6. Ast D, Finn S, McCaffrey I: The Newburgh-Kingston Caries Fluorine Study I. Dental findings after three years of water fluoridation, *Am J Public Health* 40:716, 1950.
7. Newbrun E: *Cariology,* Chicago, 1989, Quintessence.
8. Klein H, Palmer C, Knutson J: Studies of dental caries. I. Dental status and dental needs of elementary school children, *Public Health Rep* 53:751, 1938.
9. Gruebbel A: A measurement of dental caries prevalence and treatment service for deciduous teeth, *J Dent Res* 23:163, 1944.
10. US Department of Health and Human Services: *Oral health of United States children: the national survey of dental caries in U.S. school children: 1986-1987,* Washington, DC, 1989.
11. US Department of Health and Human Services: *Oral health of United States adults: the national survey of oral health in U.S. employed adults and seniors: 1985-1986,* Washington, DC, 1987.
12. National Center for Health Statistics: *Decayed, missing and filled teeth among persons 1-74 years: United States,* Washington, DC, 1981.
13. Kaste LM et al: Coronal caries in the primary and permanent dentition of children and adolescents 1-17 years of age: United States, 1988-1991, *J Dent Res* 75(spec iss):633, 1996.
14. Graves R, Stamm J: Oral health status in the United States: prevalence of dental caries, *J Dent Educ* 49:341, 1985.
15. Newbrun E: Effectiveness of water fluoridation, *J Public Health Dent* 49(spec iss):279, 1989.
16. Levy S: Review of fluoride exposures and ingestion, *Community Dent Oral Epidemiol* 22:173, 1994.
17. Griffin S et al: Quantifying the diffused benefit from water fluoridation in the United States, *Community Dent Oral Epidemiol* 29:120, 2001.
18. Newbrun E: Current regulations and recommendations concerning water fluoridation, fluoride supplements, and topical fluoride agents, *J Dent Res* 71: 1255, 1992.
19. Brunelle J, Carlos J: Changes in the prevalence of dental caries in U.S. schoolchildren, 1961-1980, *J Dent Res* 61:1346, 1982.
20. Marthaler T: The prevalence of dental caries in Europe 1990-1995, *Caries Res* 30:237, 1996.
21. Spencer A et al: Caries prevalence in Australasia, *Int Dent J* 44(suppl 1):415, 1994.
22. Petersson H, Brathall D: The caries decline: a review of reviews, *Eur J Oral Sci* 104:436, 1996.
23. Hugoson A et al: Caries prevalence and distribution in 3–20-year-olds in Jonkoping, Sweden, in 1973, 1978, 1983, and 1993, *Community Dent Oral Epidemiol* 28:83, 2000.
24. Brunelle J, Carlos J: Recent trends in dental caries in U.S. children and the effect of water fluoridation, *J Dent Res* 69:723, 1990.
25. Ripa L: Nursing caries: a comprehensive review, *Pediatr Dent* 10:268, 1988.
26. Ismail A, Sohn W: A systematic review of clinical diagnostic criteria of early childhood caries, *J Public Health Dent* 59(3):171, 1999.
27. Horowitz H: Research issues in early childhood caries, *Community Dent Oral Epidemiol* 26(suppl 1):67, 1998.
28. Reisine S, Douglass J: Psychosocial and behavioral issues in early childhood caries, *Community Dent Oral Epidemiol* 26(suppl 1):32, 1998.
29. Douglass J et al: Dental caries patterns and oral health behaviors in Arizona infants and toddlers, *Community Dent Oral Epidemiol* 29:14, 2001.
30. Seow W: Biological mechanisms of early childhood caries, *Community Dent Oral Epidemiol* 26(suppl 1):8, 1998.
31. Bowen W: Response to Seow: biological mechanisms of early childhood caries, *Community Dent Oral Epidemiol* 26(suppl 1):28, 1998.
32. Drury T et al: Diagnosing and reporting early childhood caries for research purposes, *J Public Health Dent* 59(3):192, 1999.

33. Karjalainen S et al: A prospective study on sucrose consumption, visible plaque and caries in children from 3 to 6 years of age, *Community Dent Oral Epidemiol* 19:136, 2001.
34. Milgrom P et al: Dental caries and its relationship to bacterial infection, hypoplasia, diet, and oral hygiene in 6- to 36-month-old children, *Community Dent Oral Epidemiol* 28:295, 2000.
35. Winn D et al: Coronal and root caries in the dentition of adults in the United States, 1988-1991, *J Dent Res* 75(spec iss):642, 1996.
36. Brown L, Swango P: Trends in caries experience in U.S. employed adults from 1971-1985: cross-sectional comparisons, *Adv Dent Res* 7:52, 1993.
37. Downer M: Changing trends in dental caries experience in Great Britain, *Adv Dent Res* 7:19, 1993.
38. Hugoson A et al: Caries prevalence and distribution in 20–80-year-olds in Jonkoping, Sweden, in 1973, 1983, and 1993, *Community Dent Oral Epidemiol* 28:90, 2000.
39. DePaola P, Soparkar P, Kent RJ: Methodological issues relative to the quantification of root surface caries, *Gerodontology* 8:3, 1989.
40. Aherne C, O'Mullane D, Barrett B: Indices of root surface caries, *J Dent Res* 69:1222, 1990.
41. Beck J: The epidemiology of root surface caries: North American studies, *Adv Dent Res* 7:42, 1993.
42. Banting D: Diagnosis and prediction of root caries, *Adv Dent Res* 7:80, 1993.
43. Fejerskov O, Baelum V, Ostergarrd E: Root caries in Scandinavia in the 1980s and future trends to be expected in dental caries experience in adults, *Adv Dent Res* 7:4, 1993.
44. Katz R: A method for scoring and reporting root caries in epidemiologic studies, *J Dent Res* 58:389, 1979.
45. Katz R: Prevalence and intraoral distribution of root caries in an adult population, *Caries Res* 16:265, 1982.
46. Lawrence H et al: Five-year incidence rates and intraoral distribution of root caries among community-dwelling older adults, *Caries Res* 30:169, 1996.
47. Nordblad A: Changes in epidemiologic pattern of dental caries in cohorts of schoolchildren in Espoo, Finland, during a 3-year period, *Community Dent Oral Epidemiol* 14:126, 1986.
48. Winter G: Epidemiology of dental caries, *Arch Oral Biol* 35(suppl):1S, 1990.
49. Winter G: Prediction of high caries risk diet, hygiene and medication, *Int Dent J* 38:227, 1988.
50. Grindefjord M et al: Stepwise prediction of dental caries in children up to 3.5 years of age, *Caries Res* 30:256, 1996.
51. Krasse B: Biological factors as indicators of future caries, *Int Dent J* 38:219 1988.
52. Alaluusua S: Salivary counts of mutans streptococci and lactobacilli and past caries experience in caries prediction, *Caries Res* 27(suppl 1):68, 1993.
53. Holbrook W, de Soet J, de Graaff J: Prediction of dental caries in pre-school children, *Caries Res* 27:424, 1993.
54. Thibodeau E, O'Sullivan D: Salivary mutans streptococci and incidence of caries in preschool children, *Caries Res* 29:148, 1995.
55. Reisine S, Litt M, Tinanoff N: A biopsychosocial model to predict caries in preschool children, *Pediatr Dent* 16:413, 1994.
56. van Houte J: Microbial predictors of caries risk, *Adv Dent Res* 7:87, 1993.
57. Demers M et al: A multivariate model to predict caries increment in Montreal children aged 5 years, *Community Dental Health* 9:273, 1992.
58. Stamm J et al: The University of North Carolina assessment study: final results and some alternative modelling approaches. In Bowen WH, Tabak LA, editors: *Cariology for the nineties,* Rochester, NY, 1993, University of Rochester Press.
59. Navia J: Carbohydrates and dental health, *Am J Clin Nutr* 59:719s, 1994.
60. Hunter P: Risk factors in dental caries, *Int Dent J* 38:211, 1988.
61. Pitts N: Risk assessment and caries prediction, *J Dent Educ* 62(10):762, 1998.
62. Szpunar S, Eklund S, Burt B: Sugar consumption and caries risk in schoolchildren with low caries experience, *Community Dent Oral Epidemiol* 23:142, 1995.
63. Scheinin A et al: Multifactoral modeling for root caries prediction: 3-year follow-up results, *Community Dent Oral Epidemiol* 22:126, 1994.
64. Joshi A et al: The distribution of root caries in community-dwelling elders in New England, *J Public Health* 54:15, 1994.
65. Loe H: Periodontal diseases: a brief historical perspective, *Periodontology 2000* 2:7, 1993.
66. Jeffcoat M: Prevention of periodontal diseases in adults: strategies for the future, *Prev Med* 23:704, 1994.
67. Armitage G: Development of a classification system for periodontal diseases and conditions, *Ann Periodontol* 4(1):1, 1999.
68. American Academy of Periodontology: Consensus report: dental plaque–induced gingival diseases, *Ann Periodontol* 4(1):18, 1999.
69. Genco R: Classification and clinical and radiographic features of periodontal disease. In Genco RJ, Goldman HM, Cohen DW, editors: *Contemporary periodontics,* St Louis, 1990, Mosby.
70. Ranney R: Classification of periodontal diseases, *Periodontology 2000* 2:13, 1993.

71. American Academy of Periodontology: Consensus report: aggressive periodontitis, *Ann Periodontol* 4(1): 53, 1999.
72. American Academy of Periodontology: Consensus report: chronic periodontitis, *Ann Periodontol* 4(1):38, 1999.
73. Loe H et al: Natural history of periodontal disease in man, *J Clin Periodontol* 13:431, 1986.
74. Loe H, Anerud A, Boysen H: The natural history of periodontal disease in man: prevalence, severity, and extent of gingival recession, *J Periodontol* 63:489, 1992.
75. Page R: Milestones in periodontal research and the remaining critical issues, *J Periodontol Res* 34:331, 1999.
76. Russell A: The periodontal index, *J Periodontol* 38:585, 1967.
77. Ramfjord S: The periodontal disease index, *J Periodontol* 38:602, 1967.
78. Beck J, Loe H: Epidemiological principles in studying periodontal diseases, *Periodontology 2000* 2:34, 1993.
79. Brown L, Loe H: Prevalence, extent, severity and progression of periodontal disease, *Periodontology 2000* 2:57, 1993.
80. Ainamo J et al: Development of the World Health Organization (WHO) Community Periodontal Index of Treatment Needs (CPITN), *Int Dent J* 32:281, 1982.
81. Ainamo J, Ainamo A: Validity and relevance of the criteria of the CPITN, *Int Dent J* 4:527, 1994.
82. Pilot T, Miyazaki H: Global results: 15 years of CPITN epidemiology, *Int Dent J* 4:553, 1994.
83. Papapanou P: Periodontal diseases: epidemiology, *Ann Periodontol* 1(1):1, 1996.
84. American Academy of Periodontology: Consensus report: periodontal diseases: epidemiology and diagnosis, *Ann Periodontol* 1(1):216, 1996.
85. Loe H, Silness J: Periodontal disease in pregnancy. I. Prevalence and severity, *Acta Odontol Scand* 21:533, 1963.
86. Loe H: The gingival index, the plaque index and the retention index systems, *J Periodontol* 38:610, 1967.
87. Cinacio S: Current status of indices of gingivitis, *J Clin Periodontol* 13:375, 1986.
88. Brown L, Brunelle J, Kingman A: Periodontal status in the United States, 1988-91: prevalence, extent, and demographic variation, *J Dent Res* 75:672, 1996.
89. Ranney R: Differential diagnosis in clinical trials of therapy for periodontitis, *J Periodontol* 63:1052, 1992.
90. Fleming N: Periodontitis, *Ann Periodontol* 4(1):32, 1999.
91. Oliver R, Brown L, Loe H: Variations in the prevalence and extent of periodontitis, *J Am Dent Assoc* 122:43, 1991.
92. Drury T, Garcia I, Adesanya M: Socioeconomic disparities in adult oral health in the United States, *Ann N Y Acad Sci* 896:322, 1999.
93. Saxen L: Prevalence of juvenile periodontitis in Finland, *J Clin Periodontol* 7:177, 1980.
94. Saxby M: Prevalence of juvenile periodontitis in a British school population, *Community Dent Oral Epidemiol* 12:185, 1984.
95. Lopez N et al: Prevalence of juvenile periodontitis in Chile, *J Clin Periodontol* 18:529, 1991.
96. Neely A: Prevalence of juvenile periodontitis in a cirumpubertal population, *J Clin Periodontol* 19:367, 1992.
97. Loe H, Brown L: Early onset periodontitis in the United States of America, *J Periodontol* 62:608, 1991.
98. Michalowicz B: Genetic and heritable risk factors in periodontal disease, *J Periodontol* 65:479, 1994.
99. Hart T: Genetic risk factors for early-onset periodontitis, *J Periodontol* 67:355, 1996.
100. Page R: Critical issues in periodontal research, *J Dent Res* 74:1118, 1995.
101. Wolff L, Dahlen G, Aeppli D: Bacteria as risk markers for periodontitis, *J Periodontol* 65:498, 1994.
102. Genco R, Loe H: The role of systemic conditions and disorders in periodontal disease, *Periodontology 2000* 2:98, 1993.
103. Page R, Beck J: Risk assessment for periodontal diseases, *Int Dent J* 47(2):61, 1997.
104. Page R et al: Rapidly progressive periodontitis: a distinct clinical condition, *J Periodontol* 54:197, 1983.
105. Kornman K, Loe H: The role of local factors in the etiology of periodontal diseases, *Periodontology 2000* 2:83, 1993.
106. Haber J et al: Evidence for cigarette smoking as a major risk factor for periodontitis, *J Periodontol* 64:16, 1993.
107. Bergstrom J, Preber H: Tobacco use as a risk factor, *J Periodontol* 65:545, 1994.
108. Research Science and Therapy Committee of the American Academy of Periodontology: Position paper: tobacco use and the periodontal patient, *J Periodontol* 67:51, 1996.
109. Hashim R, Thomson W, Pack A: Smoking in adolescence as a predictor of early loss of periodontal attachment, *Community Dent Oral Epidemiol* 29:130, 2001.
110. Beck J: Methods of assessing risk for periodontitis and developing multifactoral models, *J Periodontol* 65:468, 1994.
111. American Academy of Periodontology: Position paper: epidemiology of periodontal disease, *J Periodontol* 67(9):935, 1996.
112. Haffajee A, Oliver R: Periodontal diseases working group: summary and recommendations. In Bader JD, editor: *Risk assessment in dentistry,* Chapel Hill, NC, 1990, University of North Carolina Dental Ecology.
113. Weintraub J, Burt B: Oral health status in the United States: tooth loss and edentulism, *J Dent Educ* 49:368, 1985.

114. Marcus S et al: Tooth retention and tooth loss in the permanent dentition of adults: United States, 1988-1991, *J Dent Res* 75:684, 1996.
115. Brown L: Trends in tooth loss among U.S. employed adults from 1971 to 1985, *J Am Dent Assoc* 125:533, 1994.
116. Ainamo J: Changes in the frequency of edentulousness and use of removable dentures in the adult population of Finland, 1970-1980, *Community Dent Oral Epidemiol* 11:122, 1983.
117. Grabowski M, Bertram U: Oral health status and need of dental treatment in the elderly Danish population, *Community Dent Oral Epidemiol* 3:108, 1975.
118. Swallow J et al: A survey of edentulous individuals in a district in Amsterdam, the Netherlands, *Community Dent Oral Epidemiol* 6:210, 1978.
119. Clarkson J, O'Mullane D: Edentulousness in the United Kingdom and Ireland, *Community Dent Oral Epidemiol* 11:317, 1983.
120. Katz R, Gustavsen F: Tooth mortality in dental patients in a U.S. urban area, *Gerodontics* 2:104, 1986.
121. Hunt R et al: Edentulism and oral health problems among elderly rural Iowans: the Iowa 65+ rural health study, *Am J Public Health* 5:1177, 1985.
122. Heft M, Gilbert G: Tooth loss and caries prevalence in older Floridians attending senior activity centers, *Community Dent Oral Epidemiol* 19:228, 1991.
123. Douglass C et al: Oral health status of the elderly in New England, *J Gerontol* 48:M39, 1993.
124. Eklund S, Burt B: Risk factors for total tooth loss in the United States: longitudinal analysis of national data, *J Public Health Dent* 54:5, 1994.
125. Bailit H, Braun R: Is periodontal disease the primary cause of tooth extraction in adults? *J Am Dent Assoc* 114:40, 1987.
126. Oliver R, Brown L: Periodontal diseases and tooth loss, *Periodontology 2000* 2:117, 1993.
127. Corbet E, Davies W: Reasons for tooth extractions in Hong Kong, *Community Dental Health* 8:121, 1991.
128. Ong G: Periodontal reasons for tooth loss in an Asian population, *J Clin Periodontol* 23:307, 1996.
129. Klock K, Haugejordan O: Primary reasons for extraction of permanent teeth in Norway: changes from 1968 to 1988, *Community Dent Oral Epidemiol* 9:336, 1991.
130. Ekanayaka A: Tooth mortality in plantation workers and residents in Sri Lanka, *Community Dent Oral Epidemiol* 12:128, 1984.
131. Bouma J, Schaub R, van de Poel A: Periodontal status and total tooth extraction in a medium-sized city in the Netherlands, *Community Dent Oral Epidemiol* 13:323, 1985.
132. Baclum V, Fejerskov O: Tooth loss as related to dental caries and periodontal breakdown in adult Tanzanians, *Community Dent Oral Epidemiol* 4:353, 1986.
133. Manji F, Baelum V, Fejerskov O: Tooth mortality in an adult rural population in Kenya, *J Dent Res* 67:496, 1988.
134. Johansen S, Johansen J: A survey of causes of permanent tooth extractions in South Australia, *Aust Dent J* 22:238, 1977.
135. Reich E, Hiller KA: Reasons for tooth extraction in the eastern states of Germany, *Community Dent Oral Epidemiol* 21:379, 1993.
136. Kay E, Blinkhorn A: The reasons underlying the extraction of teeth in Scotland, *Br Dent J* 160:287, 1986.
137. Hawkins R, Main P, Locker D: The normative need for tooth extractions in older adults in Ontario, Canada, *Gerodontology* 14(2)75, 1998.
138. Chestnutt I, Binnie V, Taylor M: Reasons for tooth extraction in Scotland, *J Dent* 28:295, 2000.
139. Micheelis W, Baauch J: Oral health of representative samples of Germans examined in 1989 and 1992, *Community Dent Oral Epidemiol* 24:62, 1996.
140. Bergman J, Wright F, Hammond R: The oral health of the elderly in Melbourne, *Aust Dent J* 36:280, 1991.
141. Marcus S, Kaste L, Brown L: Prevalence and demographic correlates of tooth loss among the elderly in the United States, *Spec Care Dent* 14:123, 1994.
142. Greenlee R et al: Cancer statistics, *CA Cancer J Clin* 51:15, 2001.
143. Muir C, Weiland L: Upper aerodigestive tract cancers, *Cancer* 75:147, 1995.
144. Ostman J et al: Malignant oral tumors in Sweden 1960-1989—an epidemiologic study, *Oral Oncol Eur J Cancer* 31B:106, 1995.
145. McCarten B, Crowley M: Oral cancer in Ireland 1984-1988, *Oral Oncol Eur J Cancer* 29B:127, 1993.
146. Ries L et al: *SEER cancer statistics review, 1973-1997,* Bethesda, MD, 2000, National Cancer Institute.
147. Franceschi S et al: Comparisons of cancers of the oral cavity and pharynx worldwide: etiological clues, *Oral Oncology* 36:106, 2000.
148. US Department of Health and Human Services: *Cancers of the oral cavity and pharynx: a statistics review monograph 1973-1987,* Atlanta, 1991, Centers for Disease Control and Prevention.
149. Morse D et al: Trends in the incidence of lip, oral, and pharyngeal cancer: Connecticut, 1935-94, *Oral Oncology* 35:1, 1999.
150. Reid B et al: Head and neck in situ carcinoma: incidence, trends, and survival, *Oral Oncology* 36:414, 2000.
151. Parker S et al: Cancer statistics, *CA Cancer J Clin* 46:5, 1996.
152. Preventing and controlling oral and pharyngeal cancer: recommendations from a national planning conference, *MMWR Morb Mortal Wkly Rep* 47(RR14):3, 1998.

153. Blot W et al: Smoking and drinking in relation to oral and pharyngeal cancer, *Cancer Res* 48:3282, 1988.
154. Marshall J et al: Smoking, alcohol, dentition and diet in the epidemiology of oral cancer, *Oral Oncology Eur J Cancer* 28B:9, 1992.
155. Mashberg A et al: Tobacco smoking, alcohol drinking, and cancer of the oral cavity and oropharynx among US veterans, *Cancer* 72:1369, 1993.
156. Day G et al: Racial differences in risk of oral and pharyngeal cancer: alcohol, tobacco, and other determinants, *J Natl Cancer Inst* 85:465a, 1993.
157. Graham S et al: Dentition, diet, tobacco, and alcohol in the epidemiology of oral cancer, *J Natl Cancer Inst* 59:1611, 1977.
158. Kabat G, Hebert J, Wynder E: Risk factors for oral cancer in women, *Cancer Res* 49:2803, 1989.
159. Wynder E, Stellman S: Comparative epidemiology of tobacco-related cancers, *Cancer Res* 37:4608, 1977.
160. Brugere J et al: Differential effects of tobacco and alcohol in cancer of the larynx, pharynx, and mouth, *Cancer* 57:391, 1986.
161. Kabat G, Chang C, Wynder E: The role of tobacco, alcohol use, and body mass index in oral and pharyngeal cancer, *Int J Epidemiol* 23:1137, 1994.
162. Winn D et al: Snuff dipping and oral cancer among women in the southern United States, *N Engl J Med* 304:745, 1981.
163. Morse D et al: Smoking and drinking in relation to oral epithelial dysplasia, *Cancer Epidemiol Biomarkers Prev* 5:769, 1996.
164. Winn D: Diet and nutrition in the etiology of oral cancer, *Am J Clin Nutr* 61:437S, 1995.
165. LaVecchia C et al: Epidemiology and prevention of oral cancer, *Oral Oncology* 33(5):302, 1997.
166. DeStefani E et al: Diet and risk of cancer of the upper aerodigestive tract. II. Nutrients, *Oral Oncology* 35:22, 1999.
167. Boyle P et al: European school of oncology advisory report to the European Commission for the Europe Against Cancer Programme: oral carcinogenesis in Europe, *Oral Oncology Eur J Cancer* 31B:75, 1995.
168. US Department of Health and Human Services: *The health consequences of using smokeless tobacco: a report of the advisory committee to the Surgeon General*, Bethesda, MD, 1986, US Department of Health and Human Services.
169. Winn D: Smokeless tobacco and cancer: the epidemiologic evidence, *CA Cancer J Clin* 38:236, 1988.
170. Use of smokeless tobacco among adults—United States, 1991, *MMWR Morb Mortal Wkly Rep* 42(14): 263, 1993.
171. Youth tobacco surveillance—United State, 1998-1999, *MMWR Morb Mortal Wkly Rep* 49(SS10):5, 2000.
172. Tomar S et al: Oral mucosal smokeless tobacco lesions among adolescents in the United States, *J Dent Res* 76(6):1277, 1997.
173. Velly A: Relationship between dental factors and risk of upper aerodigestive tract cancer, *Oral Oncology* 34:284, 1997.
174. UNAIDS/WHO: *AIDS epidemic update: December 2000*, Geneva, 2000, UNAIDS/WHO.
175. Centers for Disease Control and Prevention: *HIV/AIDS surveillance report*, Atlanta, 2000, Centers for Disease Control and Prevention.
176. US Department of Health and Human Services: *HIV/AIDS surveillance report*, Atlanta, 1995, Centers for Disease Control and Prevention.
177. Davis S et al: Prevalence and incidence of vertically acquired HIV infection in the United States, *JAMA* 247:952, 1995.
178. Greenspan D, Greenspan J: Oral manifestations of human immunodeficiency virus infection, *Dent Clin North Am* 37:21, 1993.
179. Itin P et al: Oral manifestations in HIV-infected patients: diagnosis and management, *J Am Acad Dermatol* 29:749, 1993.
180. Chigururpati R, Raghavan S, Studen-Pavlovich D: Pediatric HIV infection and its oral manifestations: a review, *Am Acad Pediatr Dent* 18:106, 1996.
181. Kline MW: Oral manifestations of pediatric human immunodeficiency virus infection: a review of the literature, *Pediatrics* 97(3):380, 1996.
182. Phelan J: Oral manifestations of human immunodeficiency virus infection, *Med Clin North Am* 81(2):511, 1997.
183. Patton L et al: Changing prevalence of oral manifestations of human immunodeficiency virus in the era of protease inhibitor therapy, *Oral Surg Oral Med Oral Pathol Oral Radiol Endod* 89:299, 2000.
184. Barasch A et al: Oral soft tissue manifestations in HIV-positive vs. HIV-negative children from an inner city population: a two-year observational study, *Pediatr Dent* 22:215, 2000.
185. Leggott P: Oral manifestations of HIV infection in children, *Oral Surg Oral Med Oral Pathol* 73:187, 1992.
186. Ficara G, Eversole L: HIV-related tumors of the oral cavity, *Crit Rev Oral Biol Med* 5:159, 1994.
187. Lamster I et al: New concepts regarding the pathogenesis of periodontal disease in HIV infection, *Ann Periodontol* 3:62, 1998.
188. Winkler J et al: Periodontal disease in HIV-infected and uninfected homosexual and bisexual men, *AIDS* 6:1041, 1992.
189. Winkler J, Robinson P: Periodontal disease associated with HIV infection, *Oral Surg Oral Med Oral Pathol* 73:145, 1992.
190. American Academy of Periodontitis: Consensus report: necrotizing periodontal diseases, *Ann Periodontol* 4(1):78, 1999.

191. Masouredis C et al: Prevalence of HIV-associated periodontitis and gingivitis in HIV-infected patients attending an AIDS clinic, *J Acquir Immune Defic Syndr* 5:479, 1992.
192. Riley C, London J, Burmeister J: Periodontal health in 200 HIV-positive patients, *J Oral Pathol Med* 21:124, 1992.
193. Laskaris G et al: Gingival lesions of HIV infection in 178 Greek patients, *Oral Surg Oral Med Oral Pathol* 74:168, 1992.
194. Ramos-Gomez F et al: Classification, diagnostic criteria, and treatment recommendations for orofacial manifestations in HIV-infected pediatric patients, *J Clin Pediatr Dent* 23(2):85, 1999.
195. Cohen M: Etiology and pathogenesis of orofacial clefting, *Oral Maxillofac Surg Clin North Am* 12(3):379, 2000.
196. Mitchell L: Genetic epidemiology of birth defects: nonsyndromic cleft lip and neural tube defects, *Epidemiol Rev* 19(1):61, 1997.
197. Robert E, Kallen B, Harris J: The epidemiology of orofacial clefts. 1. Some general epidemiological characteristics, *J Craniofac Genet Dev Biol* 16:234, 1996.
198. Derijcke A, Eerens A, Carels C: The incidence of oral clefts: a review, *Br J Oral Maxillofac Surg* 34:488, 1996.
199. Bender P: Genetics of cleft lip and palate, *J Pediatr Nurs* 15(4):242, 2000.
200. Carlsson G, LeResche L: Epidemiology of temporomandibular disorders. In Sessle B, Bryant P, Dionne R, editors: *Temporomandibular disorders and related pain conditions: progress in pain research and management,* Seattle, 1995, IASP Press.
201. Dworkin S et al: Epidemiology of signs and symptoms in temporomandibular disorders: clinical signs in cases and controls, *J Am Dent Assoc* 120:273, 1990.
202. Mosses A: Scientific methodology in temporomandibular disorders. I. Epidemiology, *J Craniomandibular Pract* 12:114, 1994.
203. Clark G, Delcanho R, Goulet JP: The utility and validity of current diagnostic procedures for defining temporomandibular disorder patients, *Adv Dent Res* 7:97, 1993.
204. Marbach J: Reaction paper. In Sessle B, Bryant P, Dionne R, editors: *Temporomandibular disorders and related pain conditions: progress in pain research and management,* Seattle, 1995, IASP Press.
205. Dworkin S, LeResche L: Research diagnostic criteria for temporomandibular disorders: review, criteria, examinations and specifications, critique, *J Craniomandibular Disorders* 6:301, 1992.
206. De Kanter R et al: Prevalence in the Dutch adult population and a meta-analysis of signs and symptoms of temporomandibular disorder, *J Dent Res* 72:1509, 1993.
207. National Institutes of Health: Management of temporomandibular disorders, *NIH Technol Statement Online* 18:1, 1996.
208. Von Korff M: Health services research and temporomandibular pain. In Sessle B, Bryant P, Dionne R, editors: *Temporomandibular disorders and related pain conditions: progress in pain research and management,* Seattle, 1995, IASP Press.
209. Lipton J, Ship J, Larach-Robinson D: Estimated prevalence and distribution of reported orofacial pain in the United States, *J Am Dent Assoc* 124:115, 1993.
210. Goldstein B: Temporomandibular disorders, *Oral Surg Oral Med Oral Pathol Oral Radiol Endod* 88:379, 1999.
211. Antczak-Bouckoms A: Epidemiology of research for temporomandibular disorders, *J Orofacial Pain* 9:226, 1995.
212. Dworkin S, LeResche L: Research diagnostic criteria for temporomandibular disorders: review, criteria, examinations and specifications, critique, *J Craniomandibular Disorders* 6:301, 1992.
213. Dworkin S: Behavioral characteristics of chronic temporomandibular disorders: diagnosis and assessment. In Sessle B, Bryant P, Dionne R, editors: *Temporomandibular disorders and related pain conditions: progress in pain research and management,* Seattle, 1995, IASP Press.
214. Greene C, Laskin D: Temporomandibular disorders: moving from a dentally based to a medically based model, *J Dent Res* 79(10):1736, 2000.
215. Fejerskov O, Thylstrup A, Larsen M: Clinical and structural features and possible pathogenic mechanisms of dental fluorosis, *Scand J Dent Res* 85: 510, 1977.
216. Rozier R: Epidemiologic indices for measuring the clinical manifestations of dental fluorosis: overview and critique, *Adv Dent Res* 8:39, 1994.
217. Ripa L: A half-century of community water fluoridation in the United States: review and commentary, *J Public Health Dent* 53(1):17, 1993.
218. Pendrys D, Stamm J: Relationship of total fluoride intake to beneficial effects and enamel fluorosis, *J Dent Res* 69(spec iss): 529, 1990.
219. Heller K, Eklund S, Burt B: Dental caries and dental fluorosis at varying water fluoride concentrations, *J Public Health Dent* 57(3):136, 1997.
220. Pendrys D, Katz R, Morse D: Risk factors for enamel fluorosis in a nonfluoridated population, *Am J Epidemiol* 143:808, 1996.
221. Szpunar S, Burt B: Fluoride supplements: evaluation of appropriate use in the United States, *Community Dent Oral Epidemiol* 20:148, 1992.

222. Pendrys D, Katz R: Risk factors for enamel fluorosis in optimally fluoridated children born after the US manufacturers' decision to reduce the fluoride concentration of infant formula, *Am J Epidemiol* 148:967, 1998.
223. Pendrys D, Katz R, Morse D: Risk factors for enamel fluorosis in a fluoridated population, *Am J Epidemiol* 140:461, 1994.
224. Osuji O et al: Risk factors for dental fluorosis in a fluoridated community, *J Dent Res* 67:1488, 1988.
225. Riordan P: Dental fluorosis, dental caries and fluoride exposure among 7-year-olds, *Caries Res* 27:71, 1993.
226. Pendrys D: Risk of fluorosis in a fluoridated population: implications for the dentist and hygienist, *J Am Dent Assoc* 126:1617, 1995.
227. Pendrys D: Risk of enamel fluorosis in nonfluoridated and optimally fluoridated populations, *J Am Dent Assoc* 131:746, 2000.
228. Mascarenhas A: Risk factors for dental fluorosis: a review of the recent literature, *Pediatr Dent* 22:269, 2000.
229. Barnhart W et al: Dentifrice usage and ingestion among four age groups, *J Dent Res* 53:1317, 1974.
230. Ekstrand J, Ehrenebo M: Absorption of fluoride from fluoride dentifrices, *Caries Res* 14:96, 1980.
231. Beltran E, Szpunar S: Fluoride in toothpastes for children: suggestion for change, *Pediatr Dent* 10:185, 1988.
232. Horowitz H: The need for toothpastes with lower than conventional fluoride concentrations for preschool-age children, *J Public Health Dent* 52:216, 1992.
233. Riordan P: Fluoride supplements in caries prevention: a literature review and proposal for a new dosage schedule, *J Public Health Dent* 53:174, 1993.
234. ADA Council on Access Prevention and Interprofessional Relations: Caries diagnosis and risk assessment, *J Am Dent Assoc* 126(spec suppl):195, 1995.
235. Committee on Nutrition, American Academy of Pediatrics: Fluoride supplementation for children: interim policy recommendations, *Pediatrics* 95:777, 1995.
236. Feigal R: Recent modification in the use of fluorides by children, *Northwest Dentistry* 62:19, 1983.
237. Johnson J, Bawden J: The fluoride content of infant formulas available in 1985, *Pediatr Dent* 9:33, 1985.
238. VanWinkle S et al: Water and formula fluoride concentrations: significance for infants fed formula, *Pediatr Dent* 17:305, 1995.
239. Levy S, Kiritsky M, Warren J: Sources of fluoride intake in children, *J Public Health Dent* 55:39, 1995.

CHAPTER

9

THE IMPACT OF TRANSMISSIBLE DISEASE ON THE PRACTICE OF DENTISTRY

Helene Bednarsh • Bennett Klein

ACQUIRED IMMUNODEFICIENCY SYNDROME

No single factor has affected the practice of dentistry since the early 1980s more than acquired immunodeficiency syndrome (AIDS). "Once upon a time, no one in the world had ever heard of the acquired immunodeficiency syndrome (AIDS). Neither was the human immunodeficiency virus (HIV) known. That state of innocence has ended forever."[1] In 2000 Larry Kramer, the co-founder of the AIDS Coalition to Unleash Power (ACT UP), reminded the world that the AIDS crisis is more devastating than ever: "Even if we were to find a cure tomorrow, millions and millions of people will die. You were all told this before it was too late. Now it is too late. So sit back and watch the destruction of the world."[2] This may appear melodramatic; however, the message was confirmed at the International Conference on AIDS in South Africa in 2000, where concerns over the expansion of the epidemic were discussed. The United Nations Programme on HIV/AIDS (UNAIDS) estimates that globally, nearly 22 million have died of AIDS and more than 36 million are living with HIV or AIDS. "HIV disease is reversing decades of public health progress."[3] The emphasis of the conference was more on reducing stigma and increasing access to care than on biomedical research.

Dealing with the HIV epidemic and its consequences may prove to be the greatest challenge ever faced by the dental profession. The manner in which dentistry responds to this challenge may, to a large degree, shape dentistry's future. This ribonucleic acid (RNA) virus has forced dentistry to reassess its ethics, legal obligations, and ability to protect dentists, staff, and patients from transmissible disease. It has exposed innermost fears and prejudices and clouded the ability to distinguish fact from fiction.

HIV is an epidemic that must be understood within its historical perspective. In June 1981 the Centers for Disease Control and Prevention (CDC) reported through its *Morbidity and Mortality Weekly Reports* (MMWR, the disease status and policy reports of the CDC) that five young homosexual men had required treatment for *Pneumocystis carinii* pneumonia, an opportunistic infection previously seen almost exclusively in immunodeficient patients such as transplant recipients and those under treatment for cancer. Its occurrence in five previously healthy individuals without a clinically apparent underlying immunodeficiency was unprecedented. These men also had cytomegalovirus (CMV) infection and oral candidiasis, further indications that they had a "cellular-immune dysfunction relative to a common exposure that predisposes individuals to opportunistic infections."[4] One month later the CDC reported the occurrence over a 30-month period of an uncommon malignancy, Kaposi's sarcoma, "among (26) previously healthy homosexual men."[5] The CDC noted that the clinical characteristics of these cases differed from those usually seen with Kaposi's sarcoma, which had generally been regarded as a disease of elderly men. Again, the situation suggested a common underlying factor—immune suppression.[6]

In 1984 evidence implicated a retrovirus as the etiologic agent of AIDS, and two prototypes were isolated: lymphadenopathy-associated virus (LAV) in France and human T-cell lymphotropic virus type III (HTLV-III) in the United States, which were later shown to represent the same virus. In 1985 a serologic test became available to detect the presence of antibody to HTLV-III/LAV.[7] The availability of this test had varied consequences. First, it permitted investigation of the prevalence of the virus, and these studies demonstrated that infection with the virus itself was more common than the clinical illness (AIDS) in populations with an increased incidence of AIDS. Second, serologic testing gave an opportunity to study the progression of the disease within populations. Third, with the ability to detect antibodies, it became possible to screen blood and plasma donations for the virus. Surveillance of health care workers exposed to the virus also became possible.

Thus in June 1982 there was a hypothesis that a sexually transmitted infectious agent was causing disease in homosexually active men.[8] Since then, the landscape has changed considerably. There is an identified agent, a case definition, and a realization that groups other than men who have sex with men (MSM) are being affected. Because of this realization, the focus of prevention has changed from risk groups such as MSM and intravenous (IV) drug users to risk behaviors such as MSM, IV drug use, and multiple sex partners. Clinically well-defined signs and symptoms exist, some of which are oral. Markers are available for the disease, treatments exist, and tests have been developed to measure viral load. Unfortunately, no cure or vaccine exists.

In 1993 the CDC proposed a change in the case definition of AIDS to more realistically measure the extent of disease. The new case definition was defined by a T-cell count of 200 or less and the presence of specific AIDS-defining conditions. These were expanded from the original definition to include, for example, cervical cancer and other conditions that would capture groups without previously recognized symptoms. Although this was important from a surveillance standpoint for tracking disease, it was also important to individuals in terms of becoming eligible for medical benefits that required an AIDS diagnosis. Therefore the increase in AIDS cases in that year was more a product of a change in reporting than an overall increase in HIV incidence.[9]

The HIV antibody test was licensed in 1985.[10] This test detects the presence of antibodies to HIV, not the virus itself. The test thus indicates only that infection with HIV has occurred, with no implications as to health status. A person who has antibodies to HIV is referred to as seropositive, and one without detectable antibodies is termed seronegative. Seroconversion is said to have occurred when an individual's test becomes positive after some time previous to which test results had been negative. It is important to note that there is a window period during which a person may be infected but during which the body has not yet responded to the virus with detectable antibody response. This time period can range from 3 to 12 weeks after infection, although reports of 6 months or more have been made. The screening test used is the enzyme-linked immunosorbent assay (ELISA). If a specimen has a positive result, a repeat ELISA is generally performed. A persistent positive result is confirmed by a Western blot test. Although both the ELISA and the Western blot test for antibody, the Western blot is considered a more sensitive assay. Therefore persons testing negative on the ELISA are considered seronegative (at least for that point in time), and persons with a positive test confirmed by a Western blot are considered seropositive. For those in whom the results are indeterminate, the tests are repeated.

The Food and Drug Administration (FDA) approved the first antigen test kit in 1996 for use in screening blood donations.[11] Although it may take up to 3 months or more to detect antibodies to HIV, antigens, the virus's own protein, may be detected an average of 6 days earlier. Transfusion-related HIV infection is low. Current tests fail to detect only 1 in 450,000 to 660,000 HIV-positive donations. This represents approximately 18 to 27 donations per year. Use of antigen testing prevents 5 to 10 cases (approximately 25% of current cases of transfusion-associated HIV) per year. Antigen testing is approved only for blood screening and not as a diagnostic tool. Nucleic acid testing can detect minute amounts of viruses such as HIV and hepatitis C virus even earlier and allow detection of contaminated blood in less than 20 days.[12]

In 1996 the FDA licensed the first home test for HIV antibody.[13] Some controversy surrounds this test because in a majority of states and under the professional recommendations, testing should not occur without appropriate counseling before and after the test. That first test was an over-the-counter specimen collection kit in which the user mails a dried blood sample to a laboratory for analysis, with results available after 1 week by telephone. The reported sensitivity is 99.9% and the specificity close to 100%. Therefore 1 in 1000 false-positive results and almost no false- negative results would be expected. Also licensed by the FDA in 1996 is the first saliva-based HIV test. The accuracy of this test is close to that of tests using blood samples.

The FDA has also approved tests that measure the concentration of HIV in the blood, a more appropriate predictor of the progression of disease than previously available tests such as those that measured CD4 counts. Studies on these viral load tests have shown that individuals with levels below 10,000 viral units per milliliter of serum were more likely to survive the 6-year study period than were those with higher levels of virus. The FDA is also reviewing rapid testing for HIV, but no product is yet approved. The CDC has called for faster FDA approval because earlier results may reduce the rate of new infections. The failure of many individuals to return for HIV test results could be minimized by a rapid test. Approximately one fourth of those tested, or 10,000 people annually, do not return for their results.[14] A phenotypic HIV drug resistance test exists that can detect the emergence of drug resistance before significant increases in viral loads of patients in treatment. The clinical significance is that modifications in treatment can be made earlier as signs of treatment failure are detected. This could become a standard monitoring tool.[15]

As of December 1999, more than 733,734 cases of AIDS and 438,795 deaths had been reported to the CDC, and the estimate of those infected with HIV (HIV seropositive without signs and symptoms of AIDS) is 600,00 to 900,00 in the United States, approximately 20,000 of whom are unaware of their infection.[16] It took 9 years for the first 100,000 cases to be reported but less than 2 years for the second 100,000 cases. By the end of 1992, 100,000 people had died of AIDS, and there is an AIDS death approximately every 15 minutes. Although the HIV epidemic still affects men who have sex with men more than other groups, the spread of disease into the heterosexual population is becoming more evident. In 1992 the number of women infected through heterosexual contact exceeded the number infected by IV drug use. In 2000 40,000 new cases were reported, and 30% of the new cases were among women. Among men, 60% of the new cases were in men who have sex with men and 15% in heterosexual men. Although the number of new cases steadily declined in the past few years, the slowdown has been reduced for reasons such as complacency about prevention and poor access to treatment. The CDC national goal is to reduce the number of new infections to 20,000 by 2005.[17]

Newly released figures from the United Nations indicate that 34.3 million people worldwide are either HIV positive or have an AIDS diagnosis. Africa accounts for more than two thirds of the global epidemic, and transmission there is primarily heterosexual.[18] It has been suggested that the HIV pandemic ranks as "one of the most destructive microbial scourges in history."[19] Approximately 16,000 new infections occur daily, and more than 95% of these occur in developing countries.

Epidemiologic studies have shown an increase in infection rates among IV drug users and disproportionate rates among minority groups. In *Living with AIDS,* the National Commission on AIDS reported, "As of June 1991, women accounted for 10% of all AIDS cases . . . cases among women are growing faster than AIDS cases among men."[20] The rate of new infections has increased in women and individuals of color, who now represent 67% of newly diagnosed AIDS cases, 62% of those living with AIDS, and 69% of new HIV infections. The highest rates are in African-American men and women. African-American and Latina women account for approximately 80% of cases among women.[21]

Children are becoming infected as well. Nearly 70% of all pediatric AIDS cases are related to the mother's exposure to the disease. Clinical trials reported in 1994 demonstrated that the use of zidovudine (AZT) can reduce by two thirds the risk of HIV transmission from women to their unborn children. The perinatal transmission rate for women taking AZT was 8.3% compared with 25.5% for those taking a placebo. Vertical transmission rates have steadily declined from more than 20% between 1985 and 1990 to 6.5% between 1990 and 1997. This decline is attributed to the routine treatment of pregnant women with zidovudine. Estimates in 1994 were that between 6000 and 7000 women infected with HIV gave birth in the United States each year and that 1500 to 2000 of the infants were infected. An FDA advisory panel has recommended that AZT be given to all HIV-infected women during specified prenatal and postnatal periods.[22] This also has implications for postexposure management in those dental health care workers (DHCW) who are pregnant, although no recommendations have been proposed.

GUIDELINES AND REGULATIONS REGARDING TRANSMISSIBLE DISEASES

What does all this mean for dentistry? Several salient concepts emerge from the data provided by prevalence studies using the HIV antibody tests. First, the concept of "risk groups" is of diminishing usefulness for evaluating who may be at risk. Second, the majority of persons with serologic evidence of infection have no symptoms of infection. Third, 9 of 10 infected persons are unaware that they are infected. Thus, while risk groups become less distinct, the asymptomatic population continues to grow and increasingly consists of individuals unaware of their status. It follows that dentists are treating many unknown HIV-seropositive patients. With this knowledge, it becomes obligatory that all patients be treated as potentially infectious for HIV. There is simply no scientific rationale (or legal precedent) for selecting certain patients or groups of patients to be subject to particular infection-control procedures. These arguments provide the basis for the use of universal rather than selective precautions in infection control.

Universal Precautions have the added advantage of being effective against other viruses transmitted by blood and saliva during the course of oral health treatment. Infectious diseases are not a new threat in dentistry. Although HIV disease carries with it stigmas and fears that are a new phenomenon, hepatitis B virus (HBV) has always been an occupational hazard. Hepatitis C virus is also recognized as a potential occupational hazard. State, federal, and local regulatory and advisory agencies have caused DHCWs to change the way they practice and to alter the environment in which they place themselves, their staffs, and their patients.

In 1970 Congress passed the Occupational Safety and Health Act, creating, within the Department of Labor, the Occupational Safety and Health Administration (OSHA).[23] The charge to OSHA was to protect workers and ensure healthful working conditions for every worker in the United States. This act required all employers to provide to all employees "a workplace that is free from recognized hazards that are causing or likely to cause death or serious physical harm." Before finalizing the bloodborne pathogens rule on December 6, 1991, OSHA relied on this general duty clause to enforce the use of recommended guidelines to control the spread of bloodborne disease among health care workers.[24] OSHA is a regulatory agency with enforcement authority and an ability to make citations and impose fines or penalties for failure to comply with established standards, especially when this failure results in illness, injury, or death.

CENTERS FOR DISEASE CONTROL AND PREVENTION

The CDC is an advisory agency with an intent to protect and promote the health of the public. The CDC has no regulatory authority, and the guidelines issued are for the most part voluntary, although over time these guidelines become standards of practice and, in some cases, the basis for regulation by agencies such as OSHA. Once the CDC published its first infection control guidelines in 1982, standards of care evolved for the dental profession.[25] The early guidelines did not specifically address dental care but outlined suggested precautions to be used when dealing with patients with AIDS, such as the use of gloves, refraining from bending or recapping needles, the use of gowns, and the use of extraordinary care to prevent injury. In general, early in the epidemic the CDC, reasoning by analogy, recommended use of procedures already known to be appropriate for persons infected with HBV. The first actual recommendations for DHCWs in 1983 stated the following:

1. Personnel should wear gloves, masks, and protective eyewear when performing dental or oral surgical procedures.
2. Instruments used in the mouths of patients should be sterilized after use.[26]

State-of-the-art infection control guidelines for dentistry did not emerge until April 18, 1986, when the CDC published "Recommended Infection Control Practices for Dentistry."[27] These recommendations were based on the use of a common set of infection-control strategies to be used routinely in the care of all patients in dental practices. This represented a shift to Universal Precautions from selective precautions. Of special interest is the editorial note that "all DHCWs (dental health care workers) must be made aware of sources and methods of transmission of infectious diseases."[27] It was emphasized that disease transmission in either direction (patient to DHCW or DHCW to patient) could be minimized by following the infection-control guidelines. In addition, vaccination for HBV was strongly recommended for dental personnel as a supplement to, not a replacement for, strict adherence to Universal Precautions.

The guidelines for dentistry, updated and released in July 1993, represent a logical progression of knowledge in the emerging science of infection control and exposure management.[28] The new recommendations emphasize behavior-driven components of exposure control and issues of patient safety, including providing a clear understanding of disease transmission mechanisms and associated risk. The overall premise is the same as in 1986, that "dental patients and DHCWs may be exposed to a variety of microorganisms via blood or oral respiratory secretions. . . . Infection via any of these routes requires that all three of the following conditions be present: a susceptible host; a pathogen with sufficient infectivity and numbers to cause infection; and a portal through which the pathogen may enter the host. Effective infection control strategies are intended to break one or more of these links in the chain, thereby preventing infection."[28] In addition, there is a shift from the earlier emphasis on bloodborne disease transmission to now include airborne disease concerns, such as *Mycobacterium tuberculosis* and other upper respiratory illnesses. These new recommendations are intended to provide direction where there is no current regulation from OSHA.

Other major guidelines for infection control were released in 1987 and 1988 from the CDC and referred, in part, to all health care workers but also, in part, specifically to DHCWs.[29,30] The CDC now made note of the fact, cited previously, that the antibody status of most patients would not be known; therefore these recommendations were to apply to all patients and all health care workers who performed or assisted in invasive procedures. The 1987 guidelines were the first to introduce the concept of Universal Precautions. All previous recommendations were selective precautions. The recommendations included the wearing of gloves and other personal protective barriers such as masks and eyewear, the handling of needles and other sharp instruments in such a manner as to prevent injury, and the management of specific exposure incidents with a potential for disease transmission. In the recommendations specific to dentistry it was emphasized that gloves were to be regarded as single-use items. Handwashing; the use of masks, protective eyewear, and gowns where indicated; disinfection of environmental surfaces; and sterilization of instruments were more fully defined. The precautions recommended for dentistry began to recognize that blood, saliva, and gingival fluid should be considered infective. Handpiece sterilization and infection control procedures for dental laboratory cases emerged as important issues for dentistry. All of these recommendations became the basis for the OSHA bloodborne pathogens standard.

RISK TO DENTAL HEALTH CARE WORKERS

The first case of occupationally acquired HIV infection, by a needlestick, was reported in Africa in 1984. It also became apparent during this period (1988 to 1990) that DHCWs were themselves susceptible to becoming infected.[31] Indeed, two dentists were reported to have most likely seroconverted as a result of occupational exposure.

As of December 31, 1999, 56 health care workers had been reported to the CDC as having a documented occupational transmission of HIV, through a special study set up to monitor health care workers.[32] Documented means that seroconversion occurred after an occupational exposure to blood known to be infected with HIV. The exposed DHCW must also have had a baseline HIV test that was negative at the time of exposure, and seroconversion must have occurred 3 to 6 months later. Among the documented cases, 48 reported percutaneous exposures; 5 reported blood splashes to the eyes, nose, or mouth; 2 reported percutaneous and mucocutaneous exposure; and 1 reported an unknown route. Forty-nine were exposed to blood of an HIV-infected person, 1 to visibly blood-contaminated bodily fluid, 3 to an unspecified fluid, and 3 to concentrated virus in a laboratory. Subsequently, AIDS has developed in 24 of these health care workers.

This report may not represent the total number of exposed and infected health care workers because it may not include those not reporting an occupational exposure or infection. No DHCWs have been reported through this surveillance system as a documented occupational infection. Reporting occupational incidents to agencies is important in tracking not just seroconversion but the routes and circumstances of the injury as well. The CDC has two programs for voluntary reporting. For incidents related to known HIV-infected source individuals, the report is to the National Center for Infectious Disease's Hospital Infections Program. To report documented HIV seroconversion, contact the local or state health department, which in turn reports to the CDC. In addition, reports of medical device failures that may have facilitated the injury should go to the FDA Medwatch program. This program is designed for health care workers to report adverse events and product problems.

One hundred thirty-eight health care workers have been reported to the CDC as a "possible occupational transmission," and among these are six dental workers. These health care workers have been investigated and are "without identifiable behavioral or transfusion risks; each reported percutaneous or mucocutaneous occupational exposures to blood or body fluids, or lab solutions, but HIV seroconversion specifically resulting from an occupational exposure was not determined."[32] Occupational exposure control is a serious issue. In February 1995, OSHA issued a guide to dental employer obligations as a follow-up to the bloodborne pathogens standard in regard to occupational exposure.[33] These detail, in a step-by-step guide to compliance, the recommendations and regulations regarding management of exposure incidents in oral health facilities (Fig. 9-1). The employer is obligated to provide, not perform, a confidential medical evaluation and follow-up by a licensed health care professional at no cost to the employee.

Among the medical services that the employee must be offered are counseling, collection and testing of the employee's blood, postexposure prophylaxis (in accordance with U.S. Public Health Service recommendations), and evaluation of reported illnesses. The employer is obligated to pay only for the cost of treating the incident and not the cost of the subsequent disease should seroconversion occur. All exposure incidents are recordable for purposes of OSHA's record-keeping requirements. Testing of source patients is in accordance with state laws and with consent of the patient. The U.S. Public Health Service did not officially recommend zidovudine for HIV postexposure prophylaxis until recently. OSHA therefore did not require the employer to pay for it.[34] It would be prudent to assume that OSHA would expect the employer to now pay for the antiviral regimen because there have been changes in the U.S. Public Health Service recommendations. Previously the U.S. Public Health Service neither recommended nor advised against the use of zidovudine for postexposure prophylaxis. However, the agency did recommend offering it to an exposed health care worker. Findings released by the CDC in December 1995 associate the use of zidovudine with a lower risk for HIV transmission after studying its use in health care workers who sustained percutaneous injuries to blood known to be infected with HIV.[35] The data suggest that use of zidovudine postexposure may be protective for health care workers. The study investigated factors associated with HIV transmission, such as exposure to a large quantity of blood, a deep injury, a visibly contaminated device, and terminal illness in the source patient. Risk for HIV infection among health care workers who used zidovudine was reduced approximately 79% with other factors controlled. These results prompted the U.S. Public Health Service to evaluate the data and to propose revisions for postexposure management (PEM) on the basis of the severity of an injury and the HIV status of the source patient. Newly released recommendations for PEM of individuals exposed to blood known to be infected with HIV include the use of antiretrovirals, either as monotherapy or in combination as determined by source individual and injury information.[36] The current U.S. Public Health Service recommendation is that health care workers who are exposed to HIV on the job should, in many cases, take zidovudine and other antiretroviral drugs after exposure to reduce their risk of becoming infected.

Injury data on DHCWs has been derived from observational, retrospective, and prospective studies (including self-reported data). In 1987 dentists reported approximately 1 injury per month (12 per year). By

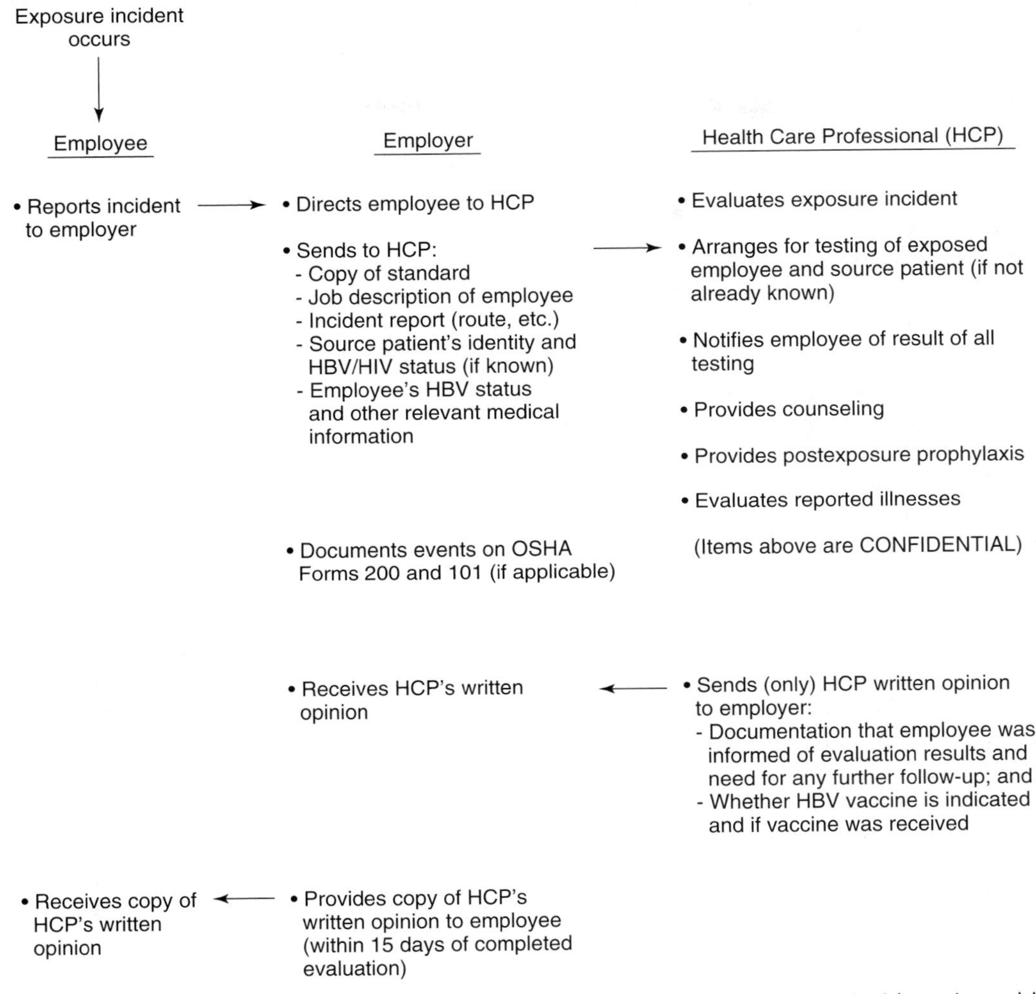

Fig. 9-1. Recommendations and regulations regarding management of exposure incidents in oral health facilities. (From *Postexposure evaluation and follow-up requirements under OSHA's standard for occupational exposure to bloodborne pathogens: a guide to dental employer obligations,* Washington, DC, 1995, Department of Labor, Occupational Safety and Health Administration.)

1991 dentists reported 0.3 per month, or approximately 3 to 4 per year. More recent data from the CDC indicate a further decline to approximately 0.18 per month, or 2 to 3 per year. This supports the assumption that most injuries are preventable with appropriate administrative, engineering, and work practice controls. Most percutaneous injuries occurred outside the patients' mouth, most on the hands of the dentist. Burs were the most common source (37%), followed by syringe needles (30%), sharp instruments (21%), and orthodontic wires (6%). The CDC stated that "the rate of percutaneous exposures among dental workers . . . is probably less than among general surgical personnel.

Most injuries are outside the mouth, involve the fingers and hands and are self-inflicted."[37]

Data on 104 percutaneous injuries reported to the CDC national surveillance of occupational injuries for DHCWs between June 1995 and March 2000 confirm that the majority of injuries are without significant risk of transmission according to criteria identified by the CDC. The purpose in collecting these data is to establish the likelihood that occupational exposures put DHCWs at risk for bloodborne disease transmission and to determine the proportion of injuries that may have been prevented. Of the injuries assessed, 44% were among dentists, 33% among oral surgeons, 19% among dental assistants, and 8% among dental hygienists. Twenty-two percent were superficial, 75% were moderate, and only 3% were deep puncture wounds. The presence of visible blood was reported for 45%, no visible blood for 33%, and unknown for 22%. Fifty-four of the injuries occurred during device use, 37% after use but before disposal, 7% during or after disposal, and 2% unknown. Forty-four percent were patient related and nonpreventable, 18% may have been prevented with the use of a safety device, and 27% may have been prevented by a safer work practice. Overall, it appears that DHCWs were exposed to small volumes of blood.

Of a total population of more than 213,357 professionally active dentists and dental hygienists, the current estimate of dentists and dental hygienists with AIDS is only 467, of which approximately 374 have died.[16] There are possibly more than 2000 DHCWs with HIV. The best estimates of risk to health care workers is 0.3% for HIV transmission from percutaneous exposures and 0.09% for mucous membrane exposures (even less for skin contacts), 3% to 10% for hepatitis C virus (HCV), and 30% for HBV transmission after percutaneous injury from an infected patient.[38] From the data available, it appears that the risk of HIV infection to DHCWs is extremely low. Health care workers represent approximately 5% of the general population and approximately 5% of reported AIDS cases, indicating that they are not overrepresented.

RISK TO PATIENTS

DHCWs had already recognized the potential to transmit disease in either direction. HBV transmission had been well documented from dentists to patients, as well as herpes transmission from dental hygienists to patients. Transmission of HBV from dentists to patients has not been reported since 1987. Health care workers, primarily physicians and dentists, have a threefold to fivefold higher prevalence of HBV than the general population does. However, transmission from HIV-infected dental health care workers to patients had not yet been reported. Since the early 1970s, when serologic testing became available for HBV, the CDC had reported on 20 clusters of HBV transmission to more than 300 patients from infected health care workers. In 12 of the clusters the health care worker did not routinely use gloves, and some reported skin lesions that could have promoted the transmission. Nine of these clusters were linked to dentists or oral surgeons. Many of the transmissions could have been prevented by strict adherence to current Universal Precautions. Most of the reports were before the acceptance of Universal Precautions. The CDC suggested that "the limited number of reports of HBV transmission from HCWs [health care workers] to patients in recent years may reflect the adoption of Universal Precautions and increased use of HBV vaccine."[39]

Previous experience with HBV transmission suggested that the performance of invasive procedures was more likely to contribute to disease transmission, that the use of Universal Precautions was likely to reduce the risk of transmission, and that this transmission would be expected to "occur only very rarely."[40] Therefore routine testing of health care workers was not recommended. Recent reports of HBV transmission from a health care worker to patients during performance of invasive, exposure-prone procedures are not among dentists, but refer to a surgeon who is HBeAg positive and had not been vaccinated against HBV. Approximately 1% of surgeons are infected with HBV, and transmission is thought to be rare.[31] In 1992 a female patient was diagnosed with HBV, and transmission was associated with cardiac surgery. No deficiencies in infection control were detected and no specific events could be identified. HBV was transmitted to at least 19 patients studied, and epidemiologic and laboratory evidence "support the surgeon as the source of infection." Factors of transmission were more likely related to irritations on the surgeon's fingers, and virus, which may have escaped through tiny holes in the gloves, was found in the glove washings. Health care workers who are positive for HBeAg are more infectious, and reports of transmission of HBV since the early 1970s have been associated with this state.

Hepatitis C virus (HCV) transmission in health care facilities has also been documented. In a study conducted from 1992 to 1994, five patients of a cardiac surgeon were identified in whom infection may have been transmitted by the surgeon. All were infected with the same HCV genotype. The surgeon reported one serious percutaneous exposure from a patient with HBV and was treated for this exposure. Overall, the surgeon reported a rate of approximately 20 percutaneous injuries per 100 procedures, most of which went unnoticed until after the procedure.[41] This resembles reports of HBV transmission in surgical and dental settings as a cluster of cases. Simultaneous transmission of HIV and HCV to a health care worker who sustained a deep needlestick injury from an HIV/HCV-infected source patient in 1990 was reported. Use of zidovudine was declined. This is the first report of simultaneous transmission.[42] Researchers at the International Conference on Emerging Diseases convened in 2000 reported that health care workers had a 20 to 40 times greater risk of contracting HCV from an accidental needlestick than HIV. A study of 66 hospitals in South Carolina indicated that 5.2% of health care workers were infected with HCV compared with 2.3% with HIV.[43]

When the inevitable became the actual with the first report of transmission of HIV from an infected health care worker to a patient during an invasive procedure, it was indeed in dentistry.[44] The first report of a "possible" transmission to "patient A" came in the July 1990 issue of the CDC's *Morbidity and Mortality Weekly Report*.[45] By January 1991 the transmission was no longer considered merely possible, and the report then read, "Update: Transmission of HIV Infection during an Invasive Dental Procedure."[46] The concept of transmission from health care worker to patient had progressed from highly improbable to possible to probable in less than a year, and the involvement had increased from one to six patients.[47] These events, leading up to the death of patient A, Kimberly Bergalis, left an indelible imprint on dentistry.

GUIDELINES FOR HUMAN IMMUNODEFICIENCY VIRUS/ HEPATITIS B VIRUS–INFECTED DENTAL HEALTH CARE WORKERS

The public outcry over the "first real victim of AIDS" was deafening. Conservative congressmen called for stiff measures, from jailing infected health care workers who continued to practice to mandatory testing of all health care workers. One of the most serious possible consequences of this event for the health care field in general could be the loss of the professional control over the future of health care workers. At a minimum, proposals ranged from reviewing the health status of infected health care workers (HIV and HBV) by expert review panels to mandatory testing and patient notification. By an act of Congress in October 1991, states were given 1 year in which to adopt the CDC "recommendations for preventing transmission of human immunodeficiency virus and hepatitis B virus to patients during exposure-prone invasive procedures" or else to come up with their equivalent and have it approved by the CDC; all states have complied.[48] In essence, the CDC recommendations cited by Congress are based on a series of assumptions as to the likelihood of transmitting disease from infected providers to patients:

1. Infected health care workers who adhere to Universal Precautions and who do not perform invasive procedures pose no risk for transmitting HIV or HBV to patients.
2. Infected health care workers who adhere to Universal Precautions and who perform certain exposure-prone procedures pose a small risk for transmitting HBV to patients.
3. HIV is transmitted much less readily than HBV.

The key phrase is "exposure-prone procedures," and the problem is how to define them and how and when to restrict their practice by infected health care workers. The task may have seemed simple at first, with the plan being to have the professions determine a list of exposure-prone procedures. It proved, however, to be far from a simple matter, and professional organizations either refused to produce a list, were unable to come up with lists, or thought that it was not in their best interest to list these procedures. Data from the CDC were challenged during public testimony by, for example, the American Dental Association and the University of Texas Health Science Center at San Antonio, which presented testimony offering that the rates of injury were lower than those estimated by the CDC and that therefore their assumption that 13 to 128 patients were infected with HIV and 406 to 4057 with HBV by surgeons and DHCWs during an invasive procedure was incorrect (*The Nation's Health,* April 1991).

A more accurate measure of provider-to-patient transmission potential is not possible until a much larger sample of patients on whom exposure-prone invasive procedures were performed can be studied. Looking back at more than 22,032 patients of 63 HIV-infected providers (including 33 dentists or dental students), no other case of transmission of HIV has been discovered.[49] In 15 years only one cluster of cases has been linked to provider transmission. The CDC cites the risk from an infected health care worker, more specifically, a dentist, to transmit HIV to a patient as between 1 in 263,100 to 1 in 2,631,000 dental procedures. More than two billion dental procedures have been performed in the United States since the beginning of the AIDS epidemic without a single documented case of occupationally acquired HIV infection among DHCWs. Limitations exist in these retrospective studies, but the data are consistent with the assessment that the risk for HIV transmission from infected health care workers is exceedingly low.

Whatever plan a state adopts, it must be in compliance with statutes and court actions on discrimination and disability such as Section 504 of the Rehabilitation Act of 1973, the Americans with Disabilities Act of 1990, and any pertinent state laws. All states have submitted plans to the CDC or verified that they will comply with existing CDC guidelines. The literature suggests that a majority of states rejected mandatory testing in favor of voluntary testing, rejected patient notification, recommended the use of expert review panels, and emphasized the importance of education, training, and the use of Universal Precautions. Findings from a research project by a dental intern from Harvard University School of Dental Medicine in conjunction with the Boston Public Health Commission, HIV Dental Ombudsperson Program, indicate that of states validated as being in compliance with CDC guidelines, 100% rejected mandatory testing, 96% rejected patient notification, 71% recommended the use of expert review panels for HIV-positive DHCWs and 63% for HBV-positive DHCWs who are HbeAg positive, 90% emphasized the importance of education and training, and 98% recommended the use of Universal Precautions. Furthermore, 86% stated that currently available data provide no basis for recommendations to restrict HIV- or HBV-positive DHCWs who perform invasive procedures.[39] These guidelines are currently under revision as a result of evidence that the overall risk of bloodborne virus transmission is very low and that the health of infected workers has improved from advances in medical treatment. Revised guidelines would have to include HCV. The literature indicates that bloodborne viruses are more likely to be transmitted from patient to health care worker than from health care worker to patient or from patient to patient. Transmission between health care workers and patients is most often caused by a percutaneous injury. The majority of patient-to-patient transmission has involved breaches in recommended infection control practice.

OCCUPATIONAL SAFETY AND HEALTH ADMINISTRATION REGULATIONS

The recommendations of the CDC are not regulatory, only advisory. Although they may set professional standards, they do not have full legal force behind them. However, these recommendations became, for OSHA, the basis for the final rule on occupational exposure to bloodborne pathogens, issued on December 6, 1991. As an OSHA administrator remarked, "We are providing full legal force to universal precautions—employers and employees must treat blood and certain body fluids as if infectious. Meeting these requirements is not optional. It's essential to prevent illness, chronic infection and even death."[24] The U.S. Department of Labor expects this standard to protect more than 5.6 million workers and prevent more than 200 deaths and 9200 bloodborne infections each year.

The purpose of the OSHA standard is to minimize occupational exposure to blood or other potentially infectious body fluids or materials that pose a risk of transmission of bloodborne disease in a health care setting. It covers any employee exposed, or potentially exposed, during the performance of his or her duties, to blood, body fluids, or potentially infectious materials. Health and safety are recognized as one aspect of practice administration. Although OSHA obligates the employer to provide for the employee, free of charge, a series of hazard abatement measures to diminish the risk of exposure, these measures are in the best interest of each DHCW and will pay for themselves by ensuring a safe dental practice. Some costs are one-time improvements (e.g., an eyewash station) and preventive measures (HBV vaccination), whereas others, such as gloves and masks, are recurring costs. OSHA estimates the annual cost per dental establishment, of which there are 100,174, to be approximately $873. The highest-cost area is personal protective equipment, followed by vaccination and postexposure follow-up. Some costs may vary, depending on the length of employment, turnover, and actual office experience with injuries.

The hazard abatement measures include mandating the use of Universal Precautions (Standard Precautions), emphasizing engineering and work practice controls, providing and requiring employees to use personal protective equipment, making available the hepatitis B vaccination (and associated tests and boosters) at no cost to the employee, making available specific procedures for employees who sustain an occupational exposure (including confidential medical evaluation and follow-up), and the communication of hazards to employees by warning signs and labels. OSHA further mandates that the training provided relate specifically to information about the standard itself, the particular office exposure control plan contemplated, and information about the transmission of bloodborne disease. Requirements exist on identifying at-risk employees and their tasks within the context of a written exposure control plan. This plan must be specific as to how the office will comply with the standard. Employers have record-keeping requirements, including written schedules for housekeeping, plans for waste management, and exposure management.

Some states have their own occupational safety and health plans that may differ from the federal standard. DHCWs should become familiar with their state plan or the federal standard, as appropriate. It will also be necessary to review individual state and local regulations on infectious and hazardous waste management and disposal because there is no federal standard on dental waste as yet. The Environmental Protection Agency did have a pilot medical waste tracking act and will consider whether to make it national in scope.

The OSHA bloodborne standard is not the only regulation from the Department of Labor of concern to dentistry. In 1987 OSHA extended the hazard communication standard to the health care industry.[50] The standard became final for the health care industry in 1989. The intent of this standard is to protect health care workers from hazards associated with the use of chemical agents during the course of employment. The standard is based on the simple concept that employees have a need and a right to know the hazards and identities of the chemicals to which they are exposed. Employers are obligated to identify and list hazardous chemicals in their workplaces; obtain material data safety sheets (MDSSs) for these chemicals; develop and implement a written hazard communication program; and communicate hazard information to their employees through labels, MDSSs, and formal training programs. Employees must understand what personal protective equipment is necessary to prevent illness or injury and how to manage an exposure incident or an emergency. Unlike the bloodborne standard, training in hazard communication must occur before an initial assignment. Training in both bloodborne exposure and chemical hazard exposure must be renewed whenever the hazard changes. Training is required to be specific to the agents used by an employee.

In 1999 OSHA issued a new compliance directive, "Enforcement Procedures for the Occupational Exposure to Bloodborne Pathogens (CPL2-2.44D)," which updates all previous directives.[51] This directive does not place new requirements on employers, but it recognizes advances made in technology and science. The seven key revisions include annual review of the exposure plan, engineering and work practices, FDA device approval evidence, multiemployer worksites, CDC guidelines on vaccinations and postexposure management, effective training and education, and update of appendices. Within the engineering controls revision is the emphasis on use of safer medical devices. OSHA considers engineering controls as a first-line defense against injury.

In 2000 Congress passed the Needlestick Safety and Prevention Act, which requires medical and dental facilities to use "safer" devices. Under the legislation, health care facilities must provide safety devices, involve health care workers in their selection, provide training, and keep a detailed log of needle-related injuries. Enforcement is through OSHA.[52] The estimated impact is the potential of an 80% decrease in the estimated 800,000 needlesticks that occur annually. The Needlestick Safety and Prevention Act has four major categories: modification of definitions of engineering controls, revision and updating of the Exposure Control Plan, involvement of employees in selection of devices, and record keeping. Twenty states had previously passed needlestick safety bills or had bills under consideration.

TRANSMISSIBLE DISEASES

The oral cavity harbors microorganisms with potential to transmit a wide spectrum of infectious agents. Dental professionals are therefore at risk for any orally transmissible disease from the blood or saliva of the patients they treat. In addition, the trauma of some dental procedures and the mixing of blood and saliva enhance the risk of bloodborne disease transmission. Any patient's blood or saliva is potentially infectious and puts the DHCW at risk.

Before the HIV epidemic there was concern over the transmission of disease in dental settings, and HBV drove the model for infection control. Although HBV is still the basis of infection control procedures, HIV drives many of the evolving regulations and guidelines. The transmissible diseases currently of greatest concern to the dental professional are HBV, HIV, HCV, and *M. tuberculosis*, although the list of transmissible diseases is more widely encompassing. Each of these diseases is discussed in terms of etiology, tests available for diagnosis, risk of transmission, and recommendations for prevention in the professional context.

HEPATITIS B

The disease is produced by a virus known as the Dane particle. This intact virus consists of an inner core antigen (HBcAg) and an outer coat surface antigen (HBsAg) and is highly infective. As little as 0.00000001 ml of blood can transmit the disease. Initial symptoms may include vague abdominal discomfort, myalgia, diarrhea, jaundice (30% of cases), lack of appetite, and low-grade fever. However, approximately 80% of individuals infected with the virus are asymptomatic and unaware that they are infected. People who are infected with the virus can transmit HBV whether or not they manifest clinical signs and symptoms. HBV is one of the most common reportable diseases in the United States and is "primarily a disease of young adults, with about 75% of cases occurring in persons aged 15 to 39."[53] Cases reported underestimate the rate of true infection because of the subclinical state. Health care providers also underreport cases despite laws that mandate reporting. The CDC estimates, after correcting for underreporting, that approximately 300,000 HBV infections occur in the United States each year. The most serious consequence is not acute infection but chronic carrier states that occur in approximately 6% to 10% of adults, more in children. These carriers also represent a population at risk of spreading infection.

"HBV infection is the major infectious occupational hazard to health care workers."[53] Health care workers represent approximately 2% to 6% of reported cases, and this recognition, along with the availability of the HBV vaccine, was the driving force behind the development of the OSHA bloodborne pathogens standard.

Fortunately for dental professionals, a vaccine has been developed to immunize recipients against HBV. Three doses are given to confer immunity: an initial dose, followed by a second dose at 1 month, and then a third dose 6 months after the first. Given dental personnel's high risk of contracting HBV, it is strongly recommended that all dental professionals be immunized. Indeed, great emphasis exists on vaccination in the OSHA bloodborne pathogens standard where the employer is obligated to provide the vaccination free of charge to potentially exposed employees with a specific waiver to be signed by an employee who declines the vaccine. The risks associated with HBV include not only the morbidity of the acute phase of the disease but also the possible sequelae of the chronic carrier state, including cirrhosis of the liver or primary hepatocellular carcinoma. There are no current recommendations for a booster dose of the vaccine. In 1997 the CDC revised its recommendations on postvaccination titer testing to determine if an immune response is evident. The current recommendation is that titer testing is indicated in health care workers who have blood or patient contact and are at ongoing risk for percutaneous injuries. Knowledge of antibody response will assist in postexposure therapy decisions.[54] OSHA follows current U.S. Public Health Service recommendations for immunization under the bloodborne pathogens standard. Although the vaccine is successful in more than 90% of individuals, some do not initially respond, do not develop HBsAg, and therefore are not protected; however, in a majority of these cases an additional dose is effective. A very small percentage never respond, and immunity cannot be ensured in these individuals.

Approximately 86% of DHCWs have been vaccinated.[55] Before the vaccine, approximately 250 health care workers died per year as a result of complications from HBV. After compliance with the vaccination recommendations, the estimate dropped to approximately 100 per year. Vaccination should be received before exposure occurs or it will be of no benefit.

Serologic testing is available to determine

the presence in the blood of HBV antigens and antibodies to those antigens. The presence of hepatitis B core antigen (HBcAg) is associated with active viral infection and infectivity. The hepatitis B surface antigen (HBsAg) appears before acute illness and usually disappears quickly. Anti–hepatitis B core antibody (anti-HBcAb) is not protective, appears early in the illness, and decreases in titer in those who become immune. Persistent high titer indicates ongoing infectivity. HBsAb does not appear for several months and then rises to a high titer in those who become immune. The e antigen (HBeAg) is associated with higher risk of chronic liver disease and higher risk of infectivity. Also of concern is delta hepatitis (HDV), a single-stranded circular RNA virus. Often referred to as the "delta agent," this is a defective virus that relies on HBV for its pathogenicity. It is a piggyback virus that cannot infect on its own but depends on the presence of HBV for infectivity. The combination results in a "supervirus" and a more fulminant course of disease. Vaccination against HBV will prevent HDV coinfection, as long as the person has not already become an unknown HBV carrier. For an estimated 1% of health care workers who are HBV carriers, prevention of HDV would be difficult. Essentially, prevention relies on strict compliance with Universal Precautions and practicing in such a manner as to avoid injury or exposure. Research is being conducted on the use of interferon-α and other antiviral agents.

Hepatitis C

Hepatitis viruses that were not A and not B became known as non-A, non-B (NANB) in the early 1970s. Diagnosis was not based on identification of an agent but by mode of transmission, for example, whether it was serologic or enteric. In 1989 one of the NANB viruses was identified as hepatitis C (HCV), a single-stranded RNA virus that appears to have cytopathic activity. HCV is implicated in viral hepatitis and is of concern to DHCWs. Transmission is similar to HBV in the parenteral routes identified and mostly is associated with intravenous drug use or administration of blood products, less with sexual or vertical transmission. HCV has been found in saliva. As with HBV, acute infection is usually asymptomatic and may go undetected.[56] Studies indicate that HCV may be responsible for 90% of post-transfusion hepatitis and approximately 60% to 70% of sporadic NANB hepatitis. The community prevalence of anti-HCV has ranged from 1% to 3% in the United States. Approximately 170,000 people become infected each year, and the number of deaths is estimated at 8000 to 10,000 per year. The clinical course of the disease is similar to that of HBV. At least 85% will, however, have chronic hepatitis, and 20% of these chronic carriers will have cirrhosis or even hepatocellular carcinoma.

Blood transfusions had been thought to be the most efficient route of transmission. A screening test for HCV antibody was developed in 1990; however, the test fails to detect all infections and has a low predictive value in populations with low prevalence. A supplemental or confirmatory test comparable to that available for HBV is needed to eliminate false-positive and identify true-positive results. However, this was not available with first-generation tests and only by specific physician request with second-generation tests. Third-generation tests are being released, and more data are needed to determine their efficacy. These tests also fail to differentiate between active HCV infection, immunity to HCV, or a carrier state.[56] Screening of blood donors has reduced the risk of transmission associated with transfusions by approximately 80% in studies conducted in the early 1990s. Fewer than 5% of cases now reported to the CDC are related to transfusions. The majority of new cases reported are among IV drug users, and there are reports of sexual transmission. Only 30% to 40% of newly infected persons show symptoms; when they occur, it is within 3 to 20 weeks after exposure and symptoms are mostly mild and intermittent. HCV RNA can now be detected in blood within 1 to 3 weeks after exposure. Antibodies appear within 15 weeks in approximately 80% of infections, within 5 months in 90% of cases, and within 6 months in 97% of cases. The prevalence estimate is approximately 3.9 million, of whom 2.7 million are chronically infected.

No vaccine or postexposure prophylaxis is available; therefore prevention is paramount. Compared with HBV, HCV is less transmissible after a single exposure. The average risk of infection after a needlestick injury is approximately 1.8%.[40] This falls between risk estimates of HBV and HIV transmission. In terms of acute infections annually, HBV is most prevalent and HCV next; however, higher rates of chronic infection and death are reported with HCV.[37] HCV seroconversions are more likely to occur where there are breaches of infection control. The CDC stresses that bloodborne pathogens, wherever they are and whatever the titer, can be transmitted in either direction. The most important steps a DHCW can take is the appropriate use of recommended hazard abatement procedures to prevent exposure. The FDA recently approved combination therapy of ribavirin and interferon alfa to treat chronic HCV disease. This therapy was previously used only in patients who had relapsed or not responded to monotherapy. Studies indicate sustained response with the use of this therapy. There are serious side effects, which require close monitoring by a physician. Among the side effects are adverse reproductive effects, so it is advised that women not become pregnant while on this therapy and for 6 months after.

It does not appear that health care workers (including dentists) have a disproportionate rate of HCV infection. Results of a voluntary study suggest that the rate of infection of health care workers may be less than that found in voluntary blood donors.[57] As expected, the risk is more evident in health care workers frequently exposed to large quantities of blood. In one study, the highest infection rate was among housekeeping staff.[56] Among health care workers in the early 1970s, as detection became available, HBV rates were as high as 17%, whereas HCV rates were significantly lower. This low risk estimate is validated by at least one needlestick study wherein HCV developed in only 4% after injury from blood known to be HCV positive, and in only three health care workers was seroconversion demonstrated. Other studies have shown anywhere from 0% to 1.3% seroprevalence of anti-HCV in health care workers. There appear to be significant differences between HBV and HCV in terms of transmission risk to health care workers. However, there are very few studies of DHCWs.

Tuberculosis

Although the major infectious diseases of greatest concern to dentistry are HBV, HCV, and HIV/AIDS, other diseases pose a risk to the health care worker. Of emerging concern is tuberculosis (TB), which made a comeback in direct proportion to AIDS cases.

"Tuberculosis is a recognized risk in health-care settings."[58] A 1990 report by the

CDC was prompted by outbreaks of TB in recent years, including some multidrug-resistant strains. Transmission is most likely from patients without recognized disease, not from those receiving anti-TB therapy. Environmental factors, such as inadequate ventilation and contact with patients in small, enclosed areas, can play a part in transmission. Estimates are that for every active TB case there are 15 asymptomatic yet infected people. The risk of disease progression after infection may be heightened in persons with HIV disease.

In April 1994 OSHA issued a notice of proposed rule making for a standard to regulate indoor air quality, which is currently in a comment and review period. The standard is designed for nonindustrial workplaces; the effect on dental facilities is undetermined, but it may consider the effects of aerosolized dental unit water. Also, in 1992 OSHA was petitioned, much in the same fashion as with the Bloodborne Pathogens Standard, for a national compliance directive on occupational exposure to TB. When no action was taken, the Secretary of Labor was petitioned in August 1993 to initiate rule making to promulgate a national standard on TB. As a result, on October 20, 1993, OSHA issued "Enforcement Guidance in the Face of Increased Exposure to Tuberculosis," which is based on guidelines issued by the CDC in 1990 for preventing the transmission of tuberculosis in health care settings. In October 1994, the CDC issued the final version of "Guidelines for Preventing the Transmission of *Mycobacterium tuberculosis* in Health-Care Facilities." The intent is to emphasize the importance of a hierarchy of control measures to reduce the risk of exposure. The fundamentals of TB infection control are not based on Universal Precautions but require the application of a selective hierarchy of controls to identify, isolate, and treat TB. The three levels of control include administrative measures, engineering controls, and personal respiratory equipment. Measures recommended are based on community and facility risk of exposure to TB. Most oral health care facilities fall into the minimal or very low risk determinations. The CDC provides specific guidance for dental facilities depending on the setting. At a minimum, a risk assessment must be done annually; there must be a written TB infection control plan; protocols should be in place for identifying and managing patients who have active TB; DHCWs must be educated, trained, and screened; and a method of evaluating problems must be established. With specific regard to oral health care facilities, the CDC states, "In general, the symptoms for which patients seek treatment in a dental care setting are not likely to be caused by infectious TB. Unless a patient requiring dental care coincidentally has TB, it is unlikely that infectious TB will be encountered in the dental setting. Furthermore, it has not been demonstrated that oral health care procedures generate TB droplet nuclei. Therefore, the risk for transmission of *M. tuberculosis* in most dental settings is probably quite low." More specifically, the CDC recommends that patient medical histories include questions on TB and that those with suggestive symptoms be referred for medical evaluation. Such patients should not remain in the dental care facility any longer than required for a referral and should wear masks and be instructed to cover their mouths and noses when coughing or sneezing. Elective dental treatment should be deferred until a physician confirms that the patient does not have infectious TB. If urgent care is required, such care should be rendered in a facility that can provide TB isolation. DHCWs providing care in these circumstances should use respiratory protection. DHCWs symptomatic for TB should be evaluated and not return to the workplace until a diagnosis of TB has been excluded or until the DHCW is on therapy and determined to be noninfectious.

The Institute of Medicine released a report indicating that health care workers and others are not as likely to contract active TB occupationally because of decreases in new cases and improved infection control practices. The rates reported for health care workers were similar to those for non–health care settings. The report noted that workers are not "risk free" and it is important to follow precautions to prevent the transmission of TB in health care settings.[59]

PREVENTION: INFECTION CONTROL

Because treatment of HBV, HCV, HIV/AIDS, and other transmissible diseases is symptomatic at best, prevention is the most important aspect in the discussion of these diseases. Even if a cure were available, protection from the untoward effects and discomfort of each disease would be desirable. Because many diseases can go undetected for long periods of time, the focus must be on preventing disease transmission from providers to patients, from patients to providers, and between patients and families. Again, it is important to emphasize that one of the most important personal barriers is the HBV vaccine, and as a result the CDC has recommended its inclusion in the childhood vaccination series.[53]

In 1993 the CDC updated all previously published recommendations relative to infection control in dental facilities.[28] The following recommendations should be used routinely in the care of all patients in dental practice to control the spread of infection.

Medical History

A complete medical history should always be obtained. Specific questions about lymphadenopathy, recent weight loss, and infections should be included. All positive responses should be followed up. An individual may not be aware of an infectious state, so diagnostic acumen may be required.

Vaccinations

Vaccines for vaccine-preventable diseases are indicated for all DHCWs. OSHA recommends that all health care workers with potential for exposure be offered the HBV vaccination at no charge.

Protective Attire and Barrier Techniques

Protective attire and barrier techniques should be used wherever the potential exists for contacting blood, blood-contaminated saliva, or mucous membranes. This includes, but is not limited to, the use of appropriate personal protective equipment such as gloves, masks, chin-length face shields, and protective eyewear when involved in procedures likely to generate splashing or splattering of blood or other potentially infectious materials, as is the case in most dental procedures. These should be changed when visibly contaminated or compromised and between patients. They should be removed when leaving the patient area. Protective clothing is indicated when contamination is likely. Appropriate maintenance and disposal should be in accordance with OSHA and CDC recommendations. In 1997 the National Institute for Occupational Safety and Health (NIOSH) issued an alert on preventing allergic reactions to natural rubber latex

(NRL) in the workplace. NIOSH recommends the selection of products and work practices that reduce the risk of allergic response, including worker education. DHCWs at risk for a latex reaction should be screened to detect symptoms. Handwashing and the use of powder-free latex gloves may assist in reducing exposure. Alternatives to latex gloves are available. The FDA has also issued latex labeling requirements for all items made from or containing NRL. Products containing NRL that come in contact with humans should state the following: "Caution: This product contains natural rubber latex, which may cause allergic reactions." Medical devices containing dry natural rubber must also have labels indicating presence in the device. Additionally, the term *hypoallergenic* must be removed from products containing natural rubber.[60]

Environmental barriers are indicated for surfaces that are difficult to clean and disinfect and that may become contaminated during oral health care procedures. These should be removed and replaced between patients in accordance with state and federal recommendations. Use of rubber dams, high-velocity evacuation, and proper patient positioning will minimize aerosolization. The Healthcare Infection Control Practices Advisory Committee (HICPAC) draft guidelines support these recommendations.[61]

Handwashing and Care of Hands

Handwashing is indicated before and after patient care, at any time hands become contaminated (even if gloved), and after touching surfaces likely to be contaminated. Handwashing with plain soap is adequate for examinations and nonsurgical procedures. Antimicrobial surgical hand scrubbing is necessary with surgical procedures. Gloves compromised by a puncture or tear should be removed as soon as patient safety permits, hands should be thoroughly washed, and new gloves should be used when continuing patient care. Note: The CDC recommends that "DHCWs who have exudative lesions or weeping dermatitis, particularly on the hands, should refrain from all direct patient care and from handling dental patient-care equipment until the condition resolves."

Use and Care of Sharp Instruments and Needles

Any sharp instrument, contaminated or not, should be considered potentially infectious and handled in a manner that will prevent injuries. Needles should not be recapped or otherwise manipulated with both hands, nor should a technique that involves directing the point of a needle toward any part of the body (the operator's or someone else's) be used. A one-handed technique or a mechanical device designed to isolate a needlestick hazard should be used. Disposal of all sharp instruments, including needles, scalpel blades, and other items or instruments, should be in puncture-resistant containers located as close as practical to their area of use. Removal of needles from nondisposable syringes should not be attempted if uncapped, and recapping only by approved methods with one hand should be used.

Sterilization or Disinfection of Instruments

Reprocessing of instruments used in dental practices should follow the classifications of *critical* (used to penetrate soft tissue or bone and require sterilization), *semicritical* (do not penetrate, but have contact with oral tissues and should be sterilized if capable of withstanding the process or undergo at least high-level disinfection), and *noncritical* (contact skin and require intermediate or low-level disinfection). Appropriate cleaning and use of appropriate personal protective equipment during reprocessing are necessary. CDC guidelines should be reviewed for reprocessing. Critical and semicritical heat-stable instruments should be routinely sterilized by autoclave, dry heat, or chemical vapor, with appropriate packaging and in biologically monitored units. Use of high-level disinfection should be according to manufacturers' directions with Environmental Protection Agency–registered agents. CDC guidelines, including draft guidelines by HICPAC, should be reviewed.[61]

Cleaning and Disinfection of Dental Unit and Environmental Surfaces

All surfaces that become contaminated should be appropriately maintained according to schedules recommended in the guidelines with Environmental Protection Agency–registered tuberculocidal hospital disinfectants.[16] General housekeeping in keeping with the guidelines may be accomplished through the use of low-level Environmental Protection Agency–registered chemical agents. These agents are not recommended for critical or semicritical instruments.

Disinfection in the Dental Laboratory

Manufacturers' guidelines should be reviewed for appropriate cleaning and disinfection of materials before they are manipulated in the laboratory, after handling, and before placement in the patient's mouth. At least an intermediate-level disinfectant is recommended. The dental facility and laboratory should review the guidelines and establish communication.

Use and Care of Handpieces, Antiretraction Valves, and Other Intraoral Dental Devices Attached to Air and Water Lines of Dental Units

All high-speed dental handpieces, low-speed components used intraorally, and reusable prophy angles should be sterilized between patients by a heating process capable of sterilization. Manufacturers' directions should be reviewed. Surface disinfection is not acceptable. Retraction valves should be used to prevent fluid aspiration and reduce the potential for transmitting infectious material. Routine maintenance is required. Flushing of water lines and discharging water and air from high-speed handpieces are indicated. The guidelines should be consulted for details.

Single-use Disposable Instruments

Single-use disposable instruments are not designed or intended for reuse and should be appropriately handled and disposed of properly.

Use of Extracted Teeth in Dental Education Settings

Extracted teeth should be considered infective and handled with Universal Precautions in the same manner as a biopsy specimen. Workers in contact with extracted teeth should be vaccinated against HBV. Guidelines should be reviewed for cleaning and disinfection. Extracted teeth given to a patient are not considered regulated waste.

Disposal of Waste Materials

State, local, and federal guidelines should be reviewed and waste disposed of according to the requirements and published recommendations.

Boil Water Advisories

The CDC has suggested measures appropriate to dental offices during boil water advisories. This may be in addition to those issued by state or local authorities. While such advisories are in effect, public water should not be delivered to a patient through any equipment attached to the dental unit. Patients should not use public water to rinse. DHCWs should not use public water for handwashing; instead the use of nonwater agents or towelettes is recommended. When the advisory is canceled, incoming lines from the public water system should be flushed. All faucets in the dental setting should be turned completely on for 30 minutes, including dental unit water lines. After flushing, lines should be disinfected. The manufacturer of the dental unit should be consulted for the appropriate methods to disinfect the unit. Alternative water sources cleared by the FDA may be used.[62]

Dental Unit Water Quality

Dental unit water line (DUWL) contamination has been reported in the literature for more than 30 years. Although there is no evidence of a public health risk, infection control principles are indicated. In 1995 the American Dental Association adopted a statement on this issue based on the premise that "water delivered to most dental patients was of poor microbiologic quality."[1] The goal is to provide water with less than 200 colony-forming units (CFU) of heterotropic mesophilic bacteria per milliliter. This is a standard for hemodialysis units. Draft guidelines from the CDC's HICPAC released in March 2001 also address DUWLs and recommend cleaning water systems according to system manufacturers' instructions. The specific recommendations are to flush all dental instruments that use water, including high-speed handpieces, for several minutes before the start of each clinic day; to ensure that water in DUWLs meets nationally recognized drinking water standards (less than 500 CFU/ml for heterotrophic plate count) at a minimum; and to consult with manufacturers to determine suitable methods and equipment to obtain good water quality. Further, the guidelines state that routine sampling of water systems for biofilms is not warranted. However, if an epidemiologic investigation implicates the water as a possible source of infection, sampling should be considered.[61] Because these are draft guidelines and are under professional and public review, it is prudent to consider the following CDC interim recommendations:

- Run source water through the water lines with handpiece attached for several minutes at the beginning of the day.
- Run high-speed handpieces to discharge air and water for 20 to 30 seconds after each patient.
- Follow manufacturer's instructions for proper water line maintenance.
- Consider commercial options.
- Use sterile saline or sterile water for surgical procedures (cutting of bone).

Infection Control in Public Health Settings

The CDC notes that "with adequate maintenance of hygienic conditions, oral health surveys and screenings should present few, if any, opportunities for bloodborne disease transmission."[63] Instruments and devices used for survey purposes are generally limited to explorers, probes, and mouth mirrors, which have little risk of bleeding associated with their use. The CDC has identified three levels of contact:

- Contact level I: contact anticipated with patient's mucous membranes, blood, or saliva
- Contact level II: contact anticipated with patient's mucous membranes but not blood or saliva
- Contact level III: contact not anticipated with patient's mucous membranes, blood, or saliva

The guidelines are based on principles of infection control that include actions to stay healthy, avoidance of blood contact, limiting the spread of blood, and making instruments and equipment safe for use. In terms of actions to stay healthy, levels I and II are similar in the recommendation for HBV vaccination and consideration of other immunizations. Handwashing is a vital component of actions to stay healthy, and for these levels handwashing before and after examinations, before and after gloving, and between subjects is indicated. Antimicrobial soaps are not necessary, but waterless products that contain antimicrobials may be useful. Although level III does not require handwashing based on the nature of contact, it is still prudent to wash or use towelettes.

To avoid contact with blood requires the use of protective coverings such as gloves, masks, and protective eyewear (the latter if splashes may occur), and they are indicated for levels I and II, but not for level III as long as instruments can be managed without contact with contaminated surfaces and spattering is not expected. Use of protective clothing is recommended for level I, advised for level II if contamination may occur, and optional for level III. Avoiding injuries is related to levels I and II, where sharps may be used, but not for level III, where sharps are not in use. Proper attention to environmental surface contamination and waste is dependent on the level of contamination. For all levels, contaminated instruments must be appropriately managed and, if not managed immediately, stored for transport in a rigid, covered container.[63]

Other Recommendations

Written protocols and training should be in place in all dental facilities. In addition, research into factors that may contribute to the risk of transmission of bloodborne pathogens and other infectious agents is necessary to assess risk and offer suggestions to reduce risk. The CDC has introduced Standard Precautions in addition to Universal Precautions as a broader infection control strategy that includes all the elements of Universal Precautions and reinforces basic principles of infection control.

These guidelines are meant to provide the reader with an awareness of the precautions that should become a routine part of the daily practice of dentistry. Variations on these basic precepts may exist within certain school, clinic, or hospital settings. However, common sense and good judgment will help each professional determine the best preventive techniques for each environment. Because the art and science of infection control is continually evolving, practitioners must make every effort to remain up to date through continuing education and by reviewing journals and other resources. For example, in addition to recently updated or draft guidelines, the CDC is also revising the 1993 infection control document for dental facilities.

AIDS and HIV disease have generated a new set of professional standards for infection control, a series of federal obligations to meet these standards, and other federal regulations to deal with the chemicals we use in controlling infection. However, HIV disease has also presented dentistry with the insidious issue of discrimination. In their 1990 report on AIDS discrimination, the American Civil Liberties Union noted that the most frequent complaints were against dentists and nursing homes.[64] "Dentists turn AIDS patients away," noted Mitchell Karp, a supervising attorney for the New York City AIDS Discrimination Unit. A recent analysis of dental discrimination identified three major factors associated with negative attitudes of dentists toward persons with HIV: (1) fear of infection, (2) concerns about the competence to treat patients with HIV safely or effectively, and (3) business-based concerns about the effect of treating patients with HIV on other patients and staff.[65] The first two factors are reduced by education and experience, but business-based concerns remain significant. Many other reasons are given for refusal to treat: low reimbursement rates by Medicaid, a lack of understanding about the disease, fear of transmission, fear of becoming known as an "AIDS dentist," prejudice, and more.

LEGISLATION AND LITIGATION

Refusals to treat people with HIV/AIDS by dentists and other health care professionals may well be the most common and blatant form of discrimination against people with HIV today. In a survey of U.S. dentists in 1995, only 50% of male dentists and 38% of female dentists believed that a private dental office was an acceptable location in which to treat people with HIV.[66] During the first 3 years, 1990 to 1993, of the HIV Dental Ombudsperson Program (a Ryan White CARE Act program in Boston), 12% of all callers indicated that they had experienced discrimination by a dentist. Approximately 20% of callers throughout the duration of the program indicated that they were uncomfortable seeking dental care out of a concern over discrimination.[67]

STATE AND FEDERAL DISABILITY DISCRIMINATION LAWS

People with HIV (or other disabilities) are protected under state and federal disability discrimination laws, the Americans with Disabilities Act (AWDA), and the Rehabilitation Act of 1973. Most state statutes and both federal statutes define disability as having the following:

1. A physical or mental impairment that substantially limits one or more of the major life activities of such individual
2. A record of such impairment
3. Being regarded as having such impairment

Courts have uniformly found that people with HIV are protected by disability discrimination laws. The legislative history of the AWDA and interpretive guidelines written by the U.S. Department of Justice specifically provide that people with asymptomatic HIV are substantially limited in numerous major life activities, including procreation and intimate sexual relations, and are therefore covered by the AWDA. In addition, these individuals are covered by the "regarded as" prong of the definition even if they are not limited in any major life activity.

When Congress passed the Rehabilitation Act of 1973, it was an effort to provide some national protection against discrimination on the basis of a "handicap." The Civil

Rights Restoration Act of 1987 added a clarifying position to section 504, "which implicitly acknowledged this act's coverage of HIV infection" (including asymptomatic HIV).[68] Section 504 prohibits discrimination against people with disabilities from agencies or programs that receive federal funds, including private dental or medical offices and hospitals that accept Medicare or Medicaid.

In 1990 Congress passed the AWDA, which extended disability discrimination protection to private places of public accommodation. A place of public accommodation is any place that is open to and accepts the general public, including the professional offices of dentists and physicians. Section 504 was limited in its scope of application to those receiving federal assistance.

Most states also have laws that prohibit discrimination in places of public accommodation that do not receive federal assistance. Many states have similar civil rights laws, which vary in their scope of protection. In addition, most states have regulatory boards that license and discipline DHCWs and can pursue complaints of discrimination. Although each state law is different, the AWDA is the most specific and comprehensive disability discrimination law affecting dental offices.

The AWDA of July 26, 1990, "is perhaps the most sweeping civil rights legislation passed since the enactment of the Civil Rights Act of 1964 nearly 30 years before."[69] The AWDA is "to provide a clear and comprehensive national mandate for the elimination of discrimination against individuals with disabilities" and picks up where Section 504 left off, that is, to extend coverage to those not receiving federal assistance. Titles I and III of the AWDA hold the most significance for dental offices. Title I prohibits employment discrimination and Title III prohibits discrimination by a "place of public accommodation," which explicitly includes the "professional office of a health care provider."

Title III of the Americans with Disabilities Act

Title III is specific in the type of discriminatory conduct that is prohibited. As applied to the delivery of oral health services, it is illegal to do the following:

1. Deny an HIV-positive patient the "full and equal enjoyment" of dental services or deny an HIV-positive patient the "opportunity to benefit" from dental services in the same manner as other patients
2. Establish for the privilege of receiving dental services "eligibility criteria" that tend to screen out patients who have tested positive for HIV
3. Provide "different or separate" services to patients who are HIV positive or fail to provide services to patients in the most "integrated setting"
4. Deny equal services to a person who is known to have a "relationship" or "association" with a person with HIV, such as a spouse, partner, child, or friend

Although the AWDA has specific prohibitions against discrimination by places of public accommodation, it does permit the denial of services to an individual where there is a "direct threat to the health and safety of others." The AWDA defines the term *direct threat* as a "significant risk to the health and safety of others that cannot be eliminated by a modification of policies, practices, or procedures." The assessment of whether an individual poses a direct threat is made on the basis of reasonable judgment that relies on current medical knowledge or on the best available objective evidence to ascertain (1) the nature, duration, and severity of the risk; (2) the probability that the potential injury will occur; and (3) whether reasonable modifications to policies, practices, and procedures will mitigate the risk.

Abbott v Bragdon, 912 F. Supp. 580 (D. Me. 1995), a case litigated in federal district court in Bangor, Maine, involved a dentist who had a written policy stating that he did not treat any patient with an active infectious disease, including HIV, in his office. The dentist argued that the performance of invasive dental procedures on a patient with HIV was such a "direct threat" because of the potential for blood-to-blood contact. The plaintiff presented evidence that it is safe to provide routine dental care to persons with HIV. The CDC testified through Donald Wayne Marianos, DDS, MPH, Director of the Oral Health Division, that people with HIV may be safely treated in a private dental office with use of Universal Precautions (Standard Precautions) for all patients. This testimony is of particular importance because the U.S. Supreme Court has specifically ruled that courts addressing the issue of whether discrimination against a person with a contagious disease is justified by a health or safety risk "should normally defer to the reasonable medical judgments of public health officials" unless those judgments are "medically unsupportable."[70] The court deferred to the judgment of the CDC in deciding that it is safe to treat patients with HIV and ruled that Dr. Bragdon had not been able to counter that judgment with any admissible evidence about the significance of the risk. Of all facts considered, the court gave the most weight to the "probability" of HIV transmission in dentistry, stating that neither the duration nor the severity of HIV infection "outweigh the evidence as to how the disease is transmitted and the slight probability of transmission."[71]

The U.S. Court of Appeals for the First Circuit upheld the trial court's ruling on March 5, 1997. Like the trial court, the appeals court ruled that each of Dr. Bragdon's claims about a "significant risk" of HIV transmission from patient to dentist was "too speculative or too tangential" to establish a "direct threat" under the AWDA.[72] The court relied on guidelines from the CDC and the American Dental Association to conclude that it is safe for a dentist to provide routine dental care in a private dental office to a patient with HIV. The court concluded that Dr. Bragdon violated the AWDA by refusing to provide routine dental care in his office to a patient with HIV. Several state public health departments and national public health associations submitted a friend of the court brief indicating that not only is it safe to provide routine dental care to patients with HIV but that a decision for Dr. Bragdon would result in a public health disaster.[73] The American Dental Association filed a brief in support of the dentist arguing, in spite of its policy that a dentist ethically must treat patients with HIV, that people with asymptomatic HIV should not be covered by disability discrimination laws. To date, every court has ruled that it is illegal for a dentist to refuse to treat a patient on the basis of HIV status. It is important to remember, however, that HIV instills fear and discomfort in judges who are ruling on these cases.

Illegal Referrals

Another common form of discrimination by dentists is automatic referral of patients with HIV on the assumption that routine dental treatment of an HIV-positive patient requires a specialist. The U.S. Department of

Justice has issued regulations that provide that a health care worker may refer a patient with a disability such as HIV in the following cases:

1. The treatment being sought is outside the referring provider's area of specialization.
2. If, in the normal course of operations, the referring provider would make a similar referral for an individual without HIV who seeks or requires the same treatment.[74]

In *United States v Morvant,* a 1995 federal court decision, the court rejected the notion that dental treatment of patients with HIV requires specialization.[75] The court agreed with the extensive testimony that no special training or expertise is necessary to provide such care and that there is no medical or scientific basis to refer all patients with HIV. Of particular importance is that the court rejected the dentist's argument that he had not kept up with the literature and training necessary to understand HIV. The court specifically noted the extensive educational materials available to dentists and said that Dr. Morvant "chose to ignore the information and in doing so ran afoul of the law as it now stands."[75]

Other Decisions

Under Title III of the AWDA the Department of Justice recently settled a complaint against a dentist in East Hartford, Connecticut, for allegedly refusing to treat a patient with AIDS. The dentist agreed to implement a policy that would not discriminate on the basis of HIV/AIDS. In addition, he paid the estate of the complainant $20,000 in compensatory damages and $9,000 in civil penalties.[72]

In Houston a large chain of dental offices agreed under a consent decree to pay $80,000 in compensatory damages for refusal to treat an HIV-positive patient. In addition, the owner of Castle Dental and its management company each agreed to pay $10,000 in civil penalties to the federal government. The agreement includes staff training on nondiscrimination and requirements to provide "equal services" to persons with HIV/AIDS and "send periodic reports to the DOJ [Department of Justice] so that compliance can be monitored."[76]

Also under the AWDA, a federal court in New Jersey ruled that a dentist violated the AWDA and New Jersey state law by refusing to treat a patient with HIV and referring him to a "special clinic for HIV . . . better suited to take care of [his] needs." The court ruled the referral "a pretext for discrimination because no specialized skills are required to treat patients who are HIV positive."[75] In addition to paying compensatory damages of $25,000 and punitive damages of $25,000, the defendants were ordered to institute and maintain a policy of nondiscrimination on the basis of HIV status and to post this policy prominently in the waiting room.*

THE FUTURE

Even after 20 years of the epidemic and more than 15 years of promoting Universal Precautions as procedures to minimize the risk of disease transmission from DHCW to patient, patient to DHCW, or patient to

*The material in this chapter necessarily simplifies complex legal issues and is not intended as legal advice. Dental health care workers with specific questions about legal rights and obligations should consult an attorney.

patient, confusion and questions still persist. During the 1996 World Congress of the American Dental Association, members who questioned the efficacy of Universal Precautions were soundly defeated by the scientific community reaffirming the effectiveness of Universal Precautions. Policies on professional judgment and designated centers to treat persons with HIV/AIDS were also debated. Courts have decided that it is safe to provide oral health services to persons with HIV/AIDS, but appeals to these decisions will determine the future role of the profession, the protection of the HIV infected (both patient and provider), and the safety of providing oral health care services.

REVIEW QUESTIONS

1. What are three results of serologic testing for the presence of HIV?
2. What are Universal Precautions? Give an example of how to apply them to a dental procedure.
3. If a DHCW is not protected by active or passive immunity and is exposed to blood containing either HBV, HCV, or HIV, what is the risk associated with the transmission of each of these viruses?
4. Has any documented case of an HIV-infected DHCW transmitting HIV to a patient ever occurred?
5. How does a dental patient with HIV, HBV, or HCV, who has no visible signs of illness, fit within the AWDA's definition of "disability"?
6. How do courts assess whether a dental patient with HIV can be excluded from a dental office or treated differently based on the "direct threat" defense contained in the AWDA? How would a dentist's decision to treat patients with HIV only as the last appointment of the day be analyzed under that test?

REFERENCES

1. As AIDS epidemic approaches second decade, report examines what has been learned, *JAMA* 264:431, 1990.
2. Aids activist Larry Kramer is still gay gadfly no. 1, *Times Out New York*, 256, Aug 17-24, 2000.
3. Fauci AS, National Institutes of Health, NIAID: *World AIDS Day statement*, Dec 2000.
4. Pneumocystis pneumonia—Los Angeles, *MMWR Morb Mortal Wkly Rep* 30:250, 1981.
5. Kaposi's sarcoma and pneumocystis pneumonia among homosexual men: New York City and California, *MMWR Morb Mortal Wkly Rep* 30:305, 1981.
6. Follow-up on Kaposi's sarcoma and pneumocystis pneumonia, *MMWR Morb Mortal Wkly Rep* 30:40, 1981.
7. The HIV/AIDS epidemic: the first 10 years, *MMWR Morb Mortal Wkly Rep* 40:22, 1991.
8. A cluster of Kaposi's sarcoma and pneumocystis carinii pneumonia among homosexual male residents of Los Angeles and Orange Counties, California, *MMWR Morb Mortal Wkly Rep* 31, 1982.
9. *Centers for Disease Control and Prevention AIDS case definition change,* Atlanta, 1993, Centers for Disease Control and Prevention.
10. Diagnostic tests for evidence of HIV infection (supplement on testing) PIPerspective: a publication of Project Inform, San Francisco, October 11, 1988.
11. US Department of Health and Human Services: FDA approves first test for HIV antigen screening of blood donors, press release, March 14, 1996.
12. Nucleic testing reduces risk of HIV infection, McClam Associated Press, July 19, 2000.
13. US Department of Health and Human Services: FDA approves first home kit to test for HIV, press release, May 14, 1996.
14. Rapid HIV tests: CDC urges quicker FDA approval, *Kaiser Daily HIV/AIDS Report,* June 14, 2000.
15. Phenotypic testing can predict HIV, *AIDS Weekly Plus,* January 8, 2001, p. 131.
16. USPHS, DHHS, CDC: *HIV/AIDS Surveillance Report, Year End Edition* 11(2):5, June 2000.
17. AIDS in the US: infection rates leveling off at 40,000 per year, *Sunday Times,* South Africa, July 9, 2000.
18. AIDS complacency rising among American homosexuals, Agence France-Presse, July 10, 2000.

19. Fauci AS: The AIDS epidemic: considerations for the 21st century, *Global Issues, an Electronic Journal of the U.S. Department of State* 5:2, July 2000.
20. National Commission on Acquired Immune Deficiency Syndrome: *Living with AIDS,* Washington, 1991, US Government Printing Office, Superintendent of Documents.
21. Anastos K: Re-examining treatment recommendations for women, *Bulletin of Experimental Treatments for AIDS,* Summer 2000, p. 4.
22. Bednarsh H, Eklund K: AZT reduces perinatal HIV transmission, *Access* 8(7):4, 1994.
23. Public Law 91-596, 91st Congress, S.2193, Washington, 1970, Department of Labor, OSHA.
24. Occupational exposure to bloodborne pathogens, final rule, Washington, 1991, Department of Labor, OSHA, Part II, 29 CFR Part 1910.1030.
25. Acquired immunodeficiency syndrome (AIDS): precautions for clinical and laboratory staffs, *MMWR Morb Mortal Wkly Rep* 31, 1982.
26. Acquired immunodeficiency syndrome (AIDS): precautions for health care workers and allied professionals, *MMWR Morb Mortal Wkly Rep* 32, 1983.
27. Recommended infection control practices for dentistry, *MMWR Morb Mortal Wkly Rep* 35:15, 1986.
28. Recommended infection control practices for dentistry, 1993, *MMWR Morb Mortal Wkly Rep* 42:RR-8, 1993.
29. Recommendations for prevention of HIV transmission in health-care settings, *MMWR Morb Mortal Wkly Rep* 36:2S, 1987.
30. Update: universal precautions for prevention of transmission of HIV, HBV, and other bloodborne pathogens in health care settings, *MMWR Morb Mortal Wkly Rep* 37:24, 1988.
31. Klein RS et al: Low occupational risk of human immunodeficiency virus infection among dental professionals, *N Engl J Med* 318:86, 1988.
32. USPHS, DHHS: CDC Surveillance of HCWs, April 2000.
33. *Post-exposure evaluation and follow-up requirements under OSHA's standard for occupational exposure to bloodborne pathogens: a guide to dental employer obligations,* Washington, 1995, Occupational Safety Health Administration, Department of Labor.
34. Bednarsh H, Eklund K: Prevention and management of bloodborne occupational exposure incidents—it's not as easy as 1,2,3. . ., *Access* 8(9):6-15, 1994.
35. Case control study of HIV seroconversion in health care workers after percutaneous exposure to HIV-infected blood—France, United Kingdom, and United States, January 1988–August 1994, *MMWR Morb Mortal Wkly Rep* 14(50):929, 1995.
36. Update: provisional public health service recommendations for chemoprophylaxis after occupational exposure to HIV, *MMWR Morb Mortal Wkly Rep* 45:22, 1996.
37. Centers for Disease Control and Prevention, ACGIH: Frontline healthcare workers. National Conference on Prevention of Sharps Injuries and Bloodborne Exposures, August 14-16, 1995, Atlanta.
38. *Estimates of the risk of endemic transmission of HBV and HIV to patients by the percutaneous route during invasive surgical and dental procedures,* draft, January 30, 1991, Centers for Disease Control and Prevention.
39. Recommendations for preventing transmission of HIV and HBV to patients during exposure prone invasive procedures, *MMWR Morb Mortal Wkly Rep* 40:RR-8, 1991.
40. Harpaz R et al: Transmission of hepatitis B virus to multiple patients from a surgeon without evidence of inadequate infection control, *N Engl J Med* 334(9):549, 1996.
41. Estebon J et al: Transmission of hepatitis C virus by a cardiac surgeon, *N Engl J Med* 334(9):555, 1996.
42. Ridzon K et al: Simultaneous transmission of both human immunodeficiency virus (HIV) and hepatitis C virus (HCV) with delayed seroconversion in a healthcare worker (HCW), abstract, Proceedings of the Thirty-Fifth Interscience Conference on Antimicrobial Agents and Chemotherapy, American Society for Microbiology.
43. FrontLine Healthcare Workers National Conference on Prevention of Sharps Injuries and Bloodborne Pathogens, Washington, DC, August 2000.
44. Gerbert B et al: Possible health care professional to patient HIV transmission: dentists' reactions to a Centers for Disease Control and Prevention report, *JAMA* 265:1845, 1991.
45. Possible transmission of human immunodeficiency virus to a patient during an invasive dental procedure, *MMWR Morb Mortal Wkly Rep* 39:489, 1990.
46. Update: Transmission of HIV infection during an invasive dental procedure—Florida, *MMWR Morb Mortal Wkly Rep* 40:21, 1991.
47. Update: investigations of persons treated by HIV-infected health-care workers—United States, *MMWR Morb Mortal Wkly Rep* 42:17, 1993.
48. Davenport R, Bednarsh H: Unpublished data on an analysis of state plans regarding HBV and HIV infected health care workers, 1996.
49. Robert LM et al: Investigations of patients of healthcare workers infected with HIV: the Centers for Disease Control and Prevention database, *Ann Intern Med* 122:653, 1995.

50. OSHA hazard communications, final rule, standards only, Department of Labor, OSHA, 29, CFR, August 24, 1987.
51. DOL, OSHA, CPL2-2.44D, Enforcement Procedures for the Occupational Exposure to Bloodborne Pathogens, November 5, 1999.
52. DOL, OSHA, 29 CFR Parts 1904 and 1952, Occupational Injury and Illness Recording and Reporting Requirements, Final Rule.
53. Kane M et al: Hepatitis B infection in the United States, *Am J Med* 87(suppl 3A):11S, 1989.
54. CDC: Recommendations of the Advisory Committee on Immunization Practices (ACIP) and the Hospital Infection Control Practices Advisory Committee (HICPAC), *MMWR,* 46:RR-18, 1997.
55. Cleveland J: Division of Oral Health, Centers for Disease Control and Prevention, personal communication, August 1996.
56. Molinari J: Hepatitis C virus infection, *Dent Clin North Am* 40(2):309, 1996.
57. Cooper B et al: Seroprevalence of antibodies to hepatitis C virus in high-risk hospital personnel, *Infect Control Hosp Epidemiol* 13(2):82, 1992.
58. Guidelines for preventing the transmission of tuberculosis in health care settings with special focus on HIV related issues, *MMWR Morb Mortal Wkly Rep* 39:RR-17, 1990.
59. Garret L: HIV alarm in city, survey finds worst rise in gay black males, *Newday,* January 24, 2001.
60. US FDA: *Medical Bulletin, Natural Rubber Latex Allergy,* 27:2, Summer 1997.
61. USPHS, DHHS, CDC: Healthcare Infection Control Practices Advisory Committee, draft guideline for environmental infection control in healthcare facilities, NIOSH publication #97-135, 2001.
62. USPHS, DHHS, CDC: Suggested procedures for dental offices during boil-water advisories, December 23, 1998.
63. Summers C et al: Practical infection control in oral health surveys and screenings, *J Am Dent Assoc* 125: 1213, 1994.
64. Epidemic of fear, American Civil Liberties Union, 1990.
65. Burris S: Dental discrimination against the HIV-infected: empirical data, law and public policy, *Yale J Regul* 13(1):1, 1996.
66. Kunzel C, Sadowsky D: Assessing HIV related attitudes and orientations of male and female dentists, *J Am Dent Assoc* 126:866, 1995.
67. Boston Public Health Commission: Ryan White CARE Act, Title I.
68. Public Law No. 100-259, 56 U.S.L.W. 46 (Apr. 5, 1988); 134 Cong. Rec. H587-8 (daily ed. Mar. 2, 1988).
69. US Department of Justice, Office of Justice Programs, National Institute of Justice: The Americans with Disabilities Act and criminal justice: an overview, Sept 1993.
70. *School Board of Nassau County v Arline,* 480 U.S. 273 (1987).
71. *Abbott v Bragdon,* 912 F. Supp. 580 (D. Me. 1995).
72. *Abbott v Bragdon,* No. 96-1643, U.S. Court of Appeals for First Circuit (March 5, 1997), Slip Opinion at 31.
73. *Abbott v Bragdon,* No. 96-1643, U.S. Court of Appeals for First Circuit. Brief of Amici Curiae, Rhode Island, Dept. P.H., Commonwealth of Massachusetts, Bureau of Health, Maine Department of Human Services, APHA, ASTDD, ASTHO.
74. Bednarsh H, Eklund K, Klein B: Courts strike down HIV discrimination in dental offices, *Access* 10(3):12-16, 1996.
75. *United States v Morvant,* 898 F. Supp. 1157 (E.D. LA. 1995).
76. US Department of Justice: *Enforcement highlights: fighting discrimination against persons with HIV/AIDS,* Washington DC, Civil Rights Division.

CHAPTER

10

EFFECTIVE COMMUNITY PREVENTION PROGRAMS FOR ORAL DISEASES

Myron Allukian, Jr. • Alice M. Horowitz

An ounce of prevention is worth a pound of dental cure.
—Olde Dental Public Health Proverb

Oral diseases have been referred to as "the neglected epidemic" because they affect almost the total population, with many people having new diseases each year.[1] For example, at age 6 years only 5.6% of U.S. schoolchildren have had tooth decay in their permanent teeth. However, by age 17 years, 84% have had the disease with an average of eight affected tooth surfaces (for more information about the epidemiology of dental caries, see Chapters 2 and 8).[2] For vulnerable populations, such as those with low incomes, minorities, the developmentally disabled, and persons with acquired immunodeficiency syndrome (AIDS), the extent of oral disease is even greater. The national goal for oral health as stated in *Healthy People 2010* is to "prevent and control oral and craniofacial diseases, conditions, and injuries and improve access to related services."[3] The oral health objectives shown in Box 10-1 are intended to prevent, decrease, or eliminate oral health disparities in the U.S. population. Yet our country has not made oral health a priority.[4] Further, the United States does not have a national oral disease prevention program, despite an estimated $65 billion annual dental bill.[5] Compounding the problem, a 1996 study of children eligible for Medicaid reported that only one out of five, or 20%, received dental treatment, and a 2000 study showed that most dentists do not participate in Medicaid.[6,7] Despite the progress made in the prevention of oral diseases in the last several decades as a result of community water fluoridation, use of other fluorides, and greater emphasis on prevention in general, much more remains to be done.

PREVENTION

Prevention of premature death, disease, disability, and suffering should be a primary goal of any society that hopes to provide a decent future and a better quality of life for its people. *Primary prevention,* or preventing

BOX 10-1

Healthy People 2010 Oral Health Objectives

21-1 Reduce the proportion of children and adolescents who have dental caries experience in their primary or permanent teeth
21-2 Reduce the proportion of children, adolescents, and adults with untreated dental decay
21-3 Increase the proportion of adults who have never had a permanent tooth extracted because of dental caries or periodontal disease
21-4 Reduce the proportion of older adults who have had all their natural teeth extracted
21-5 Reduce periodontal disease
21-6 Increase the proportion of oral and pharyngeal cancers detected at the earliest stage
21-7 Increase the proportion of adults who, in the past 12 months, report having had an examination to detect oral and pharyngeal cancers
21-8 Increase the proportion of children who have received dental sealants on their molar teeth
21-9 Increase the proportion of the U.S. population served by community water systems with optimally fluoridated water
21-10 Increase the proportion of children and adults who use the oral health care system each year
21-11 Increase the proportion of long-term care residents who use the oral health care system each year
21-12 Increase the proportion of low-income children and adolescents who received any preventive dental service during the past year
21-13 (Developmental) Increase the proportion of school-based health centers with an oral health component
21-14 Increase the proportion of local health departments and community-based health centers, including community, migrant, and homeless health centers, that have an oral health component
21-15 Increase the number of states and District of Columbia that have a system for recording and referring infants and children with cleft lips, cleft palates, and other craniofacial anomalies to craniofacial anomaly rehabilitation teams
21-16 Increase the number of states and District of Columbia that have an oral and craniofacial health surveillance system
21-17 (Developmental) Increase the number of the tribal, state (including the District of Columbia), and local health agencies that serve jurisdictions of 250,000 or more persons that have in place an effective public dental health program directed by a dental professional with public health training
1-8.1 In the health professions, allied and associated health profession fields, and the nursing field, increase the proportion of all degrees awarded to members of underrepresented racial and ethnic groups
3-6 Reduce the oropharyngeal cancer death rate
5-15 Increase the proportion of persons with diabetes who have at least an annual dental examination

Numbering in box indicates the chapter and objective number as listed in *Healthy People 2010.*

From the US Department of Health and Human Services: *Healthy People 2010: with understanding and improving health objectives for improving health,* ed 2, Chapters 1, 3, 5, and 21, Washington, DC, US Government Printing Office.

a disease before it occurs, is the most effective way to improve health and control costs. *Secondary prevention* is treating or controlling the disease after it occurs, such as placing an amalgam restoration. *Tertiary prevention* is limiting a disability from a disease or rehabilitating an individual with a disability, such as providing dentures for those who have lost all their teeth.

Prevention may be accomplished at the

Table 10-1. Three Levels of Caries Prevention by Individual and Community Approaches

	Levels of Prevention				
	Primary		Secondary	Tertiary	
Preventive Services Provided by the	Health Promotion	Specific Protection	Early Diagnosis and Prompt Treatment	Disability Limitation	Rehabilitation
Individual Approach					
Individual patient (self-administered)	Diet planning; demand for preventive services; periodic dental visits	Appropriate use of fluoride: • Fluoridated water • Fluoride prescriptions • Fluoride dentrifice • Oral hygiene	Self-examination and referral; use of dental services	Use of dental services	Use of dental services
Dental professional	Patient education; plaque control program; diet counseling; recall reinforcement; dental caries activity tests	Topical fluoride; fluoride supplement/rinse prescription; pit and fissure sealants	Complete examination; prompt treatment of incipient lesions; preventive resin restorations; simple restorative dentistry; pulp capping	Complex restorative dentistry; pulpotomy; root canal therapy; extractions	Removable and fixed prosthodontics; minor tooth movement; implants
Community Approach					
Community	Dental health education programs; promotion of research, policy, and legislation	Community or school water fluoridation; school fluoride mouth rinse or tablet program; school sealant program	Periodic screening and referral; provision of dental services	Provision of dental services	Provision of dental services

Modified from Dunning JM: *Principals of dental public health,* ed 4, Cambridge, MA, 1986, Harvard University Press; Mandel I: What is preventive dentistry? *J Prev Dent* 25, 1974; Leske GS, Ripa LW, Callanen VA: Prevention of dental diseases. In Jong AW, editor: *Community dental health,* St. Louis, 1993, Mosby.

individual or community level. On the individual level a procedure is either provided by a professional on a one-on-one basis, for example, a dental hygienist providing dental sealants for a child patient, or it is self-administered, that is, the patients perform the procedure themselves, such as toothbrushing. An individual procedure also may be a combination of actions of an individual patient and a dental professional, such as the prescription by a dentist of a systemic fluoride that is taken daily by a patient. Table 10-1 shows the three levels of prevention for dental caries at the individual and community level or approach.

This chapter focuses on primary preventive measures that are science based and that have been shown to be effective in preventing oral diseases with a community- or population-based approach. There are many ways to prevent oral diseases with the individual approach. The community approach, however, helps ensure a greater impact at a lower cost for a larger number of individuals, especially vulnerable populations, such as low-income and minority groups. Self-responsibility by individuals for prevention also is important and is discussed as an adjunct to effective community prevention programs.

DEFINITIONS

To put "effective community prevention programs" in perspective with how prevention is often considered, the following definitions are used for this chapter:[8]

Effective—1. having an effect: producing a result; 2. producing a definite or desired result (efficient); 3. in effect: operative, active; 4. actual, not merely potential or theoretical

Community—1. all the people living in a particular district, city, etc.; 2. a group of people living together as a smaller social unit within a larger one, and having interests, work, etc., in common

Prevention—1. the act of preventing . . . prevent; 2. to keep from happening: make impossible by prior action; hinder

Program—1. orig. (a) a proclamation, (b) a prospectus or syllabus. . . . 2. a plan or procedure for dealing with some matter.

In essence, an "effective community prevention program" is a planned procedure that prevents the onset of a disease among a group of individuals. Stated another way, *effective community prevention programs are those that work for groups of individuals.* A group may be as small as a school classroom or as large as a nation. Although many different oral diseases and conditions exist, this chapter focuses on methods of preventing dental caries, gingivitis, unintentional oral-facial injuries, and oral and pharyngeal cancers.

DENTAL CARIES

Dental caries, or tooth decay, is both a universal and a lifelong disease. This disease is universal in the sense that the prevalence or percent of the population affected increases with age, ultimately affecting almost the entire population. All of us are at risk for caries as long as we have our natural teeth. Thus it is lifelong and may occur as early as the first year of life as early childhood caries (ECC) (sometimes referred to as nursing or baby-bottle tooth decay; see Chapter 7), continue throughout childhood and young adulthood, and continue in adults as root surface caries. During adolescence and into adulthood, the incidence of dental caries continues depending on the level of community, personal, and professional protection; genetic influences; and dietary habits. Approximately 99% of adults have had tooth decay by age 40 to 44 years, with an average of 30 affected tooth surfaces.[9] For adults over age 75, nearly 60% had root surface caries with 3.1 affected tooth surfaces.[10] Recurrent decay can occur at any time throughout the life cycle. Thus it is important to prevent the onset of the disease because once a tooth has been restored the restoration must be replaced over time, and each restoration becomes larger and larger. Ultimately, costly crowns, root canals, or extractions may be needed.

Prevention of Dental Caries

Because dental caries is nearly ubiquitous, treating this disease is costly in terms of health, time, and money. On the basis of what we now know, dental caries can be controlled or nearly eliminated when science-based, preventive measures are applied appropriately. Because caries can continue throughout life, preventive measures must be a part of everyone's lifestyle. Many different approaches to preventing caries exist. The most cost-effective method is use of a community- or population-based approach.

FLUORIDES

The use of fluorides has made a significant impact on preventing dental caries in the United States. Fluoride is a naturally occurring compound of the element fluorine, which is never found in its free state in nature. It is the thirteenth most abundant element in the earth's crust and is found at different concentrations in all water supplies and most foods. Everyone's diet contains some fluoride, but not necessarily enough to prevent dental caries. The caries-preventive benefit of fluoride was first discovered by Dr. Frederick McKay, who was trying to determine the cause of "Colorado brown stain" (fluorosis, sometimes referred to as mottled enamel) in the 1920s. Dr. H. Trendly Dean subsequently demonstrated the relation between dental fluorosis, the concentration of fluoride in the water, and caries prevention with his classic epidemiologic studies in the 1930s. The first controlled study of adjusted fluoride level in a public water supply began on January 25, 1945, in Grand Rapids, Michigan.

Fluoride is now used in many different ways to prevent dental caries. Table 10-2 shows individual and community preventive measures that have been shown to be effective, the primary mode of application, and the target population. Initially it was believed that the primary anticaries benefit from fluoride was systemic, when the fluoride ion was ingested and became part of the developing tooth, before the tooth erupted in the mouth. The exact mechanisms of action of fluorides are not yet known. There are both preeruptive and posteruptive benefits from fluoride. A recent study from Australia reconfirms the preeruptive benefits from community water fluoridation.[11] Major benefits also are a result of posteruptive fluoride levels in plaque, saliva, and gingival exudate that continuously bathe the teeth and increase the remineralization of demineralized enamel caused by acids produced by cariogenic bacteria.

COMMUNITY WATER FLUORIDATION

Community water fluoridation was first implemented in the United States in 1945. Since then, millions of Americans have enjoyed the health and economic benefits of this prevention measure. According to *Healthy People 2010*, community water fluoridation "is an ideal public health method because it is effective, eminently safe, inexpensive, requires no cooperative effort or direct action, and does not depend on access or availability of professional services. It is equitable because the entire population benefits regardless of financial resources."[3]

Further, the Centers for Disease Control and Prevention (CDC) has recognized community water fluoridation as "one of the great public health achievements of the 20th century."[12] Community water fluoridation should be the foundation of oral disease prevention or treatment programs in communities with a central water supply. *Community water fluoridation* is defined as the adjustment of the concentration of fluoride of a community water supply for optimal oral health. Fluoridation is often referred to as nature's way to help prevent tooth decay. The recommended level of fluoride for a community water supply in the United States ranges from 0.7 to 1.2 parts per million (ppm) of fluoride, depending on the mean maximum daily air temperature over a 5-year period.[13] Thus in a warm climate the fluoride level would be lower, and in a cold climate it would be higher. In the United States most communities are fluoridated at approximately 1 ppm, which is equivalent to 1.0 mg of fluoride per liter of water. To put this concentration in perspective, consider that one part per million is equivalent to 1 inch in 16 miles, 1 minute in 2 years, or 1 cent in $10,000. At this level fluoridated water is odorless, colorless, and tasteless.

Natural Fluoridation. All water contains at least trace amounts of fluoride. In the United States in 1992 approximately 10 million people lived in 1924 communities with 3784 water systems that are fluoridated naturally at 0.7 ppm or higher.[14] The eight states with the most people served with natural fluoridation—6.6 million in 662

Table 10-2. Effective Community and Individual Preventive Measures for Dental Caries Prevention

Measure	*Method of Application*	*Target*	*Period of Use*
Community Programs			
Community water fluoridation	Systemic	Entire population	Lifetime
School water fluoridation	Systemic	Schoolchildren	School years
School fluoride tablet program	Systemic	Schoolchildren	Age 5-16 yr
School fluoride rinse program	Topical	Schoolchildren	Age 5-16 yr
School sealant program (professionally applied)	Topical	Schoolchildren	Age 6-8 and 12-14 yr
Individual Approach			
Prescribed fluoride tablets or drops	Systemic	Children	Age 6 mo-6 yr
Professionally applied fluoride treatment	Topical	Individual need	High-risk populations
Over-the-counter treatments	Topical	Individual need	High-risk populations
Fluoride toothpaste	Topical	Entire population	Lifetime
Professionally applied dental sealants	Topical	Children	Age 6-8 and 12-14 yr

communities—are shown in Table 10-3. Texas has the highest, with almost 3 million people in 284 communities.

In Alaska, Rhode Island, Maine, Tennessee, Pennsylvania, Vermont, and the District of Columbia, no one is served with a naturally fluoridated water supply at the recommended level (0.7 to 1.2 ppm). The next three lowest states are Massachusetts, Hawaii, and West Virginia with 659 communities. The five states with the highest proportion of their populations having access to naturally fluoridated water are Idaho (28.5%), Texas (16.7%), Colorado (23.4%), Montana (11.6%), and New Mexico (18.2%). In 2000, an estimated 11 million people lived in communities naturally fluoridated at the recommended level.

Table 10-3. Eight Highest-Ranking States by Number of Persons and Communities Served with Natural Water Fluoridation, 1992

State	*Number of Persons*	*Number of Communities*
Texas	2,955,995	284
Florida	929,105	35
Colorado	811,024	106
Illinois	442,714	127
California	414,798	29
South Carolina	386,940	2
Louisiana	359,906	31
Arizona	345,266	48
TOTAL	6,645,748	662

Adjusted Fluoridation. In 1992, 134.6 million Americans had access to adjusted community water fluoridation in 8572 communities with 10,567 water systems compared with approximately 151 million Americans in 2000.[14,15] Fig. 10-1 shows the national fluoridation rank of states with the percentage of the population served by adjusted and natural community water fluoridation in 2000. Adjusted fluoridation is accomplished "by adding fluoride chemicals to fluoride deficient water: by blending two or more sources of water naturally containing fluoride, or partial de-fluoridating, that is removing naturally occurring excessive fluoride to obtain the recommended level."[14] There is no difference between adjusted or natural fluoridation in safety or preventive benefits. A fluoride ion is a fluoride ion, whether it occurs naturally in the water supply or whether it is placed or added by a water engineer. The three major fluoride compounds used for fluoridation in 1992 with the population served and number of water systems are given in Table 10-4. The type of compound used depends on the size and type of water facility and the preference of the water supply engineer.[16]

Table 10-4. Population and Number of Public Water Supply Systems Served by Major Fluoride Compounds, 1992

	Population	*%*	*Number of Water Systems*
Hydrofluosilic acid (fluosilic acid)	80,019,175	62.2	5876
Sodium silicofluoride (sodium fluorosilicate)	35,084,896	28.2	1635
Sodium fluoride	11,701,979	9.1	2491
TOTAL	127,806,050		

NOTE: Fluoride compound used was not indicated for all systems, so these data do not reflect national total.

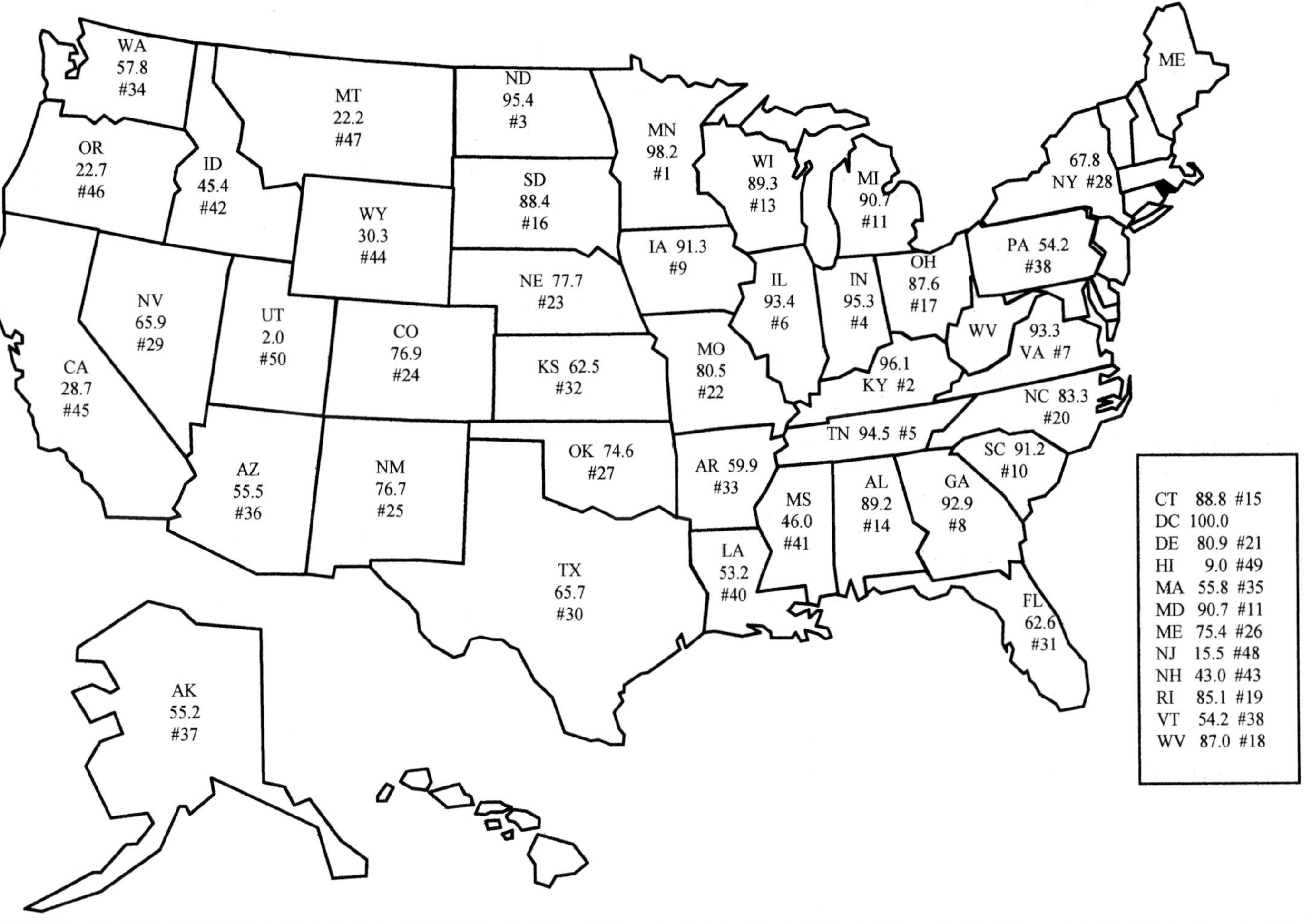

Fig. 10-1. Percentage of state populations on public water systems using fluoridated water and state rank, 2000. (From Centers for Disease Control and Prevention, http://www.cdc.gov/nccdphp/oh)

The United States has more people served by fluoridation than any other country in the world. Consider the following data. In 2000, 162 million Americans, or 65.8% of the 246.1 million on public water supplies, had fluoridation compared with 144.2 million Americans, or 62.1% of the 232 million on public water supplies in 1992.[14,15] This is approximately 57.5% of the total U.S. population. More than 119 million Americans did not have access to fluoridation, of whom approximately 35 million were not served by a public water system. Federal government policy requires fluoridation of water supplies on military installations. In 1992, a total of 133 military installations had adjusted fluoridation, serving 1.36 million residents with another 78,528 served by natural fluoridation.[14]

Of the 50 largest cities in the United States, all but eight have a fluoridated water supply. These eight cities, which have a combined population of approximately 5.4 million people, are San Diego, San Jose, and Fresno, California; Portland, Oregon; San Antonio, Texas; Tucson, Arizona; Honolulu, Hawaii; and Wichita, Kansas. Three of these cities are in California, which passed a statewide fluoridation law in October 1995 requiring fluoridation of all public water systems with at least 10,000 service corrections, depending on available funding. San Diego and San Antonio, respectively, ordered and voted for fluoridation in 2000, but have not yet implemented it. Fresno is partially fluoridated. Tucson, which is partially fluoridated naturally, voted for fluoridation in 1992, but it has yet to be implemented.[17]

Safety. The safety of fluoridation has been well documented by numerous studies over the years.[18-22] Soon after fluoridation became known as a public health measure, beginning in the 1950s, a variety of diseases and conditions, including premature death, have been alleged to be caused by fluoridation. All have been shown to be false. The following is a partial list of some of the more common conditions *falsely* attributed to fluoridation: AIDS, allergies, Alzheimer's disease, bone disease, cancer, chromosomal damage, pregnancy, gastrointestinal damage, heart disease, infertility, kidney disease, Down syndrome, and sterility.

Those opposed to fluoridation for a variety of reasons have had a tendency to use any argument possible to capture the public interest to oppose fluoridation. The arguments range from "being a communist plot" to "causes rusty pipes" in the 1950s and 1960s to cancer, AIDS, and Alzheimer's disease in the 1970s, 1980s, and 1990s, respectively. A misuse of facts and quoting from studies lacking scientific rigor are often used to support these allegations.[23-25] The safety of fluoridation has been time-consuming and costly to document because of the range of allegations made by the opponents, or "antifluoridationists," over the years. As a result, fluoridation is one of the most well researched public health measures. Concomitantly, the safety of this preventive measure has been relatively easy to document because millions of Americans have for generations lived in communities with naturally fluoridated water. In addition, many communities in the United States and other countries have a fluoride level that is naturally much higher than the recommended level, so that it is much easier to do studies to disprove these false allegations. The safety and effectiveness of water fluoridation as a public health measure is well established for the scientific and health communities; thus most national organizations representing these disciplines, such as the American Medical Association, the American Public Health Association, the American

Association of Public Health Dentistry, and the American Dental Association, have endorsed or supported fluoridation (Box 10-2).

Effectiveness. The effectiveness of fluoridation in preventing dental caries has been well documented.[26] Early controlled studies of adjusted fluoridation demonstrated that 50% to 70% of caries in the permanent teeth of children was prevented.[27-30] Since 1980, because of the widespread use of fluorides in the United States, the measurable effectiveness of water fluoridation is now approximately 20% to 40%.[26] This phenomenon is due, in part, to the fact that many other fluoride-containing products are now available, such as dietary fluoride supplements, rinses, toothpaste, professionally applied treatments, and dilution and diffusion effects, which are described here.

A comprehensive review of fluoridation states that fluoridation prevents caries in primary teeth by 30% to 60% for children 3 to 5 years of age, 20% to 40% for children with a mixed dentition (ages 6 to 12 years), and approximately 15% to 35% for adolescents and adults.[18,31] Fluoridation also helps prevent root caries in senior adults by 17% to 35%.[31] In countries or communities where there is no widespread use of fluorides, the effectiveness would be expected to be similar to that in early studies conducted in the United States. A recently reported study documented this phenomenon.[32]

Dilution and Diffusion Effects. Water fluoridation is as effective now as it was in the past. Because of the widespread use of fluorides in the United States in both fluoridated and nonfluoridated communities, however, the measurable benefits of fluoridation are lower in the United States. This phenomenon is called the *dilution* effect. Communities without fluoridation also benefit from foods and drinks processed in communities with fluoridation and sold or used in communities without fluoridation. This factor is called the *diffusion* effect and it also affects the measurable benefits of water fluoridation.[26] A recent study showed that in nonfluoridated communities that had a high diffusion effect from fluoridated communities, there is less dental caries.[33] Diffusion effects also can occur when individuals who live in communities without fluoridation work or go to school in a community that has optimal fluoridation. In contrast, the effects of the increased use of bottled water and filters for tap water are not known.

Cost. Of all the measures used to prevent dental caries in the United States, water fluoridation is the most economical and cost-effective. In 1989 the weighted average cost of fluoridation was estimated to be $0.51 per capita per year for the United States, with a range of $0.12 to $5.41, depending on the size of the community and the complexity of the water system.[34] In 1999 dollars, this would translate to an average per capita cost of $0.72 per year with a range of $0.17 to $7.62.[35] For larger communities the cost of fluoridation is usually less and for smaller communities it is more, as shown here in 1999 dollars:

Annual Cost per Capita	Community Population
$0.84–$7.62	Less than 10,000
$0.25–$1.05	10,000 to 200,000
$0.17–$0.29	Greater than 200,000
Weighted average: $0.72	

For approximately 85% of the population in fluoridated communities, the average annual cost per capita was $0.12 to $0.75 in 1989 dollars[36] or $0.17 to $1.05 in 1999 dollars. A recent study showed that Medicaid-eligible children who lived in

BOX 10-2

National and International Organizations That Recognize the Public Health Benefits of Community Water Fluoridation

Academy of Dentistry International
Academy of General Dentistry
Academy of Sports Dentistry
Alzheimer's Association
American Academy of Allergy, Asthma and Immunology
American Academy of Family Physicians
American Academy of Oral and Maxillofacial Pathology
American Academy of Pediatrics
American Academy of Pediatric Dentistry
American Academy of Periodontology
American Association for the Advancement of Science
American Association for Dental Research
American Association of Community Dental Programs
American Association of Dental Schools
American Association of Endodontists
American Association of Oral and Maxillofacial Surgeons
American Association of Orthodontists
American Association of Public Health Dentistry
American Cancer Society
American College of Dentists
American College of Physicians—American Society of Internal Medicine
American College of Prosthodontists
American Council on Science and Health
American Dental Assistants Association
American Dental Association
American Dental Hygienists' Association
American Dietetic Association
American Federation of Labor and Congress of Industrial Organizations
American Hospital Association
American Medical Association
American Nurses' Association
American Osteopathic Association
American Pharmaceutical Association
American Public Health Association
American School Health Association
American Society of Clinical Nutrition
American Society for Dentistry for Children
American Society for Nutritional Sciences
American Student Dental Association
American Veterinary Medical Association
American Water Works Association
Association for Academic Health Centers
Association of Maternal and Child Health Programs
Association of State and Territorial Dental Directors
Association of State and Territorial Health Officials
British Dental Association
British Fluoridation Society
British Medical Association
Canadian Dental Association
Canadian Dental Hygienists Association
Canadian Medical Association
Canadian Nurses' Association
Canadian Paediatric Society
Canadian Public Health Association
Chocolate Manufacturers Association
Consumer Federation of America
Delta Dental Plans Association
Dental Health Foundation (of California)
European Organization for Caries Research
FDI World Dental Federation
Federation of Special Care Organizations in Dentistry
- Academy of Dentistry for Persons with Disabilities
- American Association of Hospital Dentists
- American Association for Geriatric Dentistry

Health Insurance Association of America
Hispanic Dental Association
International Association for Dental Research—International Association for Orthodontics
International College of Dentists
Institute of Medicine
National Academy of Sciences
National Alliance for Oral Health

Continued

BOX 10-2

National and International Organizations That Recognize the Public Health Benefits of Community Water Fluoridation—cont'd

National Association of County and City Health Officials
National Association of Dental Assistants
National Confectioners Association
National Council Against Health Fraud
National Dental Assistants Association
National Dental Association
National Dental Hygienists' Association
National Down Syndrome Congress
National Down Syndrome Society
National Foundation of Dentistry for the Handicapped
National Kidney Foundation
National PTA
National Research Council
Society of American Indian Dentists
U.S. Department of Defense
U.S. Department of Veterans Affairs
U.S. Public Health Service
  Centers for Disease Control and Prevention (CDC)
  Health Resources and Services Administration (HRSA)
  Indian Health Service (IHS)
  National Institute of Dental and Craniofacial Research (NIDCR)
World Federation of Orthodontists
World Health Organization (WHO)

fluoridated communities in Louisiana had approximately 50% lower dental bills than Medicaid-eligible children who lived in nonfluoridated communities.[37] For every dollar spent on water fluoridation there is an estimated $25 to $80 savings in treatment costs based on community size, costs, and different study methodologies.[38,39] This is an excellent cost-benefit ratio and is the highest for all the caries preventive measures used in the United States.

Practicality. Fluoridation is the most practical preventive measure in dentistry. No individual effort is needed. Everyone who lives in a community with fluoridation and consumes the water or uses it to prepare foods will receive some benefit, irrespective of age, sex, race, lifestyle, or level of education or income. Those individuals who are born in such a community and live there for their entire lives accrue maximum benefits because they receive both systemic and topical benefits for a lifetime.

The concentration of fluoride in a water supply must be monitored on a routine and systematic basis. Thus it is important for water operators to have the appropriate training in fluoridation and to maintain and monitor the concentration of fluoride as recommended.[13,40]

Antifluoridationists. Individuals who are opposed to community water fluoridation are termed *antifluoridationists.* Reasons used for opposing fluoridation include safety, individual rights, government mistrust, home rule, and religious freedom. None of the arguments against fluoridation has any merit based on scientific knowledge and public health experience. Further, none of the arguments has any merit on the basis of state or federal laws. The U.S. Supreme Court has denied a review of fluoridation cases 13 times between 1954 and 1984.[41] The primary reasons antifluoridationists have had some limited success are mainly due to an uninformed public, weak or uninformed decision makers, and a weak or poorly organized program to promote and implement fluoridation. A number of significant fluoridation battles have occurred over the years; however, with more than 55 years of health and economic benefits for millions of Americans, the arguments against fluoridation become weaker and weaker. This reality does not mean antifluoridationists have given up or ever will.

Antifluoridationists attempt to appeal to the emotions of the public and elected officials and promote fluoridation as a political issue rather than a public health program. Most communities in the United States make their decisions to fluoridate administratively on the basis of public health expertise. From 1989 to 1994, 337 communities in the United States decided to fluoridate the water supply, and 318, or 94%, were decided by administrative decisions from a city council or commission.[42] Of the 32 referenda or public votes that occurred during that time, 19 (61%) supported fluoridation. In fall 2000 there were 23 fluoridation referenda in different communities throughout the United States. Of these, there were 9 (39%) wins for fluoridation and 14 (61%) losses. However, the 9 winning communities had a population of approximately 3.9 million people compared with approximately 366,347 for the losing communities, more than a tenfold difference.[43] When the public is forced to vote on a complex public health program such as fluoridation, the antifluoridationists usually use deceptive, misleading, and incorrect information to confuse the public so that they vote for the status quo, to their own detriment. Compounding this problem is the fact that we have failed to educate the American population about how fluorides work and who benefits from their use. Numerous studies have shown that, in general, the U.S. public is not knowledgeable about fluorides and does not know that the use of fluoride is the best approach to caries prevention.[44,45] Fluoridation battles still occur in some communities; however, if the political and professional will is present and the public and decision makers are well informed, the implementation of fluoridation will be successful.[46-51] For example, in 2000 three major U.S. communities—Clark County (Las Vegas), Nevada; Salt Lake County (Salt Lake City), Utah; and San Antonio, Texas—had public votes in support of fluoridation, after extensive educational efforts in these communities.

Community Support. The key to achieving fluoridation in most communities is through organized community support, which is the essence of dental public health, defined by the American Board of Dental Public Health as "the science and art of preventing and controlling dental diseases and promoting dental health through organized community efforts."[52] Just as community water fluoridation should be the foundation of any caries prevention program, educating the public is the key to achieving and maintaining community water fluoridation or any other public health measure. Box 10-3 includes basic concepts about fluorides that everyone should know and understand.

A planned educational program for community leaders, organizations, agencies, and institutions is important, beginning with health and human services leadership and then including all other community groups. Once there is widespread community support for fluoridation or any other type of population-based program, it is much easier to implement, support, and sustain. As part of such an educational effort, dentists and physicians also should educate their patients, especially those who are community leaders, about the benefits of fluoridation for the community. It is beyond

BOX 10-3

What Everyone Should Know about Preventing Oral Diseases

DENTAL CARIES

FLUORIDE

- What fluoride and fluoridation are
- How fluorides work to protect teeth from decay
- Methods of application
- Safety, effectiveness, and cost of each procedure
- Who needs them
- Recommended frequency of use and duration

PIT AND FISSURE SEALANTS

- What dental sealants are
- How they work to protect teeth from decay
- Who needs them and when
- Monitoring and reapplication

ORAL CANCERS

- Risk factors for oral cancers
- Signs and symptoms of oral cancers
- What comprises a thorough oral cancer examination and recommended frequency
- Need for oral cancer examination
- Protective factors against oral cancers

GINGIVITIS

- What dental plaque is
- Role of dental plaque in oral diseases
- How to remove plaque
- Frequency of plaque removal
- Recommended types of toothbrushes and floss

the scope of this chapter to detail how to organize an educational campaign for fluoridation. Many states and large cities have dental directors who have had experience with implementing and monitoring fluoridation. Further, the dental literature has many articles on fluoridation campaigns that may be helpful.[46-51,53-59]

National Fluoride Plan. In 1996 a national fluoride plan to promote oral health in the United States was developed by the U.S. Public Health Service.[60] The purpose of this plan was to determine what must be done to reach the water fluoridation or fluoride-related objectives of *Healthy People 2000* and to respond to the recommendations of the U.S. Public Health Service report *Review of Fluoride: Benefits and Risks.*[18] The plan was organized into four areas: policy, research, surveillance, and education. A status report for each area was given with recommendations for future strategies of action, which should include the following:

1. Promote and support effective coalition building to ensure the appropriate use of fluorides and the community adoption of water fluoridation
2. Develop "on-site" field expertise and "steering committees" in states with large numbers of nonfluoridated communities
3. Encourage research in areas related to fluorides and water fluoridation
4. Provide a collateral strategy for the surveillance and quality of water fluoridation to ensure that community water systems consistently supply water with fluoride within recommended ranges, as outlined in the CDC Engineering and Administrative Recommendations for Water Fluoridation, 1995
5. Promote the effective, proper, and safe use of fluorides and community water fluoridation through education; training; publications; endorsements; and broadcast, print, electronic, and visual media coverage

The national fluoride plan addressed the need to provide fluoridation and fluoride to the more than 100 million Americans who do not live in communities with a fluoridated water supply. In addition, the plan encouraged continued studies of fluorides, especially with regard to the increase in fluorosis. An ongoing national fluoridation plan with appropriate resources is key to improving the oral health of all Americans.

Dental Fluorosis. In recent years an increase in dental fluorosis has occurred in the United States in both fluoridated and nonfluoridated communities as a result of inappropriate uses of fluorides.[18,35] Dental fluorosis is the hypomineralization of enamel and the disruption of enamel development from excessive fluoride intake. It occurs in primary and permanent teeth, but in the United States it is less common in primary teeth. The severity of fluorosis depends on the amount of excess fluoride consumed over a period of time while teeth are developing, between ages 6 months and 6 years. One study suggests that the maxillary central incisors are at greatest risk for fluorosis from 15 to 24 months of age for males and from 21 to 30 months for females.[61] Once teeth have erupted, fluorosis cannot develop. Most dental fluorosis in the United States is considered a cosmetic problem, not a health problem. Very mild and mild fluorosis may occur in 10% to 15% of children reared in a community with fluoridated water.[18] In its mild form, usually only dental personnel will notice the bilateral white chalky appearance. In its more severe form, which occurs most often in communities in which the concentration of fluoride is naturally at much greater than the recommended level, there may be pitting and discoloration of teeth. Most of the increase in fluorosis in the United States is of a very mild or mild form.

The increase of fluorosis is caused by inappropriate prescribing and use of dietary fluoride supplements, ingesting fluoride toothpaste, prolonged use of infant formula made from powder and mixed with fluoridated water, and the fluoride concentration of the water supply. Authorities have estimated that only a twofold increased risk of fluorosis exists in an optimally fluoridated community today compared with an eighteenfold increase in the 1930s because of the increased risk in nonfluoridated communities.[62] A recent study showed that in nonfluoridated communities, 65% of the fluorosis was caused by fluoride supplementation under the pre-1994 protocol and 34% was the result of children under age 1 using more than a pea-size amount of fluoride toothpaste.[63] In fluoridated communities, 68% of the fluorosis resulted from more than a pea-size amount of fluoride toothpaste being used by children under age 1, 13% was caused by inappropriate fluoride supplements, and 9% resulted from the use of powdered concentrate infant formula.[63]

Teeth with dental fluorosis are less susceptible to dental caries. In 1994 the American Dental Association's Council on Scientific Affairs recommended a new dosage schedule that reduced the dosage for dietary fluoride supplements[64] (Table 10-5). Physicians and dentists can help prevent fluorosis by prescribing dietary fluoride supplements appropriately (according to the current dosage schedule) and only for children living in communities without fluoridation. Parents should be educated by their health providers on the appropriate use of infant formula and to use only a pea-size amount of fluoride toothpaste for children younger than 6 years old and to monitor their children closely to help prevent the ingestion of toothpaste.[35]

Comparison of Effective Community Prevention Programs. In the United States, five effective community prevention programs for dental caries are used (Table 10-6). Of the five

Table 10-5. Supplemental Fluoride Dosage Schedule, 1994*

	Concentration of Fluoride in Drinking Water (ppm)			
Age of Child	*<0.3*	*0.3-0.6*	*>0.6*	*Preparation*
6 mo-3 yr	0.25 mg	0	0	Drops
3-6 yr	0.50 mg	0.25 mg	0	Tablets
6-16 yr	1 mg	0.50 mg	0	Tablets

*Recommended by American Dental Association, American Academy of Pediatric Dentistry, and American Academy of Pediatrics.

NOTE: Amounts represent milligrams of fluoride per day.

Table 10-6. Comparison of Five Effective Community Prevention Programs for Dental Caries*

Program	*Effectiveness (%)*	*Adult Benefits*	*Cost per Year*	*Practicality*
Community fluoridation	20-40	Demonstrated	$0.51 per capita[‡] $0.72 per capita[†]	Excellent; most practical; no individual effort necessary
School fluoridation	20-30[§]	Expected but not demonstrated	$0.85-$9.88 per child[‡] $1.19-$13.83 per child[†]	Good; if there is no central community water supply, no individual effort necessary
School dietary fluoride	30	Expected but not demonstrated	$0.81-$5.40 per child[‡,‖] $1.13-$7.56 per child[†]	Fair, continued school regimen Daily supplement program required for 8-10 yr
School fluoride mouth rinse program	25-28[§]	Not expected	$0.52-$1.78 per child[‡,‖] $0.73-$2.49 per child[†]	Fair; continued daily or weekly school regimen required
School sealant program	51-67[¶]	Expected but not demonstrated	$13.07-$28.37 per child[‡] $18.30-$39.72 per child[†]	Good; primarily done for children ages 6-8 yr and 12-14 yr

Data from Burt B: Proceedings of the workshop. Cost-Effectiveness of Caries Prevention in Dental Public Health, *J Public Health Dent* 1989:49(5, spec iss): Allukian M: Oral diseases: the neglected epidemic. In Scutchfield FD, Keck WC, editors: *Principles and practices of public health.* Albany, NY, 1996, Delmar.

*This table is a simplified comparison of these prevention programs. A thorough analysis of the literature should be done to understand the relative merits of these programs.

[†]In 1999 dollars.

[‡]In 1989 dollars.

[§]This range may now be high; no recent studies.

[‖]Includes use of volunteer personnel.

[¶]First molar chewing surfaces only over 5-year period.

programs, community water fluoridation is not only the most cost-effective and practical but also the only community preventive measure that has demonstrated benefits for adults. Although salt fluoridation has been used successfully in other countries, it has not yet been used in the United States; therefore it is not included in the list. Table 10-6 applies to the United States only because the fluoride dilution and diffusion effects decrease the measurable benefits of fluoride. In other countries where there are fewer communities with fluoridation and other fluoride products, the effectiveness would be comparable to the 50% to 70% reduction in caries found in the 1950s to 1970s in the United States. Table 10-6 shows the relative differences among these preventive measures. Studies are needed on effectiveness and cost because of the diffusion and dilution effects of fluoride. A thorough analysis of the literature also would be helpful to appreciate the differences in these prevention regimens.

School-Based Programs. When a community does not have a public or central water supply or does not yet have fluoridation for whatever reason, another approach is to use a caries-preventive regimen in schools. This approach is logical in that most children in the United States attend school regularly. Preventive regimens provided in schools can be one of three types: (1) a community type, such as school water fluoridation; (2) self-applied, which refers to any health activity that is performed by an individual student, such as fluoride mouth rinse conducted in a school setting; or (3) operator applied, which refers to any health activity that is performed by a health care provider for a student, such as the application of pit and fissure sealants in a school setting.

Increasingly, school-based health centers are being viewed as an effective approach to improve access to health, including oral health, and social support services for underserved populations.[65] The number of school-based health centers was estimated to be 1380 in 1999–2000; however, the number with a dental component may be low.[66] Interestingly, in 2001 the Robert Wood Johnson Foundation announced a new program, Caring for Kids: Expanding Dental and Mental Health Services, through expanded services organized by school-based health centers. They will fund up to six oral health projects.[67] (For more information about school-based educational programs, see Chapter 11.)

SCHOOL WATER FLUORIDATION

School water fluoridation was developed and tested in the United States in the 1960s for use in rural schools with an independent water supply, preferably those schools that included grades kindergarten through 12. Fluoridation of water supplies of individual schools is similar to community water fluoridation in that no direct action is required of beneficiaries other than direct consumption of or use of the water in food preparation. The major difference is that the recommended concentration for school water fluoridation is 4.5 times the concentration of fluoride recommended for community water supplies in the respective geographic area. The higher concentrations are recommended to compensate for part-time exposure because children spend only part of their time at school.[68]

Effectiveness. Studies conducted on school fluoridation have shown that a 20% to 30% reduction in caries can be expected when children have consumed school water fluoridation for 12 years.[68,69] Despite the higher fluoride concentration, no dental fluorosis has been produced. A primary reason for this lack of fluorosis is because of the age of children when they start school, 5 or 6 years, when dental fluorosis is less likely to occur. There are disadvantages to school water fluoridation in that there is both delayed and part-time exposure. Further, it benefits only the children attending school and the adults who work there. Finally, unlike community water fluoridation, we do not know whether there are retained benefits after a child leaves a fluoridated school environment and goes to a community in which the water is not fluoridated. In the 1980s there were approximately 600 schools in the United States whose water was fluoridated. In 1992 there were 332 schools with 117,430 children in 12 states that had access to school water fluoridation.[14] The number has diminished for several reasons. Some rural schools with an independent water supply previously using school water fluoridation have been incorporated into major, central water systems that are now optimally fluoridated, thus eliminating the need for a school water fluoridation system. One state discontinued the school water fluoridation program because state officials determined that children were receiving ample fluoride from other sources.

Cost. In 1989 school water fluoridation was estimated to cost between $0.85 and $9.88 per child per school year.[34] In 1999 dollars, this would be $1.19 to $13.83 per child per school year.

Practicality. The practicality of school water fluoridation is good when a community does not have a central water supply. All the children benefit with no individual effort required on the part of the recipient. Monitoring the concentration of fluoride in the water must be conducted daily. The role and responsibility for monitoring must be worked out between the school and health and water departments. The individual responsible for monitoring the school fluoridation equipment must be well trained.

FLUORIDE TABLETS

Another method for administering systemic fluoride in school settings is the daily use of dietary fluoride supplements in the form of tablets. Table 10-5 shows the currently recommended fluoride dosage schedule, which should be adhered to whether the supplement is used at school or home. This procedure is most often identified as one to use at home when a health care provider prescribes a fluoride supplement with or without vitamins. Because the compliance required for this regimen—daily for 16 years—may be more than most parents can achieve, this procedure often is used in schools. The usual procedure is for an adult to distribute the tablets to each participating student and then under supervision the tablet is chewed for approximately 30 seconds. The resultant solution is then swished between the teeth for another 30 seconds and then swallowed.[69] Thus this procedure provides both systemic and topical benefits. A supervising adult maintains a record of when each child takes a tablet. Supervised, self-administered use of fluoride tablets is a well-established regimen that has been used in the United States and abroad for more than 40 years.

Effectiveness. Although it is not the most popular school-based fluoride regimen used in the United States, this method is well documented with research and has been shown to be effective. Studies conducted in this country have shown that the daily use of fluoride tablets on school days will provide up to a 30% reduction in new carious lesions.[70]

Cost. The average cost of a school-based fluoride tablet program in 1989 was approximately $2.53 per child per school year with a range of $0.81 to 5.40, depending on whether paid personnel or volunteers are used to supervise the procedure.[34] In 1999 dollars, this would be $3.54 per child with a range of $1.13 to $7.56.

Practicality. The daily consumption of fluoride tablets in school settings is an excellent method to use in areas where the water is fluoride deficient. This procedure can be supervised by a classroom teacher or volunteer with minimal training. It takes only a few minutes of classroom time and it is highly accepted by students, faculty, and parents. A major drawback to this method is that it is a daily procedure. Therefore the practicality is fair. Only children with parental consent may participate. Table 10-7 compares the advantages of using either a school-based fluoride tablet or mouth rinse regimen.

FLUORIDE MOUTH RINSE

Fluoride mouth rinse has been used in schools in the United States for approximately three decades, and it is the most popular school-based fluoride regimen in the United States.[69] Fluoride rinsing is generally supervised in classrooms by teachers or adult volunteers. In some cases health or teacher aides are responsible for this activity. For children in grades 1 and above the procedure consists of distributing a paper napkin and a paper cup with 10 ml of solution to each participating student. In unison, the students empty the contents of the cup into the mouth and rinse the solution vigorously for 60 seconds. The supervising adult times the procedure; at the end of 60 seconds students are requested to empty the contents of the mouth into the cup and to place a tissue into the cup to absorb the liquid. The materials are then collected and disposed of properly.[69] The supervising adult also maintains a record for each child who rinses.

The rinse procedure for children in kindergarten is the same as that for older students except they are advised to use only 5 ml of the solution. The rationale for this

Table 10-7. Comparison of School-Based Fluoride Regimens

Fluoride Mouth Rinse	*Fluoride Tablets*
Safe and effective	Safe and effective
Inexpensive	Inexpensive
Easy to learn and do	Easy to learn and do
Nondental personnel can supervise	Nondental personnel can supervise
Well accepted by participants	Well accepted by participants
Little time required—5 minutes *weekly*	Little time required—3 minutes *daily*
Provides topical benefits	Provides systemic and topical benefits
	No waste materials
	Suitable for preschool children

Modified from Horowitz AM: Community-oriented preventive dentistry programs that work, *Health Values* 8(1):21, 1984.

recommendation is that younger children tend to swallow some of the solution, which may contribute to fluorosis if this practice continues over time among children 6 years old or younger. Practice sessions with plain water are recommended, especially for younger children.

Effectiveness. Numerous studies have demonstrated that dental caries can be reduced by approximately 25% to 28% by rinsing daily or weekly in school with dilute solutions of fluoride.[34] Because rinsing weekly with a 0.2% neutral sodium fluoride (NaF) solution requires fewer supplies and less time than daily rinsing with a 0.05% NaF solution, weekly school-based rinse programs are more common. Further, studies have shown that when used in school, there is little difference in caries protection between daily and weekly use.[71] This procedure is usually not used in schools in communities that have been fluoridated for three or more years. Table 10-8 shows appropriate fluoride programs for use in grades 1 through 12.

Cost. The cost of this procedure in 1989 ranged from $0.52 to $1.78 per child depending on whether paid or volunteer adult supervisors were used.[34] In 1999 dollars, it would cost $0.73 to $2.49.

In addition, the cost varies depending on whether a unit dose (individual, premixed serving) is used or whether packets of NaF are purchased and mixed with water and dispensed into cups. The premixed unit dose is more convenient and requires less time, but the materials cost more.

Practicality. The practicality of this measure is fair because it is performed once a week. It is somewhat more practical in terms of frequency than the use of fluoride tablets, but it is less practical in that the children should not swallow the rinse; thus close monitoring is required and the used products must be collected and disposed of properly.

DENTAL SEALANTS

The appropriate use of fluorides is the best approach to preventing caries. Fluoride, however, is believed to be least effective on the occlusal or chewing tooth surfaces. Most decay among school-age children now occurs on the chewing surfaces. Thus the use of fluorides and pit and fissure sealants is needed to provide nearly total caries prevention.[72] In the United States the

Table 10-8. Appropriate Self-Applied Fluoride Programs for Use in Grades 1 through 12

Fluoride in Water Supply (ppm)	*Tablets (Daily)*	*Mouth Rinse (Weekly)*	*Grade*	*Recommended Procedure*
<0.3	1 mg fluoride		1-8	Fluoride tablets
	1 mg fluoride	or 0.2% NaF	9-12	Fluoride tablets or fluoride mouth rinse
0.3-0.6	0.5 mg fluoride	or 0.2% NaF	1-8	Fluoride tablets or fluoride mouth rinse
>0.6	Dietary fluoride tablets should *not* be provided	0.2% NaF	1-12*	Fluoride mouth rinse*

*For high-risk children or youths in a fluoridated community.

application of dental sealants must be performed by a dentist, a dental hygienist, or a dental assistant, depending on individual state practice acts. The application procedure is relatively simple; however, it is operator dependent. Because sealant material is extremely susceptible to saliva contamination, the procedure must be done with great care.[72]

Oral health objectives in *Healthy People 2010* specify that 50% of children should have their permanent molars sealed by ages 8 and 14.[3] Unfortunately, the most recent data show that only approximately 23% of 8-year-olds and 15% of 14-year-olds have had this preventive procedure.[73] Unlike other countries, for example, Finland, where 85% of children have pit and fissure sealants on the permanent molars, practitioners in the United States have basically ignored this procedure. Concomitantly, the public (parents) have not been educated about the existence of and need for sealants; thus most do not have enough knowledge about them to request this preventive procedure for their children.[74]

Effectiveness. This procedure was first demonstrated to be effective in studies conducted approximately 30 years ago. Their effectiveness has been reported to be in the range of 51% to 67%.[34]

Cost. The 1989 estimated cost for dental sealants ranged from $13.07 to $28.37, depending on whether a dentist or dental auxiliary placed the sealant, whether they were paid or volunteer, and the type of equipment used.[34] In 1999 dollars, the cost would be from $18.30 to $39.72.

Practicality. Numerous states have school-based sealant programs, which, in itself, speaks for their practicality. Sealant programs focus on children 6 to 8 years old and 12 to 14 years old because the first and second permanent molars usually erupt during these years. These two molars are the teeth most often sealed in school-based programs. Some programs use mobile dental vans that are sent to schools, and children receive sealant application in the van. Other programs use portable equipment that is transported from school to school where it is set up in whatever space is available and students are brought to the designated room for the procedure. A few schools have dental clinics where they provide this service as well. The process is well accepted by students, parents, faculty, and staff and has been shown to reduce racial and economic disparities in sealant prevalence among school children.[75] As with all school-based caries-preventive measures, parental consent is required. Box 10-3 includes concepts about dental sealants, about which parents and children should be educated.

Community-Based Programs Used in Other Countries

For a variety of reasons, several different approaches to preventing dental caries are available and have supporting research but are used rarely or not at all in the United States. A few of these preventive approaches are salt fluoridation, fluoride varnishes, and atraumatic restorative treatment.

SALT FLUORIDATION

Salt fluoridation is the controlled addition of fluoride during the manufacturing of salt for use by humans. Sodium or potassium fluoride is usually used. Salt fluoridation is generally not recommended in countries that are using community water fluoridation. Adding fluoride to salt was first suggested by Wespi, who recognized the value of adding iodine to salt to prevent goiter. Recognized as an expert on iodized salt, he urged health authorities in Switzerland to add fluoride to iodized salt. Zurich was the first canton to authorize the sale of fluoridated domestic salt in 1955. By 1966 fluoridated salt accounted for 65% of the domestic salt market in Switzerland. The generally recommended concentration is roughly the equivalent of 1 ppm; however, each country must determine its needs on the basis of the consumption of salt and the concentration of fluoride in the local water supply.[76] Many other countries also have adopted Switzerland's innovative approach; these countries include France, Germany, Costa Rica, Jamaica, and Uruguay. The Pan American Health Organization (PAHO) has a major initiative to promote salt fluoridation in eight countries in the Region of the Americas, Belize, Bolivia, Dominican Republic, Honduras, Nicaragua, Panama, Paraguay, and Venezuela.[77]

Effectiveness. Fluoridated salt has been demonstrated to be as effective as community water fluoridation, when all domestic salt is fluoridated.[78] Domestic salt refers to that salt sold in markets and salt sold in bulk to restaurants, bakeries, hospitals, schools, and other institutions and companies that process foods. In Jamaica a caries reduction study among 1120 children showed a 69% decrease in caries experience for 15-year-olds and an 87% decrease for 6-year-olds after 8 years of salt fluoridation. Fluorosis was negligible.[79]

Cost. Generally, salt fluoridation is as effective as community water fluoridation but costs less. Authorities estimate that in some Latin American countries the potential saving may be as high as $391 for dental expenditures, with an average of $172, for each dollar invested in the regimen. The cost-benefit ratio range for seven countries in the Americas was 1:18 to 1:391.[77] On average the cost is approximately $0.08 to $0.12 per kilogram of salt.[77]

Practicality. Salt fluoridation provides a choice to consumers that community water fluoridation does not, sometimes a major issue in initiating this procedure. There has been some opposition to salt fluoridation by individuals who are concerned about the need to reduce salt consumption; however, this concern is not justified for several reasons. Although excess salt consumption over a lifetime is linked to higher blood pressure, the use of salt does not increase when fluoride is added. Further, the amount of fluoride added to salt can be adjusted. Another concern that is often cited is the question about distribution of salt in a country, state, or canton where some water has natural concentrations of fluoride that range from 0.6 to 1.2 ppm and higher. This situation, of course, is true for most countries and can be accommodated by educating the salt manufacturers and the food distributors and the public at large. In countries where fluoridated salt is sold, containers are not only labeled but are also usually color coded, a procedure also used to distinguish iodized salt from plain salt. Further, salt manufacturers ship fluoridated salt only to communities with specified lower concentrations of fluoride in the water supply. This effort does not preclude the fact that an uninformed consumer could go to a market in another community and inadvertently purchase fluoridated salt. Overall, this approach to offering a preventive regimen has been given little notice in North America, where community water fluoridation is well established.

However, many rural locations, for example, Native American reservations in Canada and the United States and states such as Alaska, might benefit dramatically from the use of this preventive procedure.

FLUORIDE VARNISHES

Fluoride varnishes were developed in Europe more than 35 years ago and remain in wide use there. They are operator applied, and biannual application is the usual recommendation. In Finland varnishes are used in 92% of the community preventive programs for children.[80] Most of the clinical studies, with the exception of one Canadian trial, were conducted in Europe.[81] The original purpose for their development was to increase the uptake of fluoride by enamel, when it was thought that this factor would lead to greater caries protection. Fluoride varnishes do increase the fluoride concentration in saliva for a longer period of time than do other professionally applied fluoride products.[82] The U.S. Food and Drug Administration recently approved the marketing of DuraFlor (formerly Duraphat), which has been hailed by some as a giant step forward.[83]

Effectiveness. Numerous studies have shown that there is a wide range of efficacy, between 7% and 75%. Fluoride varnishes are as efficacious as other caries-preventive agents.[84] Studies have been conducted mostly on children, but there is no reason the product could not be studied and used on adults. This kind of fluoride may be especially useful to prevent root surface caries among the growing number of older adults who have gingival recession. In addition, fluoride varnishes may be especially attractive for use with disabled children and bed-bound patients who still have their own teeth. More recently, fluoride varnishes have been used in demonstration programs to help prevent infant or early childhood caries among children in some Women, Infants, and Children (WIC) and Head Start programs. North Carolina and Washington State allow physicians to apply fluoride varnishes to the teeth of young children to prevent early childhood caries. In 2001 the Nevada Medicaid program began reimbursing physicians, physician assistants, and nurse practitioners for applying fluoride varnish.

Practicality. The use of fluoride varnishes is as practical as any operator-applied fluoride treatments.

ATRAUMATIC RESTORATIVE TREATMENT

In recent years research has provided an increased understanding of the process of dental caries, how to prevent it, and better approaches to treating the disease. Keeping a tooth healthy and intact through appropriate use of fluorides and pit and fissure sealants helps to prevent costly repairs.[85] In many developing countries, and for some populations within highly industrialized countries, dental caries is a widespread problem and treatment often is available only for the affluent. When the caries process is left untreated, the only choice of treatment often is extraction of the tooth. A new method for treating caries is atraumatic restorative treatment (ART).[86,87] ART is a secondary preventive measure. This procedure offers treatment to disadvantaged populations and consists of caries removal with use of hand instruments only and then the application of adhesive restorative material. No electricity, water, drill, or expensive dental equipment is necessary. This procedure is used in at least 25 countries, including Zimbabwe, China, Thailand, and Cambodia. Further, the World Health Organization endorses its use. A growing body of research supports the use of this procedure, and additional studies are underway.[86,87]

Practicality. ART is extremely practical in that only hand instruments are used along with an adhesive dental material. Thus the equipment and materials are easy to pack, carry, or mail. This procedure may have applicability for bed-bound patients and others who are physically challenged. Although ART has yet to be used in the United States, the procedure could be beneficial for the disadvantaged, especially children, who have no way to finance dental treatment. ART is closely related to the application of pit and fissure sealant material in that similar dental material is used and both are minimal intervention methods. The major difference, of course, is that sealants are used to prevent caries, whereas ART is used to treat the disease.

Periodontal Disease Prevention

Periodontal diseases consist of a variety of inflammatory and degenerative conditions of the supporting structures of the teeth. The two most common types are gingivitis and periodontitis. There is ample evidence to demonstrate the relationship between the presence of bacterial plaque and gingivitis. These diseases are insidious and can affect children and adults, although more severe types are more likely to be found among adults. Gingivitis—inflammation of the soft tissue surrounding teeth—can be prevented or controlled by thoroughly removing dental plaque periodically.[88]

Although no studies clearly define the necessary frequency of thorough plaque removal to prevent gingivitis, it is generally recommended that plaque should be removed at least daily. Generally, thorough plaque removal is accomplished mechanically with a toothbrush and dental floss or tape.[88] Dental plaque also can be controlled with the use of antimicrobial products such as chlorhexidine.[89] In community-based programs, however, only mechanical plaque removal has been used. At one time, school-based plaque removal regimens were popular. These toothbrushing drills often did not include the use of a fluoride dentifrice, thus severely limiting their value. Today, toothbrushing in classrooms is not used as much as it was two decades ago. Instead, children often are shown in school how to remove plaque with a toothbrush and sometimes dental floss or tape. These procedures may or may not include actual use of the implements. In either case, a toothbrush and floss are sometimes sent home with instructions to use them on a routine basis. If toothbrushing is to take place in a school environment, a fluoride dentifrice should be used so that both dental caries and gingivitis prevention are addressed. Dental floss or tape should be used only after proper instructions, so that the gingival tissues are not injured. All students should be taught the concepts listed in Box 10-3 regarding the prevention of gingivitis.

EFFECTIVENESS

Studies conducted in the 1970s and early 1980s showed that regular, thorough plaque removal under supervision could reduce gingivitis among schoolchildren.[90] In one study, however, in which examinations were conducted at the beginning and at the end of each school year, it was observed that much of the gain achieved in reducing gingivitis over the school year disappeared or at least was reduced over the summer when plaque removal was not supervised.[90]

COST

An estimated cost for this procedure for use in schools is not known, but it is relatively expensive because of the expense of toothbrushes, dentifrice, floss (if used), and various paper products if a sink is not used. In addition, teachers' time must be taken into consideration.

PRACTICALITY

Although toothbrushing in classrooms is possible, most public school teachers are less than enthusiastic about its practice. Much of this reluctance is understandable in that the procedure is invariably messy when dealing with younger children. Further, not all classrooms have sinks, thus making it necessary to use multiple types of paper products including paper cups, towels, or napkins. Moreover, the toothbrushes must be stored in a place where they can be kept clean and the waste products must be properly disposed of.

Brushing in school-based programs is found more frequently in Head Start classes where teachers appear to be more accepting of spills and the need to clean up than in public schools. The purpose is to teach the children how to brush, to help instill the need for routine toothbrushing and the feel of a "clean, fresh mouth," and, in some cases, to provide the only toothbrush the child has owned.

HIGH-RISK OR VULNERABLE POPULATIONS

Some groups of individuals are more vulnerable, more susceptible, or at higher risk for oral diseases and conditions than others because of their knowledge, attitudes, behavior, education, income, occupation, sex, age, health status, residency location, race, ethnicity, culture, or minority status.[3,4,52,91-94] These individuals have been called high-risk, vulnerable, underserved, special needs, or disadvantaged populations. Effective community prevention programs for dental caries are either for the whole community, such as fluoridation, or a specific age group, such as school prevention programs. However, a school prevention program such as dental sealants may be targeted to higher-risk children, maximizing access to limited services.[75,95] Also a school dental program may be targeted for those schools where there are children either at higher risk for disease or at higher risk for being unable to obtain treatment. Effective community prevention programs for dental caries can also be supplemented with an individual approach for children who are at high risk, such as use of home fluoride gels or rinses for individuals undergoing orthodontic treatment or taking medications that decrease salivary flow.[64] Populations also may be at "high risk" because of beliefs, behavior, or cultural patterns. Early childhood caries may be high in groups of children whose mothers or other caregivers put sugar or juices in their baby bottles, and oral cancer is high among persons who smoke and drink alcohol excessively.

When a community prevention program is being planned, the needs of high-risk populations must be considered. A high-risk group in one culture, neighborhood, or community may not be at high risk in another. For example, low-income children in the United States usually are at high risk for dental caries. However, low-income children in a developing country, especially in rural areas, usually are at low risk for dental caries because they do not have access to candies and other sweets.[91] Examples of some high-risk or vulnerable populations are as follows: bed bound, chemically dependent, cultural minorities, dentally indigent, developmentally disabled, elderly, ethnic minorities, children in Head Start programs, homebound, homeless, institutionalized, linguistic minorities, medically compromised, migrants, Native Americans, persons with human immunodeficiency virus or AIDS, rural populations, and teenagers.

The diversity of high-risk populations requires an understanding and appreciation of their needs, attitudes, knowledge, and behavior to develop an effective prevention program. These high-risk populations often have the greatest dental needs, the least resources and access to care, the least knowledge about preventing diseases, and few or no fact-finding skills, making primary prevention of disease even more important.

UNINTENTIONAL ORAL-FACIAL INJURIES

Oral-facial injuries may be intentional or unintentional. Intentional oral injuries may occur from abuse, domestic violence, self-mutilation, or violence in general. Dental personnel have a role in and responsibility for early detection, treatment, and referral for these patients. This section discusses the prevention of unintentional injuries that usually occur from contact sports, recreational activities, motor vehicles, and daily living.

Unintentional injuries result in more than 92,000 deaths per year, with motor vehicle crashes accounting for approximately half of these deaths, followed by other unintentional injuries, falls, poisonings, suffocation, and drownings.[3] For persons age 1 to 34 years, unintentional injuries are the major cause of death. Injury costs are estimated to be more than $441 billion a year, and approximately 29 million people per year go to emergency wards as a result of unintentional injuries.[3] Unintentional oral-facial injuries may result in broken and avulsed teeth, facial bone fractures, concussion, permanent brain injury, temporomandibular joint dysfunction, blinding eye injuries, and even death.[96] Although no national data exist on the extent of oral-facial injuries, the following is known:

- Approximately 25% of the U.S. population ages 6 to 50 years has had incisal tooth trauma.[97]
- Almost half of abused children have oral-facial trauma.[98]
- Approximately 25 million children in the United States participate in competitive school sports and approximately 20 million play in organized sports outside of school.[99]

PREVENTION OF UNINTENTIONAL ORAL-FACIAL INJURIES

No single mechanism or program can prevent all the different types of unintentional injuries. An organized community effort is needed that includes many different disciplines, such as health, education, transportation, law, engineering, architecture, and safety services.[3] Although not directly related to dentistry, support by the dental profession of the following injury prevention programs on community and individual levels may result in fewer oral-facial injuries:

- Increased use of mass transit
- Drunk driving prevention programs
- Seat belt and child safety seat laws and programs
- Improved pedestrian safety
- Motorcycle and bicycle helmet laws and programs
- Safe playground equipment

- Protective bars on upper-story windows
- Home fire safety measures
- Protective mouthguards and headgear for sports
- Home environment modifications
- Timely emergency medical services

Although no national data for the various causes of oral-facial injuries exist, sports appear to account for a significant proportion, with some estimates as high as 33%.[100,101] More than 14 million of the 20 million school-age children in the United States who participate in sports do so in at least one sport listed in Table 10-9, which does not include basketball. More than 25% of these children participate in two sports.[96] Baseball and softball are the most popular sports, played by 24% of school-age children, followed by 12.8% of children for soccer and 10% for football.[96] The highest number of unintentional injuries from product-associated sports treated in emergency departments in 1995 were from basketball, followed by bicycling, football, baseball, soccer, and softball (Table 10-10).[102] In a recent nationwide study of parents whose 5- to 14-year-old children play at least one of six organized team sports (soccer, football, basketball, baseball, softball, or T-ball), 53% of the parents stated that they do not worry much about injuries. In contrast, 30% of these children were injured at least once, with football (28%) and soccer (22%) having the most injuries, followed by the batting sports (18%) and basketball (15%).[103]

Protective headgear and mouthguards have been demonstrated to prevent unintentional injuries in sports. Approximately 50% of all high school football injuries were to the face and mouth before 1962, when protective oral-facial devices became required by the National Alliance Football Rules Committee.[104] One in 10 players had a chance of receiving such an injury during the playing season.[104] With the use of face guards and mouth protectors, there has been a dramatic reduction in oral-facial injuries in football since 1962.[104] Currently, only five amateur sports require mouth-

Table 10-9. Estimated Number and Percentage of Children Who Played Organized Sports in the United States, 1991

Sport	Number of Children	%
Baseball/softball	9,338,980	24.4
Soccer	4,906,134	12.8
Football	3,824,708	10.0
Karate/judo	977,180	2.6
Wrestling	960,763	2.5
Field/ice hockey	603,008	1.6
Lacrosse	141,480	0.4
Boxing	144,380	0.4
Rugby	52,686	0.1

Data from Nowjack-Raymer RE, Gift HC: Use of mouthguards and headgear in organized sports by school-aged children, *Public Health Rep* 111:82, 1996.

Table 10-10. Estimated Number of Sports Injuries Treated in U.S. Hospital Emergency Departments by Age, 1995

Sport	Number of Cases	Percentage by Age		
		0-4 yr	5-14 yr	15-24 yr
Basketball	692,386	0.3	30.5	48.0
Bicycling	549,988	7.4	56.3	15.1
Football	389,463	0.3	45.9	43.5
Baseball	210,395	4.0	50.3	23.2
Soccer	156,960	0.3	44.9	38.6
Softball	155,669	0.9	23.0	27.5

Data from National Safe Kids Campaign: *Sports injury fact sheet*, Washington, DC, 1996.

guards during games and practice: boxing, football, ice hockey, lacrosse, and women's field hockey.[105]

Mouth protection is needed in other sports. One statewide study showed that nearly 31% of high school basketball players sustained an oral-facial injury during the varsity basketball season, and 22% of these injuries required professional attention.[106] Only 4% of these players wore mouth protectors, and the injury rate for those without mouth protection was nearly seven times greater. In a study in another state of high school athletes, 9% of all players had some form of injury and 3% reported loss of consciousness.[107] Approximately 40% of the injuries were in baseball and basketball, with 75% occurring in players not wearing mouth protection. There also were fewer concussions in those athletes wearing

Table 10-11. Percentages of Children Who Wear Headgear and Mouthguard while Playing Baseball or Football by Selected Variables

	Baseball		*Football*	
	Headgear	***Mouthguard***	***Headgear***	***Mouthguard***
Total	35%	7%	72%	72%
Gender				
Male	40	8	77	77
Female	25	5	15	15
Grade level				
Elementary school	35	6	52	52
Middle school	36	9	80	79
High school	35	12	88	88
Race				
Black	33	17	74	71
White	35	6	72	72
Ethnicity				
Hispanic	33	11	46	52
Non-Hispanic	36	7	77	75
Poverty level				
Below	24	11	54	54
At/above	36	6	77	75
Parent's education				
<HS/HS	34	8	68	69
>HS	36	6	78	75

From Nowjack-Raymer RE, Gift HC: Use of mouthguards and headgear in organized sports by school-aged children, *Public Health Rep* 111:82, 1996.

HS, high school.

mouth protection. In a recent state survey of five sports (boys and girls soccer, boys and girls basketball, and wrestling) at seven high schools, only 6% of the athletes reported mouthguard use. The seasonal incident rate for at least one oral-facial injury per athlete was 28% in soccer, 72% in wrestling, and 55% in basketball, with 10% of athletes sustaining dental injuries.[108] In a national study of high school students who played baseball or softball, only 35% wore headgear and 7% mouthguards all or most of the time.[96] Approximately 40% of the males wore headgear compared with 25% of the females. Approximately 12% of these ballplayers wore mouthguards compared with 7% of soccer players and 72% of football players.[96] Table 10-11 shows the comparison of headgear and mouthguard use for baseball and football by gender, grade level, race, ethnicity, and socioeconomic level.

Studies also show that more children are injured in sports outside of school (60%) than when in school, and more injuries occur during practice (60%) than during games.[99,109] Protective sportswear usually is used much less often in sports outside of school and in practice. In *Healthy People 2010* one of the national prevention objectives is to "increase the proportion of public and private schools that require use of appropriate head, face, eye, and mouth protection for students participating in school-sponsored physical activities."[3]

Promotion of regulations, requirements, and guidelines for the use of effective protection in sports should include the mouth. Custom-fitted mouthguards allow for easier breathing and better speech; therefore compliance is much better than with stock mouthguards. Referees, coaches, parents, school officials, the dental profession, athletic organizations, and local and state health departments should all play a role in protecting the health and safety of children and athletes.[110-112]

PREVENTION AND EARLY DETECTION OF ORAL AND PHARYNGEAL CANCERS

Annually, nearly 30,000 Americans are diagnosed with oral and pharyngeal cancers, which translates into the fact that about one person dies each hour, nearly 8000 annually, as a result of these cancers. More Americans die from oral cancers than from cervical cancer.[113] Oral cancers can occur in all sites of the oral cavity, including the tongue, floor of the mouth, soft palate, tonsils, salivary glands, back of the throat, and lips. Of these, the floor of the mouth and the tongue are the primary sites. Nearly 90% of all oral cancers are squamous cell carcinoma.[114] In the United States, oral cancer is more prevalent among males than females and is most often diagnosed among persons age 45 years and older.

Oral cancers in advanced stages cause pain, loss of function, and frequently disfiguring impairment that can cause social isolation. The 5-year relative survival rate for oral cancers is 58% for whites and 34% for blacks. Oral cancers have one of the lower 5-year survival rates of the major cancer sites.[115] When oral cancers are detected early, prognosis for survival is much better than for most other cancers. Dentists, physicians, nurse practitioners, and other primary care providers can play a significant role in oral cancer prevention and early detection.[116]

Primary risk factors for oral cancers in the United States are use of tobacco and alcohol products and, for lip cancers, unprotected exposure to the sun. Tobacco and alcohol use account for 75% of all oral and pharyngeal cancers.[114-116] Dietary factors also may play a role. Similar to other cancers, such as colorectal cancer, eating fruits and vegetables that contain essential vitamins (A, C, and E) and other nutrients may provide protection against the development of oral cancers.[117] Variations of use of betel nut combined with tobacco, which is used in many other countries and now is found in the United States, also is a risk factor for oral cancers. In addition, certain viruses and marijuana have been identified as risk factors for these cancers.[118,119]

Despite available knowledge about risk factors for and signs and symptoms of oral cancers, the American public is ill informed about these matters.[120-122] Further, recent data show that only 13% of U.S. adults 40 years of age and older have had an oral cancer examination in the past 12 months, the periodicity recommended by the American Cancer Society.[3] Additionally, data suggest that dentists, dental hygienists, physicians, and nurse practitioners are not as knowledgeable about oral cancer prevention and early detection as they might be.[123-127] Complicating the problem is the fact that approximately 25% of U.S. dental schools use health history forms that are deficient in determining a patient's high-risk behaviors related to oral cancers—use of tobacco and alcohol products.[128] During the 1996 National Strategic Planning Conference for the Prevention and Control of Oral and Pharyngeal Cancer, it became apparent that comprehensive educational interventions directed at all health care providers and the public at large should be implemented.[129-130] Recently, several states have begun these kinds of activities.[131] Box 10-3 contains basic information that everyone should know and understand for the prevention and early detection of oral cancers.

In addition to well-planned educational interventions, community-based supports such as policy, legislation, and ordinances are critically needed for prevention and early detection of oral cancers.[129,131] In the United States there is a trend to use public policy to help decrease or prevent behaviors that contribute to diseases. For example, "no smoking" policies in schools, hospitals, worksites, and restaurants help curtail smoking and make it socially unacceptable. These policies may be especially influential among youth, who are the ones most likely to become addicted to tobacco products. Further, enforcing ordinances and laws make it more difficult for underaged youth to purchase tobacco or alcohol products, thus providing strong support for decreasing the initiation of their use. Concomitantly, enforcing fines and other disciplinary actions against individuals who sell or give these products to youths are equally necessary. A recent report by the Surgeon General evaluates the scientific evidence of educational, clinical, regulatory, economic, and comprehensive approaches to reduce tobacco use.[132] The bottom line is that there is more than enough information to act now and that comprehensive programs (i.e., programs that include all approaches) provide the best results.

Other policies might be directed at health care providers. For example, dental and dental hygiene schools could require students to have exit competence in oral cancer examinations.[129] No state or regional dental board currently requires applicants to demonstrate competence in providing an oral cancer examination. Thus dental examining boards could require that applicants perform an oral cancer examination for licensure. Further, relicensure could require that applicants take a refresher course in oral cancer prevention and early detection—a strategy used in other content areas.[129]

School-based drug interventions frequently begin in primary grades and often focus on developing self-esteem, building skills to resist peer pressure, and urging children to remain free of tobacco, alcohol, and other drugs. These school-based efforts often are implemented in conjunction with other community-based activities aimed at preventing children and youths from starting the habit and urging users to stop. Unfortunately, these kinds of educational interventions often do not identify tobacco products as risk factors for oral cancers. Similarly, efforts focusing on alcohol use as a risk factor for fetal alcohol syndrome, cirrhosis of the liver, and liver cancer usually do not identify alcohol as a risk factor for oral cancers.[120]

NEED FOR HEALTH PROMOTION IN ORAL DISEASE PREVENTION

Today, we know how to prevent or control most oral diseases. With the appropriate use of fluorides and pit and fissure sealants, dental caries can be nearly eliminated among children. Also, with thorough and frequent plaque removal by an individual and periodic appointments with a dental care provider, most periodontal diseases can be prevented. Further, and most important, risk factors for and signs and symptoms of oral cancers have been established and there is an oral cancer screening examination for early detection. The knowledge resulting from scientific studies, however, is superfluous if it is not applied by appropriate lay and professional users. No matter how effective a preventive measure may be, the public cannot benefit if the procedure is unknown and not used appropriately. There are enormous gaps between what we know about preventing oral diseases and what we do.[133] It is now accepted that health promotion influences knowledge and behaviors at all levels of social organization. Health promotion helps bridge the gap between the knowledge generated by scientific studies and its appropriate application.[134]

Over the past 30 years interest in health promotion and disease prevention has increased significantly. At least three factors are responsible for this trend. First, ever-increasing expenditures for health care, most of which pay for the treatment of diseases or conditions, have taken an ever larger proportion of the U.S. gross national product. Second, a growing body of data has confirmed that many chronic diseases result from lifestyles that, theoretically, could be changed, resulting in better health. Third, and very important, a body of scientific literature in health education and promotion has accumulated. Today, health promotion is recognized as a viable approach to preventing diseases and disorders and promoting health. To better understand health promotion, health education must be addressed.

HEALTH EDUCATION

Health education is "any combination of learning experiences designed to facilitate voluntary actions conducive to health."[135] These actions or behaviors may be on the part of individuals, families, institutions, or communities. Thus the scope of health education may include educational interventions for children, parents, policy makers, or health care providers. Education is necessary at all stages of designing, implementing, evaluating, and continuing appropriate oral health programs. Education of all relevant groups is a critical factor in the process to gain acceptance and use of preventive measures, although education alone cannot function as a method to prevent disease. Knowledge is an important aspect of

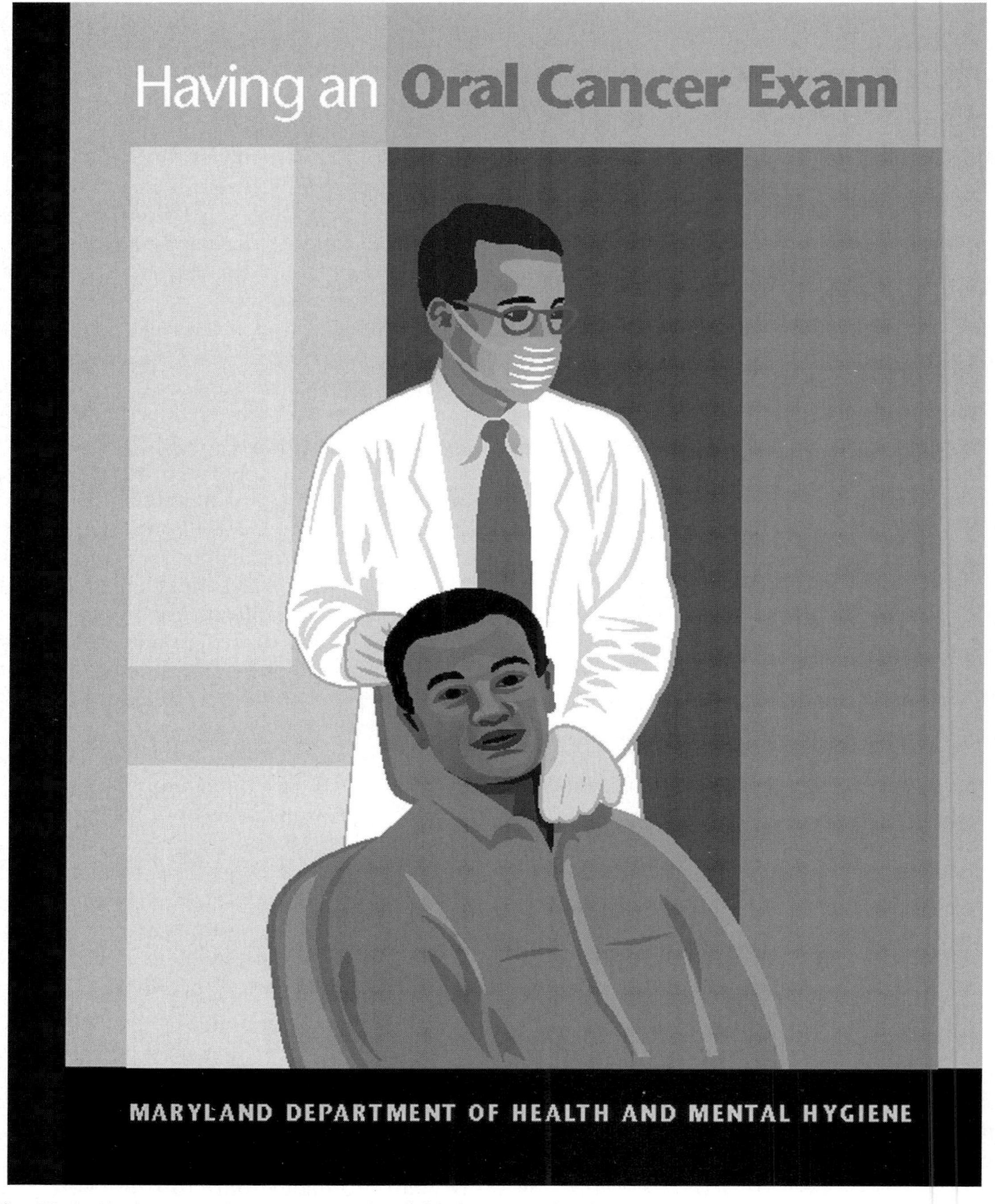

Fig. 10-2. Having an oral cancer exam. (Available from Maryland Department of Health and Mental Hygiene, Office of Oral Health, 201 West Preston St., Baltimore MD 21201.)

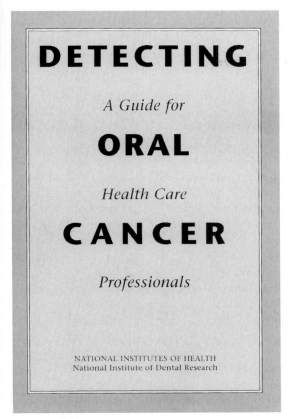

Fig. 10-3. Detecting oral cancer. (Available from the National Oral Health Information Clearinghouse, 1 NOHIC Way, Bethesda, MD 20892-3500.)

empowerment.[134-137] Without appropriate knowledge, individuals can neither make nor be expected to make intelligent decisions about their oral health or, in the case of decision makers, for the oral health of their constituents. Box 10-3 lists content areas that all relevant publics need to know to attain and maintain optimal oral health. Figures 10-2, 10-3, and 10-4 are examples of printed materials that might be used. It must be understood, however, that simply handing out a brochure on water fluoridation or a poster about the evils of tobacco use does not constitute a comprehensive educa-

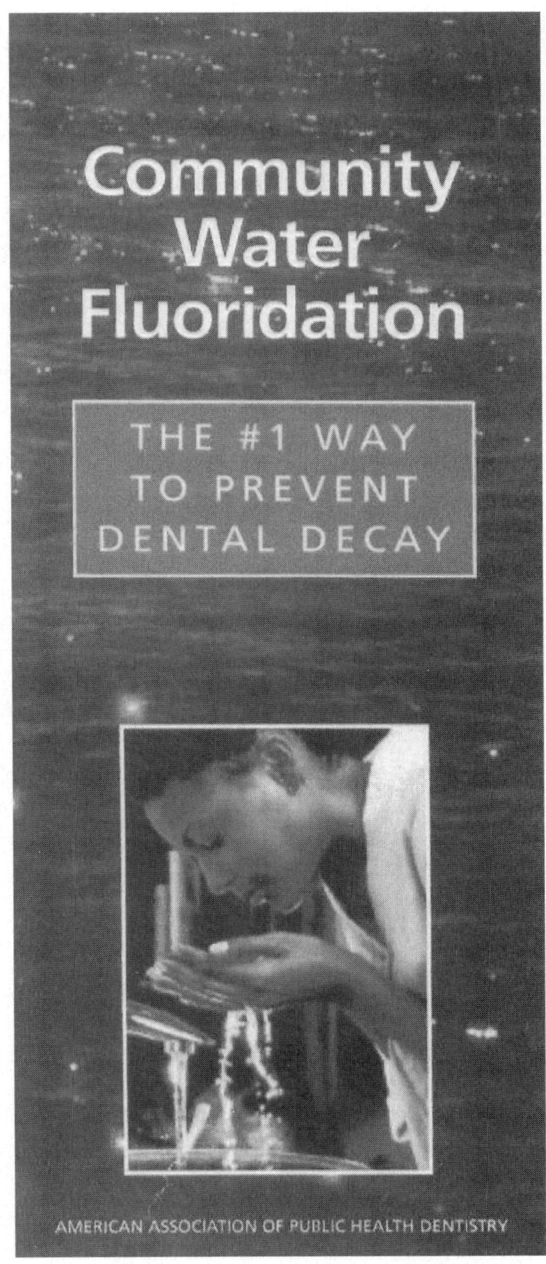

Fig. 10-4. Fluoridation leaflet. (Available from the American Association of Public Health Dentistry, 1224 Center West, Suite 200B, PO Box 7389, Springfield, IL 62791-7389.)

tional program. It is clear that simply having information or knowledge does not automatically mean that appropriate actions or behaviors will follow. Thus education is necessary, but not sufficient, to prevent oral diseases and conditions. However, without such information, the likelihood of taking appropriate actions is severely diminished.

HEALTH LITERACY

Health literacy is the degree to which individuals have the capacity to obtain, process, and understand basic health information and services needed to make appropriate health decisions. Increasing health literacy also is one of the *Healthy People 2010* objectives.[3] Frequently people with the greatest health burdens have the least access to information about their condition, appropriate care, and supporting social services. Increasing health literacy may help decrease health disparities by enabling individuals to know more about their condition and how to navigate the health care system.[138]

HEALTH PROMOTION

Health promotion is "any planned combination of educational, political, regulatory, and organizational supports for actions and conditions of living conducive to the health of individuals, groups or communities."[135] Supports alter a person's environment in a way that will improve health in the absence of individual actions (water fluoridation) or enable the individual to take advantage of preventive procedures by removing barriers to their use. An example is making dental sealants available to children, especially those in low-income groups or in school settings. Health promotion is the process used to transfer research results to appropriate users to improve health.[137]

SUMMARY

Oral diseases are a "neglected epidemic" because they affect almost the total population, with millions of people having new disease each year. By age 17 years 84% of youths have had tooth decay, with an average of eight affected tooth surfaces, and, by age 40 to 44 years, 99% of adults have had tooth decay with an average of 30 affected tooth surfaces. For vulnerable populations, including low-income persons, minorities, the developmentally disabled, the homebound, and those with AIDS, the extent of the problem is even greater. Although approximately $65 billion is spent annually in the United States for dental care, only one of five children receiving Medicaid, or 20%, receive dental care. Unfortunately, oral health is not a priority in this country, and we do not have a national oral disease prevention program.

Prevention of disease, disability, and suffering should be a primary goal of any society that hopes to provide a decent quality of life for its people. Primary prevention is the most effective way to keep people healthy and to control costs because the disease is prevented before it occurs. Secondary prevention treats the disease after it occurs, and tertiary prevention limits or rehabilitates a disability from disease. Prevention on the community or population-based level is the most cost-effective approach and has the greatest impact on a community, whether it is a school, neighborhood, or nation. Community prevention programs should be used only when they have been shown to be effective by well-designed clinical studies. The use of fluorides, the thirteenth most abundant element in the earth's crust, has made a significant impact on preventing caries in the United States.

Community water fluoridation should be the foundation of oral disease prevention and treatment programs. Fluoridation is the most cost-effective prevention measure in dentistry. Water fluoridation at 1 ppm prevented tooth decay by 50% to 70% in the early controlled studies, and now, as a result of the widespread use of fluoridation and other fluoride products in the United States, it prevents caries in primary teeth by 30% to 60% and in mixed dentition by 20% to 40% and 15% to 35% for adolescents and adults, respectively. It also prevents root caries in older adults by up to 35%.

In 2000 more than 162 million Americans, or 65.8% of the 246 million people on public water supplies, had fluoridation, nearly 57.5% of the total population. Approximately 11 million Americans live in communities that are naturally fluoridated at the recommended level. The safety and legality of fluoridation has been well documented since the first controlled studies in 1945. A well-planned educational program for community leaders and decision makers is important to help them understand all the benefits of this public health measure. This education must continue over time. A well-educated community is the best strategy against antifluoridation activities.

School-based fluoride programs are an alternative when community water fluoridation is not available. These programs may include school water fluoridation, dietary fluoride supplements, or fluoride rinses. School dental sealant programs are effective on the occlusal (biting) surfaces of the teeth of children ages 6 to 8 and 12 to 14 years when the first and second molars erupt.

Periodontal disease (gingivitis) prevention programs on a community level have been shown to be effective when supervised, but they are not very practical. Everyone, however, needs to practice proper oral hygiene and have a prophylaxis or mechanical plaque removal periodically.

Unintentional oral-facial injuries may result in broken teeth, facial fractures, concussions, and temporomandibular dysfunction. More than 25 million U.S. children participate in competitive school sports and 20 million in organized sports outside school. Protective headgear and mouthguards have reduced dramatically the number of oral-facial injuries in football. Other sports such as basketball, baseball, wrestling, and soccer should have regulations and promotion for effective head, face, eye, and mouth protection.

Approximately 30,000 Americans are diagnosed with oral cancer each year. More Americans die from oral cancers than from cervical cancer, approximately 8000 persons yearly. Oral cancer has one of the lower 5-year survival rates of the major cancer sites because of late detection. Tobacco and alcohol account for 75% of all oral and pharyngeal cancers. Community-based incentives for policy, legislation, and ordinances to prevent and control tobacco use are important. Dentists, physicians, and other primary care providers can play a significant role in oral cancer prevention and early detection.

Health promotion, which includes health education and health literacy, is pivotal to implementing primary effective community prevention programs. Effective community prevention programs for oral diseases must be the foundation for responding to this neglected epidemic if we are to have a healthy society.

REVIEW QUESTIONS

1. Define an effective community oral prevention program and give three examples.

2. Cite three advantages of an effective community prevention program and describe the major differences between a prevention program on the community versus individual level.
3. How would you define community water fluoridation? Provide three reasons why it is the most cost-effective preventive measure in dentistry.
4. Describe three different school-based prevention programs and give the major advantages and disadvantages of each.
5. Give three examples of how the dental profession may help prevent oral-facial injuries for the public at large.
6. Differentiate health education from health promotion and health literacy and give one example of each.
7. Describe the differences between primary, secondary, and tertiary prevention and give one example of each.

REFERENCES

1. Allukian M: The neglected epidemic and the Surgeon General's Report: a call to action for better oral health, *Am J Public Health* 90:843, 2000 (editorial).
2. National Institute of Dental Research: *Oral health of United States children: the National Survey of Dental Caries in U.S. School Children: 1986-1987,* DHHS pub, NIH 89-2247, Bethesda, MD, 1989, US Department of Health and Human Services.
3. US Department of Health and Human Services: *Healthy People 2010: with understanding and improving health objectives for improving health,* ed 2, 2 vols, Washington, DC, 2000, US Government Printing Office.
4. US Department of Health and Human Services: *Oral health in America: a report of the Surgeon General,* Rockville, MD, 2000, US Department of Health and Human Services, National Institute of Dental and Craniofacial Research, National Institutes of Health.
5. Health Care Financing Administration, Office of Actuary: National health expenditure amounts and average change by type of expenditure: selected calendar years 1980-2010, June 14, 2001. Available at www.hcfa.gov/stats/NHE-Proj/Proj/2000/tables/t2.htm.
6. Office of Inspector General, Children's Dental Services Under Medicaid: *Access and utilization,* OBI-09-93-00240, Washington, DC, 1996, US Department of Health and Human Services.
7. US General Accounting Office: *Oral health factors contributing to low use of dental services by low-income populations,* GAO/HEHS-00-149, 2000, US General Accounting Office.
8. *Webster's new world dictionary of American English,* ed 3, New York, 1993, Prentice Hall/MacMillan.
9. National Institute of Dental Research: *Oral health of United States adults: the National Survey of Oral Health in US Employed Adults and Seniors: 1985-1986,* DHHS pub, NIH 87-2868, Bethesda, MD, 1987, US Department of Health and Human Services.
10. Winn DM et al: Coronal and root caries in the dentition of adults in the United States, 1988-1991, *J Dent Res* 75(spec iss): 642, 1996.
11. Sing KA, Spencer JA, Allister JH: Pre- and posteruption exposure to fluoridated water and caries prevention of permanent teeth in Australian children, *J Public Health Dent* 60:100, 2000 (abstract).
12. Centers for Disease Control and Prevention: Fluoridation of drinking water to prevent dental caries, *MMWR Morb Mortal Wkly Rep* 48:933, 1999.
13. Centers for Disease Control and Prevention: Engineering and administrative recommendations for water fluoridation, *MMWR Morb Mortal Wkly Rep* 44(RR-13):1, 1995.
14. Centers for Disease Control and Prevention: *Fluoridation census: 1992,* Atlanta, 1993, US Public Health Service, US Department of Health and Human Services.
15. Centers for Disease Control and Prevention: Populations receiving optimally fluoridated drinking water—United States, 2000, *MMWR Morb Mortal Wkly Rep* 51(07):144-147, 2002.
16. Reeves TG: Technical aspects of water fluoridation in the United States and an overview of fluoridation engineering worldwide, *Community Dent Health* 13(suppl 2):21, 1996.
17. Easley M: *National Center for Fluoridation Policy and Research, Buffalo, NY,* personal communication, April 4, 2001.
18. *Review of fluoride: benefits and risks,* Washington, DC, 1991, US Public Health Service.
19. Kaminsky LS et al: Fluoride: benefits and risk of exposure, *Crit Rev Oral Biol Med* 1(4):261, 1990.
20. National Research Council: *Health effects of ingested fluoride,* Washington, DC, 1993, National Academy Press.
21. American Dental Association: *Fluoridation facts,* Chicago, 1999, American Dental Association.

22. Institute of Medicine, Food and Nutrition Board: *Dietary reference intakes: calcium, phosphorus, magnesium, vitamin D and fluoride,* 1997, Washington National Academy Press.
23. Wolf CA et al: *Abuse of the scientific literature in an antifluoridation pamphlet,* Baltimore, 1985, American Oral Health Institute.
24. Hunt J et al: Putting Yiamouyannis into perspective, *Br Dent J* 179:121, 1995.
25. Horowitz HS: Why I continue to support community water fluoridation, *J Public Health Dent* 60:67, 2000.
26. Ripa LW: A half-century of community water fluoridation in the United States: review and commentary, *J Public Health Dent* 53:17, 1993.
27. Arnold FA Jr et al: Fifteenth year of Grand Rapids fluoridation study, *J Am Dent Assoc* 65:780, 1962.
28. Hillboe HE et al: Newburg-Kingston caries-fluorine study: final report, *J Am Dent Assoc* 52:290, 1956.
29. Blayney JR, Hill IN: Fluorine and dental caries, *J Am Dent Assoc* 74(spec iss):233, 1967.
30. Brown HK, Poplove M: The Brantford-Sarnia-Stratford fluoridation caries study: final survey, 1963, *Can J Public* Health 56(80):319, 1965.
31. Newbrun E: Effectiveness of water fluoridation, *J Public Health Dent* 49(spec iss):279, 1989.
32. Tsutsui A, Yagi M, Horowitz AM: The prevalence of dental caries and fluorosis in Japanese communities with up to 1.4 ppm of naturally occurring fluoride, *J Public Health Dent* 60:147, 2000.
33. Griffin SO et al: Quantifying the diffused benefit from water fluoridation in the United States, *Community Dent Oral Epidemiol* 29:120, 2001.
34. Burt B: Proceedings of the workshop: Cost-Effectiveness of Caries Prevention in Dental Public Health, *J Public Health Dent* 49(spec iss):250, 1989.
35. Centers for Disease Control and Prevention: Recommendations for using fluoride to prevent and control dental caries in the United States, *MMWR Morb Mortal Wkly Rep* 50(RR-14):1-42, 2001.
36. Centers for Disease Control and Prevention: *Fluoridation census 1989: summary,* Atlanta, 1991, US Public Health Service, US Department of Health and Human Services.
37. Centers for Disease Control and Prevention: Water fluoridation and costs of Medicaid treatment for dental decay: Louisiana, 1995-1996, *MMWR Morb Mortal Wkly Rep* 48:753, 1999.
38. Griffin S, Jones K, Tomar S: An economic evaluation of community water fluoridation, *J Public Health Dent* 61:78, 2001.
39. Centers for Disease Control and Prevention: Public health focus: fluoridation of community water systems, *MMWR Morb Mortal Wkly Rep* 41(2):372, 1992.
40. Lalumandier JA et al: US drinking water: fluoridation knowledge level of water plant operators, *J Public Health Dent* 61:92, 2001.
41. Block LE: Antifluoridationists persist: the constitutional basis for fluoridation, *J Public Health Dent* 46:188, 1986.
42. Neenan ME: Obstacles to extending fluoridation in the United States, *Community Dent Health* 13(suppl 2):10, 1996.
43. American Dental Association, Council on Access, Prevention and Interprofessional Relations: Unpublished data, November 7, 2000, American Dental Association.
44. Gift HC, Corbin SB, Nowjack-Raymer RE: Public knowledge about prevention of dental caries and symptoms of gum disease—1990 NHIS, *Public Health Rep* 109:397, 1990.
45. O'Neill HW: Opinion study comparing attitudes about dental health, *J Am Dent Assoc* 109:910, 1984.
46. Allukian M, Steinhurst J, Dunning JM: Community organization and a regional approach to fluoridation of the greater Boston area, *J Am Dent Assoc* 104:491, 1981.
47. Allukian M, Ackerman J, Steinhurst J: Factors that influence the attitudes of first-term Massachusetts legislators toward fluoridation, *J Am Dent Assoc* 104:494, 1981.
48. Boriskin JM, Fine JI: Fluoridation election victory: a case study for dentistry in effective political action, *J Am Dent Assoc* 102:486, 1981.
49. Easley MW: The new antifluoridationists: who are they and how do they operate? *J Public Health Dent* 45:133, 1985.
50. Smith KG, Christen KA: A fluoridation campaign: the Phoenix experience, *J Public Health Dent* 50:319, 1990.
51. Frazier PJ: Priorities to preserve fluoride uses: rationales and strategies, *J Public Health Dent* 45:149, 1985.
52. Executive summary: application for continued recognition of dental public health as a dental specialty, *J Public Health Dent* 46:35, 1986.
53. Allukian M: Fluoridation—a continual struggle in Massachusetts, *Harvard Dent Alum Bull* 28:77, 1968.
54. Collier DR: The statewide fluoridation program of Tennessee through the voluntary process, *J Am Dent Assoc* 93:837, 1976.
55. Clark DC, Hann HJ: A win for fluoridation in Squamish, British Columbia, *J Public Health Dent* 49:170, 1989.
56. Faine RC et al: The 1980 fluoridation campaigns: a discussion of results, *J Public Health Dent* 41:138, 1981.
57. Jones RB, Mormann DN, Durtsche TB: Fluoridation referendum in La Crosse, Wisconsin: contributing factors to success, *Am J Public Health* 79:1405, 1989.
58. Horowitz AM, Frazier PJ: Promoting the use of fluorides in a community. In Newbrun E, editor: *Fluorides and dental caries,* ed 3, Springfield, IL, 1986, Charles C Thomas.

59. American Dental Association: *Community organization for water fluoridation,* Chicago, 1997, American Dental Association.
60. Oral Health Coordinating Committee: *National fluoride plan to promote oral health,* Washington, DC, 1996, US Department of Health and Human Services, US Public Health Service.
61. Evans AW, Darvell BW: Refining the estimate of the critical period for susceptibility to enamel fluorosis in human maxillary central incisors, *J Public Health Dent* 55:238, 1995.
62. Pendrys DG, Stamm JW: Relationships of total fluoride intake to beneficial effects and enamel fluorosis, *J Dent Res* 69(spec iss):529,1990.
63. Pendrys DG: Risk of enamel fluorosis in nonfluoridated and optimally fluoridated populations: considerations for the dental professional, *J Am Dent Assoc* 131:746, 2000.
64. American Dental Association, Council on Access, Prevention and Interprofessional Relations: Caries diagnosis and risk assessment: a review of preventive strategies and management, *J Am Dent Assoc Spec Suppl* 126:1, 1995.
65. Morone J, Kilbreth E, Langwell K: Health affairs: back to school: a health care strategy for youth, *Project Hope,* 20:122, Jan/Feb 2001.
66. The Center for Health and Health Care in Schools: *1999-2000 survey of school-based health initiatives: number of centers and state-financing,* Washington, DC, July 6, 2000, University. Available at www.healthinschools.org/sbhcs/sbhcs_table.htm.
67. The Robert Wood Johnson Foundation: Caring for kids: expanding dental and mental health services through school-based health centers, July 6, 2001. Available at www.rwjf.org/app/rw_applying_for_a_grant/rw_app_opencfp.jsp.
68. Heifetz SB, Horowitz HS, Brunelle JA: Effect of school water fluoridation on dental caries: results in Seagrove, NC, after 12 years, *J Am Dent Assoc* 106:334, 1983.
69. Horowitz AM, Horowitz HS: School-based fluoride programs: a critique, *J Prev Dent* 6:89, 1980.
70. Stephen KW: Systemic fluorides: drops and tablets, *Caries Res* 27(suppl 1):9, 1993.
71. Driscoll WS et al: Caries-preventive effects of daily and weekly fluoride mouthrinsing in a fluoridated community: final results after 30 months, *J Am Dent Assoc* 105:1010, 1982.
72. Ripa LW: Sealants revisited: an update of the effectiveness of pit-and-fissure sealants, *Caries Res* 27(suppl 1):367, 1993.
73. Selwitz RH et al: The prevalence of dental sealants in the US population: findings from NHANES III, 1988-91, *J Dent Res* 75(spec iss):652, 1996.
74. Mertz-Fairhurst EJ: Pit-and-fissure sealants: a global lack of science transfer, *J Dent Res* 71:1543, 1992 (guest editorial).
75. Centers for Disease Control and Prevention: Impact of targeted, school-based dental sealant programs in reducing racial and economic disparities in sealant prevalence among schoolchildren—Ohio, 1998-1999, *MMWR Morb Mortal Wkly Rep* 50:736, 2001.
76. Kunzel W: Systemic use of fluoride and other methods: salt, sugar, milk, etc., *Caries Res* 27(suppl 1):16, 1993.
77. Pan American Health Organization: *Final Report to the W. K. Kellogg Foundation, project #43225. Multi-year plan for salt fluoridation programs in the region of the Americas,* Washington, DC, 2000, Pan American Health Organization, World Health Organization.
78. Marthaler TM et al: DMF teeth in school children after 18 years of collective salt fluoridation, *Caries Res* 23:428, 1989.
79. Estupinan-Day SR et al: Salt fluoridation and dental caries in Jamaica, *Community Dent Oral Epidemiol* 29:247, 2001.
80. Seppa L: Studies of fluoride varnishes in Finland, *Proc Finn Dent Soc* 87:541, 1991.
81. Clark DC et al: Results of a 32-month fluoride varnish study in Sherbrooke and La-Megantic, Canada, *J Am Dent Assoc* 111:949, 1985.
82. Horowitz HS, Ismail AI: Topical fluorides in caries prevention. In Fejereskov O, Ekstrand J, Burt BA, editors: *Fluoride in dentistry,* ed 2, Copenhagen, 1996, Munksgaard.
83. Mandel ID: Fluoride varnishes—a welcome addition, *J Public Health Dent* 54:67, 1994.
84. Beltran-Aguilar ED, Goldstein JW, Lockwood SA: Fluoride varnishes: a review of their clinical use, cariostatic mechanism, efficacy and safety, *J Am Dent Assoc* 131:589, 2000.
85. Anusavice KJ: Treatment regimens in preventive and restorative dentistry, *J Am Dent Assoc* 126:727, 1995.
86. Proceedings of the IADR symposium minimal intervention technique for dental caries, *J Public Health Dent* 56:129, 1996.
87. Frencken JE, Holmgren J: *Atraumatic restorative treatment (ART) for dental caries,* Nijmegen, 1999, Benda Drukkers.
88. Frandsen A: Mechanical oral hygiene practices. In Loe H, Kleinman DV, editors: *Dental plaque control measures and oral hygiene practices,* Washington, DC, 1986, IRL Press.
89. Mandel ID: Antimicrobial mouthrinses: overview and update, *J Am Dent Assoc* 125:2-S, 1994.
90. Horowitz AM et al: Effects of supervised daily dental plaque removal by children after 3 years, *Oral Epidemiol Commun Dent* 8:171, 1980.

91. Chen MS: Oral health of disadvantaged populations. In Cohen LK, Gift HC, editors: *Disease prevention and oral health promotion,* Copenhagen, 1995, Munksgaard.
92. Bolden AJ, Henry JL, Allukian M: Implications of access, utilization and need for oral health care by low income groups and minorities on the dental delivery system, *J Dent Educ* 57: 888, 1993.
93. Allukian M: Oral health—an essential service for the homeless, *J Public Health Dent* 55:8, 1995 (editorial).
94. Mouradian WE, Wehr E, Crall JJ: Disparities in children's oral health and access to dental care, *JAMA* 284:2625, 2000.
95. Heller KH et al: Longitudinal evaluation of sealing molars with and without incipient dental caries in a public health program, *J Public Health Dent* 55:148, 1995.
96. Nowjack-Raynor RE, Gift HC: Use of mouthguards and headgear in organized sports by school-aged children, *Public Health Rep* 111:82, 1996.
97. Kaste LM et al: Prevalence of incisor trauma in persons 6 to 50 years of age: United States, 1966-1991, *J Dent Res* 75(spec iss):696, 1996.
98. Becker DB, Needleman HL, Kotelchuck M: Child abuse and dentistry: oral facial trauma and its recognition by dentists, *J Am Dent Assoc* 97:24, 1978.
99. National Safe Kids Campaign: *Sports injury fact sheet,* Washington, DC, 1996.
100. Lephart SM, Fu FH: Emergency treatment of athletic injuries, *Dent Clin North Am* 35:707, 1991.
101. Meadow D, Lidner G, Needleman H: Oral trauma in children, *Pediatr Dent* 6:248, 1984.
102. National Injury Information Clearinghouse: *Estimates for sports injuries,* Washington, DC, 1995, US Consumer Project Safety Commission.
103. Hart PD, Research Associates: *Get into the game: a national survey of parents' knowledge, attitudes and self-reported behaviors concerning sports safety,* executive summary, conducted for the National Safe Kids Campaign and the National Athletes Trainers' Association Research and Education Foundation, March 2000.
104. Heintz WD: Mouth protection: a progress report, report of councils and bureaus, *J Am Dent Assoc* 77:632, 1968.
105. Ranalli DN, Lancaster DM: Attitudes of college football officials regarding NCAA mouthguard regulations and player compliance, *J Public Health Dent* 53:96, 1993.
106. Maestrello-deMoya MG, Primosch RE: Orofacial trauma mouth protector wear among high school varsity basketball players, *J Dent Child* 56(1):33, 1989.
107. McNutt T et al: Oral trauma in adolescent athletes: a study of mouth protectors, *Pediatr Dent* 11:209, 1989.
108. Kvittem B et al: Incidence of orofacial injuries in high school sports, *J Public Health Dent* 58:288, 1998.
109. Soporowski NJ, Tesini DA, Weiss AI: Survey of oralfacial sports-related injuries, *J Mass Dent Soc* 43:16, 1994.
110. Elliott MA: Professional responsibility in sports dentistry, *Dent Clin North Am* 35(4):831, 1991.
111. Ranalli DR, Lancaster DM: Attitudes of college football coaches regarding NCAA mouthguard regulation and player compliance, *J Public Health Dent* 55:139, 1995.
112. Winters JE: Sports dentistry: the profession's role in athletics, *J Am Dent Assoc* 127:810, 1996.
113. Jemal A et al: Cancer statistics, 2002, *CA Cancer J Clin* 52:23-47, 2002.
114. Silverman S Jr, Shillitoe EJ: Etiology and predisposing factors. In Silverman S Jr, editor: *Oral cancer,* ed 4, Atlanta, 1998, American Cancer Society.
115. Murphy GP, Lawrence W Jr, Lenhard RE Jr, editors: *Textbook of clinical oncology,* ed 2, Atlanta, 1995, American Cancer Society.
116. Mecklenburg RE et al: *Tobacco effects in the mouth: a National Cancer Institute and National Institute of Dental Research guide for health professionals,* NIH pub no 92-3330, Bethesda, MD, 1992, National Cancer Institute, US Department of Health and Human Services, US Public Health Service.
117. Potter JD et al: *Food, nutrition and the prevention of cancer: a global perspective,* Washington, DC, 1997, World Cancer Research Fund; American Institute of Cancer Research.
118. Fouret P et al: Human papillomavirus in head and neck squamous cell carcinomas in nonsmokers, *Arch Otolaryngol Head Neck Surg* 123:513, 1997.
119. Zhang Z et al: Marijuana use and increased risk of squamous cell carcinoma of the head and neck, *Cancer Epidemiol Biomarkers Prev* 8:1071, 1999.
120. Horowitz AM, Nourjah P, Gift HG: US adult knowledge of risk factors for and signs of oral cancers: 1990, *J Am Dent Assoc* 126:39, 1995.
121. Horowitz AM, Nourjah PA: Factors associated with having oral cancer examinations among US adults 40 years of age or older, *J Public Health Dent* 56:333, 1996.
122. Horowitz AM et al: Maryland adults' knowledge of oral cancer and having oral cancer examinations, *J Public Health Dent* 58:281, 1998.
123. Horowitz AM et al: Oral pharyngeal cancer prevention and early detection: dentists' opinions and practices, *J Am Dent Assoc* 131:453, 2000.
124. Yellowitz JA et al: Survey of U.S. dentists' knowledge and opinions about oral pharyngeal cancer, *Am J Dent Assoc* 131:653, 2000.
125. Syme SE, Drury TF, Horowitz AM: Maryland dental hygienists' assessment of patients' risk behaviors for oral cancer, *J Dent Hygiene* 75:25, 2001.

126. Siriphant P et al: Oral cancer knowledge and opinions among Maryland nurse practitioners, *J Public Health Dent* 61:138, 2001.
127. Canto MT et al: Maryland physicians' knowledge, opinions and practices about oral cancer, *Oral Oncology* (in press).
128. Yellowitz JA et al: Assessment of alcohol and tobacco use in dental schools health history forms, *J Dent Educ* 59:1091, 1995.
129. Horowitz AM et al: The need for health promotion in oral cancer prevention and early detection, *J Public Health Dent* 56:319, 1996.
130. Centers for Disease Control and Prevention: *Proceedings: National Strategic Planning Conference for the Prevention and Control of Oral and Pharyngeal Cancer, August 7-9, 1996, Atlanta,* Bethesda, MD, 1997, Centers for Disease Control and Prevention.
131. Alfano MC, Horowitz AM: Professional and community efforts to prevent morbidity and mortality from oral cancer, *J Am Dent Assoc* 132:245s, 2001.
132. US Department of Health and Human Services: *Reducing tobacco use: a report of the Surgeon General,* Atlanta, 2000, US Department of Health and Human Services, Centers for Disease Control and Prevention, National Center for Chronic Disease Prevention and Health Promotion, Office on Smoking and Health.
133. Horowitz AM: The public's oral health: the gaps between what we know and what we do, *Adv Dent Science* 9:91, 1995.
134. Frazier PJ, Horowitz AM: Prevention: a public health perspective. In Cohen LK, Gift HC, editors: *Disease prevention and oral health promotion,* Copenhagen, 1995, Munksgaard.
135. Green LW, Kreuter MW: *Health promotion planning: an educational and environmental approach,* ed 3, Mountain View, CA, 1999, Mayfield.
136. Glanz K, Lewis FM, Rimer BK, editors: *Health behavior and health education theory research and practice,* San Francisco, 1990, Jossey-Bass.
137. Frazier PJ, Horowitz AM: Oral health education and promotion in maternal and child health: a position paper, *J Public Health Dent* 50:390, 1990.
138. Seiden CR et al, editors: *Health literacy, January 1990 through 1999,* NLM pub no CBM 2000-1, Bethesda, MD, 2000, National Library of Medicine.

CHAPTER

11

ORAL HEALTH EDUCATION AND HEALTH PROMOTION

Nancy R. Kressin • Marianne B. De Souza

WHY IS ORAL HEALTH EDUCATION STILL IMPORTANT?

Results from a survey of the nation's oral health indicate that, although caries rates have decreased in recent years, 45% of children and adolescents still have evidence of the disease.[1] Another survey also found that 10% of adults are completely edentulous, and only one third have all 28 teeth.[2] Periodontal disease indicators showed that one third of individuals 25 to 34 years old had moderate attachment loss, as did 63% of 45- to 54-year-olds and 80% of people more than 65 years old. More severe periodontal disease was found in 15% of those surveyed.[3] These data indicate that oral disease remains a public health problem for Americans; one way this problem can be addressed is through oral health education.

Although the American Dental Association (ADA) recommends that individuals brush and floss their teeth twice a day in addition to having regular dental examinations, research suggests that many individuals do not adhere to this recommendation.[4] In a survey of Detroit-area residents, Lang, Ronis, and Farghaly[5] found that although more than 96% of the individuals surveyed did brush at least once a day, only 84% demonstrated adherence to their definition of "acceptable" brushing technique (e.g., brushing all teeth, including those that do not show when smiling). In the same study only 33% of individuals reported flossing daily, and only 22% demonstrated "acceptable" flossing technique (e.g., flossing all teeth). Because these data suggest a need for improvement in individuals' oral self-care, the need for effective oral health education remains clear.

WHAT IS ORAL HEALTH EDUCATION?

Oral health education for the community is a process that informs, motivates, and helps persons to adopt and maintain health practices and lifestyles; advocates environmental changes as needed to facilitate this goal; and conducts professional training and research to the same end.*[6-10] Health education is any combination of learning opportunities designed to facilitate voluntary adaptations of behavior that are conducive to health.[11] Health education programs are not isolated events but educational aspects of any curative, preventive, or promotional health activity. Comprehension of the multifactorial variables in dental disease and their interaction has increased the emphasis now placed on the educational process to assist in achieving desired health outcomes.

It has been well documented in dentistry and other health areas that correct health information or knowledge alone does not necessarily lead to desirable health behaviors.[12] However, knowledge gained may serve as a tool to empower population groups with accurate information about health and health care technologies, enabling them to take action to protect their health.[13] Both internal and external variables influence whether an individual or community will comply with recommended disease prevention, health maintenance, or health promotion procedures. Health promotion is any combination of educational, organizational, economic, political, and environmental supports for behavior conducive to health.[11] Health promotion refers to actions that are intended either to alter the living environment of persons to improve their health (e.g., community water fluoridation) or to enable and empower individuals to take advantage of preventive procedures or services by reducing or eliminating access barriers. Other actions might include making available—or removing financial barriers to—procedures such as the appropriate use of fluoride supplements, use of dental sealants, supervised removal of dental plaque, and effective referral and follow-up services for individuals who need treatment.[14] Education and promotion are intertwined to achieve long-term improved health for all populations within American society.

*Modified from the definition of consumer health education adopted by the 1975 National Institutes of Health Fogarty International Center and American College of Preventive Medicine Task Force on Consumer Health Education.

Procedures implemented through promotion can prevent a given disease or condition, but only education can foster informed decision making and maintenance of needed programs, services, or behaviors. Health education and promotion processes permeate all levels of individuals and groups and may include working with patients, parents, legislators, industry, and all other levels of influential policy makers, including health care providers.[14]

The oral health educator must be cognizant of available resources and demographic changes affecting social, economic, and health services environments. In addition, the educator must weigh internal and external variables in relation to clinical and behavioral research findings when designing a community program that will be effective in achieving long-term results.

Knowledge of program planning and community organization is essential, and skill development in these areas warrants inclusion in the professional preparation of the dentist and dental hygienist. To date, however, development of these skills has received little attention. The ADA and the American Dental Hygienists' Association (ADHA) have responded to the expanding role of the dentist and the dental hygienist as health educators in the clinical practice setting and in the community by developing a variety of educational resources. Professional development products include guides, brochures, posters, flyers, and videos, many of which are available in English and Spanish for individual or group education during community presentations. ADA publications, such as *Materials You Need for Your Effective Practice,* have historically covered a wide variety of educational topics, including Educating Patients, Managing Your Practice, Controlling Infection, Posters and Plaques, and Videos That Teach.[15] The ADA has developed a new two-part teaching guide called "Smile Magic" with lesson plans, activities, and activity sheets for preschool to grade 2 and grades 3 through 5. The ADA also offers a National Children's Dental Health Month Planning Guide, starter kit, and supplemental materials to promote a successful annual February observance.[15] The ADA website (www.ada.org) includes detailed information on these educational activities and provides a variety of online educational resources for children, parents, teachers, and those engaging in public speaking about dentistry.

The ADHA has developed continuing education programs and other professional development products that present the latest in theories and techniques intrinsic to successful dental hygiene practice. The ADHA also offers an array of practical guides for helping career-minded individuals and active program planners achieve success in community outreach programs and public relations and legislative action skill development.[16] At the ADHA website (www.adha.org), additional information about current professional products for patient or consumer information is available, as well as oral health educational information for individuals of all ages.

Most professional training revolves around learning specific technical procedures and working with patients on a one-to-one basis. In this situation individual patient motivation is the primary objective of oral health education and unfortunately constitutes only a small component of the overall treatment plan.[15] Ideally, the dentist's or hygienist's relationship with the patient allows the dental practitioner to tailor the preventive prescription to each individual patient's needs, and patients can identify their own short- and long-term oral health goals. Through this process the dental professional is able to help those patients amenable to prevention to internalize the value of good oral health and to practice preventive measures. However, Chambers[6] has concluded that strong evidence suggests that only a limited number of Americans are amenable to an at-home program of controlling plaque. A principal factor suppressing this number is that habits of healthy living are not supported by deep-seated cultural values. The role of the health educator becomes an essential component in the management of dental disease and in helping patients assume responsibility for their own oral health maintenance.

In most cases the same skills that were developed in working with patients on a one-to-one basis are carried over to the community setting. As a result, community oral health programs are usually conducted in much the same manner as individual patient education. Specific educational efforts focus on presenting oral health information and on trying to change an individual's attitudes and behaviors with regard to oral hygiene habits and diet rather than on emphasizing an organized community approach to prevention and control of disease. Emphasis is placed on correct brushing and flossing techniques to help prevent, or at least control, periodontal disease and on nutritional counseling, sealants, and fluoride therapy for caries control, use of mouth guards in contact sports, emergency management of the avulsed tooth, and antismoking and anti–smokeless-tobacco education.

Success of these primary health promotion endeavors relies on the individual's development of specific skills and their incorporation into the person's lifestyle to reduce the prevalence of caries, periodontal disease, oral injuries, and oral cancer. Although popular, when it is used alone, this approach to disease prevention has had limited success in reducing oral disease and may not be an appropriate focus for public health education.[14,17-19] Behavioral theories applicable on an individual level may not be directly transferable to solving group- and community-level health problems; theories of public health and epidemiology may be more relevant for societal change.[13,20] In each case the health educator needs to choose the framework most appropriate for addressing the problem.[21] Given Winslow's definition of dental public health—the science and art of preventing and controlling dental disease and promoting oral health through organized community efforts—an alternative approach focusing on individual behavior change would be to target health education efforts to community leaders, as suggested by Frazier.[22] This approach would redirect the educational processes to the selection of prevention and control programs that operate at the community level and do not require daily compliance on the part of the individual. Further, Frazier and Horowitz[13] suggest that focusing health education and promotion efforts on a broader range of children and parents has a positive potential for a major impact on the oral health of future generations of families in different socioeconomic groups. All parents and infant caretakers—whether male or female, young or old—need to know how to prevent oral diseases. By imparting that knowledge to the children in their care and by reinforcing good daily oral health habits, the oral health of future generations could improve dramatically. School-based health education and promotion activities are viable ways of reinforcing healthy behaviors.

The purpose of this chapter is to present an overview of the current issues and concepts in oral health education and to discuss the transition in educational activities from the traditional approach to current and suggested approaches. By examining continuing community programs and examples of other organized community efforts, the student should be able to determine which program goals are appropriate for public health education and possible ways to accomplish those goals. Areas of recent and recommended educational research are highlighted. We hope that previously held beliefs will be challenged and that the extent, complexity, and importance of community oral health education will be better understood.

Key Issues in Oral Health Education

Although much progress has been made in the status of the nation's oral health through oral health education efforts in the past, a number of important dental public health problems remain, and existing programs can benefit from giving special consideration to the unique needs of a variety of populations that may need such education. Many issues still need to be addressed by future oral health education efforts. A few of these are mentioned here to provide the reader with a general understanding of the types of problems that future oral health education should address.

WATER FLUORIDATION

The appropriate use of fluorides is the best method available to prevent the onset of dental caries. Interventions that used fluoride have been successful in preventing dental caries, averting pain and discomfort, and saving money. Water fluoridation serves as the cornerstone for community oral disease prevention and is the most cost-effective method to provide protection against dental caries for people of all ages.[23,24] As stated in the *Surgeon General's Report on Oral Health in America:* "Community water fluoridation is an effective, safe and ideal public health measure that benefits individuals of all ages and socioeconomic strata."[25] Approximately 300 million people in more than 40 countries worldwide consume fluoridated water. Water fluoridation costs between $.68 and $3.00 per person per year.[25] Yet in the United States only 145 million people, or 62% of the population on community water supplies, are receiving this preventive measure. Approximately 100 million Americans (38% of those on public water systems) currently do not have access to drinking water with optimum levels of fluoride to protect their teeth. The Centers for Disease Control and Prevention (CDC) is collaborating with state and local health departments and water districts to address this issue.[25,26] It is a challenge for all health care providers to reach the entire population with preventive interventions at the community level. Oral health educational efforts are needed to continue to inform community residents and legislators about the beneficial effects of fluoridation.

ORAL SELF-CARE BEHAVIORS

Oral self-care behaviors by individuals are still not at recommended levels.[5,27] Educational efforts aimed at individuals and communities are still needed to increase the prevalence of such behaviors to improve their oral health status. Research is necessary to assess proposed theoretic models promoting oral self-care behaviors to determine if they are evidence based and appropriate for broad application. New theoretic models for study have been developed.[28,29]

ORAL SCREENING AND RISK FACTORS FOR ORAL CANCER

The American Cancer Society (www.cancer.org) reports that the incidence of and mortality rates resulting from cancers of the oral pharynx and oral cavity are sobering and fortify the need for routine oral cancer screenings at each dental visit. In the United States, 30,200 people were diagnosed with oral cancers, and 7800 deaths were attributed to these cancers, in 2000. Oral cancers are more common than leukemia, melanoma, and cancers of the brain, liver, kidney, thyroid, stomach, ovary, or cervix. Possible sites include the tongue, lips, floor of the mouth, soft palate, tonsils, salivary glands, and nasopharynx.[30] Risk factors include use of tobacco products and alcohol, exposure to the sun (lip cancer), dietary factors, and exposure to carcinogens in the workplace.[31] Use of tobacco products has also been identified as a major risk factor for periodontal diseases relative to increased susceptibility, onset in young adults, severity and extent of disease, disease progression, and treatment failure.[32] According to the American Cancer Society, 70% of adults who have smoked began before age 18 years.[30] To reduce mortality rates from, and increase early detection of, oral cancers in accordance with the *Healthy People 2010* initiative, oral care providers should ask patients about lifestyles and risk-taking behaviors and conduct screening examinations for oral cancer. Resources are available to assist health professionals in improving the health of their patients and students by implementing smoking and tobacco education, prevention, and cessation programs in their practices and in the school curriculum.[33,34] The Internet provides wide access to current information and resources, which benefits professionals and laypersons alike. Websites are frequently linked to other sites for expanded searches. The American Cancer Society currently has three websites offering smoking cessation information and resources: www.trystop.org, www.quitnet.org, and www.cancer.org. With funds from the National Tobacco Settlement being dispersed to 22 states in the United States, many state health departments are benefiting from an infusion of needed funds, which may be used to develop comprehensive tobacco prevention, education, and treatment programs, media campaigns, and policy development and regulatory enforcement activities to reduce youth access to tobacco products and limit public exposure to secondhand smoke. The Massachusetts Tobacco Control Program has successfully developed such a statewide network using funds primarily generated in response to a voter referendum in 1992 to increase state excise taxes on tobacco products. Some funding from the settlement is also helping to fuel this ongoing initiative. In 2000 the U.S. Department of Health and Human Services updated the Public Health Service–sponsored *Clinical Practice Guideline—Treating Tobacco Use and Dependence,* incorporating new and effective clinical treatments, as well as a "quick reference guide" for clinicians.[35,36]

Several health organizations have taken action to institute tobacco control programs and recommendations. In 1995 the ADA established a new clinical service code, number 01320, "Tobacco counseling for the control and prevention of dental disease." The Institute of Medicine took action to protect children and youth by adopting policy recommendations for communities, states, and the federal government.[33]

Tobacco use remains at epidemic levels, and young people still begin to smoke and use smokeless tobacco at alarming rates.[37] Oral health education efforts by dental care practitioners, other health care professionals of all types, classroom teachers, and community health educators can help decrease these trends by emphasizing how tobacco causes oral disease and many physical health problems. Fried[38] suggests that "interventions with adolescent girls may prevent initiation and habituation of tobacco use." Children learn by what they see and how they live. Parents, caregivers, and health professionals who maintain healthy, tobacco-free lifestyles set an example that youngsters may choose to follow despite peer pressure to do otherwise.

EARLY CHILDHOOD CARIES

Early childhood caries (sometimes referred to as nursing or baby-bottle caries) is a growing problem in the United States, increasingly affecting affluent members of the population in addition to the racial and linguistic minority groups that have previously been known to be affected.[39] Oral health education efforts must be targeted to a wide range of the population, pediatric and family practice physicians, pediatric nurse practitioners, nurses, physician's assistants, parents, and caregivers so that a broad-based understanding of the causes, effects, and methods of preventing this devastating condition can be effectively communicated.

ORAL HEALTH EFFECTS OF ANOREXIA NERVOSA AND BULIMIA

The oral health effects of anorexia nervosa and bulimia may assist in the clinical diagnosis of these disorders. Health care professionals need to be aware of the oral manifestations so that they can make appropriate referrals for dental treatment. These are serious psychologic disorders that may lead to death as a result of physical complications or suicide. The National Association for Anorexia Nervosa and Associated Disorders reports that at least 8 million people in the United States suffer from eating disorders that last from 1 to 15 years. Only half of those diagnosed with long-term disorders are ever cured.[40]

Dental professionals may play a significant role in identifying patients with eating disorders on the basis of specific oral symptoms (enamel erosion, caries, periodontal disease, changes in the oral mucosa [i.e., contusions or lacerations of the soft palate associated with induced vomiting], dehydration, erythema, angular cheilitis, and swollen salivary glands).[41,42] It is the responsibility of dental professionals to be familiar with the diagnostic criteria for eating disorders. Providing appropriate treatment in a supportive environment, information, and referrals for psychologic and medical help and follow-up could save a life.

ORAL HEALTH EFFECTS OF HUMAN IMMUNODEFICIENCY VIRUS/ACQUIRED IMMUNODEFICIENCY SYNDROME

The oral health effects of human immunodeficiency virus (HIV) and acquired immunodeficiency syndrome (AIDS) need to be recognized and addressed by health care professionals. Oral health educators should play a part in communicating information about the effects of the disease on oral health. Dental professionals, especially dental hygienists, should be familiar with the primary manifestations of HIV and AIDS: candidiasis (thrush), hairy leukoplakia, recurrent aphthous ulcers and herpetic lesions, Kaposi's sarcoma, linear gingival erythema (formerly HIV-G), and HIV periodontitis.[43] The initial diagnosis of AIDS or HIV may be made on the basis of oral lesions and symptoms.[43] Although there is no documentation of HIV transmission from patient to dental care providers or from patient to patient, providers struggle with fears of HIV transmission. Passage of the Americans with Disabilities Act in 1990 has led to a number of lawsuits against dentists for refusal to treat patients with HIV. Federal courts have ruled consistently that people with HIV can be treated safely in private dental offices.[44] Ideally, the hygienist and the dentist are members of a comprehensive care team working closely with the patient's physician in the medical and support group caring for people with AIDS. These issues are discussed in greater detail in Chapters 9 and 10.

CULTURAL ISSUES INHERENT IN ORAL HEALTH EDUCATION

Because oral health education must take place within a cultural context, sensitivity to cultural issues may increase the efficacy of such efforts. Oral self-care practices, attitudes, and knowledge vary across cultural groups, and these differences are important to understand before educational interventions are designed.[45] For example, if a particular cultural group has a fatalistic view that says that health cannot be influenced by any actions taken by the individual, the suggestion to brush or floss the teeth to improve oral health might go against this deeply held cultural assumption. Kiyak[46] has suggested that several general factors may affect a particular group's health care practices, including "cultural values, the socioeconomic status of a given ethnic group, language differences, misinterpretations of verbal and behavioral cues in the health care encounter, and the previous medical experiences of a given ethnic group."

An important thing to recognize is that socioeconomic status is frequently intertwined with racial and cultural factors. In the United States members of racial minority groups frequently have lower incomes and less education than whites do. Although these socioeconomic differences are associated with different racial groups, it is important to understand that the effects of race are not the same as the effects of socioeconomic factors. For example, a recent study comparing oral self-care behaviors of African-Americans and whites found significant differences in the frequency of dental visits of the two racial groups, but when socioeconomic status was taken into account, these differences were reduced.[47] Additional information concerning cultural issues is presented in Chapter 5.

ORAL HEALTH EDUCATION FOR OLDER ADULTS

The importance of preventive oral self-care behaviors may increase in later life with the advent of age-related comorbidities or medication usage that affects oral health (causing, for example, xerostomia and root caries). Negative changes in oral health may result in inadequate dentition, potentially leading to nutritional deficits, speech problems, or threats to social interaction because of related functional impairments or cosmetic factors. Given the declines in physical health and activities that some elderly people face, activities involving the oral cavity (e.g., eating, talking) may assume increased importance at this stage of life. The maintenance or preservation of oral health may therefore be more important in late life than at any other life stage. Thus the promotion of oral self-care behaviors and the assurance of their performance by elders are key issues in gerontologic health and must be addressed by oral health educators (see Chapter 6 for more detailed information about the dental needs of older adults).

ORAL HEALTH EDUCATION FOR SPECIAL NEEDS POPULATIONS

With more than 53 million U.S. citizens physically or mentally impaired, dental professionals need the training to meet the challenge of accommodating and appropriately treating the special needs of patients with or without disabilities. Since the Americans with Disabilities Act was signed into law in 1990, many dental offices have been structurally modified to accommodate the disabled, yet little has been done to understand the psychologic needs of special patients. By eliminating discrimination against those with disabilities and impairments, standards of performance have been established that dental professionals may not be adequately trained to meet. The Americans with Disabilities Act affects our employment, the architectural design of our workplace, and the delivery of dental services. Casamassimo[48] notes that more disabled people are seeking care and that this trend is likely to continue as the population ages and as health care reforms bring capitation, portability of benefits, and extended coverage to many more people. Many people in this segment of the population continue to experience difficulty in accessing dental services. For many, the attainment of adequate oral hygiene is difficult or impossible unless a caregiver is available to assist in daily care for the prevention of oral disease, especially among individuals with mild mental retardation who may lack adequate supervision. Preventive methods are available to meet the unique requirements of the person with special needs and may include the use of adaptive aids and chemotherapeutic agents that eliminate or control microbial organisms associated with caries, gingivitis, and periodontal and other oral diseases. These measures are particularly suited for persons for whom the usual mechanical hygiene procedures of brushing and flossing present difficulties. The oral health care of special patients is intimately linked with medicine and the larger health care delivery system. Appropriate oral care is an integral part of maintaining the health and well-being of people with disabilities.

Under the leadership of dental professionals, effective oral care programs in the many special care settings in which persons with disabilities are situated can be instituted with innovative approaches to staffing and the delegation of oral care tasks. Steifel[49] states that "for no other group is the achievement of good oral health as important as for those with severe disability." For many, the mouth takes on critical importance in terms of psychologic significance and physical function; it may be the only part of the body over which the individual retains voluntary control. In the event that the dentition is lost, the disabled person may be unable to wear a denture to aid in eating or to assist in verbal or device-activated communication. Also, the disabled person may often face negative consequences in appearance, self-esteem, social acceptability, and employability. In addition, dental disease and its consequences can place the individual at serious medical risk. A comprehensive team approach that includes a continuing program of education involving patients and their families, allied health professionals and direct care staff, administrators, and dental practitioners is necessary to improve the oral health of persons with disabilities. The National Institute of Dental and Craniofacial Research, one of the National Institutes of Health, maintains the National Oral Health Information Clearinghouse (NOHIC) as a resource that focuses on the oral health concerns of special care patients. Readers are encouraged to contact NOHIC at (301)402-7364 (voice), (301)656-7581 (TTY), or via e-mail at nohic@nidcr.nih.gov.

DOMESTIC VIOLENCE IDENTIFICATION AND REFERRAL

An ethical obligation of oral care providers is domestic violence identification and referral, a situation that may be difficult for some providers to encounter. Domestic violence has been called a "horrifying epidemic" and declared a "public emergency" that occurs more often than any other crime.[50] Domestic violence or violence in the family unit, with women and children as primary victims, is a major public health problem and is a worldwide epidemic. Domestic violence threatens the lives of millions of people each year, crossing all ethnic, racial, sexual orientation, religious, and socioeconomic lines. It is estimated that 90% to 95% of domestic violence victims in heterosexual relationships are women, according to www.drkoop.com/Wellness/Domestic Violence. In January 1992 the Joint Commission on Accreditation of Healthcare Organizations (JCAHO) required all nationally accredited hospital emergency departments and ambulatory care facilities to implement a protocol to identify, treat, and refer victims of domestic violence to appropriate services.[51] In 1995 President Clinton introduced the Violence Against Women Act to prevent domestic violence and assist victims. Oral care providers should become familiar with the physical signs of domestic violence, especially because 68% of battered women's injuries involve the face, 45% the eyes, and 12% the neck.[52] Dental professionals have an ethical duty to learn to recognize evidence of domestic violence or sexual assault. It is also important to be aware of the possibility of child or elder abuse. When abuse is suspected, skills in counseling and referral are necessary. For dental care providers to obtain such skills, there is a need to expand the educational curricula and continuing education to include strategies for dental professionals to address issues of family violence. Readers are encouraged to review the list of domestic violence national information centers and the suggested readings compiled by Gibson-Howell.[53]

Basic Concepts of Oral Health Education

The content and method of health education are derived from the fields of medicine and public health and from the physical, biologic, social, and behavioral sciences. Certain concepts and theories developed in these fields have influenced the efforts and practices of health educators. In the area of oral health education, many of the proven theories of behavioral scientists have been neglected, forgotten, or unaccepted. Given that the goal of oral health education is the prevention and control of dental disease, organized efforts aimed at achieving this goal should adhere to the proven theories and concepts relevant to health education activities. Current theories of health education that research has proven to be effective are reviewed so that future dental education efforts can incorporate them.

Research has shown that a fundamental error in many oral health education activities is the assumption that increasing a patient's oral health knowledge will help change dental care behavior. This approach, based on a solely cognitive model, assumes the following sequence:

Knowledge → Attitude → Behavior change

If this relationship were true, every oral health education program that increased the participants' level of dental knowledge would have resulted in a behavioral change that improved the oral health status over a long period of time. To date, no evaluation of a oral health education program has produced such results.[6-10]

An error commonly made with this cognitive approach occurs when the educator fails to assess the learners' level of knowledge before the educational encounter and treats the individuals as if they were void of any knowledge or past experiences at all. As Yacavone[9] notes, it is important to realize "that the person is already 'behaving' when we encounter him—maybe not as we would like him to, but 'behaving.'" To influence a person's behavior through health education activities, an understanding of the dynamics of behavior is paramount.

A person's behavior is the result of both internal and external forces. Beliefs, attitudes, interests, values, needs, motives, personality, expectations, perceptions, and biologic factors, plus the influence of family, peer groups, and mass economic factors such as occupation, education, and media, shape and affect actions.[54] Sociodemographic factors such as age, race or culture, sex, occupation, education, and income have also been shown to have a strong influence on oral health practices and should be considered when designing and implementing health education strategies. The interaction of these forces has been illustrated in a model developed by Kressin (Box 11-1). Considering this model, it becomes evident that a straight-line relationship between the educator's efforts and the learner's behavior usually does not exist. To develop an effective oral health education program, the educator must be aware of the interaction of all the forces on the learner. The educator must first assess the learner or learners to develop and implement a rational educational program that will result in a sustained behavior change.

SOCIAL COGNITIVE THEORY

This perspective on health behavior says that an individual's behaviors are motivated

BOX 11-1

Factors Influencing the Dental Education Process

Aspects of the learner(s) to consider when designing dental education programs:

- Sociodemographic factors (e.g., age, sex, race/culture, income)
- Values, attitudes, beliefs
- Readiness to change behaviors
- Education

Aspects of the social environment to consider when designing dental education programs:

- Cultural norms (e.g., how much of the population smokes, how many people floss their teeth)
- Cultural values/expectations (e.g., expectation that children's teeth will have brown spots/caries)
- How supportive the environment is for behavioral change
- Possible ways in which education/information can be offered

Courtesy N. Kressin, 2001.

by both beliefs (cognitive factors) and factors in the social environment (e.g., one's community, friends, and family).[55] The specific beliefs that are viewed as most important are concerned with an individual's perceptions of self-efficacy, that is, beliefs that the individual can perform a particular behavior effectively and with good results. Aspects of the social environment important in this theory include learning how to perform a specific behavior by watching others do so and receiving support or reinforcement from others in the environment for practicing certain behaviors.

A number of studies conducted by Tedesco and associates[56,57] have demonstrated that aspects of social cognitive theory are important in the development and maintenance of oral self-care behaviors such as brushing and flossing. Individuals participating in the educational programs designed by Tedesco and associates[56,57] brushed and flossed for a longer period of time when they learned about these behaviors by practicing them as part of the educational process and when they received support and reinforcement from the dental educators about their capability to perform the behaviors. The findings from this research highlight the importance of actually practicing new behaviors as part of an educational intervention and of receiving positive feedback from dental educators for practicing the behavior correctly. Together, these factors increased the participants' self-efficacy—their belief that they could successfully improve their oral self-care.

THEORY OF REASONED ACTION

The theory of reasoned action states that an individual's behaviors are primarily determined by intentions to perform the behavior.[58] In turn, the individual's intentions are determined by attitudes and beliefs about the behavior. Specifically, attitudes about what will result from performing a certain behavior (for example, that flossing will prevent periodontal disease and that retaining natural teeth is important) are thought to influence the likelihood that the individual intends to perform and actually performs a certain behavior. Also important to understanding attitudes are beliefs about how others will respond to the behavior (e.g., that others will notice and approve of cleaner-looking teeth and gums).

Oral health education efforts based on this theory should be directed toward increasing individuals' intentions to care for their oral health by (1) emphasizing the importance and value of maintaining oral health and retaining the natural teeth, (2) educating and reassuring people that they can indeed effectively care for their oral health and prevent oral disease, and (3) changing community and societal norms so that more individuals are motivated to care for their own oral health and to support their friends and family in doing so.

HEALTH BELIEF MODEL

Developed by Rosenstock,[59] the health belief model considers a variety of factors thought to influence individuals' health behaviors. The first factor is an individual's readiness to act. Without this readiness, a person is unlikely to change a particular behavior, whether it involves quitting smoking or starting to floss the teeth daily. This readiness is considered a function of two things: the individual's perceptions about the severity of the disease and the person's susceptibility to it. If an individual does not think he or she is likely to get oral or lung cancer as a result of smoking or periodontal disease if he or she does not floss, the individual is less likely to stop smoking or start flossing.

The second factor that the health belief model considers is an individual's consideration of the perceived costs and benefits of performing a certain behavior. If a person perceives a lot of difficulty in withdrawing from nicotine and perhaps gains weight as a result of quitting, he or she may conclude that the costs of quitting smoking are too great. Similarly, if a person feels that the time and energy required to floss daily are more than can be handled, that person might be less likely to do so. Alternatively, if a person's views of the benefits of quitting smoking are strong and highlight the money saved, being able to breathe easier, and decreasing risks to physical and oral health, these perceptions might make it more likely that such individuals will quit smoking.

The last set of factors that the health belief model considers are referred to as *cues to action*. These cues prompt individuals to act by reminding them of the need to change their behaviors. These stimuli may be internal (such as pain or discomfort) or external (such as advertising campaigns reminding people of the harm done by smoking or a physician telling someone how much smoking hurts health).

From the perspective of the health belief model, a major obstacle to preventing dental disease through preventive behaviors may be the perception that the consequences of dental disease are not serious. In most cases dental disease is not life threatening, and a large portion of the population functions without their natural teeth. In a survey conducted by the Opinion Research Corporation for the ADA, the public's chief barrier to prevention of dental disease was identified as the low value many Americans place on regular preventive dental care.[60] Educational efforts designed with the health belief model in mind emphasize the fact that most individuals are vulnerable to the development of oral disease if they do not care for their teeth and that such disease may result in losing the natural teeth and that oral functions such as smiling and chewing are easier with natural teeth (emphasizing the severity of the disease and the individual's susceptibility). Further, such educational efforts should emphasize that caring for the dentition through regular flossing, brushing, and preventive care will have the long-term benefit of retaining the teeth (emphasizing the perceived benefits) and that such efforts are relatively easy and require just a few minutes of time each day (emphasizing the low costs and the ease with which perceived barriers can be overcome). Finally, oral health education based on the health belief model provides cues to action that remind people about the need to take care of their oral health.

STAGES OF CHANGE MODEL

The stages of change model of behavioral change describes common stages of change through which individuals go when trying to change health-related behaviors.[61] The first stage is *precontemplation,* which represents a time during which an individual is not actively thinking of changing a particular behavior. The next stage, *contemplation,* is when the individual begins to think about behavioral change. During this time he or she may think, read, or talk to others about changing a behavior and may become open to health education, in preparation for taking actual steps to change behaviors. The *action* stage is when an individual actually takes steps to change the behavior. Individuals are in particular need of support for their changed behaviors during this time, which may include specific training or education and social support from family and friends. Assuming that successful actions are taken, the individual moves into the *maintenance* stage, in which he or she attempts to continue the behavioral change. At this time it is helpful to identify factors that may tempt a person to relapse, so as to prevent, avoid, or learn how to deal with these factors. Relapse occurs when the individual is unable to continue to maintain the changed behavior; relapse is extremely common. The model and process is circular, however, so an individual can move on to another stage when ready to try again to change behavior.

Oral health education efforts should be mindful of the various stages of change that individuals can be in because these affect receptivity to educational efforts and the subsequent efficacy of the education. On the basis of this model, it is important to offer education to individuals who are ready to hear it (i.e., those in the contemplation, action, or maintenance stages). However, in community-based efforts where attendance is voluntary, it is likely that only individuals in these stages would attend educational programs.

CONTEMPORARY COMMUNITY HEALTH MODEL

The fourth and most current approach is the contemporary community health (or public health) model of health education, which takes into account social, cultural, economic, and other environmental factors that influence health. Rather than "blaming the victim" for noncompliant behavior and subsequent illnesses, the need for changes in influential variables such as the social, political, economic, and industrial environments is recognized. The community health model emphasizes the important role of public involvement in identifying individual and community health problems, setting priorities, and developing solutions to these problems, and it empowers population groups with accurate information about health and health care technologies. The utility of broad approaches to health education and promotion at the community level has been demonstrated in studies of other health areas.[17,62-64] However, with few exceptions, dental professionals have not yet accepted many of the community-level methods used in these demonstrations. The World Health Organization has clearly stated the need for using sound community organization and community development principles of working with focus populations, such as sharing in decision making.[65,66]

The objective of community organization is to create awareness, interest, and desire to solve a problem while working with others to solve the problem. By involving people in making decisions about regimens or programs to improve their own health, people will tend to unite and maintain the level of commitment to, and motivation for, carrying out necessary actions to solve the problems.[13,14] Readers are encouraged to review the Stanford Five City Project, which describes the communication-change framework; social marketing; the application of formative research in designing, modifying, and distributing printed educational materials; the use of mass media education; program planning; and evaluation.[62] The Stanford Five City Project is an evaluation of a community-wide approach to the control of cardiovascular disease through healthy changes in behavior. This approach may be generalizable to dental disease prevention efforts as we continue to learn to unite a variety of medical, behavioral, communication, and social science theories with demonstrated applications to solve health problems.[17]

Social Marketing. Social marketing is emerging as a new method for promoting desirable social change, by increasing the public's acceptance of social ideas or practices among target groups. Social marketing combines the use of successful advertising and marketing techniques and applies them to changing people's ideas and behaviors. In comparison with traditional marketing techniques, social marketing aims to change people's attitudes about nontangible products, including ideas, services, and practices.[67]

How does social marketing work? The first aim of this method is to understand the "customer's needs." Through market research, the audience becomes known and understood by program planners. Second, the "product" must be made available through the media or other communication channels. Program planners need to selectively choose their communication channels based on their knowledge of the targeted community or population. Third, pricing must be considered. For example, if the aim is to increase rates of brushing and flossing within a population, the price of dental floss or toothbrushes may be lowered, or such products may be given away free of cost. Fourth, those involved in social marketing need to consider the opportunity costs of adopting a new behavior or idea. For example, time spent visiting the dentist or engaging in oral self-care could be spent in other activities, and individuals need to be persuaded that such activities are worth the time they invest in them.

Social marketing has been used to decrease tobacco consumption, increase health and safety, encourage improved nutrition and increased physical activity, and enhance the effectiveness of HIV/AIDS prevention programs, and it could be a useful device for oral health education as well.[68-73]

Media Influence. Silversin and Kornacki[74] have stated that the media has a role in promoting behavioral change: "Media-based campaigns to promote oral health have been shown to be more effective if they continue over long periods of time, appeal to multiple motives, are coupled with social support, and provide training in requisite skills." In addition, product advertising may influence public opinion and behavior.

Organizations such as Action for Children's Television (ACT), the Center for Science in the Public Interest (CSPI), the National Congress of Parents and Teachers (National PTA), and the American Academy of Pediatrics (AAP) have expressed concern about the marketing of relatively nonnutritious foods to children.[75-79] A nonprofit consumer-advocacy group based in Washington, D.C., CSPI has focused on nutrition and food safety issues since its founding in 1971.[80]

In 1992 the Children's Television Act took effect, setting limits on the number of advertisements allowed during children's shows and mandating that all broadcasters carry children's educational or instructional programming as a condition for license renewal by the Federal Communications Commission (FCC). However, the FCC has concluded that this requirement can be met by citing public service announcements or short vignettes in fulfillment of the programming requirement. The American Academy of Pediatrics emphasizes that local oversight is necessary to monitor how stations meet these guidelines. The academy urged parents to take an active role in educating their children to become responsible and informed consumers and noted that media literacy should be taught to children in schools and in a variety of other settings.[78,79]

The increased use of tobacco products (smoking cigarettes and cigars and using chewing tobacco) in films and on commercial television is a cause for concern. Despite the tobacco industry's agreement with the FCC to voluntarily remove tobacco advertising from television in 1969, the tobacco industry has paid stage and screen actors to smoke while acting, claiming that smoking is essential to the character or situation. In reality, performers who may serve as significant role models for our youth may by their actions be promoting dangerous and often deadly lifestyle behaviors for personal gain and tobacco industry profits. In a nation where an estimated 3000 youngsters begin smoking each day, the print, film, and advertising media are effectively influencing the actions and ultimately the health of our children. Surveys conducted by the National Center for Chronic Disease Prevention and Health Promotion indicate that brand choices of adolescent smokers were heavily concentrated on those brands with the largest advertising budgets.[81,82] A 1991 survey in the *Journal of the American Medical Association* found that Joe Camel was as recognizable as Mickey Mouse to 6-year-olds. It is not surprising that, as a result of R. J. Reynolds's Camel campaign, which was backed by a company research program, Camel's share of the youth market jumped from roughly 3% in 1988 to 13% in 1993.[83] Cigarette advertising is an important influence on the smoking behavior of the young, with advertising sensitivity being approximately three times larger among teenagers than among adults. Cigarette advertising puts children at greater risk by influencing and distorting their perceptions of the pervasiveness, image, and function of smoking within society.[84] Media images are often blamed for children adopting risky behaviors. In March 2001 a study funded by the National Cancer Institute at the Pediatrics Department of Dartmouth Medical College was released that substantiated this relationship. Data from New England middle schoolers provided the first direct evidence linking movie exposure to smoking and alcohol use in children and adolescents. After researchers measured tobacco's actual screen time in movies based on what the children had reported seeing, they found that the youngsters who had seen the most tobacco images were five times as likely to have used cigarettes as kids with the least exposure. This relationship prompted the suggestion that parents need to view movies as a potentially "toxic" exposure that could adversely affect children's health behavior and in that respect may be little different from other environmental toxins such as lead or mercury.[85,86]

Dr. David Kessler, former Commissioner of the Food and Drug Administration (FDA), has referred to smoking as a "pediatric disease" because the average smoker begins by age 15 years and is a daily smoker by age 18 years. Although smoking levels among adults have been declining, smoking is on the rise among those under 19 years of age. Many children who start smoking every day end up as statistics a few decades later. According to Michelle Bloch of the American Medical Woman's Association, "Fully half of all long-term smokers, especially those who begin in their teenage years, will be killed by tobacco. Of those half will die early in middle age."[83]

In 1995 President Clinton announced that the FDA proposed to regulate nicotine in tobacco as a drug, despite the tobacco industry's 100-year-old claim that tobacco is neither food, drug, nor cosmetic. The FDA launched a major initiative to strictly limit tobacco advertising to youth and other measures intended to curb youth access to tobacco products. The FDA's goal was to reduce the number of children and adolescents who use tobacco products by 50% within 7 years by putting restrictions on the sale and distribution of nicotine-containing cigarettes and smokeless tobacco products and by limiting minors' access to these highly addictive products. The ADHA has stood strongly in support of public policy and legislative efforts to curb underage smoking.[87] In 1996 President Clinton signed an executive order that passed the final version of regulations proposed a year earlier. The FDA had planned to phase them in over a period of 6 months to 2 years. However, the tobacco industry, the advertising industry, and the wholesale and farm communities filed three lawsuits attempting to block the implementation of the rules. In 2000 the U.S. Supreme Court ruled that the FDA did not have the explicit authority to regulate nicotine in tobacco. Also in 2000 the historic $246 billion multistate tobacco settlement between the state attorneys general from 22 states and the major U.S. tobacco companies was enacted. This settlement was intended as restitution for state Medicaid funds expended for the treatment of citizens with tobacco-related illnesses and was intended to place restrictions on tobacco company marketing and advertising activities. However, the agreement failed to address the following matters: (1) need for comprehensive programs to prevent and reduce tobacco use in every state; (2) protecting people from secondhand smoke; (3) ban tobacco vending machines and self-service displays nationally, which would greatly reduce youth access to tobacco products; (4) need for more effective and more visible health warnings on tobacco products; (5) granting the FDA explicit authority to regulate tobacco products; (6) restriction of U.S. tobacco company marketing to youth overseas; and (7) assist U.S. tobacco farmers' transition to other forms of income. The agreement has established several restrictions on tobacco company marketing and advertising. Restrictions include the following: (1) eliminates tobacco billboards and transit ads; (2) prohibits use of cartoon characters to promote tobacco products; (3) prohibits tobacco brand-name merchandise (e.g., hats, T-shirts), except at tobacco-sponsored events; (4) prohibits tobacco brand-name sponsorship of concerts, events in which any contestants are under 18, football, baseball, soccer, and hockey (except for Brown & Williamson's continued sponsorship of the Kool Jazz Festival and the GPC Country Music Festival); (5) limits other tobacco brand-name sponsorships to one event or series per year per manufacturer (e.g., Winston Cup Race Tour); (6) permits free tobacco-product distributions only at locations where children are not permitted; (7) restricts offers of nontobacco items or gifts based on proof of purchase to adults; (8) prohibits the use of nontobacco brand names on tobacco products; and (9) reaffirms the previously agreed on prohibition on tobacco product placement in movies and on TV. Despite these concessions, the agreement still permits tobacco companies numerous opportunities to market and advertise their deadly products through unlimited advertising in newspapers, magazines, places that sell tobacco products, the Internet, and direct-mail advertising; permits unlimited tobacco-company sponsorship of events in their corporate name as opposed to brand-name advertising; and permits televising of tobacco brand-name–sponsored events. Tobacco companies can continue to advertise on buildings or property of places where tobacco is sold and at industry-sponsored events and can continue to use human images in tobacco advertising. Each tobacco company may continue single brand-name sponsorship of auto racing, rodeo, or other events, which may include an entire series of events (e.g., all NASCAR races).

Although President Clinton recommended that states receiving funds from the settlement target those funds for health-related purposes, the settlement says nothing as to how that money should be spent. During the 2001 congressional legislative session, several U.S. representatives proposed tobacco control bills to address several matters that the multistate tobacco settlement did not adequately address, as well as the authority of the FDA to regulate nicotine as a drug. If enacted, the bills will explicitly authorize the FDA to regulate tobacco products, impose financial penalties against tobacco companies if youth smoking rates do not decline, establish smoke-free indoor workplaces and public places nationwide (with few exceptions), and provide funding for tobacco control programs. For more information on tobacco-related legislation, issues, and resources, check the website developed and maintained by the CDC, www.cdc.gov/tobacco, with links to other useful sites such as www.tobacco.neu.edu (maintained by the Tobacco Control Resource Center at Northeastern University School of Law) and www.tobaccofreekids.org (maintained by the Campaign for Tobacco Free Kids).

Budgets for promoting preventive oral health interventions cannot compete with budgets for promoting products that are pushed and pulled into the marketplace with huge sums of money (e.g., tobacco, automobiles, cosmetics). The success of product advertising is based on linking personal satisfaction or enhanced self-esteem with the use of a product. Thus far, oral health promotion has not succeeded in linking preventive dental behaviors with motives other than health.[74] However, promotional advertising of in-office tooth-whitening systems by organized dentistry for the purpose of enhancing personal appearance and sexual attractiveness may prove to have a strong appeal as a social marketing tool, effectively increasing demand for dental treatment among adult smokers and nonsmokers, as well as young adults.

Parents and School Programs. Rubinson[88] has identified parents as the most pervasive intervening variable in school oral health programs. Many program developers and evaluators do not consider enlisting the cooperation of parents.[88] Rubinson[88] further states that "the parents will certainly have a direct influence on oral health habits and should be involved with programmatic efforts." The evaluation of oral health programs should be redirected to focus on efforts stressing skill acquisition and reduction of behavioral risk factors through an evaluation plan that is both plausible and realistic in the school setting. Perry and associates[64] have demonstrated the effectiveness of combined school, parent, and community approaches to child health behavior in the Minnesota Home Team Project. This case demonstrated how sharing responsibility can be accomplished, and it established the superior impact of shared responsibility between the school and the home on children's knowledge, skills, and practices with respect to dietary intake of more healthful foods.

The School Health Education Evaluation (SHEE), conducted in collaboration with the CDC from 1982 through 1984, suggests that exposure to health education curricula in schools can result in substantial changes in students' knowledge, attitudes, and self-reported practices.[89] The SHEE has provided evidence that school health education curricula can effect changes in health-related knowledge, practices, and attitudes and that such changes increase with the amount of instruction. The potential impact of these changes is significant.[89] In response to this study, many school systems are re-evaluating their health curricula and considering increased integration of health messages throughout the curriculum. Teachers will require additional training to develop greater competency on health issues. In view of budget limitations, teachers will continue to be the primary source for the dissemination of health education in our schools, with the assistance of health professionals in the community. Readers are encouraged to review the 10 basic elements that constitute comprehensive school health education as defined in the SHEE study.[90]

The complexity of the variables that must be taken into account in designing an oral health education program to motivate behavioral change for an individual has been briefly discussed. Greater detail and step-by-step procedures can be found in books devoted solely to the techniques of behavior modification and to the social sciences in dentistry.[12,91,92]

Health Education in Transition

Oral health education programs for the community have gone through, and will continue to undergo, periods of transition as further study reveals educational methods that will produce desired preventive practices. Research has shown that behavior is not transmitted; behavior is learned. In health care, learning requires active participation on the part of the learner. For this reason the primary objective of most oral health education programs is to motivate individual students to seek the goal of disease prevention and tooth conservation.

Historically, oral health education for children has been a priority for the dental profession because of the high prevalence of dental caries in this age group. As a result, the school system has emerged as the most logical and practical setting to implement large-scale oral health education programs.[93] The school-based oral health program provides an opportunity to reach the largest number of children during early stages of development when habit patterns can more easily be modified or changed.

The school setting also provides an environment conducive to learning and reinforcement for a considerable period of time and allows the teachers to use various strategies for inducing children to participate in appropriate preventive oral health actions.[94]

Early school-based oral health programs based on the cognitive learning model primarily consisted of dental professionals and students participating in short-term projects such as National Children's Oral Health Week, high school career days, and one-time visits to elementary and secondary school classrooms. These projects did not seek to incorporate oral health into the school curriculum; they were (and are, where they still exist) seen as an "add-on" activity. Administratively, one-time visits present little difficulty and are often welcomed by the teacher and administration; however, reinforcement or evaluation of the oral health lesson is not usually part of the activity. Most reports on oral health education in the classroom agree that the most effective situation is when the classroom teacher works closely with the dental professional. So, regardless of who actually makes the presentation, the teacher can augment and reinforce oral health concepts and practices. The most significant behavior for the teacher is to be an effective role model of good oral health practices.[95] Although public interest may be aroused and dentistry's image enhanced, the early school programs, passive and cognitive in nature, were not found to motivate changes in oral health attitudes and behaviors.[6,93,95] According to Raynor and Cohen,[96] research in the oral health area suggests that there must be something more than motivation per se to establish oral hygiene behavior as a habit. Learning oral hygiene must involve the acquisition of a value, or a change in a value. For adults, this involves change in cognitive structure, but for children cognitive learning is secondary to motivational learning. As a consequence of this realization, the "show and tell" approach has now evolved into programs of "show and do."

A survey of state school health programs by the American School Health Association revealed that only seven states mandate the teaching of oral health and oral hygiene.[97] Unfortunately, even in those seven states requiring instruction on specific health content areas, oral health is given a low priority on the list of required subjects. If oral health education is more than rhetoric and teachers are expected to include it in the curriculum, adequate teacher training programs are a prerequisite.[98] Oral health professionals in the community can serve as valuable resources to the school. Oral health education should be an integral component of all school health education curricula. Regrettably, the majority of oral health education programs were supported through grant funds, and many were terminated when funding expired.[99] Unless a strong constituency supports oral health programs, continued efforts may be stunted as a result of budgeting constraints.

An interesting by-product of school-based oral health education programs may be the "spread effect" or the "ripple effect."[100,101] These terms have been used to describe the impact of school-based health education programs on parents. Croucher and associates[100] conducted an investigation to assess the possible indirect influence of "Natural Noshers" (a school-based oral health education program that emphasizes home activities for skill development) on the dental behavior and knowledge of other family members. "Natural Noshers" contains two distinct oral health messages, one relating to the prevention of gum disease and the other to dental decay. Take-home literature and supplies emphasize these messages. The results of this study indicate that the parents of children who had been taught "Natural Noshers" had reported new dental information more often than the parents in the control group.[100]

In another project, a group of health educators at the University of Maine at Farmington developed a series of health-related games, the "Healthway Arcade 101". The games were used primarily for an audience of kindergarten through third grade and were structured to address several health issues. "Floss Is the Boss" was a popular follow-along story that used repetition, funny sounds, and a variety of motions to cleverly state the importance of flossing the teeth. Parental feedback indicated that this live arts format was well received and that many youngsters insisted on reciting parts of the story at home for the family. This ripple effect is another way of getting a message into the home and community.[101]

An innovative project at the University of New England was developed in collaboration with social service agencies to produce a community resource for much-needed oral health care services with funding provided by Northeast Dental Corporation that may serve as a model for other dental professionals seeking to serve community needs. In this case, a dental hygiene program at a private university and an Early Head Start Program (a federally funded program similar to Head Start) joined in partnership to develop and implement a project that was deemed mutually beneficial and highly productive. At multiple rural locations in Maine, dental hygiene students provided much-needed oral health services to families with children enrolled in the Early Head Start Program (ages newborn to 3 years), which focused on infant oral care in general with a particular emphasis on early childhood caries. One of the goals of the Early Head Start Program is to prevent destruction of the dentition and preserve the level of oral health found in early infancy. On-site oral inspections, assessments of fluoride levels in drinking water, recommendations for fluoride supplementation when appropriate, documentation of disease present in the population, and referrals for treatment were conducted. Parent education focused on their role in preventing dental disease in their children, including topics such as feeding practices, plaque removal, nutrition, importance of fluoride, and the need to maintain oral health via continuity of professional care. The challenge remains to establish referral arrangements with dentists in the community to make dental treatment accessible for this population.[102]

CORPORATE-SPONSORED SCHOOL-BASED DENTAL PROGRAMS

Bright Smiles, Bright Futures

Colgate Oral Pharmaceuticals has developed an oral health educational program to teach children about caring for their teeth through proper oral hygiene, diet, and physical activity. The program enhances children's self-esteem while giving them information about taking care of their oral health. Information about its school curriculum is available online at www.colgatebsbf.com or by phone at 800-2-COLGATE (ask for Bright Smiles, Bright Futures), including a variety of learning materials adapted for early childhood. Available materials include books, videos, posters, stickers, charts, and guides for teachers or professionals administering the program.

In several U.S. communities (Philadelphia, New York City, and Oakland), a mobile van staffed by volunteer dental professionals provides dental attention on wheels, screening children and providing referrals for additional needed treatment. This partnership with America's Promise—The Alliance for Youth aims to provide dental care and information to children at risk for dental problems.

Crest's First-Grade Oral Health Education Program

Since 1963 Procter & Gamble (P&G) has been providing the curriculum resources to schools throughout America to teach children how to fight cavities. Each year Crest kits containing toothbrushes and toothpaste samples have been provided for children in more than 20,000 classrooms throughout the United States. Teachers who register for the program also receive teacher kits including an animated video, an audio sing-along cassette, a teacher's guide, and a classroom poster, in addition to the student take-home kits. The curriculum encourages youngsters to go for regular dental checkups and invites dental professionals to participate in the classroom instruction. Contact your local P&G sales representative for a list of participating schools in your area. Materials are sent directly to the participating schools each year in time for National Children's Dental Health Month (February). P&G also offers a variety of materials for oral care professionals' use, including activity books, brochures, bookmarks, stickers, lesson plan, and a poster, annually during National Children's Dental Health Month. P&G also provides other educational materials developed for professional and patient use. More information is available online at www.dentalcare.com/png.educat.htm.

Coordinated School Health Programs

One proven strategy for reaching low-income children most at risk for dental caries is through school-based programs with supporting linkages with health care professionals and other dental partners in the community. In 1998 the National Center for Chronic Disease Prevention and Health Promotion at CDC (NCCDPHP/CDC), Division of Oral Health, provided funding support to three state education agencies with 1-year awards to develop models for school-based programs to improve access to oral health education, prevention, and treatment services for children who are at high risk for oral disease. The education agencies in Ohio, Rhode Island, and Wisconsin partnered with their state health departments to develop, expand, and evaluate school-based or school-linked models, integrating oral health into their existing Coordinated School Health Programs (CSHPs), which are funded by the NCCDPHP/CDC Division of Adolescent and School Health.

In 1999 the CDC's Division of Oral Health broadened its commitment to coordinated school health programming by providing 3-year funding to support an oral health infrastructure building initiative for planning and implementation in four U.S. states. Ohio, Rhode Island, South Carolina, and Wisconsin are currently developing models for implementation and evaluation over a 3-year period.[103] The four funded states are developing infrastructure to address oral health needs, focusing on dental sealants and oral health education using a variety of approaches. The results of these model approaches will be widely disseminated and will provide valuable information about school-based and school-linked oral health surveillance, infrastructure, and policy development. The Division of Oral Health has expressed hopes that these models will serve as a foundation for a comprehensive, integrated, and sustainable approach to address the oral health needs of school-age children throughout the United States. These models will be a topic for a future edition of this text. More information is available at the following website and links: www.cdc.gov/nccdphp/oh/child-schoolhealth.htm.

Some factors may enhance the success of oral health programs in schools: (1) determining who will be responsible for oral health education, (2) involving parents who can provide reinforcement of oral health practices at home, (3) identifying and using community health resources that can contribute expertise or materials to support oral health education efforts, and (4) evaluating the results of the program.[104]

Two large-scale teaching programs in Texas and North Carolina, based on both the social cognitive and the health belief learning models, are next described in terms of program development, philosophy and goals, implementation, and evaluation. In addition, a number of innovative community educational outreach programs are also featured. A third program, Special Olympics, Special Smiles, based on the contemporary community health model, is also described. Findings of formal research investigations as reported in the literature are presented for review. The reader is asked to keep in mind the desired properties of a good oral public health measure and the planning and implementation strategy and criteria for the prevention of dental diseases when critiquing each program in terms of public health planning. Although all details for each program have not been presented, all major concepts have been included.

Current Approaches

TEXAS STATEWIDE PREVENTIVE DENTISTRY PROGRAM: *TATTLETOOTH II—A NEW GENERATION*

Development

The Tattletooth Program was first developed in the 1970s as a cooperative effort between Texas oral health professional organizations, the Texas Education Agency, and the Texas Department of Health through a grant from the Department of Health and Human Services to the Bureau of Dental Health.[105] This program was initially implemented in its original format with approximately 500,000 children in Texas per year before the new program was completed in 1989.

In 1985 the Texas legislature mandated that the essential elements for comprehensive health education curricula identified in the School Health Education Evaluation Project be incorporated into the curriculum statewide and be taught to the state's more than 3 million schoolchildren.[89,90] Oral health is one of the required elements. This legislative action stimulated a need for the Tattletooth Program statewide.[104-106]

In 1989 the Bureau of Dental Health developed a mostly new program, *Tattletooth II—A New Generation,* for grades kindergarten through 6, so named because the characters in the artwork for grades kindergarten through 2 were from the old curriculum. In 1993 a preschool program titled "SuperBrush" was completed. The preschool curriculum was designed for use with personnel in Head Start programs, public and private child care centers, public school programs, and family day care homes. A systems approach was used to develop all educational material.[106,107]

Program Philosophy and Goals

In Texas, oral health education has long been the primary prevention effort of both the private and public dental sectors.[106] The basic goal of the program is to reduce dental disease and to develop positive dental habits to last a lifetime in participants. The major thrust of the Tattletooth Program is to convince students that preventing dental disease is important and that they can do it.[106,107]

Tattletooth Program lessons are correlated with the health and science essential elements. The material in the lesson is often integrated into other subject areas, such as language arts. References to cultural differences are made throughout each unit, and lessons are also available in Spanish (in response to the cultural and linguistic needs of the growing Hispanic population).

To satisfy the legislative requirement that student performance be assessed, the Texas Education Agency requires that the Texas Assessment of Academic Skills (TAAS) be given to students in grades 3, 5, 7, 9, and 11. The Tattletooth program is correlated with the objectives and instructional targets of TAAS, thus providing students an opportunity to practice meeting those objectives before testing.

The Tattletooth lessons incorporate all the items that could be written into lessons. A scope and sequence chart shows the teacher what is to be taught and what the teacher in the previous grade level should have taught. It also tells the teacher what the students are to learn the next year.

The Tattletooth II program embraces the six elements of effective lesson design: anticipatory set, setting the objective, input modeling, checking for understanding, guided practice, and independent practice. It emphasizes the important aspects of planning in successful teaching. Teaching decisions fall into three categories:

1. What content to teach next
2. What the student will do to learn
3. What the student will do to prove that learning has occurred.

Program Implementation

The Texas Department of Health is divided into eight public health regions and employs dental hygienists and dental assistants in the regions that implement the Tattletooth Program statewide. The hygienists instruct teachers with videotapes designed for teacher training and provide them with a copy of the curriculum. In some instances the hygienists are training lead teachers who, in turn, provide training for teachers in their schools.

Each grade level has five core lessons and two enrichment lessons. Background information for the teacher is provided at the beginning of each lesson. Educational strategies are suggested for integrating dental topics into other subject areas, such as language arts, mathematics, and science. Health promotion activities are encouraged and publicized within the school community. Teachers are encouraged to invite a dental professional to demonstrate brushing and flossing in the classroom. A field trip to a dental office is strongly recommended for kindergarten children. Each unit has a brief introduction that summarizes and gives a theme to the unit. Some units have planning notes that remind the teacher of the need for advance preparations. A unit test is provided so that the teacher will not have to write one. It can also be used as a pretest for diagnostic purposes.

Other resources include bulletin board suggestions, a book list, films, videotapes available on free loan for appropriate grade levels, a list of companies providing supplementary classroom resources, and a comprehensive glossary of vocabulary words that are used in all grade levels written for the teacher in English and Spanish. Topics covered in the curriculum include correct brushing and flossing techniques, awareness of the importance of safety, and factual information relating to dental disease and its causes and preventive techniques.

Cost of Program

The Texas Department of Health has no tangible studies to support the cost-effectiveness of the Tattletooth II program. In 1990 the regional dental director for Public Health Region Six assessed the cost for program implementation at $289.25 per workshop. Because an average of 953 children benefit from each workshop, the cost per child was estimated at $0.60.

Program Evaluation

The results of program evaluations have been positive, with teachers and students praising the teacher-student interaction that was present as a result of the format. Approximately half the teachers responding had used the previous program, and half the teachers were new to the program. Approximately 94% of the teachers believed that teaching oral health can have a positive effect on children's oral health habits. Most teachers (90%) taught oral health once per year, and the average number of hours in which oral health was taught was 4.2. The Bureau of Dental Health states that, given teaching requirements, the fact that 88.7% of the teachers spent 45 minutes to 6.5 hours teaching the Tattletooth II program is an indication that the curriculum was well received.

The curriculum materials were successful in teaching dental information and in increasing awareness of oral health practices. However, results indicate that the majority of teachers did not provide students with the opportunity to practice the skills of brushing and flossing. Toothbrushes and floss are not readily available because the dental program no longer provides them. Although teachers demonstrate dental hygiene skills, students will not master skills unless they are given an opportunity to practice them. Greater efforts must be made to provide all classroom teachers with an adequate quantity of toothbrushes and dental floss to establish and maintain daily oral care programs.

Tattletooth II—A New Generation: "SuperBrush" Preschool Curriculum

The SuperBrush curriculum is intended for teachers and caregivers who work with children 3 and 4 years old in such settings as Head Start programs, prekindergarten, or public and private child care centers. The oral health curriculum consists of seven units, and the primary purpose is to teach basic toothbrushing skills and to establish toothbrushing as a daily routine in schools or day homes. The curriculum contains (1) children-directed activities that children do largely on their own and (2) teacher-directed activities that teachers do with children in large or small groups. All learning activities are developmentally appropriate for preschool children. The curriculum includes songs, games, stories, art projects, a resource list, and videotapes to show parents. The curriculum is available in English and Spanish. The curriculum is free to teachers and caregivers who participate in the health department's training sessions on how to use the materials.

Results from an evaluation of the program indicated that, overall, teachers and children alike received the preschool oral health curriculum enthusiastically. Teachers reported that it was fun and easy to use and that it provided many options that allowed them to tailor it to the needs of the classroom and to the resources they had available. Most teachers reported satisfaction with the in-service training and the level of technical support and reported that they would use the curriculum the following year. It also appears that by introducing the curriculum early in the year as opposed to late in the year, many teachers may have more time to prepare and incorporate more of the suggested activities.

As of June 1993 approximately 10,000 preschool settings existed in Texas. Of the preschools that participated in the pilot test, the number of classrooms that received oral health instruction during spring 1993 increased by 21% for independent school districts, 5% for Head Start centers, and 33% for day care centers. Widespread availability of the program to preschool programs throughout Texas would help increase the amount and quality of dental instruction provided to children between ages 3 and 6 years. It is well recognized that the preschool setting provides an important opportunity to build a foundation for healthy mental, physical, and emotional development. The potential exists to instill in young children the importance and practice of oral health habits that will last a lifetime.[107]

Other major components of the program include a parent program; a senior citizen program; a prenatal and postnatal program; a nursing home oral health program; a pregnancy, education, and parenting program; and an oral health manual for school nurses. Additionally, the Texas Department of Health maintains the Office of Smoking and Health, whose educational efforts are geared toward tobacco education, prevention, and cessation.* The state also makes oral health training materials available through the Department of Public Health's website (www.tdh.state.tx.us). "Take Time for Teeth Oral Health Training" materials include a trainer's manual, trainee's workbook, flipcharts, and brochures, as well as an accompanying video (materials are available in English, Spanish, and some in Vietnamese).

NORTH CAROLINA STATEWIDE DENTAL PUBLIC HEALTH PROGRAM

DEVELOPMENT

North Carolina has a long history of involvement in dental public health and school oral health education. The need for a school oral health education program was realized as early as 1918 when the first scientific paper addressing this subject was presented to the North Carolina Dental Society. The society endorsed the creation of an oral public health program and sought special funds from the North Carolina State Legislature. Oral hygiene was added to the North Carolina Public Health Program. In 1918 six dentists and six nurses were hired to begin an oral public health program in

*For additional information on school-based and community outreach dental programs, contact Texas Department of Health, Bureau of Dental Health, 1100 W. 49th, Austin, TX 78756, www.tdh.state.tx, www.us/dental/tattle.htm.

Table 11-1. Schematic Presentation of Preventive Dental Health Program in North Carolina

Agencies Involved	*Target Audiences*	*Approaches*
North Carolina Department of Public Instruction North Carolina Department of Environment, Health, and Natural Resources, Division of Dental Health	1. Teachers and staff of preschool programs and elementary schools	In-service training for teachers Preservice training in teacher-training institutions Public health dental consultation Provision of educational materials
North Carolina Dental Society University of North Carolina School of Dentistry and School of Public Health North Carolina Dental Hygienist's Association North Carolina Dental Assistant's Association	2. Students in preschool and elementary grades	Fluoridation of community water supplies Fluoride mouth rinse and other programs Educational programs and materials for schools Preventive dental services for eligible children
North Carolina Association of Local Health Directors	3. Parents of students	Parent education Education such as agricultural extension clubs, 4-H, civic and community groups Use of mass media for education Partnership with public health personnel such as health educators, nurses, and public health programs such as Maternal and Child Health
	4. Dentists and auxiliaries including students	Representation on advocacy committees for dental public health
	5. Community leaders, official and lay	Professional education

From North Carolina Department of Environment, Health, and Natural Resources Division of Dental Health, Raleigh, N

North Carolina, now known as the North Carolina Oral Health Section. Since then, many supportive actions have been initiated, including fluoridation of community water supplies and comprehensive state surveys of the dental disease problems. In 1970 the North Carolina Dental Society passed resolutions advocating a strong preventive dental disease program embracing school and community fluoridation, fluoride treatments for schoolchildren, continuing education on prevention for dental professionals, and plaque-control education in schools and communities. Table 11-1 provides a brief summary of the state's preventive oral health program.

Items in Dental Public Health Program	Sources of Funds
1. Fluoridation of community water supplies 2. Appropriate use of fluorides such as mouth rinse programs	Primarily state appropriations for salaries, clinical supplies, office supplies, and educational materials
3. Dental health education in preschools and elementary schools, including preservice and in-service training for teachers and staff 4. Dental education for consumers to include parents and community leaders via agencies such as agricultural extension, industry, civic clubs, and mass media	Salaries for central office staff include 3 public health dentists, 5 dental health educators, 1 dental hygiene consultant, and other administrative staff to work with 47 field-based public health hygienists and 11 public health dentists as team for educational and clinical services and other services such as statistical assistance for research, artwork, photography, film rental or purchase
5. Support services such as a. Provision of public health dental staff, health educators, maintenance staff b. Provision of supplies and equipment for dental staff c. Production and distribution of educational training aids	Six of 100 counties in North Carolina provide local funding for dental public health programs, including the salaries and supplies for dentists, dental hygienists, and dental assistants; several other counties fund salaries of dental hygienists and dental assistants; 61 staff are employed full-time by county health departments
6. Coordinated planning among agencies such as the North Carolina Dental Society, North Carolina Committee for Dental Health, and Division of Dental Health	Federal funds augment state funds in fluoridation of community water supplies for equipment and training

In 1973 a report prepared for the North Carolina Dental Society defined the extent of the dental disease problem and resulted in the initiation of a 10-year program to reduce dental disease. The 10-year preventive dentistry plan had the approval and support of the North Carolina General Assembly. In that same year a coalition of several agencies set up a steering committee that was responsible for developing a practical plan for a program in the schools. This was the first statewide program of its magnitude and remains the largest and most comprehensive of all state public health dental programs. Continuation and expansion of the North Carolina Preventive Dentistry Program for Children (NCPDPC) according to the original plan have been made possible through incremental funding from the state legislature. Initial appropriations in 1974 funded 10% of the program. Under the original plan the program would expand annually by approximately 10% so that in 10 years the program would include the entire state. The program has not been fully funded because of several lean budgetary years. Currently, the program offers some services to all counties, but the number of services provided depends on staff availability and funding.

With the North Carolina Oral Health Survey in 1986, the Oral Health Section started the process of establishing new long-range goals for the state that reinforce and expand on those started in 1973.

Program Philosophy and Goals

The North Carolina Oral Health Section is a unique public and private partnership dedicated to the mission of ensuring conditions in which North Carolina citizens can achieve optimal oral health. Oral health is considered an important part of general health and can be achieved through the coordinated efforts of individuals, professionals, and community members.[108-111] The Oral Health Section's vision is to make North Carolina the first state with a generation of cavity-free children.

The Oral Health Section's programs are based on prevention and education. The Oral Health Section is organized to provide as many direct services to the citizens of North Carolina as possible. The majority of the staff, public health dentists, and dental hygienists are located in the counties to provide services through local health departments. Primary prevention and education are considered to be the most effective means of decreasing dental disease and promoting oral health. All program activities include educational components to modify the behavior patterns of individuals to improve their oral health habits through dietary change, toothbrushing, flossing, sealants, and fluoride varnish. School-age children are the primary focus for education because the earlier a child is reached, the greater the potential for positively affecting the child's attitudes, values, and behaviors. Fluoride and sealants are recognized as the most effective public health measures for preventing dental caries. Objectives that will facilitate attainment of the goals of the section include: (1) appropriate use of fluoride and sealants, (2) health education in schools and communities, and (3) availability of public health dental staff in all counties.

Program Implementation

Oral surveys provide epidemiologic and sociodemographic data useful for program planning, implementation, and evaluation. Oral public health program decisions in North Carolina are founded on statewide, population-based oral health surveys conducted by the Oral Health Section and the University of North Carolina School of Public Health.[112,113] In the oral health status report presented in 1973, dental disease was found to affect 95% of the total population.[113] In 1982 Rozier and colleagues[114] stated that the teenage population is at greater risk of developing dental caries than any other age group and that 45% of children and adolescents show evidence of periodontal disease, almost all of which is reversible. According to the 1986–1987 North Carolina School Oral Health Survey, 53% of children 5 to 17 years of age have never had a cavity in their permanent teeth.[115] Because of a lack of funding, this is the most recent survey.

Disease levels have been steadily decreasing since the 1960s. This trend is true for all races and for both the younger and older age groups, but in different degrees of magnitude. There has been a continuing increase in dental care for all children.

The epidemiologic and sociodemographic data from surveys provide needed information for planning, implementing, and evaluating a community-based program. The comprehensive nature of the problem's definition is reflected in the uniqueness of the program, which is designed to reach several segments of the population: young children, parents, teachers, dental professionals, and community leaders. The fiscal year 1999–2000 services delivered through the program included weekly fluoride mouth rinse for 257,232 targeted elementary children in 628 schools and screening and referral for 214,545 targeted children. Dental public health staff applied almost 9600 dental sealants, with the staff emphasis on health promotion. Oral health education was presented to more than 248,000 children and approximately 34,000 adults in addition to the development, printing, and distribution of more than 400,000 pieces of educational materials. More than 47,000 people attended and received information through the 160 point-of-contact oral health education exhibits. With 10 varied topics, state and local health care professionals used the exhibit promotion across the state.[108]

The coordinated efforts of the staff of dentists, dental hygienists, and health educators are extremely important in program implementation. The activities of the central office consultant staff (made available to all public health dentists and hygienists in the state) provide for continuity in program planning and implementation. Also, the consultants serve in a capacity that helps coordinate the individual county programs and needs of staff through statewide conferences and training, in this way retaining and promoting the philosophy of the statewide preventive oral health program. To reach children, public health dental staff provide training and consultation to those who work with preschool and school-age children and maternal and child health programs, for example, elementary school teachers, health department staff, and parents. Teachers are believed to be the key in the educational program. To improve their capability for teaching and reinforcement of sound oral health principles, they receive preservice, in-service, and follow-up training to cover oral health concepts, practice oral hygiene skills, and integrate oral health into the curriculum.

To facilitate teacher effectiveness, the Oral Health Section developed an "Alignment for Dental Public Health Education" to help teachers use the "Framework for Dental Health Education," as schools implement the 1996 curriculum for the North Carolina State Board of Education. Several additional teaching aids are available for North Carolinians, such as more than 50 different pamphlets, worksheets, and handouts on nutrition, fluoride, sealants, plaque control, routine dental visits, injury prevention, and smokeless tobacco. In addition, the film library contains approximately 30 films, videos, and slide sets on oral health, which are free on loan to any school in the state, in addition to the framework videos, which have been distributed to each county. Between 2001 and 2006, all educational materials will be evaluated and revised if needed or new materials created to meet needs of the changing and diverse population. Because of budget limitations, the materials are made available only to educators and health professionals in North Carolina.

The Oral Health Section's staff and local public health staff traditionally screen elementary school students each year for caries. Fifth-grade students are evaluated for the presence of dental sealants in their permanent teeth. In the 1996–1997 school year, the Oral Health Section implemented a technique to modify and standardize dental screenings to give a new "assessment" process. This assessment gives a simple measurement of decayed and filled teeth that was added to the public health dental hygienists' annual screenings to give an indication of the prevalence of dental disease by county. Intense training and calibration increased the comparability and accuracy, and therefore the usefulness, of the dental data so that they can be better used by the counties. This assessment technique is used annually for all kindergarten and fifth-grade children in North Carolina. These data allow county and state health personnel to use this information to develop better county profiles for program planning and funding requests, to monitor dental disease levels over time, to compare disease in one county with another, and to provide accountability for expenditure of funds for public health programs.

During 1998 the Oral Health Section in the Department of Health and Human Services (which was then the Dental Health Section) celebrated the eightieth anniversary of dental public health in the state. The anniversary theme was "Seal the State in '98". The goal of "Seal the State in '98" was to prevent dental decay in children, particularly those children at high risk for dental disease, by increasing the number of sealants on children's teeth. This anniversary celebration was a cooperative venture of the North Carolina Dental Society, citizens, government, private business, and practicing dentists in coordination with the North Carolina Citizens for Public Health, Inc., which is a unique nonprofit corporation for the promotion of public health in North Carolina. "Seal the State in '98" would not have been the success it was without the tremendous support of its contributing partners. More than $110,000 was raised through outside contributions, and $1,130,801 was given as in-kind contributions for community sealant projects. The Oral Health Section had three objectives:

1. *Sealant placement*—to have free community-based sealant promotions in every county of the state on or about February 6, 1998, for at-risk children. All 100 counties had a promotion, including the four counties that have no privately practicing dentist. Sealants were placed on 8828 children as part of "Seal the State in '98". More than 68% of the targeted children were categorized as low income. The total number of sealants placed was 39,387, an average of 4.46 sealants per child. The children categorized as low income received 21,512 sealants.
2. *Sealant education*—to deliver an education sealant message to three citizens for every child who received sealants. The education message was designed to motivate parents to take their children to the dentist for dental sealants and to highlight the need for dental sealants. This education occurred in conjunction with the local sealant placement projects, classroom education sessions, health fairs, and community groups.

Various educational tools were used to spread the dental sealant message, which included exhibits, public service announcements, posters, pencils, bookmarks, banners, rulers, newsletters, report card and payroll inserts, and public resolutions. The educational message reached 195,000 North Carolinians. "Seal the State in '98" received record-breaking media attention for public health in all the major media markets of the state. There was coverage on broadcast television, cable, and radio and in print media. The donated media coverage was worth more than $600,000. The second strategy was to educate providers about the effectiveness and underutilization of dental sealants in North Carolina. To accomplish this, the Oral Health Section held a symposium in January 1998 with national dental experts providing continuing education sessions for public and private dental professionals from across the state.

3. *Partnerships*—to strengthen dental public health partnerships, both state and local, in order to collaborate more effectively to improve the oral health of North Carolinians. There was tremendous community support from more than 8000 individual volunteers. One in three practicing dentists (916), 1 in 4.5 dental hygienists (670), and 1145 dental assistants volunteered their time. Sixty percent of the total volunteers were from outside the dental profession.

The most important benefit of "Seal the State in '98" was consciousness raising. As a result, more children and adults are aware of dental sealants, more parents want sealants for their children, and more dentists are incorporating sealants into their practices.

NORTH CAROLINA'S EDUCATION/PROMOTION INITIATIVES HIGHLIGHTING SEALANTS

The sealant initiative is designed to help the state of North Carolina meet the Oral Health Section objective to increase the number of children who have dental sealants. The primary goal of the health education/health promotion component is for every person in the state to have heard or read about dental sealants. This initiative has the following major parts:

- School-based sealant demonstration projects are targeted to children, parents, and personnel in the school setting. They are designed to educate children, parents, and others in the community about the need for sealants and to encourage them to seek sealants from their private dentists. A team of public health dentists and dental hygienists conducts the projects. These are planned with input from the school superintendent, selected principals, the health director, and privately practicing dentists. After an educational campaign involving all the children in the school, parents, and community groups, a temporary "school dental office" is set up in the school where sealants are placed on eligible children at no cost to the participants.
- Thirteen copies of North Carolina's interactive health promotion exhibit, "Common Sense and Sealants," are stra-

tegically placed across the state. These are used by dental public health staff in parent meetings, mall exhibitions, and health fairs and are targeted to middle-income parents to encourage them to ask their family dentist about sealants for their child and to provide basic information about dental sealants.

- Sealant promotion in private offices is a public/private partnership in which privately practicing dentists use their facilities to place sealants on eligible children at no cost. Several models of the partnership exist. One public/private partnership model uses the resources of private dental offices and staff with a specific number of appointment slots reserved during regular office hours. The appointments are filled with eligible children identified by public health staff. Another public/private partnership model uses the private office facility where sealants are placed on eligible children by private practitioners and public health practitioners working side by side for a designated number of days. More dentists open their private offices for sealant promotions each year.
- A statewide media campaign targeted to middle-income parents was designed to encourage parents to request sealants for their children's teeth when they visit their dentist. The first part of this campaign used a public service announcement featuring Richard Petty, well-known North Carolinian race car driver, as the spokesperson for dental sealants. Former Lt. Governor Dennis Wicker and his children were highlighted in a second public service sealant announcement. The public service announcements were distributed to stations across the state in addition to being available for dental public health staff to distribute through cable access channels. In 1995 the 15- and 30-second public service announcements received 61 minutes of air time as an in-kind contribution valued at $157,349. These were used during the "Seal the State in '98" promotion and continue to be used today.*

Program Evaluation

Evaluation has been and will continue to be a necessary, ongoing process to measure the effectiveness of the oral health program.[108-110,114,116]

1. The results of a 1968 survey of schoolchildren at the Happy Valley School in Caldwell County, North Carolina, where the school water supply had been fluoridated for 8 years, indicated a 34% reduction in decayed, missing, and filled permanent teeth for children who had 8 years' experience drinking fluoridated water at school.
2. Data collected in the 1976 replication of the 1963 Fulton-Hughes survey were used to evaluate long-range goals and objectives.
3. A 1976 survey of schoolchildren in Asheville, North Carolina, where the community's water supply had been fluoridated for 10 years, revealed a 53% reduction in decayed, missing, and filled permanent teeth for children who

*For additional information on school-based and community outreach dental programs, contact Doranna Anderson, BSED, RHED, Head, Oral Health Education and Promotion Branch, Oral Health Section, Division of Public Health, North Carolina Department of Health and Human Services, 1910 Mail Service Center, Raleigh, NC 27699-1910.

had had 10 years' experience drinking fluoridated water.

4. A 1984 survey on the use of sealants in public health dental programs demonstrated an 86% total sealant retention rate after 4 years on permanent teeth.
5. A statewide oral health survey of 7000 school-age children in 1986–1987 had the following objectives: (1) to describe the oral health status and factors associated with this status by recording the survey participants' decayed, missing, and filled teeth or surfaces for primary and permanent dentition; number of teeth sealed with dental sealants; extent of gingivitis; and restorative and exodontic treatment needs; (2) to determine the extent, type, and frequency of use of smokeless tobacco products, patterns of use, and knowledge of harmful effects; and (3) to establish a policy advisory committee to the Oral Health Section.
6. In 1994 a study was conducted to look at the effectiveness of the North Carolina school-based fluoride programs: fluoride mouth rinse and school water fluoridation. The Oral Health Section collaborated with faculty at the University of North Carolina Schools of Public Health and Dentistry and the North Carolina Dental Society. The study showed that the fluoride mouth rinse was more effective in reducing caries than the school water fluoridators. As the programs have operated in North Carolina, the fluoride mouth rinse program was also more efficient at approximately one sixth the cost per person of the school water fluoridation program. School selection for the school water fluoridators was always limited and was becoming more difficult because of technical and logistic problems. Based on the results of this analysis, the school water fluoridation program, started in 1968, was discontinued statewide. Fluoride mouth rinse continues to be provided to targeted children.

SPECIAL OLYMPICS, SPECIAL SMILES: AN EXPANDING EFFORT TO REACH OUT TO PEOPLE WITH SPECIAL NEEDS IN A NONTRADITIONAL SETTING

Program Development

For people with mental retardation and other developmental disabilities, dental care often takes a back seat to more pressing medical issues. In fact, oral health is one of the most serious concerns facing these individuals and those who care for them.

For the majority of people with mental retardation, access to dental care is severely limited or, in many cases, completely denied. Many dentists and hygienists believe that they are inadequately trained in special patient care. Because employees of group homes and other care settings are often inexperienced, underpaid, and poorly trained, oral care is not a priority. The side effects of medications and other physical and mental concerns create or complicate dental problems.

Perhaps the most significant cause of poor access to care is lack of financing. Health care for persons with mental retardation is provided by Medicaid, which offers dental care only until a child becomes an adult. Beyond that threshold, in most states even the most basic preventive care is not offered. Currently, most states do not offer adult dental services through Medicaid. In the few states that do, however, the reimbursement levels are so low that most practitioners are reluctant to participate.

In 1993 Special Olympics, Special Smiles (SOSS) was founded as a national oral health screening, education, and referral initiative for the athletes of Special Olympics International (SOI) through the efforts of Dr. Steven Perlman, Associate Clinical Professor of Pediatric Dentistry at Boston University School of Dental Medicine, and Eunice Kennedy Shriver, founder and honorary chairman of SOI. SOSS was developed collaboratively among Boston University, SOI, Oral Health America (formerly the American Fund for Dental Health), and the Academy of Dentistry for Persons with Disabilities. Initially, SOSS was sponsored with the help of many organizations and through the primary sponsorship of Colgate-Palmolive and its subsidiary Colgate Oral Pharmaceuticals.[117] The SOSS program has grown into a global oral health education, screening, and referral initiative. SOI implements programming activities via partnerships with sponsors—Colgate Oral Pharmaceuticals, Inc., Philips Oral Healthcare, and several other collaborating organizations: the ADA Health Foundation, Alpha Omega, Kodak Dental Imaging, Oral Health America, Patterson Dental Supply Company, Dentsply, Sultan Chemists, The Grottoes of North America, State Farm Insurance, and Boston University School of Dental Medicine. SOSS has become one of the largest oral health programs serving people with special needs worldwide.[117]

Program Philosophy and Goals

In 1993 a mission statement and program goals were adopted. SOSS is an oral health initiative designed to improve access to dental care for people with special needs and to raise the public's and the dental community's awareness of the oral health problems many of those with special needs face. This will be accomplished by working with SOI, its state chapters, and its national programs in a caring and supportive environment and with the firm conviction that oral health is vital to overall health.

The program goals are as follows:[118]*

1. Conduct dental screening and educational programs, collecting disease surveillance data among special athletes at Special Olympics events around the world for dissemination to agencies and state health departments to facilitate evidence-based planning in addressing the oral health needs of this population.
2. Increase dental professionals' awareness of the particular oral health concerns that people with special needs face. This will be accomplished, in part, through participation in the Special Olympics programs.
3. Provide lists of regional dental professionals who care for people with special needs to all athletes who participate in the Special Olympics dental programs.
4. Continue to update and implement dental education programs for dental professionals, dental schools, community residences, institutional facilities, and Special Olympics athletes. This will also serve to promote Special Olympics as a recreation program and reach populations that are difficult to access (particularly persons with profound retardation or severe physical handicaps).

*For more information about Special Olympics, Special Smiles, see www.SpecialOlympics.org or contact Dawn Munson, Special Olympics International, Inc., 1325 G Street, N.W., Suite 500, Washington, DC 20005-3104, phone: (202)628-3630.

5. Conduct disease surveillance among special athletes.
6. Serve as advocates on standards and equality-of-care issues.
7. By working with Special Olympics medical consultants, ensure that athletes who participate in Special Olympics dental programs have access to the most current information on medical issues.
8. Maintain a sports injury prevention program for Special Olympics athletes.
9. Promote nutritional guidelines and programs for Special Olympics athletes in collaboration with the American Dietetic Association.
10. Help develop adaptive devices and orofacial sports programs for quadriplegics.
11. Work with established programs to help dental professionals recognize and report suspected physical and sexual abuse in patients with special needs.

The objectives of Special Olympics Healthy Athlete events are to

- Improve access and health care for Special Olympics athletes at event-based health screenings
- Make referrals to local health practitioners when appropriate
- Train health care professionals and students in the health professions about the needs and care of people with mental retardation
- Collect, analyze, and disseminate data on the health status and needs of people with mental retardation

To achieve these objectives, SOI enlists the support of oral health care professionals who volunteer their time to provide services at the events, as well as funds to give more athletes the opportunity to participate in the games.

Effective summer 2001, the reader will be able to access a list of dental providers (by city, state, zip code, and country) open to accepting special needs patients in their practices (www.specialsmiles.org). Dentists may also register to participate in the referral resource network.

Program Implementation

Since 1994 SOSS has offered screening events, many in inner-city neighborhoods, at Special Olympics games around the country and has expanded globally. Dental practitioners, dental students, dental hygienists, and dental hygiene students participate in this community oral health experience. Students have an opportunity to become acquainted with people with special needs, become sensitized to the needs of the population, and enjoy personal gratification in providing a valuable community service for an underserved population. Each SOSS event includes one-on-one instruction with the athletes on proper brushing techniques and a noninvasive screening of oral health conditions. The athletes receive copies of the screening review (report card), a list of local dentists who treat patients with special needs, and a souvenir bag with toothbrush, toothpaste, educational booklet, and a commemorative gift (hat or T-shirt). In 1995 the program was offered at 11 regional Special Olympics games nationwide at sites in Miami, San Antonio, Kansas City, Philadelphia, New York, Boston, Los Angeles, New Orleans, Chicago, Atlanta, New London, Washington, D.C., and the international summer world games in New Haven, Connecticut.[118] As of 2001 SOSS had expanded to approximately 60 U.S. sites and six international sites. Nutritional counseling has also been provided to athletes at all sites. A mouth guard program for sports injury prevention was introduced at the World Games in New Haven in July 1995 and resulted in the fabrication of 2000 mouth guards for special athletes and has expanded to all sites willing to participate in this part of the program.[117]

In 1996 a continuing education course was developed for program volunteers of SOSS. The course was piloted in four locations. All sites now have access to the continuing education course/video at every SOSS event. Extensive data collection began in 1997 in collaboration with the CDC, so that a significant body of knowledge about the particular oral health problems of people with special needs would be developed.[117] This information is shared with state health departments in the United States to facilitate an evidence-based oral health needs assessment for this population and support efforts to expand necessary treatment services.

Special Smiles: A Guide to Good Oral Health for Persons with Special Needs was also developed as an educational tool in association with SOSS to help in establishing personal oral hygiene programs for persons with disabilities.[119] It was updated in 2001 to reflect the latest recommendations for caries prevention, including the use of fluoride varnishes. There are plans for future expansion of the screening events focusing on countries outside of the United States.[117]

Cost of Program

Funding is provided by the sponsors Colgate Oral Pharmaceuticals, Inc., and Philips Oral Healthcare; several other collaborating organizations cited previously; and other corporate and foundation contributions. Other community partners include local dental and dental hygiene schools, state and national dental hygiene societies and associations, national oral health associations, the CDC, and dental and dental hygiene practitioners from across the country who volunteer their services. There is significant reliance on donation of goods, funds, and volunteer services.[117]

Program Evaluation

In 2001 SOSS succeeded in partnering with 39 dental schools and 40 dental hygiene schools, as well as several state and national dental associations. Approximately 2500 dentists, hygienists, and students turn out annually to participate at the events. More than 16,000 athletes are scheduled for screenings in the 2001 season of regional and world winter games from 80 countries. According to SOI, for each athlete participating in the program at least four more people will be touched by the experience. Therefore approximately 60,000 family members, caregivers, coaches, and volunteers will be reached through SOSS participation in the current year. Data collection protocols are currently being reviewed. Further development is underway to create a more comprehensive data retrieval system, which will include site-specific data modules. This will offer greater flexibility, expand the data collection system, and facilitate monitoring of athlete referrals for access to care at all sites. Treatment referrals and follow-up will take place using a duplicate system of report cards prioritizing individuals in need of immediate care. SOSS's local events coordinators facilitate media outreach efforts to promote SOSS activities in conjunction with local dental schools using a press packet provided by SOI that continues to successfully generate pre-event, on-site, and postevent publicity for the events.[120]

SUGGESTED APPROACHES

Table 11-2 provides a brief summary of the community oral health education programs described here. Each of the community oral health education programs that has been described was chosen for three reasons: (1) they are some of the most widely known and reported in the literature, (2) they represent a variety of approaches to oral health education, and (3) they illustrate the range of success that can be expected to be achieved, given their programmatic structure and goals. With the criteria that are presented in Chapters 10 and 12, several issues for discussion should become apparent. For instance, if we assume that the goal for an oral health education program for the community is to reduce the prevalence of dental caries, which of the programs, if any, is using the most cost-effective and clinically proven preventive measures? Which of the programs is using evaluation criteria that will measure caries experience? Which of the programs has determined its priorities on the basis of the collection of data gathered through a formal needs assessment? Which programs are easily implemented and administered? Answers to these questions begin to identify the strengths and weaknesses in the programs.

Yacavone[9] has noted, "Some authorities in community health feel that prevention will only be successful when individual behavior is eliminated." If this is the case, community educational efforts must focus on those disease prevention strategies that require the least compliance on the part of the individual. This would require a reorientation to health education and its goal and redirecting the educational efforts to community leaders in an attempt to improve the oral health status through organized community efforts.[22]

This is not to say that school-based educational programs should be eliminated or are not valuable; it does, however, indicate the need for further behavioral research and the need for communities to decide which of the preventive programs and the strategies or measures now used in each program should take priority. If community leaders are expected to make these decisions, they must be given the tools to do so. This would necessitate a new role or new responsibilities for the community oral health educator. Frazier[22] states that the appropriate educational methods for this target group are those designed to (1) provide accurate information about the relative merits of various disease prevention and control measures and (2) stimulate group decision making and action regarding the adoption of effective organized programs.

If these new responsibilities are to be assumed, we must know whether community oral health educators are prepared and willing to adopt this new role. Environmental change and societal needs and expectations will necessitate that we expand functions and responsibilities to care for community health, practice prevention, and promote healthy lifestyles. In the oral health care field, dental hygienists are the preventive health education specialists and as such must prepare for new and challenging roles, both in and out of the traditional dental office, without reliance on the direct supervision of a dentist in alternative practice settings (i.e., nursing homes, school-based dental programs, health centers, etc.).[121]

In 1995 the Institute of Medicine released the report *Dental Education at the Crossroads: Challenges and Change,* which examined dental education and proposed 22 recommendations for future dental education.[122] The committee recommends the "more produc-

Table 11-2. Summary of Dental Health Education Programs in Terms of Development, Program Philosophy and Goals, Implementation, Costs, and Evaluation

	Characteristics of Program	
Name of Program	***Development***	***Philosophy and Goals***
Texas Department of Health, Tattletooth II program (Pre-K thru 6th), parent program, senior citizen program, PEP, nursing home program, school nurse training program	Texas Department of Health	Goal—reduce dental caries and develop positive dental habits to last a lifetime Program tries to convince students that preventing dental caries is important and they can do it Program focuses on dental health as part of total health
North Carolina dental public health program	North Carolina Division of Dental Health, dental organizations, Department of Public Instruction, University of North Carolina School of Dentistry and School of Public Health, plus support of general assembly Based on documented needs assessment of North Carolina citizens	Prevention and education: prevention and education are most effective methods to significantly change prevalence and incidence of dental disease and to promote, protect, and ensure oral health for citizens Priority—children Mission: ensure conditions in which North Carolina citizens can achieve optimal oral health Long-range plan for continuing use of dental health materials in competency-based curriculum "Framework for Dental Health Education"—emphasizes role of classroom elementary teacher for integrating dental health education into curriculum
Special Athletes/Special Smiles	Partnership formed between Boston University School of Dental Medicine, Oral Health America, Academy of Dentistry for Persons with Disabilities, and Special Olympics International	Provide unique opportunity to open door to dental health and fuller health for people with special needs in unconventional environment Priority—Special Olympians Mission: sensitize, educate, and encourage dental professional to assist people with special needs in obtaining dental services, enjoyment of oral health and improved quality of life; increase access to care and pool of skilled professionals to treat population

Characteristics of Program		
Methods	*Funding*	*Implementation*
Dental hygienists serve as technical consultants for school districts and promote dental education for expectant women, parents, and senior citizens Supportive materials are available for teachers and program hygienists		
Statewide implementation plan Teachers are trained to present dental health information for school-age population	Estimated at $0.60 per child; state-legislated budget	Field testing Statewide continuous monitoring of material use
Priorities are community water fluoridation; fluoride mouth rinse programs and sealants Public health dental staff provides training and consultative services to teachers, parents, professionals, and community Media campaign promoting sealants Several teaching adjuncts are available: curriculum videotapes, guides, and exhibits	State budget includes salaries	Comprehensive survey of dental disease in 1976 and 1986–1987 funded by Kate B. Reynolds Health Care Trust Survey to assess sealant retention in 1984 Survey of schoolchildren after 10 years of community water fluoridation and 8 years of rural school water fluoridation After 26 years of school water fluoridation in rural communities, 1994 study finds fluoride mouth rinse more effective, more efficient, and less costly in reducing dental caries than school water fluoridation is Survey of fifth and sixth graders to assess presence of dental sealants
Volunteer dentists, hygienists, assistants and students facilitate oral screenings, referrals, and oral health education services Priorities are to provide services for people with special needs (i.e., mental retardation and developmental disabilities); raise public and professional awareness of severity of oral health needs; offer continuing education course for Special Athletes/Special Smiles volunteers; increase access to care; data collection to better assess oral health conditions of population	Primary sponsorship provided by Colgate-Palmolive and its subsidiary Colgate Oral Pharmaceuticals; other partners: Boston University, Oral Health America, and other corporations and foundations	Oral screenings for >10,000 athletes at 11 regional events and Special Olympics World Summer Games, which attracted athletes from 143 countries in 1995 Pilot testing of continuing education course at four locations in 1996 Pilot testing oral health survey instrument 1996, revisions and further testing planned in cooperation with Centers for Disease Control and Prevention

tive use of allied dental personnel in the provision of services to underserved populations" and recognizes the need for "new and challenging roles for dental hygienists" and for "more rather than less education." This recommendation supports the ADHA's objective to expand access to care for consumers, enhance career opportunities for dental hygienists, and increase the number and types of settings in which dental hygienists practice.[123]

Although dental and dental hygiene students generally participate in school-based community programs, other types of organized community efforts should serve as viable field experience alternatives. Following are several issues that require professional support and involvement and are currently receiving national attention:

1. Water fluoridation
2. Appropriate use of fluoride mouth rinses, supplements, and topical applications, including fluoride varnish
3. Oral cancer prevention
4. Early childhood caries
5. Sealants
6. Frequency of use, types of product used, patterns of use, and knowledge about the harmful effects of smokeless tobacco
7. Efforts by consumer interest and child advocacy groups to monitor and restrict advertising of cariogenic, high-cholesterol, nonnutritious foods and tobacco advertising and violence in programming directed at children
8. Infection control measures
9. Access to care for special needs populations
10. Domestic violence identification and referral
11. Issues of cultural and linguistic diversity
12. *Healthy People 2010* national health promotion and disease prevention objectives[124]

The need for active participation in these areas cannot be overemphasized.

One of the objectives in *Healthy People 2010* is the proposed increase to at least 75% in the proportion of people served by community water systems providing optimal levels of fluoride.[124] This would require that approximately 30 million people gain access to the benefits of fluoride through the addition of community water fluoridation to the public water supply systems.[125] Visible support and action in the community, for instance, can make the difference in whether a referendum for water fluoridation is passed.[125-129]

Community water fluoridation continues to be both a legal and political issue. Statewide ballots to prohibit fluoridation have surfaced, and there have also been attempts by antifluoridationists to rescind fluoridation in communities where the water supply is currently fluoridated by promoting legislation to allow local option (home rule) for fluoridation in the eight states that currently mandate fluoridation—Connecticut, Georgia, Illinois, Michigan, Minnesota, Nebraska, Ohio, and South Dakota.[125]

Although there is broad support for water fluoridation among scientists, health professionals, and the courts as safe, cost-effective, practical, equitable, and in accord with individual rights guaranteed by the U.S. constitution, opponents have been successful in defeating fluoridation efforts by creating an illusion of controversy and inciting fear.[125]

Two examples illustrating this point are

the defeat of the referendum to continue water fluoridation in Flagstaff, Arizona, in 1978 and the passage of the referendum in Seattle, Washington, in 1973.

Fluoridation in each of these cases and in most cases has proved to be a highly emotionally charged issue. In Flagstaff, organized opponents to water fluoridation, namely, the National Health Federation (NHF), held public forums and disseminated large amounts of propaganda. The usual tactic was to link fluoridation to cancer. Other arguments—that fluoridation is unconstitutional, fluoridation is a form of medication, and fluoridation is contrary to the right of "free choice of health care"—were also cited.[130] To combat these unscientific charges and the emotional fervor with which they are made, it is incumbent on all dental professionals in the community and students during their training to familiarize themselves with the strategies of the NHF and other antifluoridation groups and with the documented evidence refuting their claims. It is also a professional responsibility to educate voters, community leaders, and agencies regarding the benefits of fluoridation and regarding movements opposed to fluoridation, which pose a danger to the oral health of the community.

In the Flagstaff, Arizona, case an initial survey indicated that the referendum would pass 2 to 1; however, the NHF was able to reverse this prediction by creating an illusion of scientific controversy. Fortunately, in Seattle, Washington, the opposition was not as active or as successful. Here the dental profession focused on building a broad base of community support; it educated people to understand the workings of the ballot and on how to vote. Fifteen days before voters went to the poll, dental and dental hygiene students along with community volunteers actively campaigned door to door for fluoridation. Communities should examine this successful strategy where fluoridation is an issue. Success at one point does not mean that at some future date the decision could not be reversed, as it was in Flagstaff. In 1980, 41 fluoridation referenda were held in the United States; of those, only eight approved fluoridation. Between 1977 and 1982, approximately 25% of the ballot measures on fluoridation were approved. Dental professionals must continue to be visible in the community to reinforce the benefits of fluoridation and the decision made by the voters. Oral health education must be provided on a continuous basis if it is to serve as a means for health promotion.[125] According to the CDC, 23 communities in the United States had fluoridation initiatives on their presidential ballots on November 7, 2000. Voters in nine communities voted in favor of taking action to fluoridate their community water supplies, whereas voters in 14 communities voted against water fluoridation.

Student activities and the degree of involvement in each of the listed areas may vary from state to state. An examination of existing legislation and accreditation standards for primary and secondary schools can provide students with "ammunition" to assist communities in improving oral health. Action taken by the Alabama Dental Association to eliminate the sale of sweets in local schools led to their discovery of the Southern Association of Schools' accreditation standard, which prohibits the sale of sweets in schools, and resulted in its enforcement. The Accrediting Division of the Department of Education was not enforcing the standard because it did not have a working definition of the word "confection." The Alabama Dental Association and the Alabama Nutrition Council were able to provide the needed definition and a list of acceptable snack foods. This effort should serve as an example of what can be accomplished, and it identifies activities in which students can become involved.[13]

As the oral health preventive education specialist, the dental hygienist is uniquely qualified to instruct patients on preventive self-examination, implement the Clinical Practice Guidelines for Treating Tobacco Use and Dependence, and implement the National Cancer Institute's "How to Help Your Patients Stop Using Tobacco" program in a variety of practice settings.[131] Knowledge of addiction, the effects of nicotine on the human body, and options for nicotine replacement therapies and tobacco treatment programs are necessary, as well as a professional/practice commitment to implement a sound tobacco intervention system. Enhancing patients' understanding of the seriousness of the effects of tobacco use may increase their receptivity to tobacco cessation advice. However, there remains a need to provide more complete and accurate information regarding tobacco and alcohol addiction and patient management issues in the dental hygiene curriculum. Dentists and dental hygienists do not routinely engage in tobacco use assessment or cessation interventions with their patients, and what could be teachable moments are frequently missed opportunities. Health educators can actively promote and support legislative action on the local, state, and national levels to address the issues of youth access to tobacco and smoking in public places, restaurants, and the workplace.

Dental professionals can also take an active role in developing school-based dental sealant programs in their communities by use of a new resource manual developed by the American Association of Community Dental Programs. *Seal America: The Prevention Invention* includes a 10-minute video and a manual that covers the following topics: selecting a target population, winning community support, program budget, funding, implementation, and evaluation.[132]

Educational experiences in these areas will afford students the opportunity to begin developing necessary organizational and planning skills. Only through working with dental and other professional societies, state and local agencies, and community leaders and decision makers can an organized community effort be effective in preventing and controlling dental disease. Efforts to increase levels of knowledge of the public and the dental profession about oral disease prevention are required to achieve national objectives for oral health.[133]

Research

Oral diseases continue to be among the most prevalent problems in our society, despite the importance of oral health to personal overall health and well-being.[133] The most promising avenue to improving oral health lies in the prevention of dental disease.

The National Institute of Dental and Craniofacial Research (NIDCR) National Caries Program conducted an 11-year study beginning in 1972 to determine the long-term effects of the combination of student-applied fluoride agents (fluoride mouth rinse, fluoride tablets, and fluoride toothpaste) among schoolchildren living in a rural area with low concentrations of fluoride in the drinking water. Participating students ingested a 1 mg fluoride tablet and rinsed weekly with a 0.2% sodium fluoride solution. The children also received fluoride dentifrice and toothbrushes for home use throughout the calendar year. In 1983 dental examinations of study participants ages 6 through 17 years, who had continuously participated in the program for 1 to 11 years depending on school grade, showed a mean prevalence of 3.12 decayed, missing, or filled surfaces, which was 65% lower than the corresponding score of 9.02 decayed, missing, or filled surfaces for children of the same ages at the baseline examinations. The preventive program inhibited decay in all types of surfaces: 54% in occlusal surfaces, 59% in buccolingual surfaces, and 90% in mesiodistal surfaces.[134]

The National Preventive Dentistry Demonstration Program (NPDDP), carried out between 1976 and 1983, was the largest, most comprehensive school-based preventive dentistry program ever conducted. Its purpose was to determine the costs and effectiveness of several types and combinations of generally accepted school-based preventive dental procedures to provide the database for developing the most effective modern school-based preventive dental program. The preventive procedures selected included five general categories: (1) fluorides (topical and systemic), (2) sealants, (3) diet regulation, (4) plaque control, and (5) classroom health education. The major findings from this program include the following:[135]

1. There was a sharp decline in the prevalence of dental caries from the late 1970s to the early 1980s.
2. The application of dental sealants was the most effective preventive measure of those used in the program.
3. Community water fluoridation was effective in reducing dental caries.
4. Classroom-based preventive measures were ineffective.

The study was reviewed and critiqued by a review committee of the American Public Health Association. Although the committee had reservations as to the specific design of the study and the analytic methods applied, their consensus was that the first three findings of the study appear to be correct. The fourth finding is considered questionable because of possible flaws in the study design. Niessen[136] forecasts that health education programs will continue to be an important component of the dental public health program.

The NPDDP suggests several elements of dental research that need improvement or greater emphasis. The profession should adopt a more conservative attitude when projecting the expected benefits from the practical application of preventive measures whose merit is supported by only a few clinical trials conducted by a limited number of investigators. Many clinical trials conducted by independent investigators should be mandated before any preventive measure is regarded as safe, effective, and efficient.

Neglecting basic research while pushing ahead with practical application is imprudent. The lack of basic research on the mechanism of fluoride action in the prevention of dental decay and in the production of enamel fluorosis was evident from this study. Several of the modes of application of the agent may have been duplicating rather than reinforcing each other.

Greater attention should be given to monitoring the prevalence of dental diseases so that up-to-date indices are available that will further delineate characteristics of populations to be studied. There is a need for maintenance of an established pool of skilled clinical investigators who would be available to take part in large-scale national clinical trials. Also, there is a need to foster new research leading to improved clinical trial methods, reduced cost, and possibly reduction in the size of groups to be studied.

As a result of this study, two additional areas of research have been identified: (1) there is a definite need to develop and apply better outcome measures for the evaluation of the effectiveness of school oral health education programs, and (2) more research is needed to identify the significant characteristics of groups susceptible to dental diseases.

In 1986 to 1987 the NIDCR conducted the National Survey of Dental Caries in U.S. School Children, which revealed that 53% of children ages 6 through 8 years and 78% of 15-year-olds had caries.[137] Further, the proportion of African-American and Hispanic adolescents with untreated decay was approximately 65% higher than for the total population. Periodontal disease was also prevalent. Results from the North Carolina School Oral Health Survey of 1986 to 1987 referenced earlier parallel much of the data from the NIDCR survey.[114]

From 1988 to 1994 the NIDCR conducted the National Health and Nutrition Examination Survey (NHANES III). These data will assist oral health providers in assessing which age and ethnic groups are in greatest need. Some of the most noteworthy survey results follow. Tooth decay in children and adolescents continues to decline, with 55% of children and adolescents with caries-free permanent teeth. African-American children had the highest caries-free rate of 61%, followed by white children at 55% and Mexican-American children at 51%. Only 33% of 12- to 17-year-olds were caries free in their permanent dentitions. Although 80% of the caries in the permanent teeth of children and adolescents had been treated, African-American children had more than twice as much untreated decay as white children did. Among 2- to 9-year-olds, 62% had no caries in the primary teeth. Among 2- to 4-year-olds, 87% of white children were caries free in the primary dentition compared with 78% of African-American children and 68% of Mexican-American children. Dental caries in the primary teeth of 2- to 9-year-old children were left untreated in 47% of the study subjects, with Mexican-American children having the highest rate of untreated teeth, 62%, followed by 59% for African-American children and 41% for white children. Since 1987 dental sealant use has more than doubled but still remains low, with only 22% of white children, 8% of African-American children, and 7% of Mexican-American children benefiting from this effective preventive treatment.[1]

Survey results relative to tooth decay and tooth loss in adults revealed that 94% of people age 18 years and over have had either untreated decay or fillings in the crowns of their teeth. On average, American adults had 22 decayed, missing, or filled coronal surfaces. Women had more caries than men (24 surfaces versus 21) but had less untreated decay. White adults had the highest rate of coronal caries (24 surfaces), followed by Mexican-American adults (14 surfaces) and African-American adults (12 surfaces). Root caries was noted in 23% of adults. Only 10% of adults are missing all their teeth. Among adults age 75 or older, 44% were missing all their teeth. Among adults age 18 to 74 years, roughly 20% wore removable dentures with 60% reporting problems with their appliances.[2]

In terms of periodontal disease in adolescents and adults, it was found that women had better periodontal health than men; white adolescents and adults had fewer periodontal problems than did African-Americans and Mexican-Americans. Moderate attachment loss of 3 to 4 mm was noted in 30% of 25- to 34-year-olds, 63% of

45- to 54-year-olds, and 80% of people more than 65 years old; 15% of those surveyed exhibited more severe loss of attachment of 5 mm or greater. The highest prevalence of bleeding gums was among adolescents (13 to 17 years old), with three fourths of those surveyed bleeding on gentle probing.[3]

NHANES III included an assessment of tooth trauma and occlusal problems, which found that 25% of Americans between ages 6 and 50 years had sustained injury to the incisors. It was also found that one fourth of children and adults ages 8 to 50 years had perfect alignment of the front teeth. Both malocclusion and orthodontic treatment were more common in whites than in African-Americans or Mexican-Americans. Eighteen percent of children and adolescents and 20% of adults had undergone orthodontic treatment.[138]

Survey statistics suggest that several challenges face future oral health care professionals. Harold Slavkin, former NIDCR director, identified the top three challenges. First is the changing patterns of disease. Birth rates are up—4.2 million live births per year, which reflects an increase of one-half million more than in 1992 to 1993. Population projections for 2010 suggest that one in five Americans will be age 65 years or older and that pressing oral health issues will focus on conditions such as chronic facial pain, temporomandibular disorders, xerostomia, and implants. These demographic changes point to access to care and managed health care as the other two top challenges. Slavkin also sees managed health care as having a direct impact on the nation's oral health primarily because of issues of quality of life and access to care, especially for children born in abject poverty and for senior citizens who are homebound or have special needs. Further, Slavkin notes that "one-third of the U.S. population has no access to oral health care. By either state and/or federal legislation and the goodwill of managed health care companies, we must meet the special challenge to get these people access to care."[139]

Given that fluoridation is highly cost-effective and requires no behavior change on the part of the individual to produce its effects, future research should explore strategies for increasing its acceptance.[74] In fluoridated areas surveys should be conducted to determine whether families are consuming fluoridated tap water versus purchased bottled water, which may lack the appropriate fluoride content. Perhaps targeting groups at high risk may be a more effective way to reach individuals affected with caries.[136]

Oral Health in America: A Report of the Surgeon General

In 2000 the Surgeon General of the United States released a landmark report on the state of oral health in America. This report includes a review of the status of oral health in America and ways to promote and maintain oral health and prevent oral disease. Specific methods to prevent oral disease in the community, as well as at the individual level, are discussed, including school-based prevention programs. Interested readers are strongly advised to review this important resource, which is discussed in detail in Chapter 2.[25]

SUMMARY

An analysis of the information presented in this chapter leads to several conclusions regarding the status and future of community oral health education programs. We have seen that the traditional educational activities based on either the cognitive or behavioral models of learning alone cannot be effective in achieving the goal of disease prevention and control. Techniques developed and refined for educating an individual patient differ from those that should be applied to the community. Behavioral research and expert opinions agree that educational methods are now available that can be successfully applied to the community at large, as demonstrated by the Stanford Five City Project and the Minnesota Home Team Project.

Are dental public health professionals ready and willing to use the public health model for contemporary health education and to foster community involvement in decision making? The challenge remains for health care professionals in the private and public sectors, for school programs, and for the news media to develop and implement a variety of relevant, culturally sensitive, and effective approaches to enhance public knowledge of the appropriate use of fluorides and dental sealants, control of gingival conditions, and the value of community water fluoridation, specifically for adults in their roles as eligible voters or parents. Will such community involvement change the perception of dental disease so that persons will seek early detection and treatment for problems? Will financial barriers continue to alienate many subgroups within American society from obtaining desired or needed dental treatment? Are we fostering public and private sector partnerships to advance health education and health promotion in a managed care environment? Are we continuing to build a strong network of support for dental public health by forming coalitions with other health care professionals, industry, legislators, parents, patients, and health advocacy organizations? Are we prepared to leave politics behind to create high-performance teams of dental professionals with expanded functions, responsibilities, and shared benefits that are highly productive, efficient, and cost-effective to meet societal needs and expectations? Are we as health professionals monitoring children's television programming and advertising to ensure that broadcasters carry children's educational or instructional programming that promotes health and well-being? Are we participating in efforts on the national, state, and local community levels to achieve *Healthy People 2010* national health promotion and disease prevention objectives?

Gift and colleagues[140] offer the following strategies to further the public's oral health: (1) changing guidelines for regulations and legislation to provide an oral disease prevention program in each state public health department and a federally sponsored health center; (2) permitting efficient and cost-effective delivery of services by oral health personnel; and (3) making policy, regulatory, or institutional changes to ensure adequate reimbursement in the public and private sectors for age-appropriate oral disease prevention strategies. In May 2000 the U.S. Surgeon General issued a call for action for policy initiatives to develop a National Oral Health Plan that will provide a framework for coordinated efforts to eliminate oral health disparities and improve the quality of life for all Americans. This goal can be achieved by forming collaborations among communities, policy makers, and health care providers who are willing to work together to increase the awareness of oral health and actions that can prevent oral diseases. Armed with the *Healthy People 2010* objectives, the *Surgeon General's Report on Oral Health in America,* and state-specific reports on the status of oral health, we are facing a unique opportunity to move the nation forward to address the problems that currently exist in oral health through grass roots advocacy.

With the significant role that dental professionals play in promoting tobacco-free lifestyles with patients of all ages, perhaps this is the time to lobby to ensure that funds from the multistate tobacco settlement are used as originally intended for tobacco prevention, education, policy development, enforcement, treatment, and health care. Oral health needs may finally be addressed as one of the pressing health care issues facing the United States. This can happen provided we hold our legislators accountable. We need to inform our legislators that diverting funds to other causes, which could be funded in many cases from state general funds, is unacceptable when oral health needs remain great.

Oral health education programs for the community should be applicable to all segments of the population and should be developed through appropriate program planning and implementation criteria to facilitate education of the public and health care providers to increase knowledge, understanding, and practices that foster improved oral health for the individual and the community.[140] A needs assessment should be conducted to define the extent of the problem and serve as baseline data and to determine program objectives and priorities, alternative solutions, and evaluation guidelines. Formative and summative evaluation must be a continuing, integral component of the plan; it must focus on measuring the program's effectiveness in terms of disease reduction, not merely increased knowledge or an improved performance level. Longitudinal behavioral studies should be conducted to validate the cost-benefit ratio and cost-effectiveness of each program. Existing curricula and field experiences for dental, dental hygiene, and dental assisting students must be reexamined and revised in light of the new responsibilities these professionals must assume in the community setting. Students should be educated in community organization; group dynamics; program planning and implementation strategies; effectiveness of community preventive measures; community decision-making processes; and the necessary communication, management, and leadership skills.

Research must continue to develop, test, and evaluate new combinations of preventive programs and to evaluate the effectiveness of any new strategies for community oral health education. More must be known about the relationship between plaque and dental caries and about the acquisition of oral health as a value. Community programs must use the approaches most likely to succeed against known barriers to receiving dental care and maintaining good oral health.

If the success of oral health education programs in schools is judged by effectiveness based on knowledge, attitudes, and skill acquisition, evaluators of such programs must be held accountable for conducting evaluation studies in a manner appropriate to these predetermined general objectives.

Oral health education in schools involves the efforts of many people. Universities and colleges charged with the responsibility of preparing school personnel must include oral health as a component of the curriculum. School districts also must explore ways of including oral health education on a permanent basis. Parents must be encouraged to support oral health activities through reinforcement at home and can also join health professionals in demanding that oral health education be a mandatory component of health education in every curriculum. We also need more professional support for proven effective preventive measures such as water fluoridation, appropriate use of fluoride supplements, and topical applications, especially fluoride varnishes and sealants.

Several major changes are taking place that will affect the dental profession and the oral health of the public: a reduction in tooth decay, an increased awareness of the prevalence of periodontal disease, infection control and dental treatment phobias associated with contraction of HIV disease, population demographics that may affect the prevalence of root caries, periodontal conditions and oral cancer in association with advancing age, an increased demand for services by people with developmental disabilities in accordance with the Americans with Disabilities Act of 1990, issues of domestic violence, and an alarming increase in the use of smokeless tobacco among American youth and the increase in oral cancer associated with tobacco use and alcohol consumption. Future planning in community oral health education will include the targeting of preventive measures for specific subgroups with documented unmet needs within the general population. Innovative programs for persons with developmental disabilities residing in the community and in state institutions and programs for the elderly (ambulatory, homebound, and institutionalized) have been developed. Homeless individuals and families, unemployed or underemployed and uninsured people, and children and adults who have HIV disease have a myriad of unaddressed needs, one of which is professional dental care. Creativity and resourcefulness in future program planning are essential in view of our finite resources, especially funding, which is so crucial to program development, implementation, and evaluation.

REVIEW QUESTIONS

1. Discuss an example of a successful dental education program from the chapter, including aspects of the program and why it should be considered successful.
2. List some of the important issues facing dental education, and describe why they are important.
3. Describe some of the theories of health-related behaviors and how they are relevant for oral health education.
4. Describe how the media is both a challenge to oral health education and a tool that can be used for this purpose.
5. What are some research findings relevant for oral health educators?

REFERENCES

1. Kaste LM et al: Coronal caries in the primary and permanent dentition of children and adolescents 1-17 years of age: United States, 1988-1991, *J Dent Res* 75:631, 1996.
2. Drury T, Brown L, Zion G: Tooth retention and tooth loss in the permanent dentition of adults: United States, 1988-1992, *J Dent Res* 75:684, 1996.
3. Brown L, Brunelle J, Kingman A: Periodontal status in the United States, 1988-91: prevalence, extent and demographic variation, *J Dent Res* 75:672, 1996.
4. American Dental Association: For the dental patient . . . , *J Am Dent Assoc* 131:1095, 2000.
5. Lang WP, Ronis DL, Farghaly MM: Preventive behaviors as correlates of periodontal health status, *J Public Health Dent* 55:10, 1995.
6. Chambers DW: Susceptibility to preventive dental treatment, *J Public Health Dent* 33:82, 1973.
7. Davis MS: Variations in patients' compliance with doctors' orders: analyses of congruence between survey responses and results in empirical investigations, *J Med Educ* 41:1037, 1966.
8. Raynor JF, Cohen LK: A position of school dental health education: behavioral influences on oral hygiene practices, *J Prev Dent* 1:11, 1974.
9. Yacavone JA: Translating research in the social and behavioral sciences for more effective use in community dentistry, *J Public Health Dent* 36:155, 1971.
10. Young MAC: Dental health education: an overview of selected concepts and principles relevant to program planning, *Int J Health Educ* 13:2, 1970.

11. Green L, Johnson K: Health education and health promotion. In Mechanic D, editor: *Handbook of health, healthcare and the health professions,* New York, 1983, Wiley.
12. Dworkin S, Ference T, Giddon D: *Behavioral science and dental practice,* St Louis, 1978, Mosby.
13. Frazier PJ, Horowitz AM: Oral health education and promotion in maternal and child health: a position paper, *J Public Health Dent* 50:390, 1990.
14. Frazier PJ et al: Quality of information in mass media: a barrier to the dental health education of the public, *J Public Health Dent* 34:244, 1974.
15. American Dental Association: *Materials you need for your effective practice,* Chicago, 2000-2001, The Association.
16. American Dental Hygienists' Association: *Professional products,* Chicago, 2000-2001, The Association.
17. Horowitz AM et al: Effect of supervised daily plaque removal by children: II. 24 months' results, *J Public Health Dent* 37(3):180-188, 1977.
18. Meskins HM, Martens LV, Katz BJ: Effectiveness of community preventive programs on improving oral health, *J Public Health Dent* 38:302, 1978.
19. Winslow CEA: The untilled field of public health, *Mod Med* 2:1920, 1920.
20. Green LW: Bridging the gap between community health and school health, *Am J Public Health* 78:1149, 1988.
21. Winnett RA, King AC, Altman DG: *Health psychology and public health: an integrative approach,* Boston, 1994, Allyn & Bacon.
22. Frazier PJ: The effectiveness and practicality of current dental health education programs from a public health perspective: a conceptual appraisal, Dental Health Section Symposium, annual meeting of the American Public Health Association, Miami Beach, FL, 1976.
23. US Department of Health and Human Services, Public Health Service: Review of fluoride benefits and risks: report of the ad hoc subcommittee on fluoride of the Committee to Coordinate Environmental and Health Related Programs, Washington, DC, 1991.
24. Office of the Surgeon General, US Department of Health and Human Services (1995), [Online]. Available: http://www.cdc.gov/nccdphp/oh/fl-surgeon.htm [2001, April 6].
25. US Department of Health and Human Services: *Oral health in America: a report of the Surgeon General,* Rockville, MD, 2000, US Department of Health and Human Services, National Institute of Dental and Craniofacial Research, National Institutes of Health.
26. National Center for Chronic Disease Prevention and Health Promotion, CDC's Oral Health At-A-Glance (2001) [Online]. Available: http://www.cdc.gov.nccdphp/oh/ataglanc.htm [2001, April 6].
27. American Dental Association: Wake up to prevention for the smile of a lifetime, *J Am Dent Assoc* 116:3G, 1988.
28. Calley K et al: A proposed client self-care commitment model, *J Dent Hyg* 74:24, 2000.
29. Darby M, Walsh M: Application of the human needs conceptual model to dental hygiene practice, *J Dent Hyg* 74:230, 2000.
30. American Cancer Society: 2001. www.cancer.org, accessed 7/15/01.
31. Horowitz AM, Nourjah P, Gift H: US adult knowledge of risk factors and signs of oral cancers: 1990, *J Am Dent Assoc* 126:39, 1995.
32. Haber J: Cigarette smoking—a major risk factor for periodontitis, *Dent Hygienist News* 8:3, 1995.
33. Wagner L: Upfront—tobacco control and counseling initiatives taken, *J Dent Hyg* 70:185, 1996.
34. Massachusetts Department of Public Health, Abt Associates, Inc.: Massachusetts Tobacco Control Program: independent evaluation of the Massachusetts Tobacco Control Program, sixth annual report, 1994 to 1999, Boston, 2000.
35. US Department of Health and Human Services, Public Health Service: *Clinical practice guideline—treating tobacco use and dependence,* June 2000.
36. US Department of Health and Human Services, Public Health Service: *Quick reference guide for clinicians—treating tobacco use and dependence,* October 2000.
37. US Department of Health and Human Services: *Preventing tobacco use among young people: a report of the Surgeon General,* 1994, Public Health Service, Centers for Disease Control and Prevention, National Center for Chronic Disease Prevention and Health Promotion, Office on Smoking and Health.
38. Fried J: Women and tobacco: oral health issues, *J Dent Hyg* 74:49, 2000.
39. Ripa LW: Nursing caries: a comprehensive review, *Pediatr Dent* 10:268, 1988.
40. National Association for Anorexia Nervosa and Associated Disorders: *Surveys on anorexia nervosa and bulimia nervosa,* 1995, Highland Park, Ill, The Association.
41. Brown S, Bonifazi DZ: An overview of anorexia nervosa and bulimia nervosa, and the impact of eating disorders on the oral cavity, *Compendium* 14:1594, 1993.
42. Brownridge E: Eating disorders and oral health, *Ontario Dentist* 71:15, 1994.
43. McGivern T: Oral manifestations and dental treatment of HIV infection, *J Pract Hyg* 3:19, 1994.
44. Bednarsh HS, Eklund KJ, Klein BH: Courts strike down HIV discrimination in dental offices, *Access Am Dent Hyg Assoc* 10:12, 1996.

45. Soh G: Racial differences in perception of oral health and oral health behaviors in Singapore, *Int Dent J* 42:234, 1992.
46. Kiyak HA: Age and culture: influences on oral health behavior, *Int Dent J* 43:9, 1993.
47. Ronis DL, Lang WP, Passow E: Tooth brushing, flossing, and preventive dental visits by Detroit-area residents in relation to demographic and socioeconomic factors, *J Public Health Dent* 53:138, 1993.
48. Casamassimo PA: Special patients aren't special anymore, *Dent Teamwork* 8:18, 1995.
49. Steifel DJ: Preface. In Tesini DA, editor: *Developing dental education programs for persons with special needs: a training and reference guide,* ed 2, Boston, 1988, Massachusetts Department of Public Health, Division of Dental Health.
50. Chez N: Helping the victim of domestic violence, *Am J Nurs* 94:32, 1994.
51. Joint Commission on Accreditation of Healthcare Organizations: *1995 accreditation manual for hospitals. Standards,* PE 1.9, 100-101, Oakbrook Terrace, IL, 1994.
52. Meskin LH: If not us, then who? *J Am Dent Assoc* 125:41, 1994.
53. Gibson-Howell JC: Domestic violence identification and referral, *J Dent Hyg* 70:77, 1996.
54. Lewin K: *Field theory in social science,* New York, 1951, Harper & Brothers.
55. Bandura A: *Social foundations of thought and action: a social cognitive theory,* Englewood Cliffs, NJ, 1986, Prentice-Hall.
56. Tedesco LA et al: Effect of a social cognitive intervention on oral health status, behavior reports, and cognitions, *J Periodont* 63:467, 1992.
57. Tedesco LA et al: Self-efficacy and reasoned action: predicting oral health status and behaviour at one, three, and six month intervals, *Psychol Health* 8:105, 1993.
58. Ajzen I, Fishbein M: *Understanding attitudes and predicting social behavior,* Englewood Cliffs, NJ, 1980, Prentice-Hall.
59. Rosenstock IM: Why people use health services, *Milbank Memorial Fund Q* 44:94, 1966.
60. American Dental Association: Ask higher dental priorities at AMA-Kennedy meeting, *ADA Leadership Bull* 7(16), 1978.
61. Prochaska JO, DiClemente CO: Toward a comprehensive model of change. In Miller DR, Healther N, editors: *Treating addictive behaviors,* New York, 1986, Plenum Press.
62. Farquhar JW et al: The Stanford Five City Project: an overview. In Matarazzo J, Weiss SM, Herd JA, editors: *Behavioral health: a handbook of health enhancement and disease prevention,* New York, 1984, Wiley.
63. Green LW, Anderson CL: *Community health,* St Louis, 1986, Mosby.
64. Perry CL et al: Parent involvement with children's health promotion, the Minnesota home team, *Am J Public Health* 78:1156, 1988.
65. World Health Organization: *New approaches to health education in primary health care,* Geneva, 1983, The Organization.
66. World Health Organization: *Prevention methods and programmes for oral diseases,* Geneva, 1984, The Organization.
67. Novartis Foundation: A short course in social marketing, 2001. www.foundation.novartis.com/leprosy/social_marketing.htm, accessed 1/31/02.
68. American Hospital Association: Reducing cigarette smoking: an opportunity for social marketing? *Journal of Health Care Marketing* 1:8, 1980-1981.
69. Guidotti T, Ford L, Wheeler M: The Fort McMurray demonstration project in social marketing: theory, design, and evaluation, *Am J Prev Med* 18:163, 2000.
70. Ressler W, Toledo E: A functional perspective on social marketing: insights from Israel's bicycle helmet campaign, *Journal of Health Communication* 2:145, 1997.
71. Rudd R, Goldberg J, Dietz W: A five-stage model for sustaining a community campaign, *Journal of Health Communication* 4:37, 1999.
72. Svenkerud P, Singhal A: Enhancing the effectiveness of HIV/AIDS prevention programs targeted to unique population groups in Thailand: lessons learned from applying concepts of diffusion of innovation and social marketing, *Journal of Health Communication* 3:193, 1998.
73. Dearing J et al: Social marketing and diffusion-based strategies for communicating with unique populations: HIV prevention in San Francisco, *Journal of Health Communication* 1:343, 1996.
74. Silversin J, Kornacki MJ: Acceptance of preventive measures by individuals, institutions, and communities, *Int Dent J* 34:170, 1984.
75. Action for Children's Television, press release, Cambridge, MA, June 3, 1991.
76. Children's television called a junk food cafeteria, press release, Center for Science in the Public Interest, Washington, DC, June 3, 1991.
77. Concern about TV advertising of non-nutritious foods to children, National PTA statement, Washington, DC, June 3, 1991.
78. Pediatricians suggest eliminating TV food ads aimed at children, criticize children's television, press release, American Academy of Pediatrics, Chicago, News Release, July 23, 1991.
79. American Academy of Pediatrics: Policy statement: the commercialization of children's television, Chicago, AAP News, July 1991.
80. Center for Science in the Public Interest: Report: content analysis of children's television advertisements, Washington, DC, June 3, 1991.

81. Centers for Disease Control and Prevention: Comparison of the cigarette brand preferences of adult and teenage smokers—United States 1989 in 10 U.S. communities, 1988 and 1990, *MMWR Morb Mortal Wkly Rep* 41:169, 1992.
82. Centers for Disease Control and Prevention: Changes in the cigarette brand preferences of adolescent smokers—United States, 1989-1993, *MMWR Morb Mortal Wkly Rep* 43:577, 1994.
83. Dreyfuss R: Tobacco enemy number 1: Joe Camel's tracks, *Mother Jones (20th Anniversary Special Iss): Inside the nicotine network* 44, 1996.
84. Pollay RW et al: The last straw? Cigarette advertising and realized market shares among youths and adults, 1979-1993, *J Marketing* 60:1, 1996.
85. Sargent J, Dalton M: Media images, *Lancet* 357:29, 2001.
86. Tickle J et al: Favorite movie stars and tobacco use in a sample of adolescents, *Tob Control* 10(1):16-22, 2001.
87. Ring T: A look at health issues in the presidential election, *Access* 10:54, 1996.
88. Rubinson L: Evaluating school dental health education programs, *J Sch Health* 52:26, 1982.
89. US Department of Health and Human Services, Public Health Service, Centers for Disease Control and Prevention: Current trends: the effectiveness of school health education, *MMWR Morb Mortal Wkly Rep* 35:593, 1986.
90. Davis RL et al: Comprehensive school health education: a practical definition, *J Sch Health* 55:335, 1985.
91. Cohen L, Gift H, editors: *Disease prevention and oral health promotion: socio-dental sciences in action,* Copenhagen, 1995, Muksgaard.
92. Winett RA, King AC, Altman DG: *Health psychology and public health: an integrative approach,* Boston, 1994, Allyn & Bacon.
93. Potshadley AG, Schweikle ES: The effectiveness of two educational programs in changing the performance of oral hygiene by elementary school children, *J Public Health Dent* 30:17, 1970.
94. Haefuer DP: School dental health programs, *Health Educ Monogr* 2:212, 1974.
95. Potshadley AG, Shannon JH: Oral hygiene performance of elementary school children following dental health education, *J Dent Child* 37:293, 1970.
96. Raynor JF, Cohen LK: School dental health education. In Richards ND, Cohen LK, editors: *Social sciences and dentistry: a critical bibliography,* London, 1971, Dentaire International.
97. Castile AS, Jerrick SJ: *School health in America,* ed 2, Atlanta, 1979, US Department of Health, Education and Welfare, American School Health Association.
98. Taub A: Dental health education: rhetoric or reality? *J Sch Health* 52:10, 1982.
99. Mulholland DN: A comprehensive dental health education program, *J Sch Health* 48:225, 1978.
100. Croucher R et al: The "spread effect" of a school-based dental health education project, *Community Dent Oral Epidemiol* 13:205, 1985.
101. Kamholtz JD, Wood B: Competing with Ronald McDonald, Cap'n Crunch and the Pepsi Generation, *J Sch Health* 52:17, 1982.
102. Beaulieu E, Dufour L, Beaudet R: Better oral health for infants and toddlers: a community based program, *J Dent Hyg* 74:131, 2000.
103. National Center for Chronic Disease Prevention and Health Promotion: CDC's oral health program, children's oral health coordinated school health programs, (2000) [Online]. Available: http://www.cdc.gov/nccdphp/oh/child-ohio.htm [2001, April 6], Available: http://www.cdc.gov/nccdphp/oh/child-rhodeisland.htm [2001, April 6], Available: http://www.cdc.gov/nccdphp/oh/child-southcarolina.htm [2001, April 6].
104. Texas Department of Health, Bureau of Dental and Chronic Disease Prevention: *Preventive dentistry program,* Austin, Tex., 1992.
105. Texas Department of Health: *Tattletooth program: statewide implementation plan,* Austin, Tex., 1986.
106. Texas Department of Health, Bureau of Dental and Chronic Disease Prevention: *Summative evaluation report for the Texas Department of Health oral health curriculum. Tattletooth II—a new generation,* Austin, Tex., 1990.
107. Hide C: *Preschool dental health curriculum evaluation,* Texas Department of Health, Dental Health Services. Report prepared for Texas Department of Health, Dental Health Services, Austin, Tex., 1993.
108. Bivins EC: *History and development of dental public health in North Carolina,* 1974. Report prepared for the North Carolina Department of Human Resources, Division of Health Services, Dental Health Section, Raleigh, NC.
109. North Carolina Department of Environment, Health, and Natural Resources, Division of Dental Health, Raleigh, NC: *Program plan,* 1991.
110. North Carolina Department of Human Resources, Division of Health Services, Dental Health Section, Raleigh, NC: *A ten-year report,* 1985.
111. North Carolina Department of Human Resources, Division of Health Services, Dental Health Section, Raleigh, NC: *Program report—FY86, program plan—FY87,* 1986.
112. North Carolina Department of Human Resources, Division of Health Services, Dental Health Section, Raleigh, NC: *1986 conjoint report,* 1986.
113. Fulton J, Hughes JT: *The national history of dental disease,* Chapel Hill, NC, 1965, School of Public Health, University of North Carolina.

114. Rozier RG et al: *Dental health in North Carolina: a chartbook,* Chapel Hill, NC, 1982, Department of Health Policy and Administration, School of Public Health, University of North Carolina.
115. Hughes JT, Rozier RG, Ramsey DL: *Natural history of dental diseases in NC: 1976-1977,* Durham, NC, 1982, Carolina Academic Press.
116. McMahan EL, Hensey ER: Celebrating 70 years of NC dental public health, 1918-1988. Looking to the Future: Exploring Community Approaches to Dental Health, 70th Anniversary Symposium Proceedings, October 26-28, 1988, Durham, NC, *J Public Health Dent* 50 (2 Spec No): 139-141; discussion 142-146, 1990.
117. Special Athletes/Special Smiles: *Mission statement, Special Olympics,* adopted 1993.
118. Special Athletes/Special Smiles: *Statement of objectives. Category C-1. Community service,* 1995, Boston University School of Dental Medicine and Colgate with Mullen Public Relations.
119. American Dental Hygienists' Association: The 2001 Special Olympics World Wide Winter Games needs your help, *Access* pp. 33-34, Nov 2000.
120. Perlman SP, Friedman C, Kaufhold G: *Special smiles: a guide to good oral health for persons with special needs,* 1996 (pamphlet). Prepared by Special Olympics Special Athletes/Special Smiles and Boston University. Supported by unrestricted grant from Colgate Oral Pharmaceuticals.
121. Nash DA: The future of allied dental education: creating a professional TEAM, *J Dent Ed* 57:621, 1993.
122. Institute of Medicine: *Dental education at the crossroads: challenges and change,* Washington, DC, 1995, National Academy Press.
123. Wagner L: Upfront—ADHA participates in development of new IQM report, *J Dent Hyg* 69:104, 1995.
124. US Department of Health and Human Services: *Healthy people 2010: understanding and improving health,* Washington, DC, 2000, US Department of Health and Human Services, US Public Health Service.
125. Dyke BC: Community water fluoridation from the past toward the year 2000, *Dent Hyg News* 8:3, 1995.
126. Frankel JM, Allukian M: Sixteen referenda on fluoridation in Massachusetts: an analysis, *J Public Health Dent* 33:96, 1973.
127. Hirakio SS, Foote F: Statewide fluoridation: how it was done in Connecticut, *J Am Dent Assoc* 75:174, 1967.
128. McNeil DR: Political aspects of fluoridation, *J Am Dent Assoc* 65:659, 1962.
129. Domoto PK, Faine RC, Rovin S: Seattle fluoridation campaign 1973—prescription of a victory, *J Am Dent Assoc* 91:583, 1975.
130. National Health Federation: *This is the National Health Federation [leaflet],* The Federation.
131. Mecklenberg RE et al: *How to help your patients stop using tobacco,* report no 93-3191, Washington, DC, 1993, US Department of Health and Human Services.
132. Wagner L: Upfront—sealant manual available, *J Dent Hyg* 70:185, 1996.
133. Gift HC, Corbin SB, Nowjack-Raymer RE: Public knowledge of prevention of dental disease, *Public Health Rep* 109:397, 1994.
134. Horowitz HS et al: Combined fluoride, school-based program in a fluoride-deficient area: results of an 11-year study, *J Am Dent Assoc* 112:621, 1986.
135. Klein SP et al: The cost and effectiveness of school-based preventive dental care, *Am J Public Health* 75:382, 1985.
136. Niessen LC: New directions: constituencies and responsibilities, *J Public Health Dent* 50:133, 1990.
137. National Institute of Dental Research: *Oral health of United States children: the national survey of dental caries in U.S. school children: 1986-1987,* report no 89-2247, Washington, DC, 1989, US Department of Health and Human Services.
138. Wagner L: Upfront—US dental health status revealed, *J Dent Hyg* 70:144, 1996.
139. Lyons S: Access extra: survey reveals nation's oral health status, *Access* 10:27, 1996.
140. Gift HC, Corbin SB, Nowjack-Raymer RE: Public knowledge of prevention of dental disease, *Public Health Rep* 109:397, 1994.

CHAPTER

12

PLANNING FOR COMMUNITY DENTAL PROGRAMS

Madalyn L. Mann

Microbiologist Rene Dubos has suggested that most of human history has been a result of accidents and blind choices.[1] When a crisis occurs, our solutions are immediate and involve piecemeal efforts rather than considered and thoughtful planning. The need to develop our ability to predict, plan, and thus prevent the same crisis from recurring should have the highest priority.

WHY PLAN?

As part of our role as health professionals, we are called on to assist health agencies and organizations in developing plans for obtaining dental care. We need to develop our own abilities to take our dental expertise and channel it into the areas of policy development, decision making, and program planning in a system more complex than the one with which we are familiar in the private dental office. This complex system may take the form of a community, an organization, a corporation, or an institution. The system can be better understood if we look on it as a patient, possessing certain needs and characteristics. Because we are dealing with more than one individual, planning a program for a community or institution requires a deep understanding and analysis of the system as a whole and of the individual members that make up the system.

PLANNING DENTAL CARE FOR THE PATIENT

The steps the dentist takes when seeing a patient for the first time can be compared with the steps a planner takes when viewing a system for the first time. A new patient who walks into the dental office is given a medical and dental history form to complete. This record provides background information on the patient's health, history of diseases, and drug reactions, as well as the patient's history of dental care. Information on the patient's ethnic background, degree of education, and financial status may indicate the patient's attitude about dental care, the type of dental care wanted, and how that care will be financed. A clinical examination with the use of radiographs further reveals the type and quality of dental care received and identifies any existing conditions or disease requiring treatment. For the dentist these steps assess the needs of the patient.

The next step is to identify and diagnose the problem or problems. Perhaps the patient requires full mouth reconstruction to restore the mouth to optimum functioning. The dentist reviews with the patient the ideal plan and acceptable alternatives based on the patient's wants and financial limitations. Once the patient accepts the treatment plan and the method of payment, the plan is ready to be implemented.

The dentist selects the appropriate person to perform the necessary services from a staff of specialists and designs a realistic timetable to coordinate who will do what first, second, and so on until treatment has been completed.

When treatment has been completed, the patient is placed on an appropriate recall schedule and returns to have an evaluation of the care that was rendered. Any modifications or adjustments are done at this time. The patient is then placed on a maintenance plan and returns periodically for a routine examination. This becomes an ongoing process for the patient and the dentist. The difference between the planning steps for an individual patient and the planning steps for a community is that dealing with more than one individual at a time requires more complex steps. Box 12-1 compares the provision of dental care for a private patient with that for a community.

Planning Dental Care for the Community

Usually a planner is contacted because a problem has been identified within the community, for example, a high incidence of early childhood caries (ECC) among children. The planner, like the dentist, begins by conducting a needs assessment of the affected children and their families. Included in the needs assessment are the population's health problems and beliefs, ethnic makeup, diet, education and socioeconomic status, number of children with ECC, and the severity of the disease.[2] Again, this information will help the planner in determining an appropriate plan.

Once the information has been gathered and analyzed, the planner, along with the community, sets priorities for dealing with the problem. The planner may decide that the first priority is to treat all existing cases of nursing bottle caries within the community, followed by reeducating the parents of these children and those individuals who recommended sweetening the contents of the children's bottles. The planner then sets a reasonable goal to reduce the incidence of ECC within that community within a specified time and proposes methods or objectives to accomplish the goal.

Next, the planner identifies resources available to the community, such as who will provide the treatment, how the care will be financed, and where the care will be provided. If constraints exist (e.g., no transportation available to bring the children to the dental office or a lack of funds necessary to provide the treatment), the planner needs to consider alternative strategies to accomplish the intended goal. The planner might identify and recruit volunteer dentists or dental students to treat the children at no cost to the community.

Once the decision is made and approved by the community, it is ready for implementation. An implementation timetable is developed to provide a schedule for putting the plan into action.

After the children have been treated, a 6-month follow-up examination is insti-

BOX 12-1

A Comparison of the Provision of Dental Care for a Private Patient and a Community

PRIVATE PATIENT
1. The dentist conducts a dental and medical history and a clinical examination of the patient.
2. The dentist diagnoses the oral health of the patient.
3. The dentist develops a treatment plan based on the diagnosis, the priorities, the patient's attitude, and the method of payment for the services.
4. The dentist obtains patient consent for treatment.
5. The dentist selects the appropriate personnel to provide the care: dentist, specialist, laboratory technician, dental hygienist, and dental assistant.
6. The dentist selects the appropriate dental service for the patient: preventive services, restorative services, endodontic services, and so on.
7. The dentist evaluates the treatment rendered to the patient: clinical examination, radiographs, patient oral hygiene, and patient satisfaction.

COMMUNITY
1. The planner conducts a survey of the community's structure and dental status.
2. The planner analyzes the survey data of the community.
3. The planner develops a program plan based on the analysis of the survey data, the priorities and alternatives, the community's attitudes, and the resources available.
4. The planner obtains community approval of the plan.
5. The planner selects the appropriate labor to implement the program: dentist, dental hygienist, dental assistant, dental technician, nutritionist, health educator, schoolteacher, social worker, health aides, and public health nurses.
6. The planner selects the appropriate activities for the community: community water fluoridation and school-based fluoride rinse programs.
7. The planner evaluates the community program: comparison of baseline survey with subsequent survey, attainment of goals and objective, cost-effectiveness of activities, appropriateness of activities, and community satisfaction.

Modified from Young W, Striffier D: *The dentist, his practice, and the community,* Philadelphia, 1969, WB Saunders.

tuted to evaluate the effectiveness of the plan. At that time the planner addresses questions such as the following: How many children identified as having ECC were treated? How many dropped out of treatment, and why? How many developed new ECC? The answers to these questions will help the planner to modify and adjust the program according to the needs of the community.[3]

Many kinds of planners exist. Some have been professionally trained or educated, whereas others have received on-the-job experience within their organization. There are two distinct approaches to planning: *internal,* planning by individuals within the system or organization; and *external,* planning by those brought in from outside.[4] A planner hired from within the system is usually an individual whose work responsibility is to plan for the system on a full-time basis. The advantage of hiring from within is that the planner already has a true understanding of the issues and operation of the system, including the subtleties of that system. This knowledge enables the planner to begin making decisions more quickly regarding appropriate action. The disadvantage, however, is that the planner may already have acquired certain biases about the system that could influence his or her objectivity.

The planner brought in from outside is usually an individual who contracts to work for the company or agency on a consulting basis for a short period. The planner's job is to assist the organization in its planning by formulating a new proposal or making recommendations for changing an existing plan. The advantage of an outside planner is that the organization may receive a fresher outlook, less bias, and a greater sense of objectivity. The drawback is that the outside planner requires more time to reach a sufficient level of understanding for effective action to take place.

One of the most important concerns for any planner is to take into consideration the human element. Statistics alone do not tell the whole story. For example, a planner who reviews the health labor statistics on a multiethnic community and who sees that, overall, sufficient numbers of practitioners work within the community may think that the community does not need any new practitioners. A closer examination of the practitioner and patient populations may reveal that the practitioners are primarily of a certain ethnic background and do not like treating patients of different ethnic backgrounds, of which there are a great number in the community. Thus large subgroups of the population may not have access to dental care, even though statistically enough dentists are available in the community.[5] Although statistics can be most useful in analyzing data, a planner must be aware of their limitations.

PLANNING: A DEFINITION

Banfield presents a basic definition of the term *planning:* "A plan is a decision about a course of action."[6] In other words, a plan is a systematic approach to defining the problem, setting priorities, developing specific goals and objectives, and determining alternative strategies and a method of implementation.

Many types of health planning exist. Each varies according to the factors affecting the health system, such as the geography of a region, the sociocultural background of the population, economic considerations, and the political situation. Some types of health planning, as outlined by Spiegel and associates,[7] include the following:

1. Problem-solving planning involves the identification and resolution of a problem. An example of problem solving was the appearance of dental fluorosis among residents of a community in Colorado. This enamel disorder was identified through a scientific study of possible causative factors.
2. Program planning entails designing a course of action for a circumscribed health problem. School-based fluoride rinse programs are an example of designing a course of action for the problem of dental caries within a community setting.
3. Coordination of efforts and activities aims to increase the availability, efficiency, productivity, effectiveness, and other aspects of activities and programs. This stage often involves an adjustment process, such as a merger or a

closing of services and facilities. An example is the closing of obstetric and pediatric wards in hospitals located in areas with a declining birth rate.
4. Planning for the allocation of resources involves selecting the best alternative to achieve a desired goal when the amount of resources is limited. Planners are called on to allocate the budget, the labor, and the facilities in a system so that it may meet existing needs and demands. An example is the decision by a state government with limited financial resources for the provision of dental services to cut services to medically indigent adults based on the cost-effectiveness of providing preventive dental care to a younger population.
5. Creation of a plan involves the development of a blueprint or proposal for action containing recommendations and supporting data. It is common for a commission or special task force to be created to prepare the plan. A state health plan that describes the health status and the distribution of health services for the population in that state is a good example of such planning.
6. Design of standard operating procedures requires planners to come forth with a set of standards of practice or criteria for operation and evaluation. This can be a result of legislation, or it can be created voluntarily by the parties concerned. Guidelines for evaluating the quality of dental care as part of a continuous quality improvement program for an insurance company is one example.

This chapter describes various types of health planning but concentrates specifically on the program-planning process. This process of program planning uses a systematic approach, as seen in Fig. 12-1, and should be used as a guide to solving a particular problem. The process can be compared with the ability of a jazz musician to take the notes of a standard musical scale and use them to create a unique melody. In a similar fashion, a planner uses the program-planning steps to create a plan that is unique for the specific situation or system. The process of planning is dynamic. Within a fluctuating and ever-changing system, the process itself must remain fluid and flexible, responsive to the presentation of new factors and issues. This chapter discusses the components of program planning and focuses on the various options available to the planner. The initial step in the planning process is to conduct a needs assessment.

There are several reasons why a planner should conduct a needs assessment. The primary reason is to define the problem and to identify its extent and severity. Second, the assessment is used to obtain a profile of the community to ascertain the causes of the problem. This information helps in developing the appropriate goals and objectives in the problem solution. Assessing the community's needs not only involves identifying existing health problems but also potential health problems and health promotion needs.[8]

A needs assessment evaluates the effectiveness of the program. This is accomplished by obtaining baseline information and, over time, measuring the amount of progress achieved in solving the specific problem.

Suppose the planner designed a program to administer fluoride tablets to all school-age children in a given community. To determine how effective a fluoride tablet program is in terms of reduction of dental caries, the planner would first establish a baseline needs assessment of the caries rate

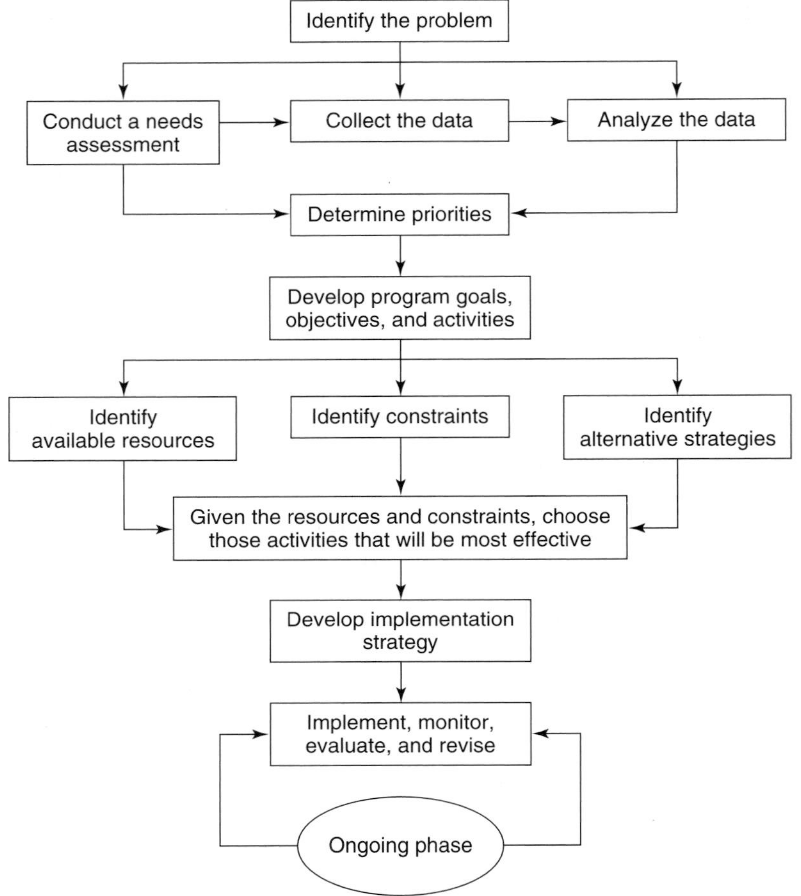

Fig. 12-1. Planning and implementation strategy flowchart.

among the school children. After the initial assessment, the program is implemented. To measure the effectiveness of such a preventive regimen, the planner would then make periodic assessments of the schoolchildren at various time intervals and compare these results with the initial assessment.

Conducting a needs assessment for a community can be a costly endeavor. If the funds are not readily available, the planner has several options. One option is to coordinate with the research activities of other agencies interested in obtaining similar health information on the given population. For example, a neighborhood health center may be involved in conducting a health survey of all the residents living in a defined geographic area.

Another method is to investigate surveys that have been done in the past by other organizations. Frequently, dental surveys are conducted through research departments of dental schools or through local and state health departments. If no surveys have ever been done, the planner may either want to solicit the assistance of these agencies and organizations or inform them that a survey will be conducted. This approach prevents overlap or duplication of activities.

Whether the planner conducts his or her own survey, combines efforts with others, or uses information from past surveys, it is important to consider what type of information is needed and how it should be obtained. Data can be obtained by various techniques such as survey questionnaires or clinical examinations or more informally through personal communications. The technique used is based on the population to be examined. Factors the planner should consider are the number of individuals, the extent and degree of severity of the problem, and the attitudes of the individuals to be surveyed. The greater the number of individuals to be examined, the more formal the survey. If the problem is clinical, as opposed to attitudinal, a clinical examination might be recommended. If the planner wants to interview a small group of individuals on their attitudes and feelings about a particular issue, a personal communication might be more appropriate.

To gather general information on a population, a population profile should be obtained. Such a profile includes the following:

1. Number of individuals in the population
2. Geographic distribution of the population
3. Rate of growth
4. Population density and degree of urbanization
5. Ethnic backgrounds
6. Diet and nutritional levels
7. Standard of living, including types of housing
8. Amount and type of public services and utilities
9. Public and private school system
10. General health profile
11. Patterns and distribution of dental disease

To gather epidemiologic data on the patterns and distribution of dental disease, the planner can use a clinical examination, review patients' dental records, or consult the National Health and Nutrition Examination Survey III (NHANES III) for data on a population residing in a similar geographic region with similar characteristics.

In addition to assessing the incidence and the distribution of dental disease, the planner needs to inquire into the history and current status of dental programs in the community. Questions to ask include the following:

1. What types of programs currently exist?
2. Are these programs oriented toward prevention, treatment, education, research, or a combination?
3. Who or what organization is responsible for the planning, implementation, and administration of the program(s)?
4. How successful have those responsible been?
5. What was the community's acceptance of such a program?

The planner must learn how policies are developed and how decisions are made within the community. The following areas should be explored:

1. Who are the financial leaders (bankers, businesspersons), and who are the political leaders (mayor, city council, other public officials)?
2. Who sets the policies for the community?

3. What is the organizational structure of the community?
4. What are the community leaders' attitudes toward oral health and community dental programs?

The planner needs to examine the types of resources available to the community. These include the funds, the facilities, and the labor. The following questions might be asked:

1. Funds
   a. What is the source of funding at the state and local level for dental care?
   b. Is third-party coverage available to the community through the workplace?
   c. Is federal funding available through special eligibility programs?
   d. Are private funds available through foundations or endowments?
2. Facilities
   a. Where is the closest major medical center?
   b. What specialty services does this center provide?
   c. What dental facilities exist, and where are they located (in public schools, health centers, hospitals)?
   d. How well are the facilities used by the population?
   e. Are the facilities easily accessible to the population served?
   f. Are the dental services provided appropriately, adequately, and efficiently?
   g. Does the facility meet the required Occupational, Safety, and Health Administration (OSHA) standards for blood-borne pathogens?
   h. Is the equipment adequate and running efficiently?
   i. How many operatories are available?
   j. How many dental laboratories are available?
3. Labor
   a. How many active licensed dentists, hygienists, and assistants are available?
   b. How many laboratory technicians are available?
   c. How many dental and dental auxiliary schools are located nearby?
   d. How many active community health aides are available?
   e. How many public health nurses are available?
   f. How many school nurses are available?
   g. How many public health hygienists, voluntary health agencies, and nutritionists are available?

When planning a preventive dental program for a community or institution, it is important for the planner to determine where the population obtains water and the fluoride status of that water. In certain regions of the country, particularly in rural areas, many persons obtain their water from either individual wells or nearby rivers, lakes, or streams. The concentration of fluoride in the water may indicate that a fluoride supplement program is not necessary for that community. If drinking water emanates from several wells, the planner needs to obtain a fluoride concentration report on each.

If a community is obtaining water from a central area, the planner needs the following information:

1. What type of drinking water is available to the community?
2. What is the fluoride content of the water?
3. Does the water contain optimum levels of fluoride?

4. What efforts, if any, have been made in the past to provide fluoridation?
5. What are the attitudes of the community, the dental profession, and decision makers toward fluoridation?
6. What are the laws with regard to fluoridation?
7. Is a referendum possible or required?
8. Are the schools' water supplies fluoridated?

To prevent duplication of fluoride administration, the planner also should inquire into the type of fluoride being administered to individuals in private offices, the schools, and the health centers. The following questions apply:

1. Do local dentists or physicians prescribe fluoride supplements to their patients?
2. Do schools (preschool, parochial, and public) have a fluoride tablet or rinse program?
3. Do the health centers or hospitals administer fluoride to their patients?
4. Do fluoride brush-in programs exist in the schools?
5. If so, how often do children brush with a fluoride toothpaste?
6. How successful have these programs been, and how are they supported?

All the information presented in this section can be obtained easily through the various survey instruments discussed. If, however, a survey cannot be conducted, the necessary information about an institution or a community also can be obtained through other means. This approach requires the planner to investigate all available sources that might have data relevant to the population or the community. Such sources include the local, state, and federal agencies and private organizations.

In a small community one can find a tremendous amount of information on the community's residents by visiting the local health department. The local health department maintains statistics on the population's health status, morbidity and mortality, general health problems, and health service use. A trip to the chamber of commerce and town hall can provide useful information on the community profile, including population distribution, age breakdown, income, educational levels, school systems, and transportation. In a larger community the state health department can also provide health-related information for all communities, cities, and towns within the state.

The federal government has large volumes of health statistics data from many of its agencies. The most familiar and widely used sources of data are the National Health Surveys and the U.S. Census Bureau. These sources provide longitudinal and comparative data regarding large population groups. Because of the magnitude of the data gathering, these surveys are usually conducted once every 10 years. Consideration of the publication date of such data and its relevancy and applicability to specific populations is important.

Other sources for obtaining such data are research studies and investigative reports. Many of these studies are funded by government agencies and are conducted by academic health centers, local organizations, research companies, or consulting groups. A considerable volume of data is usually generated from their reports. A computer literature search, such as MEDLINE, may be helpful. The National Library of Medicine provides these computer searches for a nominal fee. Most medical libraries affiliated with universities also provide this service.

Once the data are obtained, the information must be analyzed before it can be put into a plan of action. The data presented in

Analysis of Data: A Case Study

BACKGROUND

Tide Water is the fifth largest city in Massachusetts. It is situated in the southeastern section of the state on the shore of Deep Water Bay. Excellent water resources and deep-water shipping potential brought industrial growth to Tide Water, and it became the "spindle city of the world" as the cotton industry flourished. Native granite was used to construct multistory factories, some of which are still in use. This prosperity ended quickly when the cotton manufacturers moved to the South in the 1930s and 1940s. The problem of vacant mill space, in addition to the Depression, made Tide Water's economic situation one of the worst in the country. Tide Water was able to make a strong recovery with a growing garment industry, which replaced the cotton mills and other manufacturers and provided a more diversified industrial base. The available information about Tide Water is listed in the following sections.

POPULATION

2000 census: 96,988 persons

ETHNIC AND RACIAL CHARACTERISTICS

Figures reflect a large immigrant population, principally Portuguese

1. Foreign born: 16%
2. Foreign stock: 48%
3. Race: white, 99%; black, 0.5%; other, 0.5%
4. Density (persons per square mile): 2946

AGE DISTRIBUTION

	Total Male	Total Female
Under 5	4,223	4,047
5-14	8,120	7,893
15-19	378	24,028
20-64	23,992	27,458
Over 64	4,902	8,453

EDUCATION

Median number of school years completed: 8.8
Persons completing high school or more: 25.6%
Persons completing fewer than five grades: 13.3%

PERSONAL INCOME

Salary	Families
Less than $5,000	616
$5,000–$9,999	2,341
$10,000–$13,999	2,988
$14,000–$19,999	3,922
$20,000–$24,999	4,474
$25,000–$34,999	5,761
$35,000–$49,999	2,838
$50,000–$74,999	2,079
$75,000–$99,999	407
$100,000 or more	220
Total families	25,646
Median income	$18,000

TRANSPORTATION

Bus service: intracity and intercity
Taxi service: three companies, with a total of 65 radio-equipped cabs
Highways and streets: four major highways (2 north-south, 2 east-west), 600 miles of streets, 99% paved

FLUORIDE STATUS

Tide Water has a community water supply that has been fluoridated since 1995.

HEALTH RESOURCES (LABOR)

140 physicians
43 dentists

FACILITIES

Two hospitals (725-bed capacity)
One community health center (diagnosis, primary dental health care, education, and prevention; sliding fee)
Mental health centers (many facilities, inpatient and outpatient clinics, and residencies; free and sliding-scale fee)
AIDS, venereal disease, and tuberculosis programs (free)
Alcohol and drug programs (free)
15 nursing homes (1150-bed capacity, representing all levels of care)

Analysis of Data: A Case Study—cont'd

GOVERNMENT

City size: 33 square miles
Mayor (2-year term) and council (2-year term; 191 members) form of government
Democrats: 31,311
Republicans: 4,875
Independents: 10,204

EDUCATIONAL FACILITIES

20 day-care centers (50% free or sliding fee)

	Number	Enrollment
Public schools		
Elementary	32	10,007
Middle	1	982
Junior high school	2	1,852
Academic high school	1	1,948
Girls' vocational high school	1	214
TOTAL	37	15,003
Catholic parochial schools		
Elementary	15	3,379
High schools	2	992

Other
Regional/technical high school
County agricultural high school
Colleges
Community college: offers wide range of courses, many in health disciplines
Southeastern University: 4-year programs in most areas

It is important to first look into the socioeconomic structure of the community and determine the type of employment that exists. Tide Water has a large industrial garment area. This leads to the following questions: Is there a high percentage of industrial workers? If so, are they union employees? If this is the case, are they provided with a comprehensive health benefits package, including the provision of dental care? This information is important because it tells whether this population might be able to afford dental care through their jobs.

The population breakdown shows a large percentage of Portuguese living within the community. This indicates that possible cultural and language issues should be considered. In addition, the age distribution indicates that the highest proportion of people is between 20 and 60 years of age, or in the age bracket for the adult working population. There is a large population of school-age children between ages 5 and 19 years living in the community. The age distribution of a community is important to consider because it tells where the target groups are and thus sets up certain priorities for planning. For example, if the majority of the population were of middle to older age, it would not be effective to design a program that would affect only a young population, such as a schoolwide fluoride rinse program.

The educational status of a community provides two perspectives for planning. First, it tells the educational level (years of schooling) obtained by the majority of community members. Second, it may indicate what the community's values are toward obtaining an education. Planning a health awareness program centered on an educational institution would be successful only if people are attending schools and value the information they receive there.

Knowing the median income of a community is important to a health planner because it indicates the population's ability to purchase health services. If a segment of the population's income falls below the poverty level, those individuals would be eligible for federal and state medical assistance programs (provided the individual state participates in such a program), thus making health services financially accessible to these individuals.

Health care must be both geographically and financially accessible if people are going to use it. A look into the community's public transportation system provides the planner with information regarding a population's ability to get to health care services. This is especially true for rural communities where roads are unpaved and public transportation is scarce.

Looking at the health care facilities in the community tells the planner what type of services are being provided, the amount of services, and the cost of receiving those services.

The labor data give information about the number of dentists providing care. (The federal government has developed certain labor-to-population ratios that indicate whether a population is

Continued

Analysis of Data: A Case Study—cont'd

considered to be residing in a medically underserved area.) However, just looking at the number of dentists in the community will not give the planner a true picture of whether the number of dentists within the community is sufficient to provide services to the population residing there.

Although the number of dentists in the community may be adequate, the planner must question whether the dentists are available to provide the care. How long does it take to get appointments? What are the dentists' hours (e.g., do they work after 5 PM or on the weekends)? In addition to knowing the number of dentists, it is necessary to consider what types of services are being provided to whom and for what cost.

Another consideration is the type of practice. Do the dentists accept third-party payments or Medicaid payments? Do they provide comprehensive services, including preventive care? Do they provide dental health education to their patients?

Knowing the fluoride status of a community is also essential for dental planning. In the case study community profile of Tide Water, it is stated that water has been fluoridated since 1995. This indicates that those children born in 1995 and after that year will receive maximum benefits from the fluoridated water. However, it is safe to say that those children born before 1995 may need additional attention with other fluoride measures.

In most cases the politics of the community will determine the direction the program takes. A conservative government attempting to cut costs may be opposed to programs that provide prosthetic services to the medically indigent or elderly. Each local government's policies may vary in its methods of instituting new programs, allocating funds, hiring personnel, or setting priorities. In addition, the politics of the state government will also shape the overall direction taken by the communities within the state.

By looking at the educational system of a community, the planner can determine the number of schools, the enrollment for each, and the distribution of children among the schools within the community. This information can assist the planner who is developing a school-based program for the community. The public and parochial schools are the ideal settings for dental programs. Moreover, as in countries such as New Zealand, schools also serve as excellent vehicles for providing routine dental care.

The educational facilities should be designed appropriately to accommodate such programs. Teachers, parents, and school administrators should be in support of the programs, and, most important, the need must exist among the school-age population to warrant such programs. In this particular community, with its high percentage of Portuguese-American children, the schools can be a good meeting place in which to open communication channels with the families and to offer support services when needed.

If the planner is designing a dental treatment program for a specific population that is not receiving any care, methods developed by the Indian Health Service (IHS) can convert the survey data into specific resource requirements for treating the population. The IHS is a federal agency within

the following case study can be used to consider ways of developing an appropriate program.

DETERMINING PRIORITIES

"Priority determination is a method of imposing people's values and judgments of what is important onto the raw data."[7] The method can be used for different purposes, such as for setting priorities among problems elicited through a needs assessment. It also can be used for ranking the solutions to the problem.

Given the community profile and analysis of dental survey data, how are priorities established? At this point the community should be involved to assist in the establishment of these priorities. A health advisory committee or task force representing consumers, community leaders, and pro-

Analysis of Data: A Case Study—cont'd

the Public Health Service. It has been involved with extensive surveys on the oral health status of Native Americans. One method it has developed with the use of specific oral health surveys assesses the dental disease prevalence among the population and translates the data into time and cost estimates to treat the population. These surveys for disease prevalence include the decayed, missing, and filled teeth index; the periodontal index; and the simplified oral hygiene index. In addition to determining the dental need, IHS assesses treatment needs, which include prosthetic status, periodontal status, orthodontic status, oral pathology status, and restorative status.

With the use of a mathematic model, dental resource requirements can be computed and projected over a period of time. The data are then translated into time, labor, and facility requirements.

The basic measurement is time. Clinical dental services requirements and labor capability both can be expressed in time units. The IHS, to determine the amount of chair time that is necessary to complete a clinical service, has done various time requirement studies. This unit of time is called a service minute. For example:

Clinical Service	Time Required (Service Minutes)
Complete oral examination	10
Prophylaxis	17
Single-surface amalgam	10

LABOR AND FACILITY REQUIREMENTS

The number of dentists and dental auxiliaries, as well as the number of facilities and operators necessary to treat the population, is determined by obtaining the total number of service minutes required for a given population. For example, a random sample of a population was examined, and calculations showed that 70,000 service minutes per year would be required to treat approximately 60% of that population. Based on this figure, the amount of staff required to provide approximately 70,000 service minutes would be one dentist and two dental assistants.[9] The number of operators needed to accommodate this dental staff for maximum efficiency would be three.[9] The ratios (one dentist to two dental assistants to three operators) have been derived from IHS efficiency studies.

This evaluation is highly statistical. Statistics can set parameters to the problem, but the values and attitudes of persons are equally important. The planner must take into consideration the sociocultural interests or the psychologic readiness of a people to want or use health services. If the community does not agree on which of the array of statistics represents the community's priorities, little will be done to translate the need identified in the data into effective programs.

viders should be established to assist in the development of policies and priorities. Planning with community representation will aid in the program's implementation and acceptance.

Few dental public health programs meet all the dental needs of the population. With limited resources, it becomes necessary to establish priorities to allow the most efficient allocation of resources. If priorities are not determined, the program may not serve those individuals or groups who need the care most.

Certain factors should be considered in determining priorities. For example, a problem that affects a large number of people generally takes priority over a problem that affects a small number of people. However, if the problem is common colds (affecting a large number of people) competing with Lyme disease (affecting few people), the more serious problem should take priority.

If the health problem is dental disease, generally more than one population group is affected. The following are groups commonly associated with high-risk dental needs:

1. Preschool and school-age children
2. Mentally or physically disabled persons
3. Chronically ill or medically compromised persons
4. Elderly persons
5. Expectant mothers
6. Low-income minority groups (urban and rural)

If the community decides to address the problem of dental caries first, specific groups are more susceptible to dental caries, such as preschool and school-age children and low-income minority groups. The planner then begins to develop plans geared to an identifiable population group.

Once the target group has been identified (based on the dental problem), the type of program should be established. To do this, the planner begins to set program goals and objectives.

DEVELOPMENT OF PROGRAM GOALS AND OBJECTIVES

Program goals are broad statements on the overall purpose of a program to meet a defined problem. An example of a program goal for a community that has an identifiable problem of dental caries among school-age children would be "to improve the oral health of the school-aged children in community X."

Program objectives are more specific and describe in a measurable way the desired end result of program activities. The objectives should specify the following:

1. *What:* the nature of the situation or condition to be attained
2. *Extent:* the scope and magnitude of the situation or condition to be attained
3. *Who:* the particular group or portion of the environment in which attainment is desired
4. *Where:* the geographic areas of the program
5. *When:* the date by which the desired situation or condition is intended to exist

An objective might state, "By 2012, more than 90% of the population ages 6 to 17 years in community X will not have lost any teeth as a result of caries, and at least 40% will be caries free." This is known as an outcome objective and provides a means of measuring quantitatively the outcome of the specific objective. This approach helps the evaluator and the community know both where the program is and where it hopes to be with respect to a given health problem. It also aids in establishing a realistic timetable for reducing or preventing principal health problems.

Second, objectives are the specific avenues by which goals are met. Process objectives state a specific process by which a public health problem can be reduced and prevented. For example, by 2005 community X will have a public fluoride program to guarantee access to fluoride exposure via the following:

1. Fluoridation of the public water supply to the optimum level
2. Appropriately monitored fluoridation of school water supplies in areas where community fluoridation is impossible or impractical
3. Initiation of the most cost-effective topical or systemic fluoride supplement

programs available to all schools if both objectives 1 and 2 are impossible
4. Provision of topical fluoride application for persons with rampant caries and use of pit and fissure sealants where indicated[10]

Once the problem has been identified and program goals and objectives have been established describing a solution to or a reduction of the problem, the next step is to state how to bring about the desired results. This area of program planning is referred to as program activities, and it describes how the objectives will be accomplished.

Activities include three components: (1) what is going to be done, (2) who will be doing it, and (3) when it will be done. *Activity I.* Beginning January 1, 2005, two dental hygienists will be hired to administer a self-applied fluoride rinse program within the public school systems. *Activity 2.* On March 1, 8, 15, 22, and 30, 2005, a series of 2-day training workshops for parent volunteers will be conducted by the two hygienists at selected public schools in community X. In planning these program activities, it is important to carefully consider the type of resources available, as well as the program constraints.

RESOURCE IDENTIFICATION

Selection of resources for an activity, such as personnel, equipment and supplies, facilities, and financial resources, must be determined by consideration of what would be most effective, adequate, efficient, and appropriate for the tasks to be accomplished. Some criteria that are commonly used to determine what resources should be used follow:

1. Appropriateness: the most suitable resources to get the job done
2. Adequacy: the extent or degree to which the resources would complete the job
3. Effectiveness: how capable the resources are at completing the job
4. Efficiency: the dollar cost and amount of time expended to complete the job

As discussed previously, obtaining the community profile provides the planner with valuable information on available resources. The type of resources needed to develop a dental program and the sources from which they can be obtained are listed in Table 12-1.

IDENTIFYING CONSTRAINTS

When planning any program, there are usually as many reasons not to do something as there are reasons to do it. The former are usually considered to be roadblocks or obstacles to achieving a certain goal or objective.

What should be determined at this point are the most obvious constraints that are associated with meeting program objectives. By identifying these constraints early in the planning stages, one can modify the design of the program and thereby create a more practical and realistic plan.

Constraints may result from organizational policies, resource limitations, or characteristics of the community. For example, constraints that commonly occur in community dental programs include limitations of the state's dental practice act, attitudes of professional organizations, lack of funding, restrictive governmental policies, inadequate transportation systems, labor shortages, lack of or inadequate facilities, nega-

Table 12-1. Resource Identification Worksheet

Resource	*Source*
Personnel	
Sponsors or supporters	Public health organizations, professional dental organizations, dental and dental hygiene schools, industry, health consumer groups, government, labor, media, business, foundations, public schools
Clinical providers	Dentists, dental hygienists, dental assistants, dental technicians, social workers, health aides, public health nurses, physician's assistants, nutritionists
Nonclinical providers	
Planning	Health planning agencies
Clerical	Volunteers, students, parents, retirees
Educational	Professional organizations, universities, students
Analytical	Universities, consulting firms
Equipment	
Dental units and instruments	Dental supply companies, dental and dental hygiene schools, renovated public health clinics, hospitals, federal government depositories
Computers, calculators, filing cabinets	Business, industry, civic groups, hospitals
Supplies	
Office supplies	Consumer groups, industry, business, and government
Dental supplies	Dental supply companies, dental product companies
Dental Health Education	
Materials	American Dental Association, other professional organizations, public health agencies, dairy councils; local, state, or federal agencies (e.g., National Institute for Dental Research, Centers for Disease Control and Prevention)
Facilities	Hospitals, health centers, nursing homes, public schools, dental schools, public health clinics, industry, health maintenance organizations

tive community attitudes toward dentistry, and the population's socioeconomic, cultural, and educational characteristics. The community's source of water (type and location), the lack of fluoride in the water, and the community's dental health status are also viewed as constraints to program planning. In addition, the amount of time available to complete a project is considered a constraint if that time is too limited to attain the program goals.

One of the best ways to identify constraints is to bring together a group of concerned citizens who might be involved in or affected by the project. As a group that is familiar with the local politics and community structures, these individuals not only can identify the constraints but also can offer alternative solutions to and strategies for meeting the goals.

ALTERNATIVE STRATEGIES

Being aware of the existing constraints and given the available resources, the planner should then consider alternative courses of action that might be effective in attaining the objectives. It is important to generate a sufficient number of alternatives so that out of that number at least one may be considered acceptable.

The planner must be aware of those alternatives that sound good on the surface but may have certain limitations when closely examined. With limited resources, the planner needs to consider the anticipated costs and the effectiveness of each alternative. A classic example is the use of preventive measures in a community setting. If, for example, the community refused to fluoridate the central water supply, or if a community received its water from individual wells, the planner would look at the alternative preventive measures available in relation to dental caries and the cost savings in terms of needed treatment.

If the preventive measure were considered to be cost-effective, as well as practical to implement, the planner would then choose that measure as the best of the alternatives.

IMPLEMENTATION, SUPERVISION, EVALUATION, AND REVISION

This chapter has concentrated on the planning process: identifying the problem, determining priorities, defining the goals and objectives, identifying the resources and constraints, and considering the alternatives for implementation. The process of putting the plan into operation is referred to as the implementation phase. This phase is ongoing in situations where close supervision and evaluation of the program will ensure effective operations.

The implementation process, like the planning process, involves individuals, organizations, and the community. Integrating all the external variables to achieve comprehensive planning and implementation requires what Bruhn[11] terms an "ecologic" approach (Fig. 12-2). Only through teamwork between the individual and the environment can the implementation be successful.

DEVELOPING AN IMPLEMENTATION STRATEGY

An implementation strategy for each activity is complete when the following questions have been answered:

1. *Why:* the effect of the objective to be achieved
2. *What:* the activities required to achieve the objective
3. *Who:* individuals responsible for each activity
4. *When:* chronologic sequence of activities
5. *How:* materials, media, methods, and techniques to be used
6. *How much:* a cost estimate of materials and time

To develop an implementation strategy, planners must know what specific activity they want to do. The most effective method is to work backward to identify the events that must occur before initiating the activity. For example, in August 2000 Scottish Executive Publications released the text of *An Action Plan for Dental Services in Scotland.* The plan recognizes the "vital" contribution that dentistry makes to the overall health of

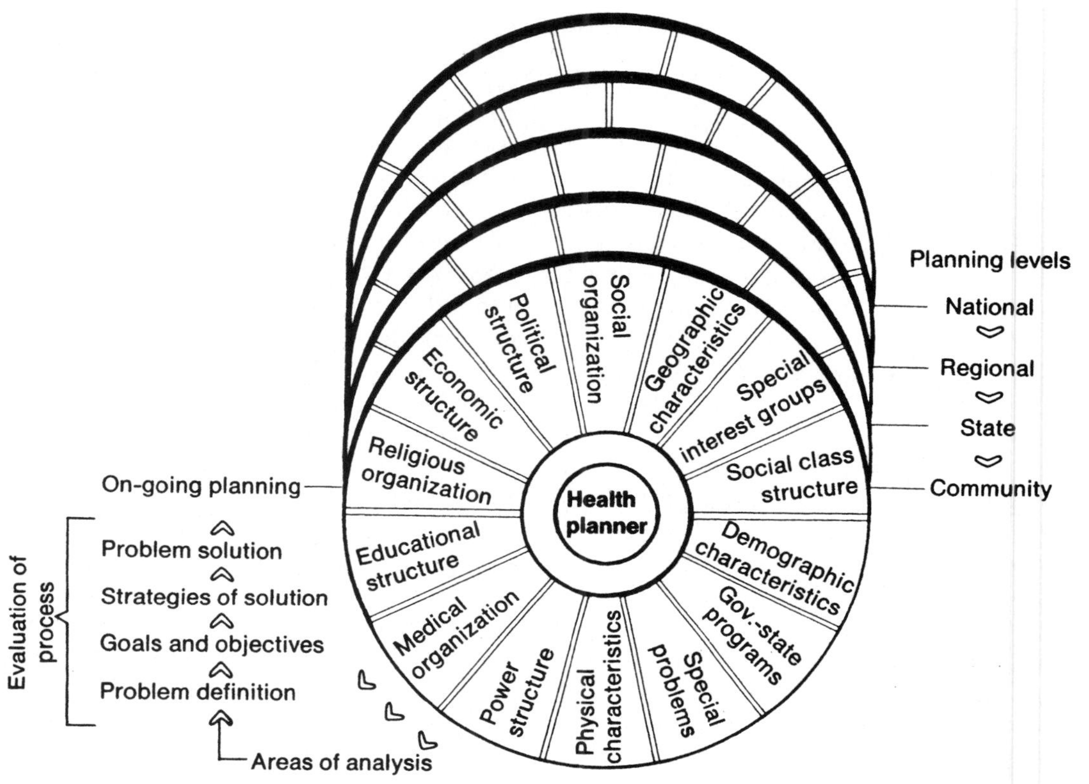

Fig. 12-2. An ecologic approach to comprehensive health planning. (From Bruhn JG: Planning for social change: dilemmas for health planning, *Am J Public Health* 63:604, 1973. © APHA)

the population and the role that dentistry plays as a component of the wider National Health Service system. The plan consists of many parts, but essentially the plan is organized around goals, objectives, and an identification of events that must take place to achieve the goals and objectives. One of the objectives under the heading of Preventing Disease acknowledges the effectiveness of fissure sealants and proposes "targeted prevention for 6- to 16-year-olds," acknowledging that although "some fissure sealant work is already undertaken in Scotland, it is not sufficiently targeted at those with the greatest need."[12]

The activities proposed include the following: (1) the early year's registration scheme will be reviewed to ensure that it continues to meet its objectives; (2) an enhanced registration payment scheme will be introduced for 6- to 8-year-olds in deprivation categories that will include the requirement for fissure sealing the first molars of these children; (3) consideration will be given to extending this scheme to second molars; and (4) proposals will be developed for oral cancer surveillance and for improved preventive services.

Once stated, the planner may specify what activities must be undertaken to im-

BOX 12-2

Rules for Implementation

1. Specify clearly the activity (who does what for whom).
2. Be sure someone is responsible for the whole activity and coordinates individuals who may carry out the different tasks.
3. Identify all the preparatory steps before doing that activity (e.g., prepare training manual, prepare materials, write article, acquire equipment, train volunteers, determine treatment protocol).
4. List steps in the order in which they must occur.
5. Check for missing steps that must be added.
6. Determine when (date) each step should begin and end.
7. Check the dates to make sure the correct amount of time has been allowed.
8. Consult with organizations affected by the activity; identify potential problems, opportunities, and so on.
9. Specify what resources will be needed and their source.
10. Specify what constraints must be addressed.
11. Make sure all people involved know what is expected of them and by when.

From National Heart, Lung and Blood Institute: *Handbook for improving high blood pressure control in the community,* Washington, DC, 1977, US Government Printing Office.

plement the activity. Box 12-2 lists rules for implementation.

Monitoring, Evaluating, and Revising the Program

Once it has been implemented, the program requires continuous surveillance of all activities. The program's success is determined by monitoring how well the program is meeting its stated objectives, how well individuals are doing their jobs, how well equipment functions, and how appropriate and adequate facilities are. Before problems arise in any of these areas, adjustments must be made to fine-tune the program.

Evaluation, both informal and formal, is a necessary and important aspect of the program. Evaluation allows us to (1) measure the progress of each activity, (2) measure the effectiveness of each activity, (3) identify problems in carrying out the activities, (4) plan revision and modification, and (5) justify the dollar costs of administering the program and, if necessary, justify seeking additional funds. Each objective should be examined periodically to determine how well it is meeting the program goals. The objective should be stated in measurable terms so that a comparison can be made of what the objective intended to accomplish and what it actually accomplished. Evaluation should address the quality of what is being done. For example, if one of the activities was placing pit and fissure sealants on specific teeth of school-age children, an evaluator would want to assess how well that sealant was placed, the appropriateness of the tooth chosen, and the time involved in placing the sealant on the tooth.

The attitudes of the recipients of the program should be examined to determine whether the program was acceptable to them. Many programs are considered successful by those who run the program; however, the people who have been the recipients of the service may have wanted something very different. Figure 12-3 illustrates this point and gives us a perspective on planning by showing the concept of the planner, the actual plan, the design, the constraints involved, the alternative strat-

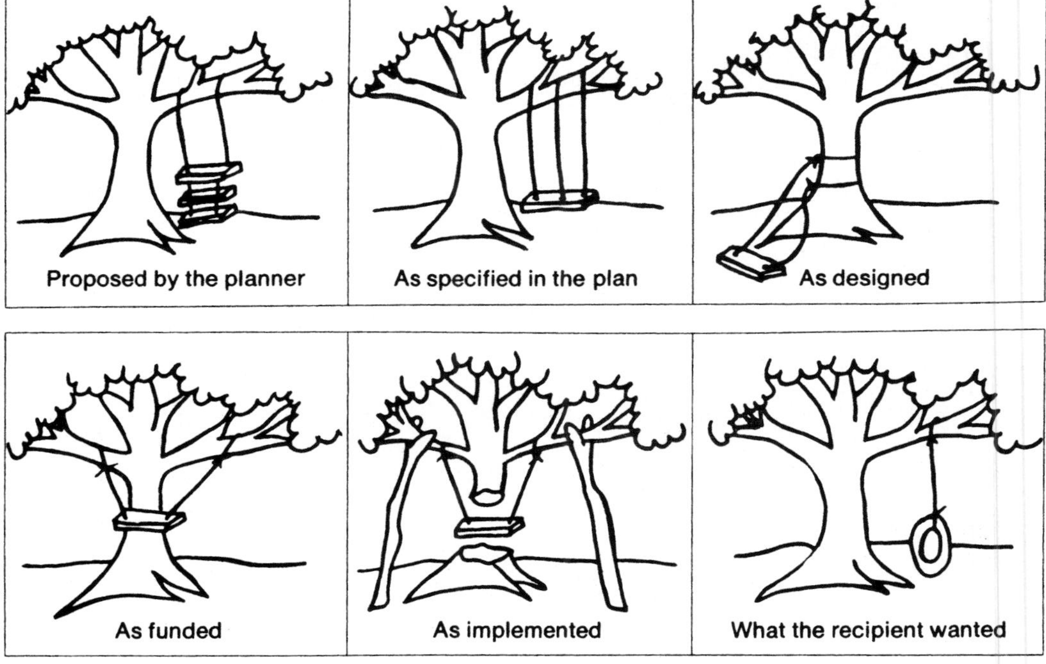

Fig. 12-3. A perspective on planning.

egy, and, finally, what the recipient wanted in the first place.

SUMMARY

The twenty-first century requires that the dental health professional, in addition to the delivery of clinical services, must demonstrate awareness of community health issues and provide leadership in the development of programs that address community needs and stress the importance of prevention. Planning is, of course, one of the activities that precedes the implementation of change. The role of the health professional is succinctly expressed in the statement of competencies by the profession of dental hygiene as approved by the house of delegates in 1999: "Dental hygienists must appreciate their role as health professionals at the local, state, and national levels. This role requires the graduate dental hygienist to assess, *plan,* and implement programs and activities to benefit the general population."[13]

REVIEW QUESTIONS

1. What steps should be considered when planning an oral health program for a community?
2. What information should be gathered when assessing the needs of a community or population?
3. How does one interpret the vast information gathered to plan an appropriate program?
4. What resources should be explored and

Proposed Community Activities for the Twenty-First Century

1. The construction of well-planned and accessible health facilities
2. The selection of appropriate, well-qualified, and sensitive health personnel
3. The provision of appropriate and effective health services
4. The time and the funds to provide the needed care
5. The active participation of representatives of those communities, organizations, and individuals who will be the recipients of the health care
6. Promotion of prevention strategies in the community
7. Planned security measures for health facilities and water supplies

what constraints should be identified in the planning process?

5. What rules should be followed when putting the plan into action?

REFERENCES

1. Dubos R: *So human an animal,* New York, 1968, Charles Scribner's Sons.
2. Striffier D: Surveying a community and developing a working policy: the administration of local dental programs, University of Michigan, School of Public Health, Proceedings from Fifth Workshop on Dental Public Health, Ann Arbor, MI, 1963.
3. Schulbert H et al: *Program evaluation in the health fields,* New York, 1969, Human Sciences.
4. Blum HL: *Note on comprehensive planning for health,* Berkeley, CA, 1968, Comprehensive Health Planning Unit, School of Public Health, University of California.
5. Provision of dental care in the community, University of Michigan School of Public Health, Ann Arbor, 1973, Proceedings from the Third Annual Course in Dental Public Health, Waldenwoods Conference Center, Hartland, MI, May 22-26, 1966.
6. Banfield EC, et al: *Politics, planning, and the public interest: the case of public housing in Chicago,* The Free Press, 1995.
7. Spiegel A et al: *Basic health planning methods,* Germantown, MD, 1978, Aspen Systems.
8. Reece SM: Community analysis for health planning: strategies for primary care practitioners, *Nurse Pract* 23(10):53-54, Oct 1998.
9. Department of Health, Education and Welfare, Public Health Service: *Dental program efficiency criteria and standards for the Indian Health Service,* Washington, DC, 1974, US Government Printing Office.
10. *Model standards for community preventive health services. A report to the U.S. Congress for the Secretary of Health, Education and Welfare,* Aug 1979.
11. Bruhn J: Planning for social change, *Am J Public Health* 63:7, 1972.
12. Guidance Note Issued by the Queen's Printer for Scotland. *An Action Plan for Dental Services in Scotland.* 2:1-5, Aug 10, 2001.
13. American Dental Hygienists Association Profile of ADHA. Available at www.adha.org/aboutadha/profile.htm.

CHAPTER 13

PROGRAM EVALUATION IN HEALTH CARE

David O. Born

PURPOSE OF PROGRAM EVALUATION

Program evaluation is concerned with finding out how well programs work by using social and behavioral science research techniques to assess information of importance to program administrators and public policy makers. The fundamental purpose of program evaluation is to provide information for decision making. Ultimately, evaluation is a judgment of merit or worth about a particular person, place, or thing.

IS EVALUATION RESEARCH?

The term *research* refers to systematic inquiry that leads one to discover or revise knowledge about a particular subject. Basic research is generally focused on discovering facts, relationships, behaviors, and underlying principles. Applied research often deals with the same phenomena, but the focus is usually less on the discovery of basic knowledge and more on the development of tools or the application of knowledge to develop solutions to actual problems. Evaluation is an example of applied research. Administrators, educators, policy makers, and others face questions (problems) about designing, implementing, continuing, and improving social, educational, health, and other programs. Evaluators assess or evaluate those programs to discover or revise knowledge about them and the problems they were designed to address so that informed judgments can be made, modifications can be implemented, and solutions can be achieved.

As researchers, program evaluators engage in scientific inquiry. They use tests, questionnaires, and other measurement devices. They collect and analyze data systematically by using common statistical procedures. Finally, they typically describe their findings in formal reports.[1]

An important difference between basic research and evaluation research is the generality of the findings. Ideally, the basic scientist is searching for basic knowledge; the more basic or fundamental, the better. Fundamental facts and principles, such as Einstein's theory of relativity, have broad applicability. They generalize across wide areas of knowledge. Most applied scientists—and program evaluators, in particular—are usually dealing with specific problems in specific settings. Their findings or conclusions can seldom be generalized to "similar" problems.

To elaborate on this distinction between the basic science researcher and the evaluator, consider the role each individual might play in the testing of a fluoride rinse. In examining the value of fluoride rinse, the basic science researcher would probably be concerned with the effects of fluoride on teeth, the strength of the solution necessary to produce a reduction in caries, and whether the conclusions could be generalized across the population. The evaluator would be more concerned with determining whether the actual mouth-rinse program, initiated to test the researcher's conclusion, was run correctly and followed the objectives that it stated. The evaluator's concern for the fluoride rinse as such is only superficial. Once the evaluator can judge whether the program is an accurate test of the fluoride rinse, the secondary results might then relate to the positive or negative effects of fluoride rinse. In other words, the particular program's operation is of prime importance to the evaluator, and the effect of fluoride is important only in terms of its results as applied to a realistic, closely monitored program.

Determining the value of things is another difference between evaluation and basic research. Evaluation eventually comes down to making a decision about what should be done or which course of action is best. Basic researchers strive only to obtain accurate, truthful information. There is no requirement to attach assessments of merit to the discovered knowledge.[1] Theoretically, the basic scientist's task does not involve making value judgments. The evaluator walks a fine line when it comes to value judgements. By its nature, evaluation research is based in a value context—the ultimate question, after all, is whether or not the subject (program) being studied is "of value." The evaluator must understand the value context within which he or she works. The best evaluation studies are those in which the evaluator is fully cognizant of this value context and is then able to "do objective science" that addresses critical questions.

FOCUS OF EVALUATIONS

Evaluation studies ultimately focus on the goals, objectives, or intent of the program or activity being studied. At the simplest level we ask, Does this program do what it was designed to do? There are, of course, many other facets to evaluation. One of the most useful frameworks for looking at the evaluation research task has been put forward by Donabedian.[2] He suggests that assessment or evaluation can profitably look at structure, process, and outcome.

Structure refers to the program setting and logistics (i.e., facilities, equipment, financing, human resources). Process refers to the techniques or methods employed in the provision of program services (i.e., delivering health care, educating children). Outcome refers to the "real world" impacts, effects, and changes brought about as a result of the program being evaluated.

Donabedian rightly sees structure, process, and outcomes as inextricably linked: the interrelationships are critical to the program's ability to meet its goals or fulfill its intent. Examining structure, process, and outcomes allows the evaluator to identify more clearly where problems and program liabilities lie and, hence, where corrections can be made if goals are to be met. Looking at goals, structure, process, and outcomes should be the primary focus for the evaluator. A second set of concerns also exists, however. These questions might be classified as "client" questions; that is, for whom and why is the evaluation research being conducted? This is not a trivial question. The researcher must understand, for example, the hierarchy of authority in the organization involved, what their interests and objectives are in requesting an evaluation, and what sorts of questions need to be asked. Often, one of the evaluator's biggest contributions lies in his or her ability to help administrators clarify their thinking about the need for and use of evaluation research.

By way of illustration, consider a situation in which a dental school implements a new curriculum for its students. An evaluator who is brought in designs and carries out a carefully planned study to determine if the program has the resources it needs (structure), how well the program is running (process), and how successful the graduates are (outcomes). Such an evaluation is appropriate if the client's interest is to determine if the curriculum is functioning properly and meeting its goals. The design would not be appropriate, however, if the client wanted to know if the graduates of the new curriculum were better-trained professionals than those of the old curriculum. The evaluator must understand the client's focus. Without such an understanding, valuable time and resources may be wasted without answering the fundamental questions and the client's needs.

Individuals interested in the results of evaluation may include program developers, program staff, program directors, policy makers (state or federal bureaucrats), program directors in other similar agencies, or epidemiologists.[3] Different groups of people have different needs and thus seek different information. Program developers seek information about ways to improve specific parts of programs that affect them directly. The director of the program is usually interested in knowing the overall effectiveness of the basic program, although he or she is generally more concerned with finding out what specific modifications will be needed to improve the organization and operation of the program. Financial issues are usually of concern to policy makers, who question whether a program should be continued as is, given more resources, or canceled. Costs and benefits are of paramount concern to them. Staff from other programs are interested in whether the program can be generalized for possible adaptation or adoption. Epidemiologists may seek to compare the effect of different program principles and generalize about the factors responsible for success.

Clearly, the evaluator faces a number of potentially competing interests. In responding to those interests the researcher must distinguish between different types of evaluation. As we have seen, Donabedian's framework allows us to focus on the critical features or components that make up a program. These factors must be taken into account if evaluation efforts are to be successful and useful. At the same time, Scriven[4] draws our attention to the fact that evaluation research may be one of two types. He uses the terms *formative* and *summative* to describe these types.

FORMATIVE EVALUATION

Formative evaluation refers to the internal evaluation of a program. It is an examination of the processes or activities of a program as they are taking place. It is usually carried out to aid in the development of a program in its early phases.

The following situation is one in which a

formative evaluation is appropriate: a fluoride rinse program is initiated at a neighborhood health center in which paraprofessionals are trained to administer three types of fluoride rinses under a strict sequence of procedures. After 3 days of operation, the work of the paraprofessionals is observed to determine the extent of adherence to a strict sequence of procedures. The observation and determination of correct or incorrect procedure sequence provide an example of examining the activities of a program as they are occurring (formative evaluation). If the sequence is incorrect, formative evaluation allows the program to make remedial changes at that point and thereby improve performance. Such a strategy is much better than waiting until the program is completed and then announcing that there were procedural errors. Formative evaluation is used primarily by program developers and program staff members concerned with whether various components of a program are workable or whether changes should be made to improve program activities.

SUMMATIVE EVALUATION

Summative evaluation, by contrast, judges the merit or worth of a program after it has been in operation. It is an attempt to determine whether a fully operational program is meeting the goals for which it was developed. Summative evaluation is aimed at program decision makers, who will decide whether to continue or terminate a program, and also at decision makers from other programs who might be considering adoption of the program.

Different evaluation designs are needed to carry out these two types of evaluation. Different types of measures and time schedules also are required. Because most programs are ongoing, with changes often being made "on the fly," a discernible end point or completion date may not exist. In such cases the dichotomy between formative and summative evaluation may not be as precise as described here, and formative evaluation may continue to be important as the program develops and matures.

Most health programs can be divided into four phases of implementation, which should occur in sequence: (1) the pilot phase, the development of which proceeds on a trial-and-error basis; (2) the controlled phase, in which a model of a particular program strategy is run under regulated conditions to judge its effectiveness; (3) the actualization phase, in which a model of the program strategy is subjected to realistic operating conditions; and (4) the operational phase, in which the program is an ongoing part of the structure. Often this ideal progression from phase 1 to phase 4 does not occur, and a program becomes lodged at one state of development. Each phase has different objectives to be met and thus different evaluation designs by which to best assess achievement of program objectives. Formative evaluation plays an important part in both the pilot phase and the controlled phase of program implementation. Summative and formative evaluations are used during the actualization phase, whereas the final operational phase is evaluated with a summative evaluation design.[5]

SPECIFYING HEALTH PROGRAM OUTCOMES AND INPUTS

One generalization that can be made of health program evaluation is that it is primarily concerned with how well a program is meeting its goals, either at some formative stage (so that the information can be fed back into the program) or at the end. The first step in evaluation, then, is to discover what the program goals are and to then restate them as clear, specific objectives written in measurable terms.

This first step is often a formidable task. Many program directors and staff members develop only general goals expressed as vague abstractions. They find it difficult to translate them into concrete specifications of the changes in behavior, attitude, knowledge, or health outcome that they hope to effect. In addition, programs often have multiple goals. Some are more important than others, some are more immediate (as opposed to long range), some are easier to study, and some may be incompatible with others. Yet all program directors and staff members must establish a sense of goal priorities if they, or external evaluators, are to assess the operation of their program. In many instances directors and staff members are unable to sort out goals, objectives, and priorities clearly, and they find it useful to bring in outside evaluators or administrative consultants to assist in this process.

Because goal statements are so often ambiguous and poorly stated, many observers have been led to speculate about the underlying reasons for this state of affairs. One view is that it usually requires support from diverse groups and individuals to get a program accepted. Program goals must be formulated in ways that satisfy the diversity of interests represented. Another speculation is that program planners lack experience with expressing their thoughts in measurable terms and concentrate mainly on the specifics of program operation. In one sense ambiguous goal statements serve a useful function: they hide differences among diverse groups by allowing for a variety of interpretations. However, such differences between groups and staff or within the staff can be disruptive when the program is implemented. Once a program has been initiated, if there is lack of true consensus as to what the program is specifically attempting to achieve, progress is difficult. Each staff member may be pulling in a different direction and trying to implement a different interpretation of the goal. As an outside agent or more objective observer, the evaluation study director can make a substantial contribution to program planning and administration in formulating goals, clarifying priorities, and reconciling divergent viewpoints related to program direction.

Ultimately, of course, evaluation attempts to measure the outcomes of a particular program. If a program's goals cannot be operationalized (stated in a precise, measurable manner), it becomes nearly impossible to determine whether the desired outcomes of a program have been achieved. In other words, without clearly stated goals and objectives, evaluation becomes an imprecise tool of questionable usefulness.

One common difficulty in specifying desired objectives is that objectives are often long range in nature, making it extremely difficult to measure success in meeting them. In the interim, evaluation is conducted by relying on surrogate measures of attitudes, knowledge, skills, or behaviors that presumably are related to the ultimate objectives.

Often, it is not until an evaluation study is started that the depth of the problem is discovered. That is, the program was implemented on the basis of important but nonetheless vaguely expressed goals that cannot be addressed effectively until they are reworked, a process that may involve administrators, boards of directors, advocacy organizations, and others. In some cases, programs may be designed to produce certain intermediate changes on the assumption that they are necessary for the attainment of ultimate goals. Probably the best that evaluation can do in such a situation is to discover whether intermediate goals are being met. Only after the more global "goals" are clearly identified and articulated can one begin the larger and more intensified research effort needed to determine the relation between these goals and desired final outcomes.

Measuring Outcomes

To evaluate the effectiveness of health programs, specific measurement instruments must be set up for systematic collection of data on the attainment of each program objective and program goal. These procedures follow accepted principles of biostatistical and research design, which are discussed in Chapters 14 and 15.

Establishment of an effective health program evaluation requires specific description and measurement of each objective and placing that information in the context of program goals. Depending on the nature of the program and the evaluation effort, some data will be collected as a part of the day-to-day operations of the program. Examples might include patient visits, staff turnover, program revenue, and supply costs. In most cases data collection instruments addressing specific objectives will also be necessary. Examples of factors to be measured by such instruments might include patient satisfaction, employee morale, sealant wear, and the mastery of skills (such as toothbrushing). Usually, multiple instruments are required. If a program has several objectives, use of a simple summary instrument is likely to be superficial and misleading. If measurement instruments that are truly relevant to program intents are available, they should be used, thus moving the evaluation process several steps ahead. Time is saved, and the program and the evaluation benefit from tested and validated instruments. Use of the same measurement instruments makes it easier to compare the relative effectiveness of one program with many other programs and adds significantly to the overall body of research knowledge. However, if existing instruments are not relevant to the program objectives, new measures constructed for the specific needs of the program must be developed.

Instrument Reliability and Validity

Measurement instruments used to assess program objectives and materials must be valid and reliable. A valid measurement instrument is one that provides a score that accurately describes the characteristics it is intended to measure. A reliable instrument consistently or repeatedly produces the same score. Validity and reliability are important because no test or other measurement instrument is perfect. Each time a test is administered, a range of scores results. We know that statistically each score contains a small amount of error because of testing and measurement procedures. If the procedure is repeated 10 times for 10 separate components of a health program, one can see how the amount of error can build, thus reducing the ability of the evaluation to assess program effectiveness accurately. The greater the reliability and validity, the more accurate the information collected during the evaluation process.

A simple example of a test that might be reliable but not valid would be the dental hygiene board examination administered to first-year dental students. Results of that test might prove to be highly reliable and consistent yet not valid. One might guess that if first-year dental students took the dental hygiene board examination several times, their individual scores would not fluctuate much higher or lower than the scores they received the first time. Thus the test would be considered highly reliable. It repeatedly produced the same or nearly the same score. This test would not be considered valid because it measured material totally foreign to the first-year dental student. The test is designed to measure skills of graduate dental hygienists, not first-year dental students. Thus the test is reliable but not valid.

As a second example, assume that a course is offered in which four tests are administered during the course of the semester. No one test was found to be perfectly reliable, thus error as a result of testing would result with each administration. Assume that student A received the following scores:

	Score	Reliability	Testing Error	Range
Test 1	80	0.80	5	75–85
Test 2	70	0.63	8	62–78
Test 3	80	0.55	12	68–92
Test 4	90	0.92	2	88–92
Average	80		73–87	

In this example student A obtained an average of 80 and probably would receive a course grade of B– or B. Yet because of normal error associated with the unreliability of the four tests, that student's true performance may be between 73 and 87. These scores indicate that student A's course grade could actually be between C– and B+, a substantial difference for most students. The more reliable the test, the smaller the error. Compare the reliability scores with the test error. The test with high reliability (0.92) has the smallest error (2), whereas the test with low reliability (0.55) has the greatest amount of error (12).

Difficulties in Obtaining Necessary Information

After consideration of what measurement instruments to use and when to measure outcomes, a final concern must be how to measure. In this area two problems are particularly important: bias and sampling. The possibility of bias is great if one evaluates his or her own work. Bias may be avoided by using objective measures (rather than subjective measures) and also by using several people (rather than a single person) to measure outcomes. Sampling is used in evaluating a health program when it is not possible or practical to obtain information from every person involved in an activity or when it is not possible to assess every activity that a program initiates.

Sample size depends on the activity to be studied. The student is advised to consult a standard research design text for a more formal discussion of bias and sampling problems related to evaluation and research.

Constant intrusions into the program for the purpose of collecting data can be a source of friction with program staff. The evaluation is a service to the program, not vice versa; therefore evaluation activities should be limited to those found essential to furthering the effectiveness of the program. One thoughtfully constructed test or questionnaire is often better than three imperfectly conceived ones. When the evaluation is clear about what is needed and why, measures can be constructed and data can be collected with a minimum of disruption.

Programs may intend to bring about changes not only in people but also in agencies, larger social systems, or the public at large. Measures must be relevant to such

Table 13-1. Component Factors of Health System Characteristics

Availability	*Accessibility*	*Cost*	*Quality*	*Continuity*	*Acceptability*
Supply of services: Existing service capacity Used capacity Supply of resources: Personnel Equipment Facilities Financial resources	Ability to obtain services in terms of these factors: 1. Economic Out-of-pocket cost Health insurance coverage and benefits Opportunity cost to patient/client, family, and others 2. Temporal Travel time Waiting time 3. Locational 4. Architectural 5. Cultural 6. Organizational 7. Informational Use of services by specified population subgroups	Service cost Costs incurred by providers Costs incurred by financing mechanisms Sources of payment for services	Structure Competence and qualifications of resources Existence and extent of review and assurance mechanisms Minimal volume of specialized services Process Accuracy of services Appropriateness of services Documentation of treatment Outcome Health status Behavior Environment	Coordination of settings among health system components and to/from other nonhealth systems Regular source of care Degree of interruptions or delays in service plan given a logical sequence of services Patient transfer Medical and health information transfer Follow-up	Consumer satisfaction with Availability Accessibility Cost Continuity Courtesy and consideration Provider satisfaction

Modified from Hadley SA, Gillespie JF Jr: Operational measures: indicators of health system performance, *Am J Health Plan* 3:44, 1978.

changes. Cost-benefit analysis is another measurement technique. This technique is not a suitable substitute for the usual methods of evaluation but a logical extension of them. Evaluation defines the program's benefits; cost-benefit analysis adds consideration of the value of the benefits. Costs of the program are compared with benefits as a way of judging whether the program is a worthwhile investment.

How does one decide which program activities to measure? Difficulties arise when theory and knowledge are inadequate to define the factors that affect success. In most program areas the general rule of thumb is that each stated objective of the program should be measured. A clearly stated objective indicates what achievement is sought, and thus such an objective will aid in the identification of what procedures to use for measuring program outcomes.

Table 13-1 presents six general factors that may serve as starting points for evaluation of health programs. Below each general factor are specific areas in which various program members would find evaluation information of interest. This list is not intended to be all-inclusive. It is designed to provide a few ideas to an individual who is not sure where to begin.

To conclude this discussion of measurement instruments, the following outline identifies three factors to consider in instrument selection: importance, statistical adequacy, and feasibility.[6]

1. Importance
   a. Is the information that is gained by administering the instrument the measure that is needed to assess health status or health program effectiveness?
   b. Does the program require this information to perform its function?
2. Statistical adequacy
   a. *Validity.* Does the instrument accurately assess what you are trying to measure?
   b. *Reliability.* Will repeated application of the computational method for the measure yield similar results? How reliable are the data used to calculate the results?
   c. *Sensitivity.* Can the instrument adequately distinguish among levels of performance?
3. Feasibility
   a. *Clarity of measure.* How precise is the measure? Is the wording understandable? Are its limitations explained?
   b. *Data availability and cost.* Does the program have the information needed to assess the objective? Are the instruments appropriate for their specific use within the program?
   c. *Compatibility.* Can data collected for this program be compared with similar data on a statewide or national basis? Can they be compared with similar data from different types of programs?
   d. *Ease of use and interpretation.* Can collection and interpretation of data for implementation of the measure be done without specialized or statistical knowledge?

STUDY DESIGNS APPROPRIATE FOR SPECIFIC PROGRAMS

In planning an evaluation study, one is immediately struck by the fact that a multitude of possible study designs exist from which to choose.[7] Choosing the best design is one of the most critical tasks the evaluator faces. In the broadest sense, evaluation research designs are divided into two groups: experimental and nonexperimental. Experimental design has long been considered the ideal for evaluation. The design requires that people, objects, and other factors be randomly assigned either to the program or to a control group. A control group is a set of individuals in an experiment whose selection and experiences are identical in every way possible to the program participants except that they are not part of the program. The control group may receive a pseudoprogram (the social science equivalent of the laboratory placebo), the standard program (the traditional rather than the innovative program), or no program at all. Relevant measurements are taken before and after the program. If the program recipients show greater positive change than the controls, the outcome can clearly be attributed to the program. Experimental design is the study design that most researchers select when given a choice.[8]

Toothbrushing studies are a perfect example of the true experimental design model. For illustration purposes the study shown in Table 13-2 demonstrates the effectiveness of a fluoride toothpaste for the reduction of new carious lesions. The study is of 3 years' duration and of longitudinal design. Both experimental and control groups brush daily under supervision. The study is double-blind; all experimental materials are color coded, and the look and the taste are identical. All participants use the same brand and model of toothbrush, with the type of toothpaste (i.e., fluoride toothpaste and nonfluoride toothpaste) being the one variable examined in the study. Results show a significant reduction in the number of new lesions, thus allowing the researcher to assume that the reduction was a result of the one differing variable (i.e., fluoride versus nonfluoride).

Table 13-2. Longitudinal Results of 3-Year Fluoride Toothpaste Study

	Randomly Assigned Groups	
	Experimental (Fluoride Toothpaste)	*Control (Nonfluoride Toothpaste)*
Baseline examination (DMFS) (before beginning testing)	97.4	97.5
After 1 yr	91.5	95.0
After 2 yr	86.3	93.4
After 3 yr	80.0	90.3
Difference	17.4	7.2

DMFS, Decayed, missing, filled surfaces.

One major problem arises when an attempt is made to implement experimental procedures in health programs. It is nearly impossible to implement the design in the busy day-to-day activities of the program. How can random services be tested on people who come to drop-in, multiservice, or neighborhood health centers? In addition, there is resistance from the program staff and difficulty resulting from the very nature of the recipient groups and from outside events that "contaminate" the controls placed on the study. These contaminations reduce the validity of the evaluation.

Two types of validity affect the ability to implement evaluation research designs according to strict experimental requirements: internal validity and external validity. These kinds of validity are different from the term *validity* used earlier in relation to measurement instruments. A program has internal validity if its outcomes result from the approach or the techniques being tested rather than from other causes that have nothing to do with the program being implemented. Internal validity determines whether the results can be accepted based on the evaluation design of the program.[2]

A program has external validity if the

results obtained can be generalized to similar programs or approaches everywhere. External validity affects one's ability to credit the evaluation results with generality based on the procedures used.[8]

By its nature the process of conducting an experimental evaluation design exercises some degree of control over the program, thus contributing to internal validity, while producing some limitations in external validity. A catch-22 situation is produced. As the circumstances of a program are controlled, the chances that what happens in the program will be exactly what the evaluator hopes to find (internal validity) increase. However, the more conditions are controlled, the less chance there is that the program will continue to work when the controls are removed (external validity).

The constant struggle between external and internal validity is an important one; external validity is of little value without some reasonable degree of internal validity to provide confidence in the conclusions. There is no advantage in being able to generalize results that are based on invalid or inconsistent program activities. The two sets of validity demands must strike a balance. There should be enough internal validity so that an experiment can be conclusive; yet it should be sufficiently realistic to be generalized. In program evaluation internal validity becomes the major concern because most programs involve only a superficial attempt to generalize results beyond their program.

Perhaps the most respected source in the area of research design is Donald T. Campbell. Campbell[9] suggests that experimental design is possible in most health programs with careful planning and administrative backing and that control groups can be used in somewhat turbulent programs.

In reality, it is often impossible to apply rules relating to internal validity fully. To evaluate programs in such situations, the evaluator must choose some approach other than experimental. If circumstances preclude experimental design, quasi-experimental designs developed by Campbell and Stanley[8] are often suitable. Campbell[9] offers three types useful in evaluation: interrupted time series, control series, and regression discontinuity designs. Although the results of these approaches do not provide the certainty and the potential for generalization of experimental designs, they guard against most of the important threats to valid interpretation. For the interested student, a standard research methods text is suggested for more comprehensive discussion of research design. It should also be noted that evaluation is concerned with making decisions about specific programs. Therefore internal validity is often more important than external validity to the evaluator.

OUTCOMES ASSESSMENT

In many social and health service sectors, attention has recently been centered on something termed *outcomes assessment.* Within the field of dentistry, this term is increasingly used in the evaluation of dental educational programs and managed care programs, among others. Although the subject of measuring program outcomes has come up throughout this chapter, the newer term *outcomes assessment* shifts the focus to a somewhat different emphasis than that of standard evaluation research; such differences as do exist tend to derive from the orientation of the evaluators involved in specifying the outcomes to be measured. Additionally, outcomes assessment tends to reflect a broader, more inclusive view of the program and the socioeconomic context within which it operates. In particular, it involves a trend toward identifying outcomes that are ultimately meaningful to the consumers of the programs being evaluated.

In the case of managed care in dentistry, providers, plan purchasers, insurers, and patients all have specific interests in the outcome of the managed care plan. Capilouto,[10] for example, points out that purchasers want lower costs and higher quality, patients want lower out-of-pocket expenses, and providers are struggling to obtain the best "price" for their services. Insurers, like purchasers, are concerned about quality and price but have an additional interest in generating profits. Other authors also have addressed the issues of outcome assessment in the highly charged atmosphere being created by the current explosion of managed care programs in dentistry.[11-13]

Although much of the work being undertaken in the development and assessment of outcome measures in dentistry is essentially evaluation research, much of it is termed *health services research.* This term suggests a broader focus than is usually attached to evaluation research. The expanded focus serves to draw our attention to the fact that with the increasing complexity of delivering and financing health care in this nation, programs must be evaluated not only in narrow terms that define their programmatic effectiveness but also in the context of their interaction with elements drawn from much wider reaches of the health arena. New political, financial, administrative, and delivery system networks and alliances are forming as active and reactive forces in the dental care marketplace. At the same time, individual patients often find their power in the marketplace diminishing as employers and insurers "wheel and deal" with enormous sums of health care dollars, shaving costs at every turn in the interest of maximizing profits.

Providers, like patients, also find their roles changing dramatically. The dynamics of the entire system have become more wide ranging, more complex, and more interconnected with nonhealth sectors of the economy. Specific dental care program evaluation (and thus outcomes assessment) must be designed to address the concerns of more and more outside agencies, individuals, and political constituencies. Therefore health services research and outcomes assessment must not only address the issues of quality of care, patient satisfaction, and other variables traditionally specified in evaluation paradigms; they also must be sensitive to and account for the influences of these more fluid, and often powerful, forces. Given these circumstances, the basic principles of good evaluation are unchanged, but the scope of the studies often must be expanded considerably.[14]

CONSTRAINTS ON USING THE RESULTS OF EVALUATION

Once the evaluation is completed, the logical expectation is that the results will be used to make rational decisions about future programming. All too often, however, the results are ignored. With all the money, time, effort, skill, and irritation that went into the acquisition of information, why do the results generally have so little impact? One reason may be that evaluation results do not match the informational needs of decision makers.

Individuals responsible for conducting evaluations should have a better understanding of decision processes and informational requirements relevant to decision making. A related issue is timing. Evaluation results should be ready in time to be considered, not after the decisions on future programming have been reached. Moreover, the evaluation results may not be relevant to the level of the decision maker who receives them. For example, overall assessments of program merit may be most useful to directors in other agencies who want to know whether a new program strategy works and, if so, under what conditions. Such people may never receive the report, or they may receive it in a nearly unreadable form.

Another constraint on the use of results may be a lack of clear direction for future programming. Results may be ambiguous, and their implications may be unclear. Results must be translated into terms that make sense for pending decisions and that delineate alternatives indicated. There seems to be a large void between the findings of program evaluation and the planning of future programs. Someone is needed to translate the evaluation results into explicit recommendations for future programs.

In practice, evaluation is sometimes undertaken for dubious reasons. Evaluation may be used by program decision makers to delay a decision, to justify a decision already made, to pass the responsibility of future decisions to others, to vindicate a program in the eyes of its observers, or to satisfy funding conditions of government or foundation agencies.[5] These noninformational reasons for evaluation are not rare, and individuals conducting an evaluation should be forewarned if they learn that one of these is the underlying purpose of evaluation. It is as important to spend enough time investigating who wants to know what and why as it is to carry out the evaluation activities. Evaluations performed for political ends or in situations in which there is no commitment to using the data for decision making might well be eliminated rather than wasting the talents of the individuals involved.[15]

External evaluators (persons called in who are not part of the program) are often reluctant to draw conclusions from their data. However, judgments and recommendations for action must be made at some point. Unless the evaluator plays a leading role in the process, this important step may not get done.

A further constraint on the use of results is that organizations are comfortable with the status quo. When organizations are presented with negative results, their prestige, ideology, and even resources are threatened. They frequently react by rejecting the results.

Campbell[9] suggests that one way out of this dilemma is for reformers to change their stance. Instead of committing themselves to new programs as though they were proven solutions, they would do better to commit themselves to seeking solutions to the problem. Then they could run a series of experimental programs until genuine solutions were found.

The prevalence of negative findings in a wide range of program fields is not something to bemoan or cover up, even when such results provoke political controversy or organizational resistance. Rather, the evidence that so many programs are having little constructive effect represents a fundamental critique of current approaches to social programming. This is a matter to which society will, in time, need to respond.

SUMMARY

Evaluation involves research into the operation and accomplishments of programs that are usually, but not exclusively, designed to have an impact on social problems. By their very nature, evaluation efforts are linked, more or less directly, to a set of values that provide the criteria for judging relative success.

In considering programs the evaluator must recognize that program structure, process, and outcomes are all interrelated and that these factors are functionally related to the program's goals and objectives. Performing a good evaluation involves formulating (or clarifying) objectives, specifying the criteria to be used in measuring success, determining and explaining the degree of observed success, and (usually) recommending modifications in program activity to improve performance.[16]

Evaluations are undertaken not simply to reveal success or failure. If that were the case, most evaluations of programs would reveal a lack of total success in attaining goals and objectives. Good evaluation does more than demonstrate the degree of attainment. It also identifies problems and points out how a structural problem, for example, links with and affects process and outcome variables.

Identified problems may also relate to ill-conceived, ill-defined, or simply misdirected goals. Ideally, good evaluations identify opportunities and ways to correct programs and to improve their efficiency. The evaluation of programs assumes that (1) programs have been planned to expend funds to enable materials to be developed and activities to be performed and (2) the activities are intended to cause the achievement of program goals.

A program may not achieve its goals for the following reasons:[17]

1. Resources were not used as planned.
2. The assumptions linking resources to activities were invalid.
3. Activities were not performed as planned.
4. The assumptions linking activities to objectives were invalid.
5. The assumptions linking objectives to the program goals were invalid.

A sixth reason, which is technically included in this list but often overlooked and thus deserving of special mention, is that the behavior of the program staff, the client population, or both may consciously or unconsciously undermine program performance. In other words, the best-designed program in the world cannot succeed if the providers and the clients do not like it and are unwilling to cooperate. Such resistance may be overt or covert but is, in either case, destructive.

If evaluation can identify the problems, subsequent program planning should proceed more effectively than it would in the absence of evaluation. Thus a successful evaluation in the hands of a thoughtful administrator can improve the planning and management of programs, thereby increasing program effectiveness.

REVIEW QUESTIONS

1. Define *program evaluation*. What is its primary purpose?
2. What is the major difference between basic research and program evaluation?
3. Describe how a researcher might test for the efficacy of fluoride rinse. Contrast this approach with that of the program evaluator.
4. Donabedian has suggested that a program be evaluated on three levels. Name and define these levels.
5. Contrast formative and summative evaluation.

6. What are the four phases of program implementation? Describe each phase.
7. Define *validity* and *reliability*.
8. Create a project to evaluate the efficacy of a school water fluoridation program. How would you evaluate the program?

REFERENCES

1. Popham JW: *Educational evaluation,* Englewood Cliffs, NJ, 1975, Prentice Hall.
2. Donabedian A: The quality of care: how can it be assessed? *JAMA* 260:1743, 1988.
3. Weiss CH: *Evaluating action programs: readings in social action and education,* Boston, 1972, Allyn & Bacon.
4. Scriven M: The methodology of evaluation. In Tyler RN, Gagne RM, Scriven M, editors: *Perspectives of curriculum evaluation,* AERA monograph series on curriculum evaluation, no 1, Chicago, 1967, Rand McNally.
5. Suchman EA: Action for what? A critique of evaluation research. In O'Toole R, editor: *The organization, management, and tactics of social research,* Cambridge, MA, 1970, Schenkman.
6. Schulberg HC, Sheldon A, Baker F: *Program evaluation in the health fields,* New York, 1969, Behavioral Publications.
7. Isaac S, Michael WB: *Handbook in research and evaluation,* San Diego, 1981, EdITS.
8. Campbell DT, Stanley JC: *Experimental and quasi-experimental design for research,* Chicago, 1966, Rand McNally.
9. Campbell DT: *Reform as experiments in evaluating action programs,* Boston, 1972, Allyn & Bacon.
10. Capilouto E: Market forces driving health care reform, *J Dent Educ* 59(4):480, 1995.
11. Bader J et al: A health plan report card for dentistry, *J Am Coll Dentists,* p 29, Fall 1996.
12. Symposium on self-reported assessments of oral health outcomes, *J Dent Educ* 60(6):485, 1996.
13. Maas W, Garcia AI: Health services research, the Agency for Healthcare Policy and Research, and dental practice, *J Am Coll Dentists* 61(1):18-24, 1994.
14. Bader J: Health services research in dental public health, *J Public Health Dent* 52(1):23, 1992.
15. Elinson J: Effectiveness of social action programs in health and welfare, assessing the effectiveness of child health services, Report of the Fifty-Sixth Ross Conference on Pediatric Research, Columbus, OH, 1967.
16. Glossary of administrative terms in public health, *Am J Public Health* 50:225, 1960.
17. Deniston OL, Rosenstock IM, Getting VA: Evaluation of program effectiveness, *Public Health Rep* 83:323, 1968.

BIBLIOGRAPHY

Anderson SB et al: *Encyclopedia of educational evaluation,* San Francisco, 1976, Jossey Bass.

Baker EL: Formative evaluation. In Popham JW, editor: *Evaluation in education: current applications,* Berkeley, CA, 1974, McCutchan.

Bloom BS, Hastings ST, Madaus GF: *Handbook on formative and summative evaluation of student learning,* New York, 1971, McGraw-Hill.

Cook TD, Campbell DT: *Quasi-experimental design and analysis issues for field settings,* Boston, 1979, Houghton Mifflin.

Dillman DA: *Mail and Internet surveys: the tailored design method,* New York, 2000, Wiley.

Donabedian A: The seven pillars of quality, *Arch Pathol Lab Med* 114:1115, 1990.

FitzGibbon CT, Morris LL: *How to design a program evaluation,* Beverly Hills, CA, 1978, Sage.

FitzGibbon CT, Morris LL: *How to present an evaluation report,* Beverly Hills, CA, 1978, Sage.

Guba EG: Development, diffusion and evaluation. In Eidell TE, Kitchell JM, editors: *Knowledge production and utilization in educational administration,* Eugene, OR, 1968, Center for the Advanced Study of Educational Administration, University of Oregon.

Guba EG: Failure of educational evaluation, *Educ Tech* 9:29, 1969.

Polit DF, Hungler BP: *Nursing research: principles and methods,* ed 2, Philadelphia, 1983, JB Lippincott.

Rosenstock IM: Evaluating health programs, *Public Health Rep* 85:835, 1970.

Rosenstock IM, Welch W, Getting VA: Evaluation of program efficiency, *Public Health Rep* 83:603, 1968.

Rossi PH, Freeman HE, Lipsey MW: *Evaluation: a systematic approach,* Newbury Park, CA, 1999, Sage.

Stufflebeam DL et al: *Educational evaluation and decision making,* Itasca, IL, 1971, FE Peacock.

Suchman EA: *Evaluation research: principles and practice in public service and action programs,* New York, 1967, Russell Sage Foundation.

Tuchman BW: *Conducting educational research,* ed 2, New York, 1978, Harcourt Brace Jovanovich.

Wholey JS et al: *Federal evaluation policy,* Washington, DC, 1970, Urban Institute.

Worthen BR: Toward a taxonomy of evaluation designs, *Educ Tech* 8:3, 1968.

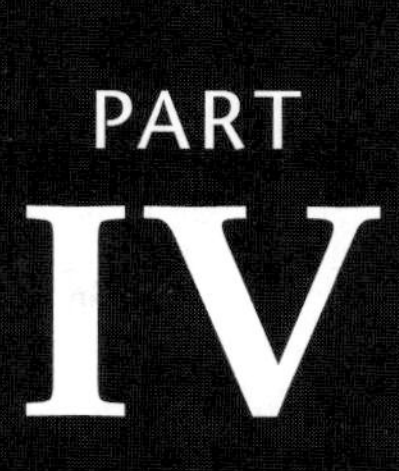

PART IV

RESEARCH IN DENTAL PUBLIC HEALTH

CHAPTER

14

OVERVIEW OF BIOSTATISTICS

Lynda Rose

Why Biostatistics?

> *Figures often beguile me, particularly when I have the arranging of them myself; in which case the remark attributed to Disreali would often apply with justice and force: "There are three kinds of lies: lies, damned lies and statistics."*
>
> —Autobiography of Mark Twain

As a practitioner and teacher of biostatistics, I have often wondered what the branch of mathematics known as statistics ever did to warrant such a contemptuous remark from Sir Benjamin Disreali, friend and confidant of Queen Victoria and prime minister of England. Disreali died in 1881, but his distrust of statistics has survived the nineteenth and twentieth centuries, and it lives today in the twenty-first. In nearly every group of biostatistics students who grace my classroom, at least one student poses the challenge: "But can't you make statistics say whatever you want them to say?" It is the goal of this chapter to introduce the reader to the sound principles of biostatistics and their proper application to dental research data. In the process, it is hoped that any lurking fear of biostatistics will be replaced with the realization that biostatistics is a powerful ally in the quest for the truth that infuses a set of data and waits to be told.

Dental health professionals have a variety of uses for data: for designing a health care program or facility, for evaluating the effectiveness of an oral hygiene education program, for determining the treatment needs of a specific population, and for proper interpretation of the scientific literature, to name just a few. In these instances, data are helpful only to the extent that these sets of data may be summarized and interpreted. Thus evidence-based decisions can be made about the results of research, program evaluation, or needs assessment. These tasks that we ask of data illustrate the two major divisions of statistics: descriptive statistics and inferential statistics. Descriptive statistical techniques enable researchers to numerically describe and summarize a set of data; inferential statistical techniques provide a basis for testing hypotheses and applying statistical results to the group of individuals or objects that form the population of interest.

DESCRIPTIVE STATISTICS

Population versus Sample

A population is any entire group of items (objects, materials, people, etc.) that possess at least one basic defined characteristic in common. Examples of populations might be all dentists, all U.S. citizens, all periodontally involved teeth, all individuals in a given school, or all patients treated at a particular private office. It is often impossible to collect information from an entire population because of the size of the population or because of such limitations as finances, time, or distance between population members. In cases in which it is impossible to collect data on the entire population, complete and reliable information can be collected from a representative portion of the population termed a *sample.* By observing and measuring a sample, it is possible to obtain information and make statements about the total population.

Statistics is a science that describes data for the purpose of making inferences about the population from which the data are obtained. When we collect a specific piece of information—data—from each member of a population, we obtain a characteristic of the population termed a *parameter.* Similarly, when we collect a piece of information from each member of a sample, we obtain a characteristic of the sample termed a *statistic.* Because most studies are conducted by using samples, statistics rather than population parameters are most commonly used. Using statistics (characteristics of a sample), we try to infer what the parameters (characteristics of a population) will be.

Random Samples

Samples, by definition, cannot have exactly the same characteristics as a population. However, a sample that is truly representative of the population can be obtained by using probability sampling methods and by taking a sufficiently large sample.

A *random sample* is defined as one in which every element in the population has an equal and independent chance of being selected. The following example illustrates two random sampling procedures: assume a population of 5000 seniors in the predental program at 50 universities. Each senior class has 100 predental students divided into five equal sections of 20 students each. The objective is to determine the grade point average (GPA) of each predental student by selecting a representative sample of 1000 students (i.e., a sampling ratio of one fifth, or 20%). A simple random sample to select the 1000 students would be completed in the following manner: a list of 5000 students must be compiled and numbered 1 through 5000. A numbered tag is prepared for each student. From the 5000 well-mixed tags, 1000 are drawn by a lottery. After each selection the tag is replaced and another tag is drawn. This is the most basic random sample approach.

A similar procedure may be applied for selecting a random sample by using a table of random numbers, which can be found in most statistics textbooks. For this example, it would be necessary to use four columns of digits in the tables so that each student, 1 through 5000, would have an equal probability of being selected. Selection would begin by blindly identifying a number on the table that corresponds to a member of the total population (1 through 5000). The selection process continues by taking numbers horizontally or vertically until the desired sample size is reached. Repeated numbers are omitted when encountered during sample selection in both procedures.

Random sampling is the procedure of choice whenever possible. It prevents the possibility of selection bias on the part of the researcher. What if GPA is related to school? A simple random sample may not ensure representation of the entire population of predental students. It may be necessary to select individuals according to certain strata or subgroups to diminish the chance of sample fluctuation. This method of selection is termed *stratified sampling*. It is accomplished by randomly selecting a proportionate number of subjects from each subgroup for the sample. In the preceding example the subgroup would be the university attended. To produce a stratified random sample, one would (1) prepare a list of students at each of the 50 universities and (2) draw at random one fifth of the students at each university. Because the sampling ratio is used in each stratum, there is a proportional allocation by school. This eliminates the possibility of sampling bias, which could result by selecting at random and giving no consideration to school.

Another type of sampling is the systematic sample. A systematic sample is not a true random sample because everyone may not have an independent chance of being selected. This type of sample is usually obtained by drawing a number and then selecting every *n*th individual, for example, having a list of names and deciding to test every even-numbered person on the list. All odd-numbered names are systematically excluded.

Two types of samples that may introduce serious bias in estimating population parameters are (1) the judgment sample and (2) the convenience sample. In a judgment sample someone with knowledge of the population may select a sample in arbitrary ways to represent the population. In a convenience sample a group is chosen because it happens to be convenient and may represent the population; for example, one classroom within a school is selected because the teacher gives permission to work with the pupils, or the patients at a particular private office are used because the dentist allows access to the patient list. Results relating to that particular classroom or that particular dentist's office may be valid, but when generalized to include the larger population of school classrooms or dentists' offices, their reliability is questionable.

Once a sample has been selected, data are collected according to the study protocol, and consideration must then be given to data analysis. As previously stated, the statistical analysis of data requires the application of the principles of descriptive statistics and hypothesis testing. Before presenting these principles, we must first answer the general question: What are data?

Scales of Measurement

In general, data are any information that can be collected. Name, address, job title, social security number, age, gender, income, height, and weight are examples of data. Though not all data are represented by numbers, this discussion is limited to numerical variables. Before one can determine the appropriate methods for summarizing and displaying data, it is necessary to understand the nature of the variable of interest, that is, its scale of measurement. The type of data also plays an important role in deciding which statistical procedures to apply in a test of a hypothesis. The two major scales of measurement are the following classifications: *categorical* (enumeration) data and *continuous* data (measurements).

CATEGORICAL DATA

Enumeration data are data that are represented by mutually exclusive categories. These data are qualitative (descriptive) and not quantitative. Categorical data are further classified into two types: *nominal scale* and *ordinal scale.*

A variable measured on the nominal scale is characterized by named categories having no particular order. For example, patient gender (male/female), reason for dental visit (checkup, routine treatment, emergency), and use of fluoridated water (yes/no) are all categorical variables measured on a nominal scale. Within each of these scales, an individual subject may belong to only one level, and one level does not mean something greater than any other level.

Ordinal scale data are variables whose categories possess a meaningful order. Severity of periodontal disease (0 = none, 1 = mild, 2 = moderate, 3 = severe) and length of time spent in a dental office waiting room (1 = less than 15 min, 2 = 15 to less than 30 minutes, 3 = 30 minutes or more) are variables measured on ordinal scales.

CONTINUOUS DATA

Continuous, or measurement, data make up the scale of measurement with which we are perhaps most familiar. Numerical values are assigned according to a systematic rule and exist on a continuum (for any two points on the scale, an intermediate value exists, at least theoretically). Some texts further characterize measurement data as interval scale (zero is only a reference point, as in temperature) and ratio scale (zero is truly "zero"). Most measurements qualify as ratio scale: blood pressure, body weight, head circumference, and number of minutes to relief of pain.

DISPLAYING DATA

FREQUENCY DISTRIBUTION TABLES

To better explain data that have been collected, the data values are often organized and presented in a table termed a *frequency distribution table.* This type of data display shows each value that occurs in the data set and how often each value occurs. In addition to providing a sense of the shape of a variable's distribution, these displays provide the researcher with an opportunity to screen the data values for incorrect or impossible values, a first step in the process known as "cleaning the data." Routinely, data analysts generate a frequency distribution table for every variable that is recorded in a research project.

The construction of a frequency distribution table is straightforward and easily accomplished with standard statistical software. The data values are first arranged in order from lowest to highest value (an array). The frequency with which each value occurs is then tabulated. The frequency of occurrence for each data point is expressed in four ways:

1. The actual count or frequency
2. The relative frequency (percent of the total number of values)
3. Cumulative frequency (total number of observations equal to or less than the value)
4. Cumulative relative frequency (the percent of observations equal to or less than the value), commonly referred to as percentile

The following example illustrates this descriptive display of data. A group of 33 dental students has taken Part I of the National Boards examinations. Their examination scores have been recorded. The dean of the dental school wishes to summarize these scores at the next school faculty meeting. Here are a few of the ways that the information could be presented.

First, an ungrouped frequency distribution table of the National Board scores is presented in Table 14-1. The variable of interest is the examination score, which is shown in the first column of the table. The examination scores for the group are listed in descending order. The next column of the table contains the frequency with which each score occurs in the data set. Next, the frequency of occurrence is expressed as a relative frequency, that is, as a percent of the total number of scores represented in the table. For example, three students scored 77 on the examination. This represents 9.1% of the group of 33 students.

Second, the data can be displayed as a cumulative frequency distribution. Table 14-1 shows the cumulative frequency and cumulative percent for the National Board scores. These descriptive measures express the frequency of occurrence of scores up to and including any given value in the data set. For example, 25 students (75.8% of the group) scored 80 or below on this examination. Also, the score that defines the 97th percentile is 88.

Instead of displaying each individual value in a data set, the frequency distribution for a variable can group values of the variable into consecutive intervals. Then the number of observations belonging to an interval are counted.

A grouped frequency distribution for the National Board scores is illustrated in Table 14-2. Note that although the data are condensed in a useful fashion, some information is lost. The frequency of occurrence of an individual data point cannot be obtained from a grouped frequency distribution. For example, seven students scored between 74 and 77, but the number of students who scored 75 is not shown here.

Table 14-1. Frequency Distribution Table for National Board Scores (NB1)

	National Boards 1			
NB1	*Frequency*	*%*	*Cumulative Frequency*	*Cumulative %*
56	1	3.0	1	3.0
57	1	3.0	2	6.1
63	1	3.0	3	9.1
65	2	6.1	5	15.2
66	1	3.0	6	18.2
68	2	6.1	8	24.2
69	2	6.1	10	30.3
70	1	3.0	11	33.3
71	1	3.0	12	36.4
72	2	6.1	14	42.4
74	1	3.0	15	45.5
75	1	3.0	16	48.5
76	2	6.1	18	54.5
77	3	9.1	21	63.6
78	2	6.1	23	69.7
79	1	3.0	24	72.7
80	1	3.0	25	75.8
81	3	9.1	28	84.8
82	1	3.0	29	87.9
83	1	3.0	30	90.9
84	1	3.0	31	93.9
88	1	3.0	32	97.0
89	1	3.0	33	100.0

Table 14-2. Grouped Frequency Distribution of National Board Scores

Scores	*Number of Students*	*%*
56-61	2	6
62-65	3	9
66-69	5	15
70-73	4	12
74-77	7	21
78-81	7	21
82-85	3	9
86-89	2	6

GRAPHS

Graphing represents another alternative in displaying data pictorially and allowing rapid assimilation of findings by the reader. A general rule for constructing graphs along the x and y axes is that the vertical y axis usually represents the frequency of scores occurring along the scale of measurement, whereas the x axis represents the scale that measures the variable of interest.

A bar graph is a two-dimensional pictorial display of data that is measured on a categorical scale, either nominal or ordinal. Each category is represented by a separate bar, and the height of the bar reflects the number or percent of observations belonging to that category. In a bar chart, the bars do not touch each other, and the order of the bars (categories) should be determined by what makes the most sense for the variable that is pictured in the chart. Figure 14-1 is an example of a graph of the distribution of a categorical variable measured on the nominal scale. Each bar displays the percent of the study's subjects who belong to each category of marital status. Because the scale is nominal, the bars can be scrambled with no loss of meaning or understanding.

A histogram is also a graphic representation formed directly from a frequency distribution table, but a histogram is used to display a continuous measurement variable. A histogram is a display in which the horizontal (abscissa) axis is a continuous number line that represents the measurement scale of the variable of interest. These values on the x axis are grouped into equal intervals, and the number of observations in each interval are counted and displayed on the vertical (ordinate) axis. Graphically, a histogram is similar to a bar graph because the frequency is also represented by the height of a bar over the interval in question. However, the bars in a histogram must touch one another because of the continuous nature of the scale of measurement. Figure 14-2 shows the histogram for the continuous variable age (in years).

As required, the x axis is divided into equal intervals, namely 5-year intervals. The midpoint of each interval is displayed in the axis labels (40, 45, 50, etc.). The number of subjects belonging to each 5-year interval is displayed on the y axis. From this histogram, one can easily determine that these patients are seniors because the majority belongs to the age intervals older than 62.5 years.

TABLES

In addition to graphs, data are often summarized in tables. When material is presented in tabular form, the table should be able to stand alone; that is, correctly presented material in tabular form should be understandable even if the written discussion of the data is not read. A major concern in the presentation of both figures and tables is readability (Box 14-1). Tables

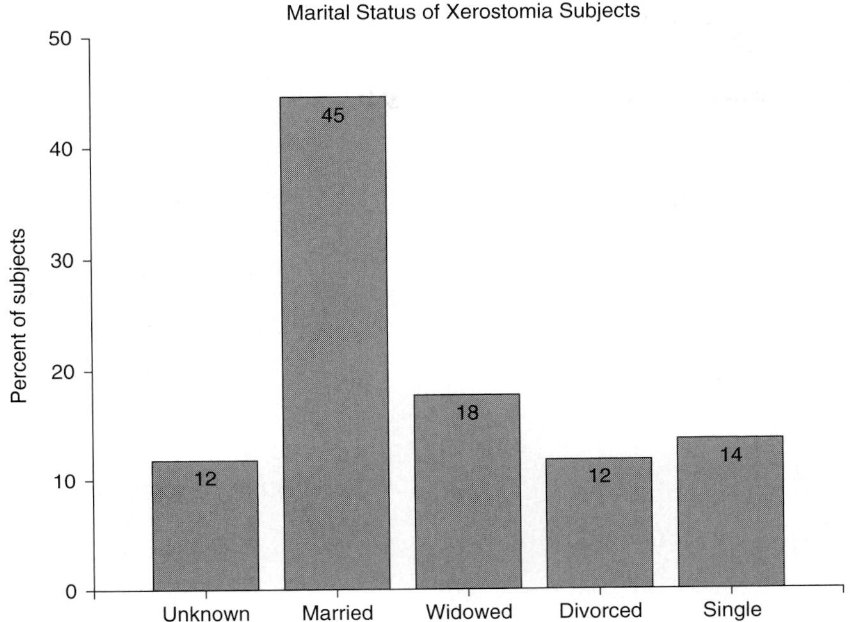

Fig. 14-1. Example of a bar chart.

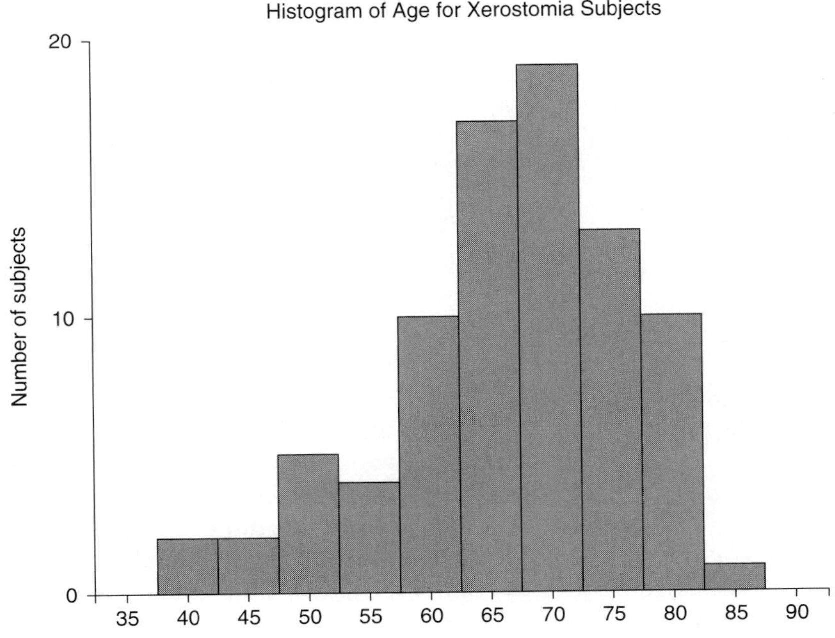

Fig. 14-2. Example of a histogram of a continuous variable.

BOX 14-1

Suggestions for the Display of Data in Graphic or Tabular Form

1. The contents of a table as a whole and the items in each separate column should be clearly and fully defined. The unit of measurement must be included.
2. If the table includes rates, the basis on which they are measured must be clearly stated—death rate percent, per thousand, per million, as the case may be.
3. Rates or proportions should not be given alone without any information as to the numbers of observations on which they are based. By giving only rates of observations and omitting the actual number of observations, we are excluding the basic data.
4. Where percentages are used, it must be clearly indicated that these are not absolute numbers. Rather than combine too many types of figures in one table, it is often best to divide the material into two or three small tables.
5. Full particulars of any exclusion of observations from a collected series must be given. The reasons for and the criteria of exclusions must be clearly defined, perhaps in a footnote.

and figures must be clearly understood and clearly labeled so that the reader is aided by the information rather than confused. The student is directed to standard biostatistics texts for a formal discussion on summarizing data in graphic and tabular form. Also, scientific writing style manuals generally contain discussions on the formal display of tables and graphs. It is also helpful to scan the existing literature for good examples of both graphs and tables.

NUMERICAL SUMMARY OF DATA

Although graphs and frequency distribution tables can enhance our understanding of the nature of a variable, rarely do these techniques alone suffice to describe the variable. A more formal numerical summary of the variable is usually required for the full presentation of a data set. To adequately describe a variable's values, three summary measures are needed:

1. The sample size
2. A measure of central tendency
3. A measure of dispersion

The *sample size* is simply the total number of observations in the group and is symbolized by the letter N or n. A measure of central tendency or location describes the middle (or typical) value in a data set. A measure of dispersion or spread quantifies the degree to which values in a group vary from one another.

MEASURES OF CENTRAL TENDENCY

The *mode* of a data set is that value that occurs with the greatest frequency. When two or more values have equally large frequencies, it is possible for a distribution to have more than one mode. For example, the distribution of scores in Table 14-1 has two modes, 77 and 81. Both occur with the equally high frequency of three. The primary value of the mode lies in its ease of computation and in its convenience as a quick indicator of the central value in a distribution. Beyond this, its statistical uses are extremely limited.

The *median* is the value that divides the distribution of data points into two equal parts, that is, the value at which 50% of the data points lie above it and 50% lie below it. Consider the following data. Patients who had received routine periodontal scaling were given a common pain-relieving drug and were asked to record the minutes to 100% pain relief. Note that "minutes to pain relief" is a continuous variable that is measured on the ratio scale. The patients recorded the following data:

Minutes to 100% pain relief:
15 14 10 18 8 10 12 16 10 8 13

By inspection, we already know two descriptive measures belonging to these data: $N = 11$ and mode = 10. Let's determine the median. First, make an array, that is, arrange the values in ascending order:

8 8 10 10 10 12 13 14 15 16 18

Next, determine which value cuts the array into equal portions. In this array, there are five data points below 12 and there are five data points above 12. Thus the median is 12.

8 8 10 10 10 12 13 14 15 16 18
⥣
Median

If the number of observations is even, unlike the preceding example, simply take the midpoint of the two values that would straddle the center of the data set. Consider the following data set with $N = 10$:

8 8 10 10 10   13 14 15 16 18
⥣

$$\text{Median} = \frac{10 + 13}{2} = 11.5$$

As we see, the median is not necessarily a member of the data set. Like the mode, the median is easy to calculate and is simple in concept, but unlike the mode, the median is used throughout the scientific literature as a descriptive measure. However, the median is not often used when making statistical decisions. Note that the median is not sensitive to extreme values in the data set. If the highest value in the group of 11 data points of time to 100% pain relief were 58 rather than 18, the median would remain unchanged.

8 8 10 10 10 12 13 14 15 16 58
⥣
Median

The median is still 12 minutes.

The measure of central tendency termed the *mean* is the quantity commonly known as the arithmetic average. The symbol for the mean is a capital letter X with a bar above it: $\overline{X}$ or "X-bar". It is calculated by summing all the values in a data set and then dividing the total by the number of observations:

$$\overline{X} = \sum X / N$$

Using the minutes to pain relief, $N = 11$ and $\sum X = 134$. Therefore

$$\overline{X} = 134/11 = 12.2 \text{ min}$$

The mean is by far the most common measure of central tendency used to describe a set of data, and the mean is often used when making statistical decisions. Unlike the median, the mean is sensitive to any change in any score in the distribution. The presence of a few extremely high or extremely low scores can change the value of the mean considerably. Let's refer again to the group of values in which one patient recorded a rather extreme, for this group, value:

8 8 10 10 10 12 13 14 15 16 58

The adjusted mean, somewhat larger than the original mean of 12.2, is calculated as follows:

$$\overline{X} = 174/11 = 15.8 \text{ min}$$

The calculation of the mean is correct, but is its use appropriate for this data set? By definition, the mean should describe the middle of the data set. However, for this data set the mean of 15.8 is larger than most (9 out of 11!) of the values in the group. Not exactly a picture of the middle! In this case, the median (12 minutes) is the better choice for the measure of central tendency and should be used. Note that reporting the median instead of the mean here involves no trickery or hidden agenda, no attempt to "get the data to say what you want." It is simply a matter of which measure is more accurate as a measure of the middle of the data set.

MEASURES OF DISPERSION

Measures of central tendency provide useful information about the typical performance for a group of data. To understand the data more completely, it is necessary to know how the members of the data set arrange themselves about the central or typical value. The following questions must be answered: How spread out are the data points? How stable are the values in the group? The descriptive tools known as measures of dispersion answer these questions by quantifying the variability of the values within a group. The range and the standard deviation are the measures of dispersion or spread used to report variability.

Formally, the *range* of a sample is defined as the difference between the largest value and the smallest value in the group: Range = Maximum − Minimum. More usual, however, is the interpretation of the range as simply the statement of the minimum and maximum values:

$$\text{Range} = (\text{Minimum, Maximum})$$

For the sample of minutes to 100% pain relief,

$$\text{Range} = (8, 18) \quad \text{or} \quad \text{Range} = 18 - 8 = 10 \text{ min}$$

The range presents the exact lower and upper boundaries of a set of data points and thus quickly lends perspective regarding the variable's distribution. Note that the range is usually reported along with the sample median (not the mean). However, the range can be deemed unstable because it is affected by one extremely high score or one extremely low value. Also, only two values are considered, and these happen to be the extreme scores of the distribution. The measure of spread known as standard deviation addresses this disadvantage of the range.

The standard deviation (SD) is a measure of the variability among the individual values within a group. Loosely defined, it is a description of the average distance of individual observations from the group mean (Box 14-2). The mathematical derivation of the standard deviation is presented here in some detail because the intermediate steps in its calculation (1) create a theme (called "sums of squares") that is repeated over and over in statistical arithmetic and (2) create the quantity known as the sample variance.

The results of steps 4 and 5 in Box 14-2 are ubiquitous terms in statistical calculations, but their usefulness in sample description is limited. Some readers may already be familiar with the term *variance,* but it, too, is generally of greater importance to statisticians than to researchers, students, and clinicians trying to understand the fruits of data collection. Note that the sample vari-

BOX 14-2

How to Calculate Standard Deviation

Step	Mathematical Term	Label
1. Calculate the mean $\overline{X}$ of the group.	$\overline{X} = \sum X / N$	sample mean
2. Subtract the mean from each value X.	$(X - \overline{X})$	deviation from the mean
3. Square each deviation from the mean.	$(X - \overline{X})^2$	squared deviation from the mean
4. Add the squared deviations from the mean.	$\Sigma (X - \overline{X})^2$	sums of squares *(ss)*
5. Divide the sums of squares by $(N - 1)$.	$ss/(N - 1)$	variance (s^2)
6. Find the square root of the variance.	$\sqrt{s^2}$	standard deviation (SD or s)

ance is a squared term, not so easy to fathom in relation to the sample mean. Thus the square root of the variance, the standard deviation, is desirable.

Table 14-3 presents the calculation of the standard deviation for our sample of minutes to 100% pain relief.

We now have two sets of complete sample description for our example.

	Sample Description 1	Sample Description 2
Sample size	$N = 11$	$N = 11$
Measure of central tendency	Median = 12 min	$\overline{X} = 12.2$ minutes
Measure of spread	Range = (8, 18)	SD = 3.31

The standard deviation is reported along with the sample mean, usually in the following format: mean ± SD. This format serves as a pertinent reminder that the SD measures the variability of values surrounding the middle of the data set. It also leads us to the practical application of the concepts of mean and standard deviation shown in the following rules of thumb:

$\overline{X} \pm 1$ SD encompasses approximately 68% of the values in a group.

$\overline{X} \pm 2$ SD encompasses approximately 95% of the values in a group.

$\overline{X} \pm 3$ SD encompasses approximately 99% of the values in a group.

These rules of thumb are useful when deciding whether to report the mean ± SD or the median and range as the appropriate descriptive statistics for a group of data points. If roughly 95% of the values in a group are contained in the interval $\overline{X} \pm 2$ SD, researchers tend to use the mean ± SD. Otherwise, the median and range are perhaps more appropriate. Once again, there is no manipulation of data here, just the application of guidelines that are grounded in the mathematical theory that defines one of the most popular and widely known distributions taken on by measurements in biology, the normal distribution.

Table 14-3. Calculation of Standard Deviation of Minutes to 100% Pain Relief

X	$X - \overline{X}$	$(X - \overline{X})^2$
15	15 – 12.2 = 2.8	$(2.8)^2$ = 7.84
14	14 – 12.2 = 1.8	$(1.8)^2$ = 3.24
10	10 – 12.2 = –2.2	$(-2.2)^2$ = 4.84
18	18 – 12.2 = 5.8	$(5.8)^2$ = 33.64
8	8 – 12.2 = –4.2	$(-4.2)^2$ = 17.64
10	10 – 12.2 = –2.2	$(-2.2)^2$ = 4.84
12	12 – 12.2 = –0.2	$(-0.2)^2$ = 0.04
16	16 – 12.2 = 3.8	$(3.8)^2$ = 14.44
10	10 – 12.2 = –2.2	$(-2.2)^2$ = 4.84
8	8 – 12.2 = –4.2	$(-4.2)^2$ = 17.64
13	13 – 12.2 = 0.8	$(0.8)^2$ = 0.64
$\Sigma = 134$	$\Sigma = 0.0$	$\Sigma = 109.64$
$\overline{X} = \sum X / N$ $= 134/11 = 12.2$		sums of squares $= ss = \Sigma\,(X - \overline{X})^2 = 109.64$ variance $= s^2 = ss/(N-1) = 109.64/10 = 10.964$ SD $= \sqrt{s^2} = \sqrt{10.964} = 3.31$

THE NORMAL DISTRIBUTION

The normal distribution is one of the most frequently occurring distributions in biomedical and dental research. The normal, or Gaussian, distribution is a population frequency distribution. It is characterized by a bell-shaped curve that is unimodal and is symmetric around the mean of the distribution. The normal curve depends on only two parameters: the population mean and the population standard deviation. In order to discuss the area under the normal curve in terms of easily seen percentages of the population distribution, the normal distribution has been standardized to the standard normal distribution in which the population mean is 0 and the population standard deviation is 1. The area under the normal curve can be segmented starting with the mean in the center (on the x axis) and moving by increments of 1 SD above and below the mean. Figure 14-3 shows a standard normal distribution (mean = 0; SD = 1) and the percentages of area under the curve at each increment of SD (in this figure, SD is denoted by s).

The total area beneath the normal curve is 1, or 100% of the observations in the population represented by the curve. As indicated in Fig. 14-3, the portion of the area under the curve between the mean and 1 SD is 34.13% of the total area. The same area is found between the mean and one unit below the mean. Moving 1 SD more above the mean cuts off an additional 13.59% of the area, and moving a total of 3 SD above the mean cuts off another 2.27%. The theory of the standard normal distribution leads

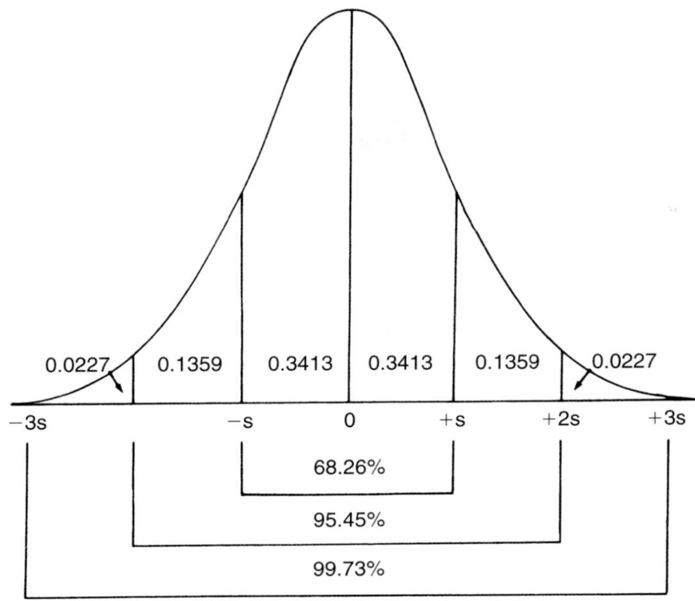

Fig. 14-3. Normal frequency curve.

us, therefore, to the following property of a normally distributed variable:

Exactly 68.26% of the observations lie within 1 SD of the mean.

Exactly 95.45% of the observations lie within 2 SD of the mean.

Exactly 99.73% of the observations lie within 3 SD of the mean.

Sound familiar? We have just derived the basis for the rule of thumb presented in the previous section on the standard deviation. It is obvious that virtually all of the observations are contained within 3 SD of the mean. This is the justification used by those who label values outside of the interval $\overline{X} \pm 3$ SD as "outliers" or unlikely values. Incidentally, the number of standard deviations away from the mean are called *Z* scores, familiar to some readers already.

INFERENTIAL STATISTICS

As stated earlier, it is often impossible to study each member of a population. Instead, we select a sample from the population and from that sample attempt to generalize to the population as a whole. The process of generalizing sample results to a population is termed *statistical inference* and is the end product of formal statistical hypothesis testing. The focus of the remainder of this chapter is hypothesis testing. The role of probability in statistical decision making, the meaning of statistical significance, and three examples of specific tests of hypotheses are presented.

THE NULL HYPOTHESIS

Statistical tests of a hypothesis begin with the statement of the hypothesis itself, but stated in the form of a null hypothesis. For example, consider again the group of patients who tested the new pain-relieving drug, drug A, and recorded their number of minutes to 100% pain relief. Suppose that a similar sample of patients tested another drug, drug B, in the same way, and investigators wished to know if one group of patients experienced total pain relief more quickly than the other group. In this case, the null hypothesis would be stated in this way: "There is no difference in time to 100% pain relief between the two pain-relieving drugs A and B." The null hypothesis is one of no difference, no effect, no association, and serves as a reference point for the statistical test. In symbols, the null hypothesis is referred to as H_0. In the comparison of the two drugs A and B, we can state the H_0 in terms of there being no difference in the average number of minutes to pain relief between drugs A and B, or H_0: $\overline{X}_A = \overline{X}_B$. The alternative is that the means of the two drug groups are not equal. This is an expression of the alternative hypothesis H_1.

Null hypothesis	H_0: $\overline{X}_A = \overline{X}_B$
Alternative hypothesis	H_1: $\overline{X}_A \neq \overline{X}_B$

PROBABILITY

When employing tests of hypotheses, we generally work with results of samples and thus need to acknowledge the variability inherent in our work. Another term for variability is *uncertainty*. An amount of uncertainty will be present in tests of hypotheses. Biostatistics deals with this uncertainty through the careful use of probability—the mathematical assumption that an event will occur according to chance a specific portion of the time. Here, probability is used to judge whether the sample's results are compatible with the H_0 or not. This probability, *p*, is the *p* value that investigators are chasing when performing statistical tests: "What is the probability *p* that the null hypothesis H_0 is true?"

STATISTICAL SIGNIFICANCE

The *p* value is the final arithmetic answer that is calculated by a statistical test of a hypothesis. Its magnitude informs the researcher as to the validity of the H_0, that is, whether to accept or reject the H_0 as worth keeping. The *p* value is crucial for drawing the proper conclusions about a set of data. So what numerical value of *p* should be used as the dividing line for acceptance or rejection of the H_0? Here is the decision rule for the observed value of *p* and the decision regarding the H_0.

If $p \leq .05$, reject the H_0

If $p > .05$, accept the H_0

If the observed probability is less than or equal to .05 (5%), the null hypothesis is rejected, that is, the observed outcome is judged to be incompatible with the notion of "no difference" or "no effect," and the alternative hypothesis is adopted. In this case, the results are said to be "statistically significant." If the observed probability is greater than .05 (5%), the decision is to accept the null hypothesis, and the results are called "not statistically significant" or simply NS, the notation often used in tables.

STATISTICAL VERSUS CLINICAL SIGNIFICANCE

The distinction between statistical significance and clinical or practical significance is worth mentioning. For example, in the statistical test of the H_0: $\overline{X}_A = \overline{X}_B$ for two drug groups, let's assume that the observed probability is $p = .01$, a value that is less than the dividing line of .05 or 5%. This would lead the investigator to reject the H_0 and to conclude that the results are "significant at $p = .01$," that is, one drug caused total pain relief significantly faster, on average, than the other drug at $p = .01$. But if the actual difference in the group means is itself clinically meaningless or negligible, the statistical significance may be considered real yet not useful.

TESTS OF SIGNIFICANCE

The science of biostatistics has given us a large number of tests that can be applied to public health data. Only a few of these are discussed in this section. Discussions here center on the chi-square test, the calculation of the coefficient of correlation, and the Student's *t*-test. Each method is best adapted to data of a certain scale of measurement and to a certain type of research question. An understanding of the tests will guide an individual toward the efficient collection of data that will meet the assumptions of the statistical procedures particularly well.

CHI-SQUARE TEST

Chi-square analysis is a test that is appropriate for categorical data only. It is used for the comparison of groups when the data is expressed as counts or proportions. For example, an investigator might wish to compare the proportion of caries-free children living in a district whose water supply is fluoridated to the proportion of caries-free children living in a nonfluoridated district. In each district, the investigator would count the number of caries-free and not caries-free children. The research question involves two categorical variables: caries status of the child (caries free or not) and fluoridation status of the district (yes/no). The question can be asked this way: Is the prevalence of caries in children contingent on the fluoridation of the district's water? Viewed in this light, chi-square is considered a *measure of association* between two categorical variables. Thus the statement of the null hypothesis is one of "no association" between the two variables.

The data for a chi-square test is displayed in an arrangement called a contingency table. The number of rows and the number of columns in the table are determined by the number of categories in the two variables of interest. The frequencies of subjects belonging to mutually exclusive categories of the two variables are called the *observed frequencies*, symbolized by the letter *O*. Let's return to the example of caries prevalence and water fluoridation. Suppose that a caries assessment was conducted in similar cohorts of children living in fluoridated and nonfluoridated districts on a well-developed Caribbean island. The number of children (ages 6 to 12 years) randomly sampled from each district was 500. The investigator reported that 62% (310 of 500) of the children from the fluoridated district were caries free, and 40% (200 of 500) of the children from the nonfluoridated district were caries free. The 2×2 (spoken as "2 by 2") contingency table for this study's observed frequencies is as follows:

	Caries Status		
Water	*Caries Free*	*Not Caries Free*	*Total*
Fluoridated:			
Yes	310	190	500
No	200	300	500
Total	510	490	1000

The arithmetic for chi-square analysis is based on the discrepancy between the observed frequencies (O) and the frequencies that one would expected to observe if the null hypothesis were indeed true. These are the expected frequencies, symbolized by the letter E. The formula for the chi-square statistic highlights the difference between the observed and expected frequencies:

$$\chi^2 = \Sigma[(O - E)^2/E]$$

For each cell in the table, the difference between O and E is squared, divided by E, and then the resulting quantities are summed to give the value for chi-square. The intermediate step of calculating an E for each O is the following: E = (Row total × Column total) ÷ Grand total. Table 14-4 illustrates the calculation of χ^2 for this example.

The H_0 (null hypothesis) for this example states that there is no association between the caries-free status of the children and the water fluoridation. In other terms, there is no difference in the proportion of caries-free children in the fluoridated and nonfluoridated areas. Now that the value of chi-square has been determined, we must decide whether our results are compatible with the H_0. This is done by comparing our calculated value of χ^2 with the critical value of χ^2 that is necessary to reject the H_0. These critical values are contained in a table that can be found in basic statistics books (not included here). The critical value is determined by the p value of .05 (the dividing line for significance) and by the degrees of freedom (df) for the test. The df for a 2 × 2 chi-square test is always 1. The critical value of χ^2 at $p = .05$ and df = 1 is 3.84. Because our calculated χ^2 is well above the critical value, we can safely reject the H_0 and conclude that there is a significant association between caries status and fluoridation of water. The proportion of caries-free children (62%) in the fluoridated district is significantly greater than the proportion of caries-free children (40%) in the nonfluoridated district.

Chi-square analysis is a popular tool in the analysis of research data, especially among researchers who collect survey data.

Table 14-4. Calculation of χ^2 for the Association of Absence of Caries with Fluoridation of Water

Category	*O*	*E*	*(O − E)*	*(O − E)²*	*(O − E)²/E*
Caries free, fluoridated water	310	$\frac{500 \times 510}{1000} = 255$	310 − 255 = 55	$55^2 = 3025$	3025/255 = 11.86
Not caries free, fluoridated water	190	$\frac{500 \times 490}{1000} = 245$	190 − 245 = −55	$-55^2 = 3025$	3025/245 = 12.35
Caries free, water not fluoridated	200	$\frac{500 \times 510}{1000} = 255$	200 − 255 = −55	$-55^2 = 3025$	3025/255 = 11.86
Not caries free, water not fluoridated	300	$\frac{500 \times 490}{1000} = 245$	300 − 245 = 55	$55^2 = 3025$	3025/245 = 12.35
					$\chi^2 = \Sigma = 48.42$

Many of the responses in survey research are categorical and thus are suitable for chi-square analysis when seeking to learn about the relationships between survey items. The example given here is for the simple case in which each variable possesses only two categories, but the analysis can easily be extended to variables that have more than two possible responses. The interpretation of chi-square results, however, becomes more difficult as the number of categories increases, and it is sometimes advisable to collapse variables into fewer categories for the purpose of analysis.

CORRELATION

As does chi-square, correlation analysis quantifies the relationship between variables, but the scale of measurement needed for correlation is continuous. The Pearson product-moment correlation coefficient is a measure of the linear association between two continuous measurement variables, both of which are normally distributed. Typical data questions answered by correlation analysis might be the following examples:

1. In a sample of elderly xerostomia patients, does the number of root caries increase with increasing amounts of sugar in the diet (number of servings per day)?
2. In a sample of patients from a large dental school clinic, is the number of years of education inversely associated with the number of decayed teeth, as a portion of the total decayed, missing, or filled teeth (DMFT) index (D/DMFT)?

In both instances, data are recorded on a single group of subjects, and each subject contributes a pair of measures (number of servings per day of sugar and number of root caries; number of years of education and D/DMFT). Commonly, any pair of variables entered into a correlation analysis is given the names X and Y.

The correlation coefficient is calculated using the raw values of the (X, Y) pairs of data. The formula is not given here, but it is simply a mixture of sums of squares calculations (as we used for the derivation of the standard deviation) for X, Y, and XY. The symbol for the correlation coefficient is r, and r takes on values from -1 to $+1$. A perfect correlation is found when $r = 1$, either positive or negative, and a scatter diagram of (X, Y) would show the coordinate points forming a straight line. The sign of the correlation coefficient is crucial in explaining the relationship between the two variables: $+r$ signifies that X and Y vary in the same direction (increasing $X \Rightarrow$ increasing Y, as in question 1); $-r$ signifies that X and Y vary in opposite directions (increasing $X \Rightarrow$ decreasing Y, as in question 2).

The relationship between two variables is easy to grasp by inspecting a scatter diagram of the coordinate points (X, Y), as in Figs. 14-4 and 14-5. If $r = 0$ (Fig. 14-4), there is no linear association between X and Y. In Fig. 14-5, however, a relation becomes apparent, not perfect but recognizable: as one variable changes, the second variable changes in the same direction.

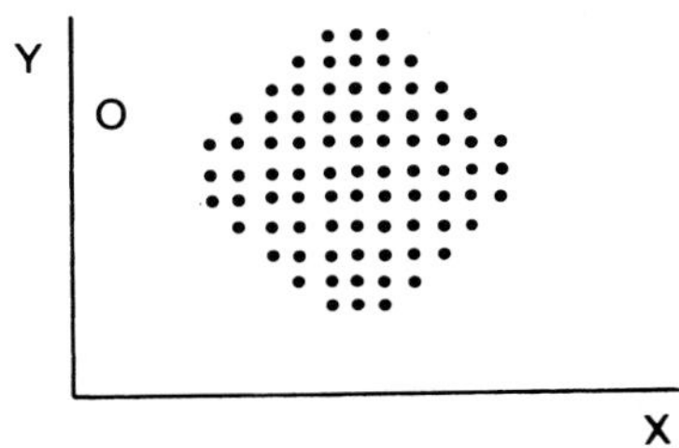

Fig. 14-4. Hypothetical scatter diagram showing correlation coefficients of 0.

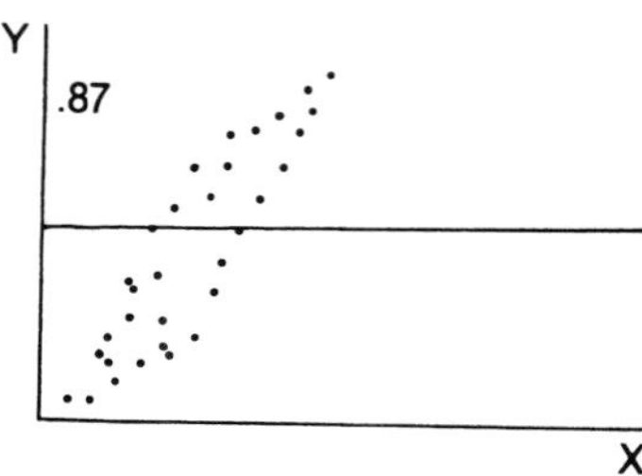

Fig. 14-5. Hypothetical scatter diagram showing correlation coefficients of +0.87.

In correlation analysis, the statement of the null hypothesis is one of no linear association between the variables *X* and *Y*. Symbolically stated, H_0: $r = 0$. As we did for the value of the chi-square statistic, the calculated *r* must be compared with a critical value so that a decision regarding the H_0 can be made. For correlation analysis, the degrees of freedom for the test of significance are dependent on the sample size *N*: $df = N - 2$, where *N* is the number of *(X, Y)* pairs. The role of the sample size is important. For example, a correlation coefficient $r = 0.88$ is needed for statistical significance ($p \leq .05$) at $N = 5$, whereas $r = 0.51$, certainly a weaker coefficient than the 0.88, would be statistically significant at $N = 15$.

It must be stressed that the correlation coefficient quantifies the degree to which two variables are related. Correlation analysis does not measure causality; a significant correlation coefficient does not give one permission to conclude that "*X* causes *Y*" or vice versa. If a researcher wishes to model one variable on another, that is, to predict the value of one variable *(Y)* from the value of the other *(X)*, the correlation analysis can be expanded to linear regression analysis.

STUDENT'S *t* TEST

Although the exploration of relationships among variables is the focus of many statistical endeavors in public health, so is the question of differences among groups of study subjects. For example, during a 9-month study of dental services utilization, female members of a dental health insurance plan underwent an average of 6.2 procedures, whereas male members underwent 4.3 services, on average. The question asked of this data is the following: Is there a difference in dental services utilization between male and female members of a dental health plan? The test of significance needed to answer this data question is the *t* test for independent samples (the nonpaired *t* test), sometimes called the Student's *t* test (Student is the pseudonym of the test's developer).

The *t* test for independent samples is reserved for the comparison of two study groups when the variable of interest is a continuous measurement that is normally distributed. The statement of the null hypothesis is one of no difference between the means of the two groups, that is, H_0: $\overline{X}_1 = \overline{X}_2$.

The following summary data can be used to illustrate the comparison of two groups using the nonpaired *t* test:

	Group 1	Group 2
N	10	10
Mean	14.8	10.8
Variance	22.84	25.96
Standard deviation	4.78	5.09

The formula for the *t* test is not given here, but these data generate a calculated $t = 1.81$. Once again, this calculated *t* statistic must be compared with a critical value of *t* at a significance level of .05 and at $df = (n_1 - 1) + (n_2 - 1) = 9 + 9 = 18$. The critical value of *t* for this test is 2.01. Because the calculated *t* does not equal or surpass the critical value, the H_0 must be accepted. The researcher therefore concludes that there is insufficient evidence to reject the null hypothesis of no difference between the means of the two groups.

Table 14-5. Overview of Biostatistics

	Data		
	Measurements (Continuous)		*Categories (Discrete)*
Research Question	*Normal Distribution*	*Nonnormal Distribution*	
Describe one sample	$\overline{X}$, SD, SE Percentiles Confidence interval (CI) around a mean	Median, range Percentiles	Counts, percents, proportion Confidence interval around a proportion
Compare two groups:			
Nonpaired	Student's t test for independent samples	Wilcoxon rank sum test	Chi-square test (2 × 2 table)
Paired	Paired t test	Wilcoxon signed rank test	CI of a difference between two proportions Fisher exact probability
Compare two or more groups	Analysis of variance (ANOVA)	Nonparametric analysis of variance	
Correlate two variables in one group	Pearson correlation coefficient r Linear regression	Spearman rank correlation r_s	
Correlate more than two variables in one group	Multiple correlation coefficient R Multiple linear regression		

Note that when more than two group means are to be compared, the t test is no longer the desired test of significance. Analysis of variance (ANOVA) is indicated. The reader is cautioned against performing multiple t tests with different combinations of means, two at a time. This is an incorrect statistical application, although it may be found in published articles and in student theses.

Parametric versus Nonparametric Tests

Both the Pearson correlation analysis and the Student's t test for independent samples are examples of *parametric* procedures. These tests assume that the measurement variables used in the test follow the normal distribution. For measurements that are interval or ratio scale variables but are not normally distributed or are categories measured on an ordinal or nominal scale, parametric procedures should not be used. Another class of statistical tests called *nonparametric* tests should be used. Nonparametric procedures are sometimes referred to as distribution-free methods because the nature of the underlying distribution of the variables is not assumed. Most elementary biostatistics texts fully explain these nonparametric tests and their proper place in statistical tests of hypotheses.

SUMMARY

This chapter offers the reader a glimpse into the orderly, principled field of applied biostatistics. There is much more to be explored, even on an introductory level, as can be seen in the overview presented in Table 14-5. Even without the reader's further pursuit of biostatistical knowledge, it is hoped that readers of this chapter will approach the analysis of their own data, and the presentation of the results of the data of other researchers, with a better understanding of the requirements for the proper handling of data and with a resolve to "do the right thing" by research data.

BIBLIOGRAPHY

Chilton NW: *Design and analysis in dental and oral research,* Philadelphia, 1967, JB Lippincott.

Colton T: *Statistics in medicine,* Boston, 1974, Little, Brown.

D'Agostino RB, Sullivan LM, Beiser AS: *Introductory applied biostatistics,* Boston, 2000, Houghton Mifflin.

Dawson B, Trapp RG: *Basic and clinical biostatistics,* ed 3, New York, 2001, McGraw-Hill.

Weintraub JA, Douglass CW, Gillings DB: *BIOSTATS data analysis for dental health care professionals,* ed 2, Chapel Hill, NC, 1985, CAVCO.

REVIEW QUESTIONS

1. In a recent survey, radiologists were asked to indicate the number of hours that they worked per week. The data were recorded in a notebook in the alphabetical order of the radiologists' last names:

   10 18 24 35 35 41 5 31 32 33
   40 40 22 20 30 28 38 38 38 50
   48 45 36 37 27

   a. The variable "hours per week worked by radiologists" is qualitative / quantitative
   circle one
   and is measured on the ratio / ordinal / nominal scale.
   circle one

   b. Examine the following statements about these data:
      A. The **mode** is greater than the **median** for this data set.
      B. The **mode** for this data set will change if the **minimum value** in the data set is dropped (omitted).

   Circle the letter of the correct observation:
   a. Statement A only is correct.
   b. Statement B only is correct.
   c. Neither statement A nor statement B is correct.
   d. Both statements A and B are correct.

2. Which measure of central tendency and which measure of spread should be used to describe a continuous variable that is
   a. not normally distributed?
   __________ and __________
   b. normally distributed?
   __________ and __________

3. A representative sample of the first-year dental student class ($N = 25$) was studied for hypertension. Each student's systolic blood pressure was measured in mm Hg, and the following descriptive measures were reported:
   $\overline{X} = 120$ mm Hg
   ss (sum of squared deviations from the mean) = 1536 mm^2 Hg
   a. Calculate the SD for this sample:
   ____
   b. Approximately 95% of the dental students have systolic blood pressure in the interval between ____ mm Hg and ____ mm Hg.

4. In a conventional test of significance for the comparison of two groups A and

B where the variable of interest is a continuous measurement that follows the normal distribution,

a. which of the following statements is an *appropriate* expression of the null hypothesis?
   A. $\overline{A} > \overline{B}$
   B. $\overline{A} = \overline{B}$
   C. $\overline{A} \neq \overline{B}$
   D. $\overline{A} = \overline{B} = 0$
b. which test of significance should be used here?
   A. Correlation coefficient
   B. Chi-square analysis
   C. Student's t test for independent samples
   D. Analysis of variance (ANOVA)
   E. Nonparametric test

5. A dental researcher has investigated the relationship between education level (expressed as the number of years of education) and four different variables of interest (the overall number of decayed, missing, or filled [DMF] teeth per person and each of the components of the DMF ratio: number of decayed teeth per person, number of missing teeth per person, and number of filled teeth per person). She reported the following:
   A. The correlation of number of years of education with number of filled teeth per person was $r = 0.75$, $p < .01$.
      a. This correlation is significant / not significant. (circle one)
      b. We can conclude that less / more (circle one) education is associated with lower / higher filled teeth (circle one) per person.
   B. The correlation of number of years of education with number of missing teeth per person was $r = -0.82$, $p < .01$.
      a. This correlation is significant / not significant. (circle one)
      b. We can conclude that less / more education is associated (circle one) with lower / higher Missing (circle one) teeth/person.

ANSWERS

1.
   a. quantitative and ratio
   b. A (median = 35 and mode = 38)
2.
   a. median and range (extremes)
   b. mean and standard deviation
3.
   a. variance = ss/$(n - 1)$ = 1536/24 = 64; SD = Square root (variance) = Square root (64) = 8
   b. 104 and 136 ($\overline{X} \pm 2$ SD: $120 \pm 2(8)$ or 120 ± 16)
4.
   a. B
   b. C
5.
   A.
      a. significant
      b. less and lower (or more and higher)
   B.
      a. significant
      b. less and higher (or more and lower)

CHAPTER

15

ACCESSING AND READING DENTAL PUBLIC HEALTH RESEARCH: EVIDENCE-BASED DENTAL PRACTICE

Van B. Afes • Eugene Hittelman

MODERN DENTISTRY IS INFORMED DENTISTRY

A revolution has taken place in health care. No longer is society willing to tolerate the health care practitioner, no matter how skilled, who relies solely on experience, personal judgment, and the training received in school to make decisions regarding patient care. It is expected that the practitioner's selection of treatment modalities, materials, and responses to patient inquiries regarding current practices and controversies in dentistry and medicine will be consistent with the best knowledge and research available in the field. As stated in the Institute of Medicine's 1995 report, *Dental Education at the Crossroads,* oral health care delivery must be an integral aspect of comprehensive health care, including primary care. "Dental education must be scientifically based and undertaken in an environment in which the creation and acquisition of new scientific and clinical knowledge are valued and actively pursued."[1] For the health care provider, learning must be a lifelong endeavor and cannot end with the attainment of a dental degree, a residency program, or specialty training.

The profession and the public expect the modern dentist to be informed and able to respond to patients' questions regarding current controversies in oral health care, public health practices, and personal oral health maintenance recommendations. Bader and colleagues[2] maintain that the incorporation of dental research findings by clinicians into their patient care is central to the maximization of treatment benefits and minimization of treatment harm.

Health policy developers in the public health sector and third-party payers in the private sector expect health care providers to be able to demonstrate the efficacy and appropriateness of their treatment decisions. Because of rising health care costs, a growing medically and dentally vulnerable aging population, and an increasing demand for health care, there is a rapidly increasing demand that practitioners demonstrate the "cost-effective" aspects of their treatment decisions.[3] The dental profession has received a great deal of criticism in the public press because of findings that enormous variations exist in treatment recommendations and health care practice. These variations have been attributed to (1) poor science underlying the clinical decisions, (2) poor quality of clinical care decisions, and (3) variations in clinical skills.[4] To counter these criticisms and to respond to the challenge of modern health care, the dentist must combine evidence-based information with practical clinical experience when engaging in the process of diagnosis, treatment planning, and treatment.

How is the dentist expected to meet this demand and continue to provide dental services in both quality and quantity adequate to meet patient demand and economic reality? The flood of new articles, books, and reports is overwhelming. Not only must information relevant to practice decisions be identified and obtained, it must also be digested, evaluated, interpreted, and prioritized for its clinical validity and practicality. In addition, the dentist, as part of the public health delivery system, must also be aware of current trends in the public health sector. Infection control, environmental intervention, public health education, and changes in strategies and regulations regarding third-party and government funding for dental services all affect daily practice.

This chapter provides some concrete suggestions for accomplishing the difficult challenge of being informed and aware of current standards of care. Basic issues and methods in dental research are discussed first. The chapter then examines current criteria for evidence in the literature and reviews the types of studies that are accepted as evidence and provides criteria for weighting their importance. The chapter concludes with a discussion of strategies for searching and identifying studies that are helpful in answering the questions important to practice decisions and relevant to patients' concerns.

THE GOAL OF RESEARCH

Research involves a systematic investigation designed to answer questions about the events we observe. The goal is to develop accurate explanations and predictions for future occurrences of these events. It is a process of discovering and documenting "regularities" in the universe. This process is intended to provide valid, consistent, and reliable predictions, explanations, and descriptions that can be used to understand, plan, and make decisions. Typically, a research study does not prove that a phenomenon or causal relationship exists but rather demonstrates that the events or population characteristics documented are not the result of an artifact created by a study but a consistent finding that can provide a basis for sound conclusions.

In most studies, a set of conditions (independent variables) is specified and then a second set of factors (dependent variables) is measured. The question posed is, "How does the dependent variable change as the values or conditions of the independent variable are manipulated or selected?" Much of research design is focused on eliminating alternative, competing explanations for observed or hypothesized relationships. The term for this effort is *capturing the variance*. Essentially, we are trying to identify the consistent percentage of the total variation in the dependent variable (effect size) that is due to the changes in the independent or causal variable. Other factors (intervening variables, including experimenter error and chance) will increase or decrease the amount of change observed. The researcher is attempting to isolate and quantify that portion of the change which is reliably (not created as an artifact or chance event that occurred in the study) affected by the variations in the independent variable. Because of this, standards of evidence emphasize the importance of replication of study findings rather than depending on the findings of a single study.

TYPES OF RESEARCH STUDIES

Dental health research, including oral public health research, can be divided into three types: descriptive studies, experimental studies, and meta-analytic studies. Box 15-1 provides examples of these three types of research.

Descriptive studies are designed to document or characterize observations resulting from data collection (e.g., surveys) and systematic observation of a target population or population sample. For example, what is the decayed, missing, and filled surfaces level in the population of children, between ages 10 and 15 years, who have not been exposed to a consistent fluoridated water supply? Documentation includes the following: epidemiologic research, in which rates (incidence and prevalence) of disease in a "target" population are documented; surveys, in which information is elicited regarding population characteristics; and demographic studies, in which the population is characterized and described in terms of the distributions of such characteristics as age, sex, economic status, education, unmet need, and oral health status.

A second type of descriptive study reports relationships between behaviors or characteristics and disease rates. Risk assessment, in which the rates of disease among individuals exposed to a particular pathogenic cause are compared with the rates of those not exposed (e.g., rates of cancer among smokers as compared with rates of nonsmokers), and correlational studies, in which rates of disease are corre-

BOX 15-1

Types of Public Health Research

I. Descriptive research
  A. Epidemiologic studies
    1. Incidence and prevalence of disease in a community
    2. Patterns of disease in a community (e.g., fluorosis studies)
  B. Descriptive epidemiology
    1. Census reports
    2. Documentation of a specific population
  C. Risk ratios and risk assessment
    1. Case-control studies
    2. Cross-sectional studies
  D. Correlational studies
    1. Cohort studies
    2. Comparison of rates of disease with population characteristics
  E. Trend analyses
  F. Economic and workforce documentation
II. Experimental research (hypothesis testing)
  A. Randomized controlled clinical trials
  B. Field experiments
    1. Natural studies
    2. Controlled studies
  C. Laboratory clinical trials
  D. Program evaluations
III. Meta-analytic studies
  A. Statistical repeated measure designs in which findings from independent studies are combined
  B. Systematic reviews and summaries of randomized controlled clinical trials

lated with characteristics such as economic status, education, and health-related behaviors, are examples of this type of study.

Experimental studies are designed to test whether a hypothesized relationship between the independent variable(s) (conditions) and a dependent or outcome variable is causally related. For example, does changing the acidity level of the saliva affect the demineralization process that is occurring in the mouth? Experimental research involves controlled studies, either in the "field" or in the laboratory, which are designed to "test" hypothesized causal relations. For example, two matched groups are compared in an experimental design in which one group is treated with an experimental drug and the second is given a placebo. The groups are then compared as to their recovery time from a particular disease. A "field experimental study" might involve a "natural experiment" in which two communities, one of which has a fluoridated water supply and the other of which has a water supply with a very low fluoride concentration, are compared over a number of years in terms of their caries incidence. A more controlled field experiment might involve a direct intervention into one community (e.g., a screening for oral cancer) and an indirect intervention into another community (e.g., an education program about oral cancer) with the goal of testing for the cost-effectiveness of a particular set of health promotion strategies. A controlled clinical study might be one in which one group uses a particular mouthwash and the other group uses another mouthwash and the two groups are compared for gingival health and calculus accumulation. The research study might occur in vivo or in vitro. The highest level of experimental research includes randomized small clinical trials in which the experiment is repeated in a variety of settings instead of in one setting with a large number of subjects.[5]

Meta-analysis involves a "secondary research method" in which a series of primary research studies is systematically explored for consistent findings across research studies. It involves the use of statistical techniques to compare and integrate the findings of a large series of independent projects.[6] Although meta-analysis was formally documented in 1976 and the statistical techniques employed have appeared in the literature over the last 60 years, the use of meta-analysis as a primary resource represents a change created by the evidence-based research movement. Meta-analysis is used to collect, analyze, and compare the results of multiple primary studies to develop an overall conclusion or summary of their findings. It not only summarizes and statistically tests the findings, but also identifies phenomena that are consistent and stable. By considering and weighting for the sample size, effect size, and research design in each study, the stability and statistical significance of the conclusions can be evaluated.[7]

Each of the research approaches considered here has value in evidence-based dentistry if conducted appropriately. Criteria for evaluating a research study are discussed later in this chapter. However, these studies can be classified in terms of their "level of evidence," or credibility. Box 15-2 provides a generalized ranking of published articles in terms of rigor and vulnerability to artifact, bias, and random effects. The lowest level of evidence comes from case descriptions, uncontrolled observational studies, and random surveys. In these studies, the researcher has not systematically controlled the conditions under which the observations occurred so that the results are often produced by the chance events sur-

BOX 15-2

Hierarchy of Studies: Evidence-based Value

I. Studies with the highest level of evidence base
   A. Studies that review multiple, double-blind, randomized design, clinical trials using clear, published selection and analytic approaches
   B. Meta-analytic studies that combine multiple, double-blind, randomized design clinical trials
   C. Multisite, randomized, small, well-designed clinical trials
II. Studies with the next level of evidence base
   A. One or more well-designed, double-blind, randomized clinical trials
   B. Experimental field studies in which subjects are randomly selected, sites are well matched, evaluators are well calibrated, and the experimental manipulations are carefully documented and systematic
III. Systematic, well-controlled, longitudinal studies with careful sampling
   A. One or more well-conducted cohort studies
   B. One or more well-conducted case-control studies
IV. Systematic, noncontrolled studies
   A. Surveys with random sampling (e.g., census)
   B. Cross-sectional studies with careful random selection and clear exclusion rules
   C. Longitudinal studies that control for attrition
   D. Field studies: descriptive and demographic studies
      1. With calibrated examiners
      2. Careful sampling techniques
      3. Natural experiments with random selection of sample
V. Dramatic uncontrolled field observations or experiments
VI. Expert committees, task forces, professional reports
VII. Studies with the lowest level of evidence base
   A. Case studies
   B. Editorials and articles in non–peer reviewed journals
   C. Opinion pieces

rounding the study. The second level of evidence comes from studies in which the researcher has taken care to control for internal biasing influences. Included in these studies are surveys based on stratified, random sampling; field studies in which the evaluators are calibrated; and longitudinal studies in which appropriate controls are used to ensure validity. In studies with a greater level of evidence, the researcher has increased the level of replication, controls for sampling error, and controls for contaminating variables (by instituting control groups, matched control groups, and random assignment to condition). The highest level of evidence is presented when the researcher combines a number of studies so that the effects and artifacts of any one study are counteracted by other studies or statistical techniques so that what remains is a stable estimate of the examined phenomena.

LEVELS OF EVIDENCE

By "evidence-based" dentistry we mean the "integration of best research evidence with clinical expertise and patient values."[8] In the appropriate application of the evidence-

BOX 15-3

Evidence Hierarchy

Level 1

Systematic replication of results from well-controlled, multiple, randomized controlled trials in which the outcomes are relatively homogeneous

Meta-analytic studies of well-designed studies in which the literature review is comprehensive and the selection criteria are explicit

Level 2

Large, multisite studies employing controls such as randomized sampling and assignment to conditions, double-blind design, and appropriate statistical analysis

Level 3

Multiple replication of studies that do not have careful controls for sampling bias

Cohort studies with minimal attrition

Retrospective studies

Level 4

Well-designed and systematic data gathering with calibrated examiners but poor sampling control

Well-designed surveys without control groups

Outcome studies and related evaluation studies

Level 5

Comparisons of selected groups (noncontrolled)

Retrospective studies

Case-control studies

Cross-sectional studies

Level 6

Unsystematic reports of observations

Noncontrolled experiments and reports

Adapted from Sutherland S: Evidence-based dentistry: part IV. Research design and levels of evidence, *J Can Dent Assoc* 67:375, 2001 and the Oxford Centre for Evidence-based Medicine Levels of Evidence, May 2001. http://cebm.jr2.ox.ac.uk/docs/levels.html.

based approach, the practitioner will combine the best evidence available, practical experience, current standards of care, and the limitations and possibilities of the specific situation to make a judicious decision. In Box 15-3, we suggest a hierarchy of research evidence authority based on the vulnerability of various types of studies to bias (validity) and chance artifacts. Later in this chapter, we will discuss strategies for reading and evaluating a research study for its rigor and design; the reader, however, must also consider the relevance, practicality, and heuristics of the study when making a final decision regarding the appropriateness of findings for use.

The strongest evidence is replication of the study findings. Independent replications provide clear evidence that the finding is not just a random event. The researcher demonstrates that the finding is not just an artifact of a single study but a consistent event. Systematic reviews of research findings (meta-analysis) represents this improved level of evidence when the guidelines for study selection and statistical compilation are followed. Systematic replication of findings using controlled studies provides evidence for the stability and validity of the reported phenomena. By combining randomized, selected studies (or the universe of available studies) from a pool of studies meeting explicit, predetermined, experimental design criteria, the researcher can counteract and eliminate bias that occurs in each individual study reviewed.

Evidence is stronger to the degree to which each research study controls internal and external contaminating influences so as to be able to identify the specific causal factors and population characteristics in question. For example, a survey may return highly biased results if only those individuals who feel strongly about a particular issue respond. If one were testing a new medication, it would be inappropriate to select for testing only patients who had a high probability of getting well while excluding those who were sicker or less responsive. These external and internal factors may be controlled statistically or by the use of experimental controls (use of systematic observation, control groups, randomized sample selection, and reliability checks on the data collected).

Ranking and selecting studies for review imply the application of rules of evidence. To the degree that the experimenter controls for bias, the study gains in validity and reliability. The experimenter can control for sample bias by using a randomized sample selection with specific stated rules for selection or rejection of the subject. The experimenter controls for experimenter bias by "blinding the experimenter" to the experimental (independent variable) conditions and by "calibrating" the observer to eliminate response bias. The experimenter controls for preexisting conditions and influences such as placebo effects, subject bias, and "maturation" by use of experimental controls. The more systematic and carefully controlled the study, the more likely the outcomes will be the result of the study process rather than of an artifact or a chance finding.

Randomized, controlled trials represent the next highest level of evidence. This level of evidence is supported by single (nonreplicated) experimental studies in which the experimental and control conditions are clearly specified and in which assignment to the experimental and control conditions is random. Epidemiologic surveys in which the population is sampled systematically (random, stratified sampling) and the observers are calibrated serve as the next level of evidence. Nonrandomized studies with controls such as case-controlled studies and field studies form the next level of evidence. Studies using historical controls but using randomized sampling or selection serve as the next level. Cohort studies in which disease risk assignments are made using correlational analysis are next in terms of evidence. Case reports and related anecdotal or descriptive evidence are next. Finally, the reports of expert committees and the opinion of experts form the lowest level of evidence.

BASIC REQUIREMENTS OF A RESEARCH STUDY

For a research study to be useful and applicable to current clinical or basic science efforts, it should satisfy the following five criteria (Box 15-4):

1. *It is based on the work of others and built on the knowledge base existent in the field.* Scientific progress is incremental. No one study can answer all questions. Each new insight or discovered regularity creates opportunities for new questions or takes on new meaning within the context of the earlier beliefs, findings, and theories. Most research either extends or clarifies the current scientific knowledge or challenges the current paradigm by suggesting modifications in the experimental method or by reformulating the research question.[9]

BOX 15-4

Basic Criteria for an Empirical Research Study

I. It is based on the work of others and builds on the knowledge base existent in the field
   A. Relevant and built on the current state of scientific research
   B. Relevant to current clinical and health policy issues
   C. Extends prior scientific findings and questions
II. It is replicable
   A. Research method is clearly described
   B. Variables are clearly defined
   C. Measurement is operationally defined
   D. Measures are reliable and valid
   E. Manageable in scope
III. It is based on currently established theory or, at least, on hypothesized relationships
   A. Data can be applied to the explanatory schema
   B. Measures and variables are based on the questions being asked
   C. Outcomes are relevant to the study hypotheses or study questions
IV. It is heuristic
   A. New questions are raised by the findings
   B. Existing paradigm is either challenged or supported
V. It is generalizable
   A. Results can be applied to the general population
   B. The clinician can apply the research to his or her own situation

For example, the discovery that periodontal disease is actually a systemic disease that can effect the patient's cardiac status has modified the dentist's responsibilities as a health care provider. Each new research study has the potential of filling in the gaps of our current knowledge base. However, work that occurs outside the knowledge stream tends, no matter how brilliant, to lie dormant until the scientific establishment enters that stream of inquiry. It is important that the research study be created within the context of the growing body of understanding that led to the formulation of the study and the interpretation of its findings.

2. *It is a replication or is replicable.* A well-designed study will describe its methods and the measurement of its variables in such a manner that future researchers can repeat or modify the study to observe whether the findings are reproducible. A study in which the findings occur only once and never again could easily be an artifact of chance or of method. Current trends in scientific research use meta-analysis to aggregate a number of studies to identify the extent and character of the phenomenon studied. This means that the use of reliable and well-defined measurement strategies and clear experimental design is essential to the building of a body of valid and usable findings.
3. *It is based on currently established theory or, at least, on current hypothesized relationships.* A good theory will guide observations and provide a structure in which to organize and explain the data collected. A theory is an organized and consistent explanatory statement that accounts for or generates hypotheses that predict the research findings. It is important to present the theory and hypotheses when generating a research study. The questions asked (the choice of which data to collect) determine

the range of possible outcomes. Research is not value free or method free; the assumptions of the researcher to a great extent effect what is discovered. By stating the assumptions and theory, which guide the study and its methodology, the researcher helps the reader understand the results that are observed.

4. *It is heuristic.* A well-designed and conceptualized study will generate future studies. Most truly valuable studies generate more questions than answers. At the conclusion of the study, the findings should help the reader to ask new and better questions about the phenomenon being explored. A study that provides an answer but does not stimulate new exploration or action is probably limited to merely providing specific demographic or descriptive information such as the "bond strength" or setting time of a particular cement or the number of individuals who have been treated in a clinic in the last month. Product information and production data are helpful but do not tend to generate new knowledge.
5. *It is generalizable.* One test of the value of a study is the extent to which its findings or knowledge generated can be applied to or exported into other situations. The fact that a particular causal relationship or association exists in a specific situation does not lead to usage. The reader wants to discover applications to his or her current issues, problems, and decisions. For the findings to have clinical implications, the sample population, design conditions, and experimental controls should be representative of the real world of the reader.

READING AND EVALUATING A RESEARCH STUDY

STANDARD FORMAT OF A RESEARCH STUDY

With little variation, most published research that appears in journal or monograph form adheres to the organization shown in Box 15-5.

- *Title.* The title of the study briefly indicates the topic and the focus of the study. Although many authors attempt to attract the reader with novelty, the text of the title should reflect or indicate the central question being posed.
- *Abstract.* The abstract, which usually appears at the head of the article and is often reproduced in the literature database, summarizes the background and focus of the study, the population sampled or objects studied, and the experimental design. It also includes a brief statement of the findings and the conclusions. In addition, the abstract may include "key words" that will allow the study to be indexed in the database. The purpose of the abstract is to allow the reader to quickly determine if the study is of interest.
- *Introduction, literature review, and hypothesis.* In the introduction, the researcher attempts to educate the reader regarding the importance and the history of the problem. Past controversies are summarized, and the question is clarified. In the literature review, the researcher provides a summary of the field to date. It is the obligation of the researcher to make the reader aware of the relevant past research and findings; to define the key issues, variables, and questions involved; and to create a context and rationale for the

BOX 15-5

Standard Format of a Research Study

I. Title of study
  A. Topic of study
  B. Focus of study
II. Abstract
  A. Topic of study
  B. Research focus or questions
  C. Methodology of study
  D. Summary of main results
  E. Conclusion of study
  F. List of key words for indexing
III. Introduction, literature review, and hypothesis (if empirical study)
  A. Importance of subject
  B. Review of major findings and key studies
  C. Statement of the current question
  D. Statement of intent, theory, or hypothesis
IV. Methodology
  A. Subject selection and sampling strategy
  B. Subject orientation: informed consent procedure if appropriate
  C. Strategy for assignment to conditions
  D. Variable definition
    1. Measurement strategy
    2. Measures
  E. Research design
    1. Controls
    2. Conditions
  F. Statistical analysis approach
V. Results section
  A. Demographics and subject characteristics
  B. Actual results from the measurements
    1. Results related to original hypotheses (primary findings)
    2. Secondary findings (post hoc findings)
  C. Statistical analysis
VI. Discussion
  A. Interpretation of results
  B. Review and summary of findings
  C. Application to hypotheses
  D. Secondary findings
  E. New hypotheses
VII. Summary and conclusion
VIII. Bibliography and references

current study. The theory being tested is stated, and the rival hypotheses are reviewed. Finally, the researcher clearly states the research question or the hypotheses being tested.

- *Methods.* The methods section organizes the research paper and allows the reader to assess the validity of the study and the reliability of the measures. In the methods section, the reader should be provided with specific and detailed information regarding how the study was conducted. From this description, the reader should be able to replicate the study. This section, combined with the next section, provides the reader an opportunity to develop an independent understanding of what this research study has found and to evaluate the legitimacy of the conclusions offered by the author at the conclusion of the report. Although the author may be tempted to interpret or extend the study findings in the discussion and conclusion sections, the reader should be able to develop an independent conclusion after reviewing the methods and results section.

The methods section usually includes four subsections:

1. The *sampling strategy* provides a description of the sampling strategy, the

sample size, and the methods for assigning samples to conditions.[10] In addition, where human subjects are involved, the reader will want to know how they were oriented and how "informed consent" was elicited. It will include a description of the population from which the sample was taken. The reader should be able, from the sampling description, to decide whether the results from the sample are appropriately attributed to the population being studied. In experimental studies, the reader will want to know if the study is conducted *in vivo* (in the organism itself) or *in vitro* (in the test tube, on extracted teeth, etc.). In addition, the reader will want to decide if the sampling methods or the sample assignment introduced *bias* into the results. Finally, the reader will attempt to determine if the sample size and selection criteria allowed the researcher to properly test the study hypotheses.

2. *Measurement strategies and measurement instruments.* How the variables are measured determines exactly what is being studied. Although the variables studied are discussed in the abstract, the introduction, and the conclusion, the actual definitions of the variables are stated in the measurement strategy. What is actually measured determines the "real" meaning of the variable. For example, if one wanted to know exactly what is meant by a carious lesion in a federal report, one might go to the instruction manual for National Institute of Dental Research field examiners and review the criteria for a carious lesion.[11] In the measurement directions, the examiner is directed to classify caries on a smooth surface when there is decalcification or a white spot and the area is determined to be soft by penetrating with the explorer or scraping away of the enamel. Visual evidence of demineralization is not enough. "Compliance" could mean keeping appointments, brushing every day, and taking medications reliably, or it could merely mean sitting still in a dental chair and accepting treatment without resistance. The careful reader will recognize that only the measurement itself can provide a clear definition of the variable; all other statements are merely assertions of meaning or descriptions of what the author intended to study. Both the validity and the reliability of the measurement involve the degree to which the measurement strategy fulfills the requirements of the experimental question involved (provides a test of the theory, the hypothetical assumptions, or the demographic question).

The reader will want to determine whether the descriptive and inferential statistics used are appropriate for the measurement scale employed to measure the independent and dependent variables. For example, the researcher may use a questionnaire in which the subjects are required to "rank" a particular item (ordinal measurement) but then incorrectly use descriptive statistics such as "means" and "standard deviations" to report the results instead of "medians" or "frequencies." This strategy is likely to add a mathematical precision to the report that did not exist in the study.

The experimenter will also need to know the degree of reliability, sensitivity, and specificity attained by the measurement. If observers or judges are utilized as examiners, the method of calibrating them should be described. If the instruments used are calibrated, standardized, or normed, this also should be documented. If the measures used in the study are new or uniquely employed, a report of how they were standardized and validated would be appropriate.

3. The *experimental design* should be presented. The experimenter should describe operationally the study design in a step-by-step sequence. The description should be sufficiently detailed so that the reader is able to replicate the study. First, the recruitment, orientation, and assignment of subjects to conditions are described. Second, the actual experimental procedure (defining the independent variable) or experimental conditions experienced by the experimental and control group, and the timing and application of the measurement tools (defining the dependent variable), must be clearly described. Third, the experimenter describes the experimental or quasi-experimental controls that are used to *rule out* alternative explanations of the findings.
4. Finally, *statistical analytic procedures* used in the study are presented. The proposed strategy for quantifying, evaluating, and analyzing the results is presented along with the actual statistical procedures proposed. In the discussion, the experimenter describes how the appropriate sample size was determined (level of *power* chosen and *effect size* criteria). The proposed statistical analytic procedures are specified, and the chosen *statistical significance* level is stated.

RESULTS

In the results section, the researcher describes the specific findings and actual outcomes of the project. The findings should be reported clearly and descriptively but not interpreted. Tables, charts, and graphs, where appropriate, are used to support the narrative, which provides a qualitative and quantitative descriptive and inferential statistical review. Subject characteristics are described and the outcomes from the measurements of the dependent variable reported. The experimenter provides, where relevant, such statistics as statistical significance, correlation, risk ratio, and effect size.

After reporting the results of the test of the hypotheses, the experimenter also provides the results of any secondary analyses undertaken, additional observations, and related findings. This "post hoc" analysis may provide important cues for future studies and explorations of the topic.

DISCUSSION AND INTERPRETATION OF THE FINDINGS

Having presented the findings objectively, the experimenter then interprets and explains the results obtained. In this section, the researcher attempts to "make sense" of the findings. The first step in this discussion would be to review the hypothesis and theory in the light of the findings. Where the study is concerned with products or epidemiologic investigations, inferences will be drawn about the material or the population and an evaluation made of the assumptions that led to the original study.

Although such findings as "statistical significance" may be reported, it will also be interesting for the researcher to speculate on the effects of the methodology, unanticipated characteristics of the subjects or of the conditions, and possible limitations of the theory. Although many readers rely on reports of statistical significance to determine the value of a study, recent commentaries in the statistical and research methodology journals have criticized this approach in favor of an approach that emphasizes "effect size" and "variance analysis."

Because research seldom genuinely "proves" or "disproves" a hypothesis, the discussion is likely to focus on the level of statistical support for the theory and the additional information provided by the secondary, or *post hoc,* analysis of the data. It is here also that the "lab notebook" (incidental and general observations) can be used to "shed light" on the research findings. Perhaps the subjects did not comply with the experimental protocol; perhaps the subjects were influenced by external conditions. The discussion session is an opportunity for the researcher to editorialize and dialogue with the reader and to propose different ways to conceptualize the outcome data and to reconceptualize the theory.

SUMMARY AND CONCLUSIONS

At the end of the article, the researcher provides a summary and interpretation of the study findings and attempts to draw conclusions related to the original theory and study question. Often, the commentary editorializes and goes beyond the actual findings to use the analysis as a basis for speculation and suggestions for future research. These speculations may go far beyond the actual findings of the study.

It is tempting for the busy clinician or student who is reviewing a large body of literature to read only the introduction and conclusions of a study. In fact, often the product brochures and the popular press report only these aspects of the studies available. However, without carefully reviewing the methods and results sections, it would be easy to be misled and to accept unsupported assertions. It is the obligation of the professional to independently and critically evaluate the discussion and conclusions in the light of what was actually performed and found. Often the reader will come to very different conclusions after careful study.

REFERENCES AND BIBLIOGRAPHY

Accurate primary references should be provided to the reader so that it will be possible to pursue the problem further and to learn more. Where established research design methodologies, instruments, observation guidelines, and statistical techniques are used, their source in the literature should be provided so that the reader can verify and follow up what is asserted. Studies and formal reviews should be documented so that the reader can draw an independent conclusion as to their content and findings.

READING CRITICALLY

SELECTING THE STUDY

For the busy dental student or clinician, the issue of what to read among the massive amounts of information available presents a daunting challenge. As a conscientious professional, the reader may wish to obtain a comprehensive view of current knowledge, but as a practical professional, the reader must recognize the limitations of time. At the end of this chapter, some suggestions, strategies, and resources (see Box 15-7) for

BOX 15-6

Steps in a Literature Search

1. Formulate a clear and focused question
2. Locate and create a bibliographic list of articles with abstracts
   a. Access relevant electronic databases
   b. Review professional journals
3. Apply a set of evidence criteria to prioritize the evidence value of the studies
4. Read selected articles critically
5. Using the bibliographic references from key articles, expand the bibliographic list of potential articles; obtain articles and their abstracts; again prioritize the evidence base of new articles
6. Critically review selected articles
7. Apply findings to the current problem
8. Evaluate the need for further evidence

locating relevant articles and related informational reports are provided. However, before beginning a search, the reader must narrow and focus the task. Box 15-6 provides suggestions for conducting this process:

1. *Formulate a clear, focused question.*[12] Beginning with a general question, the reader can narrow the search by deciding on the target population, the issue or condition of interest, and the desired outcome or problem-solving approach. As the question is clarified, it is helpful to be as specific as possible as to the type of information desired and its planned use. When looking for evidence-based answers to clinical or public health questions, the reader must ensure that the question asked is answerable rather than vague and speculative so that *key words* and *key phrases* can be selected for a bibliographic search.
2. *Create a tentative bibliographic collection.* Most electronic and bibliographic resources allow for the collection of references with short abstracts. At the end of this chapter, references and suggestions for an efficient public health search are provided. The reader should accumulate a body of references from which to select.
3. *Rank the assembled references as to evidence value.*[13] Earlier in this chapter, Box 15-3 presented a hierarchic list of evidence value. Systematic reviews and meta-analytic studies of randomized clinical trials and carefully controlled epidemiologic studies chosen using clear, stated, and valid selection criteria provide the best evidence. In these studies, the reader has the benefit of replication, minimization of chance findings, and minimization of bias and error from problems in one particular study. The second level of evidence comes from randomized, double-blind, clinical trials conducted at multiple sites and from replication studies performed at multiple sites. The third level of evidence is obtained from cohort studies and from controlled experimental studies in which the sampling strategy is specified and valid, the evaluators and subjects (where appropriate) are blind to the hypothesis, and sample size is sufficient for testing the hypothesis or predicting values in the target population. Outcomes and survey research, in which the sampling strategy is appropriate, the instruments are validated, and the statistical techniques

are appropriate, form the next level of evidence. Prospective studies tend to be stronger than retrospective studies. Case-controlled studies provide the next level of evidence. The lowest levels of evidence are provided by case reports, editorials, product announcements and advertisements from drug and equipment manufactures, and opinion pieces.

When selecting articles for review, the reader may also wish to include review articles presented by "recognized experts in the field" and committee statements from professional organizations and specialty committees. Although a specific article may not meet the criteria for an evidence-based decision, it may provide a background resource or clarification that can be helpful in resolving a problem or question.

4. *Read the chosen references critically.* Later in this chapter, we suggest a strategy for reading and evaluating a research article. A general set of guidelines for evaluating the value of an informational source would include the following: (a) Is this report valid in the light of my question? Can the results be applied to my situation and patients? (b) Is the study unbiased by either the author or the design? (c) Are the results reliable? Could the study be replicated in my situation? (d) Would application of the findings be practical (and ethical) in my situation?
5. *Use the references in the article to add to the database.* Articles that contain useful and relevant information will also contain valuable references for study. Add those references that are appropriate and interesting to the growing bibliography of your search.
6. *Select and evaluate the new articles using the criteria listed previously.* As new material is gathered, the literature search is focused and enriched. The process should continue until the reader establishes that a sufficient and comprehensive review has been accomplished.
7. *Apply the results of the review to the current problem.* At this point, the reader will be able to reevaluate the original question; focus the search, if necessary; and draw conclusions, develop a research project to build on what has been learned, or take action.
8. *Evaluate the results and determine if further exploration is needed.* All good research, including literature review, tends to be heuristic. The more that is known, the better the questions that can be formulated. Professional growth requires a constant search for clarity and a critical view of what "seems to be the case."

SEARCHING THE LITERATURE

The task of locating, accessing, and digesting the information necessary for modern, evidence-based dental practice and for maintaining an informed awareness of the trends in clinical and public health dentistry is becoming both increasingly difficult and increasingly more feasible. The amount of professional and technical information being produced is massive. It would not be possible or practical for the individual to consume this mountain of information. On the other hand, the growth in public health and scientific informatics has made it possible for the dentist to search this vast resource in an efficient and effective manner.

To stay current, the dental professional must monitor the following types of information:

1. *Peer-reviewed, scientific, and professional literature.* The dental professional should keep abreast of current findings regarding the etiology of dental disease, methods of preventing and treating disease, and strategies for maintaining individual and public health.
2. *Dental public health reports and journals.* The dental professional should be familiar with professional efforts to focus on nonclinical aspects of dental delivery such as financing health services, locating local health problems and preventing the spread of disease, health promotion strategies and campaigns, protecting against environmental hazards and toxins, and assessing and ensuring the quality and accessibility of health services.
3. *Political, professional, and social issues.* The profession is constantly involved in political and social activities related to dental public health issues. Currently the dentist must be knowledgeable about issues related to fluoridation of the public water supply, infection control, toxic wastes such as mercury and silver, infectious diseases (e.g., acquired immunodeficiency syndrome [AIDS], tuberculosis), social problems (child abuse), and access to and affordability of health care.
4. *Laws, regulations, and health standards.* The dentist must be knowledgeable about current strategies for infection control, waste disposal, and environmental protection.
5. *Product and treatment modality effectiveness.* Although manufacturers and distributors flood the dental journals and offices with news and reports of new materials every day, the dentist will want to independently discover what is available, what is acceptable, and what is effective and ineffective.
6. *Economic issues.* Currently, third-party insurance strategies and regulations are changing rapidly. The American Dental Association is actively involved in developing strategies to maintain the individual clinician's economic viability and relationships with patients. Both the government and the profession are attempting to protect patient interests in the face of rapidly changing reporting requirements and prioritizing of reimbursable dental health expenses.
7. *Local and national epidemiologic findings and current trends in dental health care.* For example, recent findings linking periodontal disease to diabetes and heart disease have placed dental practice in the center of health promotion activities. The trends in the health of the public are directly related to the economics of health care, public health planning, and distribution of the health care provider workforce.

The dentist must stay current with this massive body of information. Originally, the practicing dentist could rely on a combination of continuing education, subscribing to a small set of key professional journals, communications from supply houses and detail professionals, belonging to professional organizations and attending local and national professional society meetings, and the popular press. However, the information explosion and the speed of change quickly make the information obtained obsolete.

Over the past 15 years, new resources have become available to the dental professional for exploring professional and commercial knowledge base. Increasingly, the profession has turned to the computer and electronic media for help in accessing and exploring informational resources. Today, the professional can, with little expense, enter a vast electronic network that allows for rapid access to and interchange of information. With this electronic exchange, dentists can participate in informational links to other dentists and professional organizations, insurers, academics, biomedical libraries, and the public health sector.

In a seminal article, Friede and colleagues[14] defined public health informatics as "the application of information science and technology to public health research and practice." There are difficulties in the practical applications of public health informatics to the field of public health. This is due largely to the nature and variety of these resources. Public health information resources may be generally classified into three major categories: (1) literature, both traditional and gray; (2) statistical and epidemiologic data (vital statistics; health care utilization data; practitioner registries; disease and injury registries; disease, injury, and behavioral risk factor surveillance systems; periodic surveys; and programmatic data systems); and (3) legal and legislative material. Statistical and epidemiologic data account for the overwhelming majority of what the public health care practitioner seeks. Legal and legislative material are a distant second, and literature is a more distant third. This is true for a number of reasons but primarily because of the increasing demand for speed in identifying and retrieving information. Successful data retrieval involves the searching of numerous informational resources employing a wide array of interests and expertise. Box 15-7 is a comprehensive listing of Internet resources.

SAMPLE SEARCH

To illustrate how dental public health information is gathered, we need to look at a typical question for which dental public health professionals seek information. For the purposes of illustration, we have chosen to search for information on the following question:

- Is dental caries considered an infectious disease?

We will first search the MEDLINE database from the National Library of Medicine using the PubMed search engine. MEDLINE searches the literature published through traditionally accessible channels, such as journal articles. MEDLINE uses a controlled vocabulary, called MeSH (Medical Subject Headings) to search the literature. Controlled vocabularies are helpful to the searcher because they bring together concepts that are similar or synonymous under one searchable term and provide a consistent way to retrieve information that may use different terminology for the same concepts. Controlled vocabularies also merge variant spellings, such as British versus American English. PubMed provides a MeSH Browser that identifies MeSH terms. In our sample search, the concept of "infectious diseases" is searchable using the MeSH term "communicable diseases." This term combines both concepts into one. We can therefore use the term "communicable diseases" to search for "infectious disease," "infectious diseases," "communicable disease," and "communicable diseases." We also will use the "Explode" command. Explode will retrieve all documents containing the selected term, as well as any of its narrower terms. In other words, exploding "communicable diseases" allows us to search for other diseases considered to be of

Text continued on p. 416

BOX 15-7

Internet Resources

Traditional Literature Resources

The dentist has available a large number of informational databases that can be accessed electronically. The resources are indexed and organized to provide quick and selective access to current scientific and public health published documents:

- MEDLINE (www4.ncbi.nlm.nih.gov/PubMed/). Coverage: medicine, nursing, dentistry, veterinary medicine, the health care system, and preclinical sciences.
- NLM Gateway (http://gateway.nlm.nih.gov/gw/Cmd). The NLM Gateway is a World Wide Web–based system that lets users search simultaneously in multiple retrieval systems at the U.S. National Library of Medicine (NLM). It allows users to initiate searches from one Web interface, providing "one-stop searching" for many of NLM's information resources and databases. Coverage includes the following:

  MEDLINE (Medical Literature, Analysis, and Retrieval System Online) is NLM's premier bibliographic database that contains over 11 million references to journal articles in life sciences with a concentration on biomedicine.

  OLDMEDLINE contains citations published in the 1960 through 1965 *Cumulated Index Medicus* and the 1958 through 1959 *Current List of Medical Literature.* OLDMEDLINE covers the fields of medicine, preclinical sciences, and allied health sciences.

  LOCATORplus is NLM's online catalog and includes over 800,000 catalog records for books, audiovisuals, journals, computer files, and other materials in NLM's collections.

  AIDS Meetings (with MeSH) contains meeting abstracts from the AIDSLINE database. The meeting abstracts have been indexed with MeSH terms. (MeSH is discussed later in this chapter.) AIDS Meetings contains new meeting abstracts that are not included in the AIDSLINE database. The meeting abstracts have not been indexed.

  HSRProj provides project records for health services research, including health technology assessment and the development and use of clinical practice guidelines.

  MEDLINEplus is NLM's Website for consumer health information. It includes over 400 health topics and a guide to more than 9000 prescription and over-the-counter medications.
- Gateway access to additional NLM retrieval systems will happen over time. Among the resources to be added to the Gateway are DIRLINE, ClinicalTrials.gov, and HSTAT. Cochrane Database of Systematic Reviews (COCH) includes the full text of regularly updated systematic reviews prepared by the Cochrane Collaboration. COCH is an international network of individuals and institutions committed to preparing, maintaining, and disseminating systematic reviews of the effects of health care. In pursuing its aims, the Cochrane Collaboration is guided by six principles: collaboration, building on people's existing enthusiasm and interests, minimizing duplication of effort, avoidance of bias, keeping up to date, and ensuring access. Each issue of COCH contains new and updated reviews and protocols. COCH is unlike other "journal" or "serial" publications in that once a review is published it will appear in every issue thereafter. The COCH is published on computer disk and CD, on the Internet, and in a variety of other forms. A subscription is needed to access this resource.

Gray Literature

The Fourth International Conference on Gray Literature (GL '99) in Washington, DC, defined *gray literature* as follows: "that which is produced on all levels of government, academics,

BOX 15-7

Internet Resources—cont'd

business and industry in print and electronic formats, but which is not controlled by commercial publishers."[15] In general, gray literature publications are unconventional, volatile, and sometimes ephemeral. They may include, but are not limited to, the following types of materials: reports (preprints, preliminary progress and advanced reports, technical reports, statistical reports, memoranda, state-of-the-art reports, market research reports, etc.), theses, conference proceedings, technical specifications and standards, noncommercial translations, bibliographies, technical and commercial documentation, and official documents not published commercially (primarily government reports and documents).[16]

- GrayLIT Network (www.osti.gov/graylit/). Coverage: the gray literature of U.S. federal agencies. It taps into the search engines of distributed gray literature collections, enabling the user to find information without first having to know the sponsoring agency. The GrayLIT Network is the world's most comprehensive portal to federal gray literature. By offering a mode of communication for this hard-to-find class of literature, the GrayLIT Network enables convenient access by the American public to government information.
- HealthSTAR (http://text.nlm.nih.gov/hsrsearch/hsr.html). Coverage: health services, technology, administration, and research literature.
- HSRProj (http://text.nlm.nih.gov/hsrsearch/hsr.html). Coverage: research in progress funded by federal, state, and private grants and contracts.
- DIRLINE (http://dirline.nlm.nih.gov/). Coverage: directory of information resources (organizations, research resources, projects, databases, electronic bulletin boards concerned with health and biomedicine).
- HSTAT (Health Services/Technology Assessment Text) (http://text.nlm.nih.gov/). Coverage: Agency for Health Care Policy and Research (AHCPR) evidence reports, supported guidelines, technology assessments, and reviews; National Institutes of Health (NIH) Consensus Development Conference Statements and Technology Assessment Workshop Reports; NIH Clinical Center active research protocols, U.S. Preventive Services Task Force's guides to clinical preventive services; AIDS/HIV Treatment Service (ATIS)–approved guidelines; Substance Abuse and Mental Health Services Administration (SAMHSA) treatment improvement protocols (TIP); Substance Abuse and Mental Health Services Administration's Center for Substance Abuse (SAMHSA/CSAP) Prevention Enhancement Protocols (PEPS); Guide to Community Preventive Services.

STATISTICAL AND EPIDEMIOLOGIC DATA

For a number of reasons, but primarily because of the need for quick access to raw and summarized information for planning, the professional may need specific epidemiologic data. Data are needed not only about local communities (demographic information that can be used for deciding on where to locate an office, how to advertise, and what services to emphasize), but also about potential sources of disease and injury and about available resources in the community.

- Agency for Healthcare Research and Quality (AHRQ) (formerly the Agency for Health Care Policy and Research) (www.ahcpr.gov/). AHRQ research provides evidence-based information on health care outcomes; quality; and cost, use, and access. AHRQ supports the development of evidence reports through its 12 evidence-based practice centers and the dissemination of evidence-based guidelines through the AHRQ's National Guideline Clearinghouse.
- Centers for Disease Control and Prevention (CDC) (www.cdc.gov/). The Centers for

Continued

BOX 15-7

Internet Resources—cont'd

Disease Control and Prevention (CDC) is recognized as the lead federal agency for protecting the public's health and safety. The CDC serves as the national focus for developing and applying disease prevention and control, environmental health, and health promotion and education activities designed to improve the health of the people of the United States. The agency comprises the following organizational components:

National Center for Chronic Disease Prevention and Health Promotion (NCCDPHP) (www.cdc.gov/nccdphp/index.htm) prevents premature death and disability from chronic diseases and promotes healthy personal behaviors.

National Center for Environmental Health (NCEH) (www.cdc.gov/nceh/ncehhome.htm) provides national leadership in preventing and controlling disease, birth defects, disability, and death resulting from the interactions between people and their environment.

National Center for Health Statistics (NCHS) (www.cdc.gov/nchs/) is the principal U.S. health statistics agent. Its mission is "to provide statistical information that will guide actions and policies to improve the health of the American people." NCHS products are listed in their catalogs of electronic products and publications. The most comprehensive of these is *Health, United States,* an annual compendium on health status, health care resource use, and vital statistics. The *Vital and Health Statistics* series includes descriptions of NCHS data collection programs and methods and presents data analyses for each data collection program or family of related programs. Other NCHS publications include *Advance Data, Monthly Vital Statistics Reports, Vital Statistics of the United States, Healthy People 2010,* and *Life Tables.*

National Center for Infectious Diseases (NCID) (www.cdc.gov/ncidod/) prevents illness, disability, and death caused by infectious diseases in the United States and around the world.

National Center for Injury Prevention and Control (NCIPC) (www.cdc.gov/ncipc/ncipchm.htm) prevents death and disability from nonoccupational injuries, including those that are unintentional and those that result from violence.

National Institute for Occupational Safety and Health (NIOSH) (www.cdc.gov/niosh/homepage.html) ensures safety and health for all people in the workplace through research and prevention.

National Center for HIV, STD, and TB Prevention (NCHSTP) (www.cdc.gov/nchstp/od/nchstp.html) provides national leadership in preventing and controlling human immunodeficiency virus (HIV) infection, sexually transmitted diseases (STDs), and tuberculosis (TB).

National Immunization Program (NIP) (www.cdc.gov/nip) prevents disease, disability, and death from vaccine-preventable diseases in children and adults.

Epidemiology Program Office (EPO) (www.cdc.gov/epo/index.htm) strengthens the public health system by coordinating public health surveillance; providing support in scientific communications, statistics, and epidemiology; and training in surveillance, epidemiology, and prevention effectiveness.

Public Health Practice Program Office (PHPPO) (www.phppo.cdc.gov/) strengthens community practice of public health by creating an effective workforce, building information networks, conducting practice research, and ensuring laboratory quality.

BOX 15-7

Internet Resources—cont'd

- The CDC also provides databases that search across the entire agency to retrieve specific types of information:

  CDC Wonder (http://wonder.cdc.gov/) is an easy-to-use system that provides a single point of access to a wide variety of CDC reports, guidelines, and numeric public health data. With CDC Wonder you can search for and retrieve *MMWR* articles and prevention guidelines published by the CDC or query dozens of numeric data sets on CDC's mainframe and other computers, via "fill-in-the-blank" request screens. Public-use data sets about mortality rates, cancer incidence, hospital discharges, AIDS, behavioral risk factors, diabetes, and many other topics are available for query, and the requested data can be readily summarized and analyzed. You can also locate the name and E-mail addresses of CDC staff and registered CDC Wonder users and post notices, general announcements, data files, or software programs of interest to public health professionals in an electronic forum, for perusal by CDC staff and other CDC Wonder users.

  Epi Info 2000 (www.cdc.gov/epiinfo/EI2000.htm), used with a personal computer, allows epidemiologists and other public health and medical professionals to rapidly develop a questionnaire or form, customize the data entry process, and enter and analyze data. Epidemiologic statistics, tables, graphs, and maps are produced with simple commands such as READ, FREQ, LIST, TABLES, GRAPH, and MAP. Epi Map 2000 displays geographic maps with data from Epi Info 2000.
- The Combined Health Information Database (CHID) (http://chid.nih.gov) is a database produced by health-related agencies of the federal government. This database provides titles, abstracts, and availability information for health information and health education resources. Databases cover AIDS, STD and TB education, Alzheimer's disease, arthritis and musculoskeletal and skin diseases, cancer prevention and control, complementary and alternative medicine, deafness and communication disorders, diabetes, digestive diseases, epilepsy education and prevention activities, health promotion and education, kidney and urologic diseases, maternal and child health, medical genetics and rare disorders, oral health, prenatal smoking cessation, and weight control.
- Environmental Protection Agency (EPA) (www.epa.gov). The mission of the EPA is to protect human health and to safeguard the natural environment. The EPA's source of reference information about the definition, origin, source, and location of environmental data is the Environmental Data Registry (EDR). The EDR is a comprehensive, authoritative source of reference information about environmental data. The EDR catalogs EPA's major data collections and helps locate environmental information of interest. It does not contain the environmental data itself, but rather information that describes the data to make it more meaningful. It provides invaluable information on the definition, origin, source, and location of environmental data.
- Food and Drug Administration (FDA) (www.fda.gov). The FDA is made up of numerous centers that publish important data on public health information: the Center for Biologics Evaluation and Research, the Center for Drug Evaluation and Research, the Center for Devices and Radiological Health, the Center for Food Safety and Applied Nutrition, the Center for Veterinary Medicine, and the National Center for Toxicological Research.

Continued

BOX 15-7

Internet Resources—cont'd

- Health Care Financing Administration (HCFA) (www.hcfa.gov). The HCFA administers the Medicare and Medicaid programs. The HCFA makes a wide range of statistical information and data available, including annual statistical summaries about beneficiaries, providers, spending, and costs; downloadable public use data files; health care indicators based on analysis of recent trends in health care spending; special statistical reports and files on topics such as managed care, immunizations, mammography, enrollment, and diagnosis-related group data; and the National Health Expenditures data, including Medicare, Medicaid, private health insurance, and out-of-pocket spending.
- Health Resources and Services Administration (HRSA) (www.hrsa.gov). The HRSA directs national health programs that improve the nation's health by ensuring equitable access to comprehensive, quality health care for all. HRSA works to improve and extend life for people living with HIV/AIDS, provide primary health care to medically underserved people, serve women and children through state programs, and train a health care workforce that is both diverse and motivated to work in underserved communities. Integral to these initiatives are the Center for Managed Care, the Center for Public Health Practice, the Center for Quality, and the Oral Health Initiative.
- National Cancer Institute (NCI) (www.nci.nih.gov). The NCI leads the nation's fight against cancer by supporting and conducting groundbreaking research in cancer biology, causation, prevention, detection, treatment, and survivorship. The NCI provides cancer information through a number of online resources, including the following:

  CancerNet (http://cancernet.nci.nih.gov) provides comprehensive information about cancer by covering topics such as types of cancer, treatment options, clinical trials, genetics, causes, risk factors, prevention, testing for cancer, coping with cancer, support and resources, and cancer literature and statistics.

  CancerTrials (http://cancertrials.nci.nih.gov/index.html) is a comprehensive clinical trials site, providing access to NCI's clinical trials database, news about cancer research, and resources for patients and health care professionals about participating in clinical trials.

  Surveillance, Epidemiology, and End Results (SEER) program (www.seer.ims.nci.nih.gov) is the most authoritative source of information on cancer incidence and survival in the United States. Information on more than 2.5 million cancer cases is included in the SEER database, and approximately 160,000 new cases are added each year within the SEER catchment areas.

  Office of Cancer Complementary and Alternative Medicine (OCCAM) (http://occam.nci.nih.gov) was established in October 1998 to coordinate and enhance the activities of the NCI in the arena of complementary and alternative medicine (CAM).
- National Committee on Vital and Health Statistics (NCVHS) (http://ncvhs.hhs.gov). The NCVHS is the statutory public advisory committee to the Secretary of Health and Human Services on health data, privacy, and health information policy. NCVHS was created in 1949 at the request of the World Health Organization (WHO) as part of an international effort to build national and international health statistics. Through the years, it has contributed to the development of the International Classification of Diseases (ICD), advocated for standardization, studied and made recommendations on data aspects of pressing national health issues, and advised government

BOX 15-7

Internet Resources—cont'd

on surveys and other data collection efforts. Of particular importance to the field of public health are NCVHS activities in the areas of Core Health Data Elements and the implementation of the Health Insurance Portability and Accountability Act (HIPAA) of 1966.

- The National Guideline Clearinghouse (NGC) (www.guideline.gov/index.asp). NGC is a comprehensive database of evidence-based clinical practice guidelines and related documents produced by AHRQ, in partnership with the American Medical Association and the American Association of Health Plans. NGC is an Internet Website intended to make evidence-based clinical practice guidelines and related abstract, summary, and comparison materials widely available to health care professionals.
- National Information Center on Health Services Research and Health Care Technology (NICHSR) (www.nlm.nih.gov/nichsr/nichsr.html). The NICHSR was created to improve "the collection, storage, analysis, retrieval, and dissemination of information on health services research, clinical practice guidelines, and on health care technology, including the assessment of such technology." The overall goals of the NICHSR are to make the results of health services research, including practice guidelines and technology assessments, readily available to health practitioners, health care administrators, health policy makers, payers, and the information professionals who serve these groups; to improve access to data and information needed by the creators of health services research; and to contribute to the information infrastructure needed to foster patient record systems that can produce useful health services research data as a by-product of providing health care. NICHSR produces HealthSTAR, HSRProj, HSTAT, and DIRLINE.
- The National Institute of Dental and Craniofacial Research (NIDCR) (www.nidr.nih.gov). The NIDCR works to improve and promote craniofacial, oral, and dental health through research. The NIDCR produces and maintains the National Oral Health Information Clearinghouse.
- National Oral Health Information Clearinghouse (NOHIC) (www.nohic.nidcr.nih.gov/welcome.html). NOHIC produces and distributes patient and professional education materials, including fact sheets, brochures, and information packets. NOHIC also sponsors the Oral Health Database, which includes bibliographic citations, abstracts, and availability information for a wide variety of print and audiovisual materials. NOHIC staff members provide free custom or standard searches on specific special care topics in oral health.
- Occupational Safety and Health Administration (OSHA) (www.osha.gov). OSHA's mission is to save lives, prevent injuries, and protect the health of America's workers. OSHA provides information on workplace injury, illness and fatality statistics, approved blood lead laboratories, nationally recognized testing laboratories, and ergonomics. eCATs are OSHA's e-Compliance Assistance Tools. eCATs are illustrated, expert-based tools designed to assist businesses in identifying workplace hazards and abatements. OSHA Regulations and Compliance Links are a comprehensive and easy-to-use resource for current OSHA standards and compliance-related information.
- Office of Disease Prevention and Health Promotion (ODPHP) (www.odphp.osophs.dhhs.gov). Since 1979, ODPHP has provided leadership in stimulating, coordinating, and unifying national disease prevention and health promotion strategies among federal, state, and local agencies and major private and voluntary organizations.

Continued

BOX 15-7

Internet Resources—cont'd

Select ODPHP activities include the following:

Healthy People Initiative (www.health.gov/healthypeople) promotes health and prevents disease by establishing health improvement objectives with 10-year targets that are monitored over a decade.

Healthfinder (www.healthfinder.gov) includes almost 6000 resources on 1000 topics, which range from abstinence to wellness and include adoption, aging, AIDS, cancer, child care, heart disease, food safety, Medicare and Medicaid, nutrition, substance abuse, quality of care, and welfare.

National Health Information Center (NHIC) (www.health.gov/nhi) provides a central health information referral service for consumers and professionals using a database of more than 1700 national associations, government agencies, and other organizations.

Dietary Guidelines for Americans (www.health.gov/dietaryguidelines) has been published jointly with the U.S. Department of Agriculture (USDA) every 5 years since 1980 and is the statutorily mandated basis for federal nutrition education activities.

- The Office of the Surgeon General (www.surgeongeneral.gov/sgoffice.htm). On May 25, 2000, Surgeon General David Satcher released *Oral Health in America: A Report of the Surgeon General,* the fifty-first Surgeon General's report. These reports have helped frame the science on vital health issues in a way that has helped educate, motivate, and mobilize the public to more effectively deal with those issues. In addition to a lack of awareness of the importance of oral health among the public, the report found a significant disparity between racial and socioeconomic groups in regard to oral health and overall health issues. Based on these findings, the Surgeon General called for action to promote access to oral health care for all Americans, especially the disadvantaged and minority children found to be at greatest risk for severe medical complications resulting from minimal oral care and treatment.
- Substance Abuse and Mental Health Services Administration (SAMHSA) (www.samhsa.gov). SAMHSA is the federal agency charged with improving the quality and availability of prevention, treatment, and rehabilitative services to reduce illness, death, disability, and cost to society resulting from substance abuse and mental illnesses. SAMHSA serves as the umbrella under which substance abuse and mental health service centers are housed, including the Center for Mental Health Services (CMHS), the Center for Substance Abuse Prevention (CSAP), and the Center for Substance Abuse Treatment (CSAT). SAMHSA also houses the Office of the Administrator, the Office of Applied Studies, the Office of Program Services, and the Office of Managed Care.
- Social Security Administration (SSA) (www.ssa.gov/policy). SSA publishes information based on SSA administrative records, such as benefit and demographic data on persons receiving benefits, information about workers derived from earnings reports submitted by employers and by the self-employed, disability and retirement information, health insurance data, and Medicare and Medicaid information.
- U.S. Census Bureau (Department of Commerce) (www.census.gov). The U.S. Census Bureau provides access to numerous online sites that provide statistical information, including the following:

  American FactFinder, interactive database engine for the 1997 Economic Census, the American Community Survey, the 1990 Census, Census 2000 Dress Rehearsal, and Census 2000.

BOX 15-7

Internet Resources—cont'd

Censtats: Census Tract Street Locator, County Business Patterns, ZIP Business Patterns, Annual Survey of Manufacturers, International Trade Data, and more.

Map Stats, an easy way to view profiles of states and counties.

QuickFacts, frequently requested Census Bureau information at the national, state, and county levels.

TIGER | TIGER Map Service Info | Maps, Topologically Integrated Geographic Encoding and Referencing system.

U.S. Gazetteer, place name, and ZIP code search engine.

1990 Decennial Census Lookup allows you to create your own extract files from the 1990 summaries.

Data Extraction System (DES) allows you to create custom data extracts from Current Population Survey, 1990 Census Public Use Microdata, and more.

Ferret Data is an extraction and review tool (in collaboration with the Bureau of Labor Statistics and other statistical agencies).

- World Health Organization (WHO) (www.who.int). Health Topics and Policy (www.who.int/home/map_ht.html) has links to the following topics: communicable/infectious diseases, tropical diseases, vaccine-preventable diseases, environment, family and reproductive health, health policies, health statistics, health systems, health technology, lifestyle, and noncommunicable diseases (which includes a link to oral health).

Legal and Legislative Resources

The practitioner may need access to governmental documents that contain information about licensure requirements, local regulations, civil service and public health opportunities, and related governmental activities.

- Federal Gateway (http://fedgate.org). The Federal Gateway consolidates all the federal agencies, state and local government agencies, and nonprofit organizations into one Internet site, thereby greatly simplifying the task of acquiring U.S. federal government information.
- FirstGov (www.firstgov.com). FirstGov is a portal to U.S. government Websites that offers users access to all 20,000 government sites (with over 27 million Webpages) from a single central point. Sites are categorized principally by "interesting topics," such as Business and Economy, Healthy People, and Arts and Culture, among others. Clicking on a topic brings up a page with several featured links and numerous related links to various federal Websites.
- Search Systems (www.pac-info.com). Search Systems is created and maintained by Pacific Information Resources. This useful metasite links to a wide array of free, searchable public record databases (more than 1500). The links are organized geographically, with nationwide databases for the United States and Canada, and state databases broken down into statewide, county, and city. The number of databases listed for each state varies widely, but most include property records, court dockets and filings, professional licenses, and administrative codes. Other databases include city job postings, restaurant inspections, most wanted, inmate locator, lottery winning numbers, toxic release inventory, births and deaths, and charitable organizations.
- Quick Facts (http://quickfacts.census.gov/qfd). Quick Facts is a handy reference resource from the U.S. Census Bureau that allows users to access frequently requested Census Bureau information at the national, state, and county levels.
- State Search (https://www.nasire.org/statesearch). State Search is sponsored by the National Association of State Information Resource Executives (NASIRE) and serves as a topical clearinghouse to state government information on the Internet.
- Thomas (http://thomas.loc.gov/). Thomas is a listing of legislative information on the Internet, which includes floor activities of the House and Senate; bill summaries and status; the Congressional Record; and Committee Reports.

an infectious nature. We will also search for the term "infectious diseases" in the title and abstract fields. This is helpful in broadening the search by pulling natural language terms into the strategy. This is particularly useful in our sample search because we are looking for articles that consider dental caries to be an infectious disease even though the indexer might not have chosen "communicable diseases" as an index term. We will also truncate disease using an asterisk (*) to retrieve all instances of the term whether it is written "disease" or "diseases." We then "OR" these two concepts to create a new set that includes all the documents that contain one or the other of these terms. We then explode dental caries and search for the truncated text word "dental cavit" so that we include "cavity" or "cavities." After combining these concepts with the "OR" command, we will "AND" the two combined sets together. This will create a final set that contains only those documents that have the selected concepts in common. This narrows our search by citing the most relevant information. "AND," "OR," and "NOT" are called operators, and using them to combine terms is known as Boolean searching. The search strategy will be constructed as follows (Fig. 15-1):

(communicable diseases [MESH] OR infectious disease*) AND (dental caries [MESH] OR dental cavit*)

We first identify communicable diseases as our MeSH-supplied term by putting MeSH in brackets. We then truncate infectious disease and separate the terms by the OR, written all in capital letters. We enclose this part of the search strategy in parentheses so that the search engine knows to complete this part of the search first. We use the same process with dental caries OR dental cavity or cavities. The two parts of the search strategy are then separated by an AND.

In a database of over 11 million citations, a final set of 47 is remarkably small. This may indicate that little published research has been done on caries as an infectious disease. However, several of the relevant articles retrieved are useful background on our sample question (Fig. 15-2).

A similar search of the HealthSTAR database turns up 21 citations but no unique information. HealthSTAR was still important in our information quest because it searched the gray literature consisting of technical reports, internal documents, and other types of material that can be difficult to find and acquire.

To broaden our search and look for the information that may have been gathered on our topic but not necessarily published in the traditional formats, we turn to the statistical and epidemiologic data. This information is mostly published by governmental agencies and uses key words instead of controlled vocabularies for information retrieval. There are standard search strategies that are consistent in most governmental agency search engines. Because we have started our search in the PubMed database, from the National Library of Medicine, a governmental agency, we can use a search strategy that is only slightly modified from our PubMed search. Only PubMed uses the controlled vocabulary MeSH, so we will treat all four of our search terms as key words.

Our search strategy for the remainder of the governmental agencies will be as follows (Fig. 15-3):

(communicable disease* OR infectious disease*) AND (dental caries OR dental cavit*)

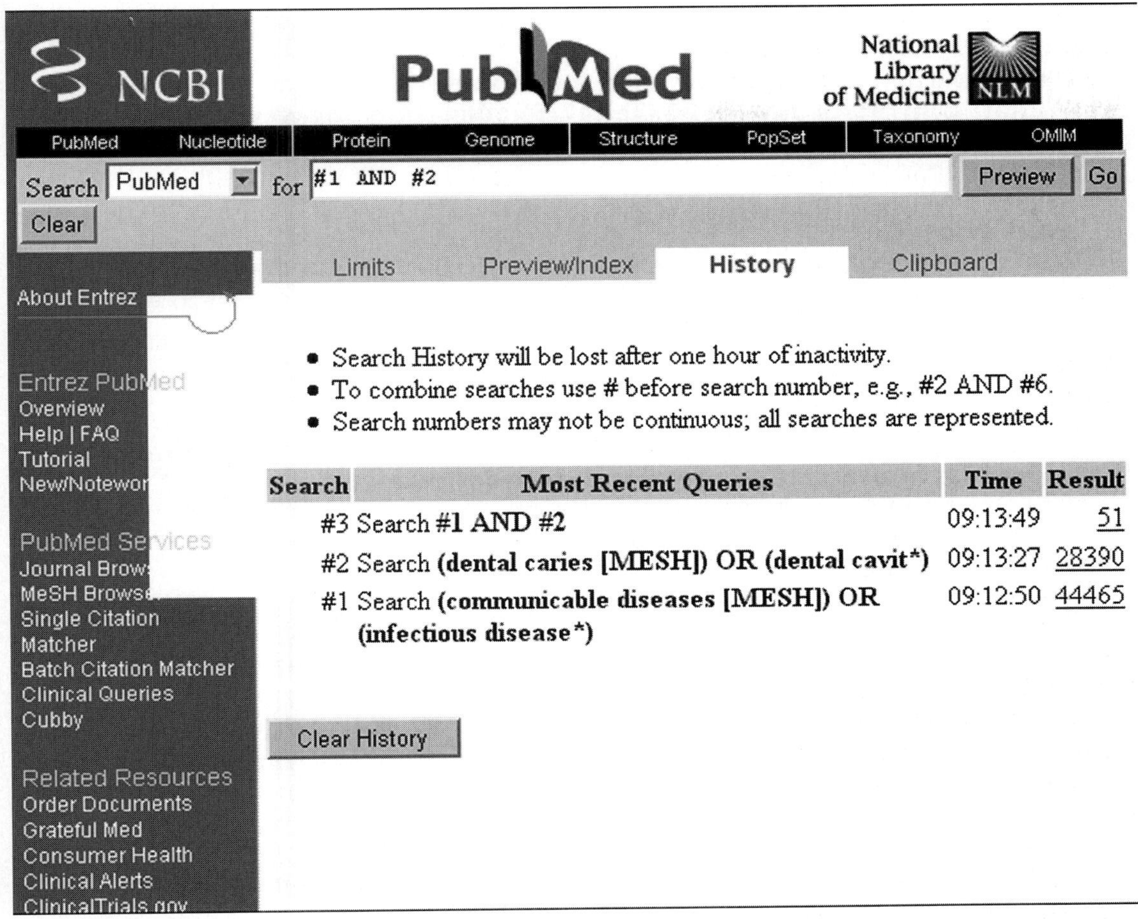

Fig. 15-1. MEDLINE search strategy.

Some governmental agencies do not provide the options to search for information using a self-constructed strategy. Information must be gathered by browsing through the Website looking for relevant links. This process is more time-consuming and less precise but still beneficial (Fig. 15-4). For example, the Health Resources and Services Administration allows you to search by "Topics A-Z." Within these topics, one finds "Oral Health." If you click on this link, you will be brought to the HRSA Oral Health Initiative. This Initiative has published a report entitled *Oral Disease: A Crisis Among Children of Poverty,* which traces the concept that dental caries in low-income children should be treated as an infectious disease pattern.

Legal and legislative material can be equally important. Some of this material is published by governmental agencies (Quick Facts and Thomas) and can be found using

Caufield PW, Griffen AL.
Dental caries. An infectious and transmissible disease.
Pediatr Clin North Am. 2000 Oct;47(5):1001-19, v. Review.
[PubMed - indexed for MEDLINE]
PMID: 11059347

Anusavice KJ.
Management of dental caries as a chronic infectious disease.
J Dent Educ. 1998 Oct;62(10):791-802. Review. No abstract available.
[PubMed - indexed for MEDLINE]
PMID: 9847883

Limeback H.
Treating dental caries as an infectious disease. Applying the medical model in practice to prevent dental caries.
Ont Dent. 1996 Jul-Aug;73(6):23-5. Review.
[PubMed - indexed for MEDLINE]
PMID: 9470624

Weinstein P.
Research recommendations: pleas for enhanced research efforts to impact the epidemic of dental disease in infants.
J Public Health Dent. 1996 Winter;56(1):55-60. Review.
[PubMed - indexed for MEDLINE]
PMID: 8667320

Tanzer JM.
Dental caries is a transmissible infectious disease: the Keyes and Fitzgerald revolution.
J Dent Res. 1995 Sep;74(9):1536-42. Review. No abstract available.
[PubMed - indexed for MEDLINE]
PMID: 7560413

Fig. 15-2. Sample citations.

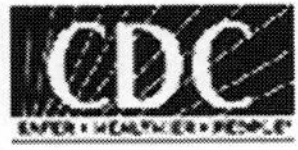

CDC Search Results

search tips

Documents bearing this logo are in Portable Document Format (PDF) and require the Adobe Acrobat Reader

Your query matched **100** documents.

---

1 0.85 **PHTN** find more like this...
Summary: Since the early days of community water fluoridation, the prevalence of dental caries has been declining in U.S. communities with and without fluoridated water. Much of the decline in areas without fluoridated water is attributable to diffusion of fluori
http://www.phppo.cdc.gov/PHTN/tenachievements/fluoride2/fl2.asp , 33048 bytes, updated 11-27-01

2 0.83 **PHTN** find more like this...
Summary: In 1931, Dr. H. Trendley Dean, U.S. Public Health Service Dental Officer, conducted pioneering research into the relationship between fluoride and dental caries. The documented effectiveness of community water fluoridation in preventing dental car
http://www.phppo.cdc.gov/PHTN/tenachievements/fluoride1/fl1.asp , 36918 bytes, updated 11-27-01

3 0.83 **PHTN** find more like this...
Summary: A series of reports was published in 1999 in CDCÆs Morbidity and Mortality Weekly Report (MMWR) regarding the 10 great public health achievements highlighted in this Web site. The MMWR Series is prepared by CDC. The data in the weekly MMWR are provision
http://www.phppo.cdc.gov/PHTN/tenachievements/mmwr/mmwr.asp , 37798 bytes, updated 11-27-01

4 0.79 **MMWR Weekly Current Volume** find more like this...
Summary: The MMWR Recommendations and Reports contain in-depth articles that relay policy statements for prevention and treatment on all areas in CDC's scope of responsibility (e.g., recommendations from the Advisory Committee on Immunization Practices). A Report
http://www.cdc.gov/mmwr/mmwr_rr.html , 39879 bytes, updated 12-22-01

5 0.78 **Health Objectives for the Nation Healthy People 2000: National Health Promotion and Disease Prevention Objectives for the Year 2000** find more like this...
Summary: Healthy People 2000 succeeds both the 1979 report Healthy People: The Surgeon General's Report on Health Promotion and Disease Prevention (2) and the 1990 health objectives published in Promoting Health/Preventing Disease: Objectives for the Nation in 198

Fig. 15-3. Search result: self-constructed strategy.

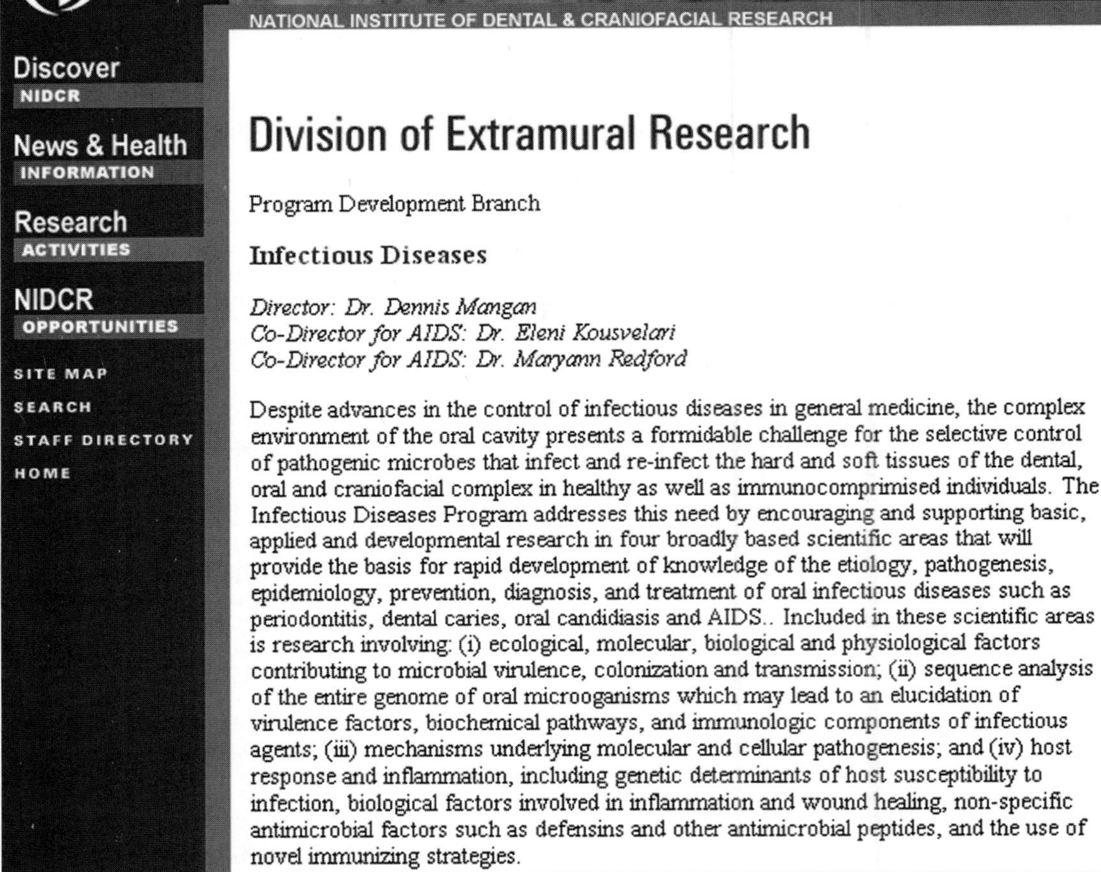
Research Activities

NATIONAL INSTITUTE OF DENTAL & CRANIOFACIAL RESEARCH

Discover NIDCR

News & Health INFORMATION

Research ACTIVITIES

NIDCR OPPORTUNITIES

SITE MAP

SEARCH

STAFF DIRECTORY

HOME

Division of Extramural Research

Program Development Branch

Infectious Diseases

Director: Dr. Dennis Mangan
Co-Director for AIDS: Dr. Eleni Kousvelari
Co-Director for AIDS: Dr. Maryann Redford

Despite advances in the control of infectious diseases in general medicine, the complex environment of the oral cavity presents a formidable challenge for the selective control of pathogenic microbes that infect and re-infect the hard and soft tissues of the dental, oral and craniofacial complex in healthy as well as immunocomprimised individuals. The Infectious Diseases Program addresses this need by encouraging and supporting basic, applied and developmental research in four broadly based scientific areas that will provide the basis for rapid development of knowledge of the etiology, pathogenesis, epidemiology, prevention, diagnosis, and treatment of oral infectious diseases such as periodontitis, dental caries, oral candidiasis and AIDS.. Included in these scientific areas is research involving: (i) ecological, molecular, biological and physiological factors contributing to microbial virulence, colonization and transmission; (ii) sequence analysis of the entire genome of oral microoganisms which may lead to an elucidation of virulence factors, biochemical pathways, and immunologic components of infectious agents; (iii) mechanisms underlying molecular and cellular pathogenesis; and (iv) host response and inflammation, including genetic determinants of host susceptibility to infection, biological factors involved in inflammation and wound healing, non-specific antimicrobial factors such as defensins and other antimicrobial peptides, and the use of novel immunizing strategies.

Fig. 15-4. Search result: category browsing.

the same search strategy created for uncovering the statistical and epidemiologic data. Commercial companies have developed other databases and search strategies unique to each system. Look for "Help" or "Search Tips" links to guide you through the process. In our sample search, there appeared to be no legislative initiatives involving dental caries as infectious disease at the time the search was constructed.

REVIEW QUESTIONS

1. In evaluating a research paper for its level of evidence-based authority, what is the reason that "replication" is considered more definitive than "statistical significance"?
2. Why does the chapter emphasize the importance of focusing on the methods

section rather than the discussion section when trying to understand the findings reported in the results section of a paper?

3. In a research study, what is the value of developing careful controls such as "randomization" and "control groups"? How do these various strategies help to improve the validity of the study?
4. In performing a search of the dental public health literature, what are the three major categories of information resources? Which category retrieves the most information? Why?
5. What is a "Boolean" search, and how is it used to construct a typical search strategy?
6. How does one retrieve information from online governmental agencies that do not provide "search" options?

REFERENCES

1. Institute of Medicine: *Dental education at the crossroads: challenges and changes,* Washington, DC, 1995, National Academy Press.
2. Bader J, Ismail A, Clarkson J: Evidence-based dentistry and the dental research community, *J Dent Res* 78(9):1480-1483, 1999.
3. Niessen LW, Grijseels EW, Rutten FF: The evidence-based approach in health policy and health care delivery, *Soc Sci Med* 51(6):859, 2000.
4. Marinho VCC, Richards D, Niederman R: Variation, certainty, evidence, and change in dental education: employing evidence-based dentistry in dental education, *J Dent Educ* 65(5):449-455, 2001.
5. Sackett D, Cook D: Can we learn anything from small trials? *Ann N Y Acad Sci* 703:25, 1993.
6. Iyengar S: Much ado about meta-analysis, *Chance* 4(1):33-40, 1991.
7. Winfred A Jr, Bennett W Jr, Huffcutt A: *Conducting meta-analysis using SAS,* Muhwah, NJ, 2001, Lawrence Erlbaum Assoc.
8. Sackett D et al: *Evidence-based medicine: how to practice and teach EBM,* ed 2, New York, 2000, Churchill Livingstone.
9. Kuhn T: *The structure of scientific revolutions,* ed 2, Chicago, 1970, University of Chicago.
10. Atchison K: Understanding and utilizing qualitative research, *J Dent Educ* 60(8):716, 1996.
11. Oral Health Surveys of the National Institute of Dental Research: *Diagnostic criteria and procedures,* Bethesda, MD, 1991, US Department of Health and Human Services, National Institutes of Health.
12. Sutherland S: Evidence-based dentistry: part I. Getting started, *J Can Dent Assoc* 67(4):204, 2001.
13. Ball C et al: Levels of evidence and grades of recommendations, *J Evidence-Based Dent Pract* 1(1):4A-5A, July 2000.
14. Friede A, Blum H, McDonald M: Public health informatics: how information-age technology can strengthen public health, *Annu Rev Public Health* 16:239, 1995.
15. Fourth International Conference on Grey Literature, GL '99. Grey Literature Network Service. Washington, DC, October 4-5, 1999.
16. Alberani V, Pietrangeli PDC, Mazza AMR: The use of grey literature in health sciences: a preliminary survey, *Bull Med Libr Assoc* 78(4):358, 1990.

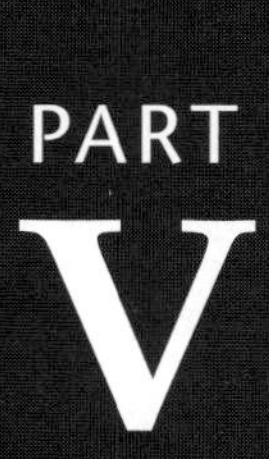

PART V

ETHICS AND THE LAW IN COMMUNITY DENTAL HEALTH

CHAPTER

16

ETHICAL ISSUES IN COMMUNITY DENTAL HEALTH

Muriel J. Bebeau • Jeffrey P. Kahn

WHAT DOES IT MEAN TO BECOME A PROFESSIONAL?

Have you been chosen by members of the dental or dental hygiene profession to become a dental professional? If so, those in the profession are telling you that they want to give you the opportunity to become their colleague. Have you thought about what it means to become a member of the dental profession? Are you aware of what distinguishes a dentist or dental hygienist from persons in other occupations or professions? Do you know what is expected of you as a student of the profession and as a future professional?

This chapter begins by describing the attributes of a profession and the implications for persons who wish to become a member of the dental profession. We describe the general moral obligations of the dental professional and then turn our attention to ethical issues that arise in community dental health. We briefly discuss the principles of biomedical ethics that apply to cases that arise in community dental health before presenting some cases to think about. We suggest that you read and discuss the cases with others before you read our analyses of them. Our hope is that this chapter will help you think more clearly about some of the problems that you are likely to encounter in your professional life. In particular, we hope this chapter will help you to think more clearly about responsibilities that extend beyond those you have to the individuals you will serve—responsibilities to the larger society. We hasten to add that we do not envision a set of professional responsibilities that are limitless. Rather, we hope to engage you in examining the nature of responsibility to others, to engage you in thinking about the limits of obligation, and to help you consider strategies that will effectively meet the profession's responsibilities to prevent disease and promote the nation's oral health.

CHARACTERISTICS OF A PROFESSION

What distinguishes a profession from some other occupation? Do certain characteristics distinguish among occupations in ways that suggest that some are held to a higher ethical standard than others? Sociologists list as many as six attributes that emerge as an occupation becomes professionalized.[1] Briefly, an occupation is given authority (i.e., to make judgments on behalf of clients or patients, to determine the standards of practice, to set standards for admission to professional school and standards for accreditation of professional schools, to self-govern, etc.) in proportion to the amount and stability of the knowledge it takes to gain access to the profession and in direct proportion to the amount of harm potentially caused by incompetent practice. Power and privilege are awarded in exchange for the profession's promise to place the rights of the client over self-interest and the rights of the society over the rights of the profession. To guide members of the profession in application of the promise, codes of ethics are developed. The canons of a code provide guidance to appropriate behavior in various circumstances and enable the profession to monitor itself. Codes are expanded as new issues emerge or as views of professional morality change. Professions value the powers and privileges granted by society and, through social organization, strive to maintain them.

Professions emerge over time, usually as a result of scientific advancement. Dentistry, for example, emerged and became more formalized in direct response to social conditions and scientific advances. In the mid-1800s some dentists made overstated claims about the benefits of treatment. The efforts to organize dentistry were based on a desire to protect the public from unscrupulous practitioners whose practices were not based on the latest scientific knowledge. The prohibitions against advertising—traced to codes of ethics developed by barristers in medieval England—were a direct effort on the part of the profession to control outrageous advertising practices and thereby make the profession more trustworthy.

The professionalization process has positive and negative outcomes. Let's consider what might be referred to as the paradox of professionalism in contemporary society. On the one hand, professionalization and organization enable standard setting that protects the public—a positive outcome. On the other hand, professionalization creates a kind of monopoly that tends to increase costs and reduce access to care—a negative outcome. The challenge for any profession is to maintain a balance between these positive and negative outcomes. Failure to do so undermines public trust in the profession's commitment—to place the interests of society above self-interest—and reduces society's interest in helping the profession maintain the powers and privileges granted.

Implications for the Professional

By considering the attributes that distinguish each occupation or profession, we notice that dentistry possesses each of the essential attributes. Society has conferred powers and privileges on dentistry commensurate with the level of power and privilege reserved for the most highly professionalized occupations (e.g., law and medicine), thereby implying that society views the provision of dental care as essential for its health and welfare.

The possession of essential attributes implies that persons who wish to become members of the profession have the following responsibilities: (1) to acquire the knowledge of the profession to the standards set by the profession; (2) to keep abreast of changing knowledge through continuing education; (3) to make a commitment to the basic ethic of the profession—that is, to place the oral health interests of the patient above the interests of the professional and to place the oral health interests of society above the interests of the profession; (4) to abide by the profession's code of ethics or work to change it if it is inconsistent with the underlying ethic of the profession; (5) to serve society (i.e., the public as a whole); and (6) to participate in the monitoring and self-regulation of the profession.

Power and privileges are granted to the profession on the basis of the assumption that each professional will take these responsibilities or obligations seriously. The profession has a right to expect that each individual who is chosen and then decides to become a dental professional will commit to these responsibilities.

Fulfilling these responsibilities is easier said than done. Professionals often find themselves in situations where personal and professional values conflict or where their professional obligations conflict. Many of the common conflicts are addressed in the American Dental Association's Principles of Ethics and Code of Professional Conduct. The field of dental ethics attempts to prepare professionals to recognize, reason about, and effectively resolve the common dilemmas of the profession. In particular, dental professionals need to develop skills in ethical reflection that enable them to make good decisions about new problems that are likely to emerge during the course of professional life. Although membership in professional organizations is not legally required, no person can participate in monitoring and regulating the profession or influence the direction the profession takes by standing on the sidelines.

Because this book is devoted to issues of community dental health, this chapter focuses specifically on the obligations of the profession and the professional to serve society. Individual dentists meet that responsibility through service to the individual patient, to the patient's family, to the community, and to the profession. The profession collectively meets that responsibility through a variety of efforts aimed at preventing disease and promoting the nation's oral health.* We not only advocate for obligations that go beyond the obligation to the individual patient, but also point out the limits of professional obligation. We are not advocating that dental professionals engage in the kind of selfless commitment to others that characterizes individuals such as Mother Teresa, but neither are we advocating that it is acceptable to exhibit the all-engrossing commitment to self exhibited by some of the more notorious examples of our time, such as inside-trader Ivan Boesky (who infamously asserted that "greed is good"). We are advocating that the dental professional has obligations to others that are somewhere on a continuum that has individuals like Mother Teresa on one end and those like Ivan Boesky on the other.

PRINCIPLES OF BIOETHICS

One way to think about the ethical obligations of dental professionals is through a popular approach focusing on three basic principles. In this approach, moral action guides are identified on the basis of duties or responsibilities to (1) show respect for persons; (2) avoid causing harm, prevent harm, remove harm, or provide benefit; and (3) act justly. These three bases for the duties are often referred to as the three principles of bioethics and are sometimes called the principle-based approach, or principlism. The principles of beneficence (including nonmaleficence) and justice were first

*For a more extensive discussion of the public duties of the professions, see Jennings B, Callahan D, Wolf SM: The public duties of the professions, *Hastings Center Report Special Supplement*, p 2, Feb 1995.

enunciated by Frankena[2] and popularized through their application to health care by Beauchamp and Childress.[3]

The distinctions among the duties to avoid harm, prevent harm, remove harm, and provide benefit are important, even though the duties may all be seen to arise out of the principle of beneficence. Frankena[2] holds that duties to avoid and prevent harm are stronger or more basic than duties to remove harm or provide benefit. These are crucial distinctions for dental health professionals, suggesting that the first duty is to avoid injuring someone through malice or incompetence. After that, the duty to prevent dental disease would be stronger than the duty to help someone who has the disease, and the duty to remove the disease would be stronger than the duty to restore oral health. In fact, some do not consider restoring oral health as a duty, but rather the discretionary act of a virtuous professional.

The principle of respect for persons is based on the contention that individuals ought to be free to determine what will happen to their bodies. In the health care setting, this principle is the basis for the practice of informed consent, by which patients are given sufficient information to make an informed decision about whether to accept a proposed treatment—and the decision itself must be well considered and voluntary. Dentists are likely to consider this principle often as they consider patient requests for particular treatments and offer patients advice and options. The principle of justice questions what kinds of treatment to provide and for which patients treatment should be provided when resources (time, effort, and budgets) are limited. The principle of justice directs us to allocate or distribute resources in ways that are fair.

These principles should not be viewed as absolute, but rather as important principles to respect and follow in making decisions about ethical issues. For example, how should a dental professional respond to a patient who requests that all his or her teeth be extracted because it would save having to brush them every day? The dental professional ought to consider the request in light of the duty to respect the decision of the patient, drawn from the principle of respect for persons, while at the same time honoring the commitment to avoid causing harm and doing what is in the best interest of the patient (doing good). This example illustrates the potential and frequent conflict between important principles. How are we to resolve these conflicts, which are what make the consideration of ethical issues both interesting and difficult? One way to resolve a conflict between principles is to ask whether any particular principle is stronger than the others at issue. In the aforementioned example, we might ask whether the principle directing us to respect a patient's request is more important (or stronger) than the principle directing us not to cause harm. A long history of protecting the right of individuals to make decisions for themselves may lead us to conclude that respect for persons takes precedent over all other ethical principles, but let's look a bit further at the example. Before respecting the decision of a patient, we must be sure that the patient fully understands, and intends to make, the decision. Another way of saying this is that the dental professional must be sure that a patient has the mental capacity to make health care decisions.* Once the dental professional determines that the patient is making a real, or autonomous, decision, a true conflict between principles exists. It is important to assess ethical situations in this way so that the ethical issues surrounding a

*For a discussion of strategies for assessing cognitive capacity and achieving consent for treatment, see Shuman SK, Bebeau MJ: Ethical and legal issues in special patient care, *Dent Clin North Am* 38(3):553, 1994.

case are addressed, rather than disagreement about the facts or other aspects of the case.

The dental professional appears to have two options in the example we have been discussing: respect the patient's decision and extract the teeth as requested or refuse to extract the teeth on the basis that the harm caused by respecting the patient's decision, even if it is autonomous, is too great. These kinds of conflicts are the source of debates about the so-called paternalistic model of the health care provider, in which the professional effectively overrides the autonomous decision of patients on the basis of a claim to superior knowledge of what is best for patients, regardless of whether the patient agrees. Such paternalism has been roundly attacked and is almost universally discredited. Nevertheless, it would be a paternalistic decision that many would support if the dental professional decided to override the autonomous decision of the patient to have all the teeth extracted. A way out may be to inform the patient that you respect his or her right of choice, but cannot violate your professional obligation to avoid actions that are harmful.

The third principle mentioned previously (i.e., the principle of justice) comes into play most frequently in considerations of allocating scarce resources, such as choosing which patients to treat when there is a shortage of dental services or dental care providers. Fair treatment is often the stated goal when such choices must be made, and reference to the principle of justice helps us decide what is fair. *Fairness* is another term for *justice,* and it can mean anything from equal treatment (the same for all) to equitable treatment (unequal but fair distribution). The principle of justice helps us to determine what method of distribution is most equitable. Methods can include distribution that is equal or based on need, merit, ability to pay, or a host of other factors. Justice requires that the method of distribution be justified and applied consistently. With these three principles, outlined here in general terms, ethical issues in dental care can be more effectively understood, examined, and, we hope, resolved. The case study analyses that follow attempt to apply these principles to real-life dental practice and the ethical issues that may arise in them.

Text continued on p. 444

CASES AND CASE ANALYSES

CASE 1

The Jeremy Lee Case

Jeremy Lee is a 33-year-old African-American man. He suffers from a heart valve disease and had an aortic valve inserted 7 years ago. Since surgery, he has been receiving antibiotic therapy intermittently for infections. He has also been taking the anticoagulant warfarin to prevent clotting of the blood. This medication is necessary to prevent clots from forming and traveling through the blood-stream to distant organs. As a result of clots that lodged in small vessels of the brain, Jeremy has had several strokes. However, to date, the strokes have not caused any substantial deficit in his neurologic abilities. In part, his difficulties are related to his failure to consistently take his medications. He has been a Medicaid recipient from time to time, is currently unemployed, and is again on Medicaid.

Continued

CASE 1

The Jeremy Lee Case—cont'd

Jeremy has five or six badly broken and neglected teeth remaining in the maxilla and about 12 teeth in the mandible. At least seven anterior teeth in the mandible are in good condition, in that they have no caries and no mobility. The gingiva is inflamed, but there is no pocketing more than 3 mm. There is some calculus, but a routine prophylaxis could improve the tissue. Jeremy has been given oral hygiene instruction but, according to the record, has shown no interest in improving his hygiene.

Because of his medical problems, Jeremy needs to be hospitalized to have his teeth removed. His health care team has to stop the warfarin, switch to heparin (which can only be given intravenously), and perform surgery under general anesthesia. After surgery, intravenous antibiotics must be continued for 48 hours and the warfarin resumed and monitored until appropriate levels are reached. The procedure requires five days of hospitalization, services of an oral surgeon (who will extract the teeth, contour the ridges, and prepare the tissues for a denture) and an anesthesiologist for 1.5 hours, recovery time, and other services, all at a cost of approximately $4,800.

Restoration of the teeth is out of the question because it would be costly and is not covered by Medicaid. As the oral surgeon, you need to decide whether to challenge the referring dentist's decision to remove all the teeth in the mandible. Perhaps you should advocate leaving the seven sound teeth. Normally, this would be preferable because wearing a full lower denture is difficult. In a person as young as Jeremy, after many years of wearing a denture resorption would occur, making it increasingly more difficult to achieve a good fit. However, if Jeremy does not change his oral hygiene habits, a partial denture could accelerate the loss of the remaining teeth. Also, any infection could further complicate his health problems, and the teeth might need to be extracted at a later date, requiring hospitalization and further expense. If Jeremy is still on Medicaid, the added expense will be borne by society. On the other hand, the experience of wearing an upper denture might influence him to change his ways to avoid having a lower denture as well.

Should you remove all the teeth? Why or why not? What reasons would you give to support your position?

ANALYSIS

Professional-Patient Issues

This dilemma raises questions about the rights of patients who are unable to pay for their own care and must rely on public assistance. Should such patients have the same rights—to be informed of alternatives, to choose the preferred treatment, or to refuse treatment—as patients who are able to pay for the treatment? Should the oral surgeon, in deciding what to do, consider the fact that Jeremy Lee seems to have difficulty complying with the directives of his health care providers? In this case, no information is provided about the patient's involvement in the treatment decision. Should we presume that the referring dentist achieved consent for the proposed treatment? The oral surgeon has a referral for extraction of all the teeth. Should the oral surgeon follow the directive of the referring dentist or overrule that decision and make a judgment as to the best interest of the patient? Although we might argue that the referring dentist should be consulted to determine whether the patient participated in the decision, it is interesting to explore whether to remove all the teeth, given the circumstances in this case.

One factor to consider is the limitations placed on Jeremy's autonomy by his lack of financial resources. As a medical assistance recipient in most states, Jeremy is provided with relief from pain, swelling, and infection, but restorative services are usually limited. For example, he may be entitled to new dentures every 5 years. Or, if the dentist decides to leave the seven sound teeth, Jeremy would be eligible for a partial denture, but more functional and esthetic restorations (e.g., crowns and bridges) typically are not covered.

Although we might argue that many people would be likely to change their health care habits after receiving an upper denture, Jeremy has a history of noncompliance, at least as it relates to his general health. Failure to take his medications has life-threatening consequences. He has experienced these consequences without improving his compliance. Although there may be important questions as to whether Jeremy understands the consequences of his actions and is making an informed decision when he fails to comply, the surgeon

CASE 1

The Jeremy Lee Case—cont'd

cannot ignore his past noncompliant behavior because it is the single best predictor of his future actions. It is important to consider the range of possible reasons for lack of compliance: (1) the patient simply lacks understanding of the consequences, in which case additional education may be effective; (2) the patient lacks understanding of the consequences and has cognitive deficiencies or beliefs that make education difficult, in which case he may need a guardian or supervision if the provider cannot achieve comprehension; or (3) the patient may be consciously or unconsciously engaging in self-destructive behaviors because of depression, mental illness, or chemical dependency. In such cases, mental health interventions are needed.

People usually do not make major changes in health habits and behaviors. The oral surgeon needs to consider prior behavior in assessment of this case, especially in view of the patient's serious medical problems.

Profession-Society/Community Issues

Conflict of Duties. One thing that makes this dilemma so difficult is that dentistry has become much more focused on preservation of tooth structure and on restoration of function, rather than on extraction of teeth. The incredible decreases in dental disease we have witnessed in the last 20 to 30 years are responsible for this change of focus.* But this has turned the focus from the prevention or removal of harm to the provision of benefit as the preeminent value of the profession. The idea that removing seven sound teeth in this case might be in the patient's best interest, given his health habits and the significant health risks associated with a second surgery, seems to fly in the face of the profession's emphasis on restoration of function and the idea that removing healthy teeth is in and of itself harmful.

In this case, it seems the surgeon would actually be "doing harm" to "prevent harm" that may come about if the teeth and surrounding tissue were left to fall victim to disease that is likely to result from the patient's continued habits.

A second conflict of duties arises between the surgeon's obligation to serve as an advocate of Jeremy's interests and his obligation to the rest of society (e.g., not to spend a disproportionate amount of public money on this patient). Many situations involving public funds are predetermined. This is one situation where the dentist may be able to argue that the patient's seven sound teeth have resisted decay and disease in the face of Jeremy's health habits and are therefore less likely to become diseased in the future.

Rights of Jeremy versus the Rights of Society. Some practitioners take the view that health care is a privilege rather than a basic right. They may believe that Jeremy should not be given any care that he cannot pay for. Other practitioners may take the view that there should be no discrimination on the basis of ability to pay and that the same benefits should be available to all irrespective of ability to pay. Such differences in views are often grounded in deeply held convictions. Rather than arguing which is the "right" view, it may be helpful to explore the beliefs that are at the root of these conflicting ideas. Many of us have been socialized to believe that anyone could take care of himself or herself, if only he or she would put forth the effort to do so. Even though we may recognize that such a view is only partially true, such ideas are rooted in concepts of individualism and the puritan ethic, values that underlie much of American history and culture.* Irrespective of personal perspective, American society currently provides basic care for those who are poor and disadvantaged, but the benefits provided do not represent optimal oral health.

Rights to Oral Health Care versus Rights to Medical Care. Medicaid programs often do not cover any adult dental care or are restricted to emergency services. Sometimes episodic procedures for relief of pain and infection are provided, but generally dental care is viewed as elective, rather

*The exception to this trend may be the recent prevalence of disease associated with excessive consumption of soft drinks. See Erickson PR et al: Soft drinks: hard on teeth, *Northwest Dent* 80(2):15, 2001.

*For a discussion of the origin of societal views about the right to health care, see Burt BA, Eklund SA: Ethics and responsibility in dental care. In *Dentistry, dental practice, and the community,* Philadelphia, 1999, WB Saunders.

Continued

CASE 1

The Jeremy Lee Case—cont'd

than as an integral part of an individual's overall primary health care. For example, before the implementation of the Oregon Health Plan in 1994, a patient could have a benign mole removed from the neck, but could not have decayed teeth restored.[4] When the Oregon Health Plan created a state-approved list of medical and dental health services by an open public process, many dental services previously excluded from the Medicaid list of benefits were suddenly included.* "Oregon now has one of the most generous dental Medicaid benefit packages in the country, including coverage for services such as endodontic treatment, scaling and root planing, along with basic preventive, restorative and prosthodontic services. Cast crowns and bridges are included with limitation. Further, over 100,000 individuals not previously covered by Medicaid were brought into the plan and provided dental coverage."[4] From the perspective of increasing access to dental care, the profession may want to reconsider the wisdom of advocating for the separation of medical and dental benefits.

Rights of Jeremy versus Other Medicaid Patients. Although we may be tempted to raise larger questions about the overall prioritization of medical and dental health benefits when society sets aside limited funding for care to the poor and disadvantaged, questions arise about the distribution of those scarce resources. For example, is it fair to use a disproportionate amount of public money on one person, if so doing diminishes the resources available to others? The following cases discuss this issue in greater detail.

*To review the Prioritized List of Medical and Dental Benefits, or the process by which the prioritized list was determined, visit the website of the Oregon Health Services Commission at www.ohppr.state.or.us.

CASE 2

The Dr. Lester Case

Dr. Jim Lester has a suburban practice that suits him fine. He lives in a Midwestern community consisting of a city of 60,000 with surrounding suburbs of approximately 40,000. He works 5 days a week for 40 hours and has time for his family and his current passion, creating a bird sanctuary outside town. His hobby is environmental protection, and he and his wife are active members of the local Sierra Club.

Dr. Lester's community has been hit hard by the economy. Two years ago, two manufacturing plants laid off large numbers of workers. Efforts have been made to attract new businesses, and many workers have stayed in the community hoping some new opportunities will develop. Many are still drawing unemployment, but medical and dental benefits expired some time ago. Several dentists have started a program through the local dental society to contribute time—mostly nights and weekends—at a downtown clinic to provide emergency and preventive care. They ask Dr. Lester to join. He refuses. He points out that he is already contributing to the community through the Sierra Club, that he feels personally fulfilled through his current practice, and that his personal goal has never been to become that involved in organized dentistry. He does a good job with suburban children and that is his interest. He has always believed that he is the kind of person who does better with a wider range of commitments.

"But, Jim," his friend Dr. Al Felding argues, "your lack of professional involvement means the rest of us have to contribute more, and lack of cooperation for this project makes us look bad at the state meetings. You're the third suburban dentist to turn me down this week."

"Look, Al," Jim counters, "you chose to do this. I'm not proselytizing you to become a member of

CASE 2

The Dr. Lester Case—cont'd

the Sierra Club. To each his own. You're fulfilling your mission in life. I'm just choosing a different track for my extracurricular activities. Come off it, will you?"

Should Dr. Lester volunteer to help? Why or why not? What reasons would you give to support your position? As you reflect on the reasons, consider reasons of self-interest for participating (or not) and reasons derived from the moral principles that might apply in this case.

ANALYSIS

This dilemma raises questions about the limits of professional obligation. Dr. Lester is already serving his community by performing dental services in his private practice 40 hours per week. He is also contributing to society through activities he enjoys—work with the Sierra Club. He does have obligations not to work so much that he is too "burned out" to give adequate time and attention to himself, his dental staff, his patients, and his family. Further, he has a responsibility to maintain a viable practice, because if he does not, he cannot serve anyone. Dr. Lester has a right to make a living, perhaps even a very good living, as long as he does not compromise his patients' right to competent care in the process. Balancing responsibilities to patients, staff, self, and family is challenging enough. But does Dr. Lester, as a health professional, also have dental responsibilities to the larger community and to the profession regardless of his activities and commitments to the environment?

Professional-Patient Issues

What if a patient tells Dr. Lester that he cannot keep his and his family's regular dental appointments because he is out of work? Does Dr. Lester have any different obligations to patients experiencing economic hardship than he has to the community and the dental profession? We can argue that he does indeed, on the basis of the relationship he has with his patients, his obligation to provide dental care, and the relative importance of those obligations to current patients compared with the community at large. Dr. Lester might argue that he has no extra time to provide free care to community members in urgent need of care because he is trying to meet demands of patients in his practice for elective or nonemergency care. We ought to then argue that Dr. Lester has an obligation to postpone some of his patients' elective work to assist his colleagues in meeting the more urgent needs of the community.

Profession-Society/Community Issues

Apparently, the local dental society is responding to an obvious need—to provide emergency and preventive dental services to members of the community whose access to care is limited by economic misfortune. Note that the dentists are providing the kind of services that meet basic needs, care that, according to one of the principles described previously, might be classified as "preventing evil or harm" or "removing evil (disease) or harm," rather than care that would "do or promote good." In this case, the local dental society and the dentists cooperating with Dr. Felding have decided to provide the kinds of care gratis that the families would be entitled to if they were eligible for medical assistance. Is the local dental society obligated to take on this responsibility, and is Dr. Lester obligated to help?

Let's take the obligation of the local dental society first. It could be argued that the obligation for emergency and preventive care rests with the community's citizens and taxpayers, rather than with the local dental society, and that dentists are responsible only to the extent that they have responsibilities as taxpayers and citizens. On the other hand, dentists are not ordinary citizens. Although all citizens are entitled to a basic education, only those with special ability are granted access to professional education. Dentists have special status in a society based on special knowledge gained through education that is subsidized, in some instances heavily subsidized, by tax dollars.*

*Despite recent increases in tuition and clinic income, in 1998 revenue from tuition and fees and clinic income covered only 36% of dental school expenditures per DDS (a weighted sum of student enrollment developed by the American Dental Association). The remainder of expenditures (64%) were met through federal, state, and local support, as well as endowments, gifts, and alumni support. See p. 558, Valachovic RW et al: Trends in dentistry and dental education, *J Dent Educ* 65(6):539, 2001.

Continued

CASE 2

The Dr. Lester Case—cont'd

On the basis of its specialized knowledge and the power given to the profession, it would seem the profession has specific responsibilities (e.g., to advise about the efficacy of public health programs, to participate in the development of public assistance dental programs, and to engage in other activities that promote the oral health of the public). Beyond that, does the profession have a moral duty to provide free dental services to those who have no access to care? After considering these issues, the dental society decided to take on this project.

It could be argued that Dr. Lester, as part of the professional society, has a responsibility to his peers to support the group's decision in some way. The burden for those who have volunteered would be less and the number of affected families would be greater if each dentist in the community and surrounding areas participated in the group's access program. But if we cannot argue that it is obligatory for Dr. Lester to help his colleagues, are there other compelling reasons to do so?

Is it in Dr. Lester's interest to help out in his community? When there is a downturn in the economy, dentists are likely to be among the first to notice. People tend to view dental care as expendable or as a need that can be postponed. The economic downturn seems not to have affected Dr. Lester's suburban practice—at least not yet—but the interdependence of business and service in most communities suggests that unless the community works together to attract other sources of employment for laid-off workers, there may be far-reaching consequences. Suburban residents may not feel the economic pinch as quickly as those who have lost their jobs, but in time the effects may reach Dr. Lester's dental practice.

Aside from the potential, and possibly eventual, negative consequences to the economic health of Dr. Lester's dental practice, he might also think about the positive consequences of helping his community and his colleagues in time of need. The most important asset any dentist has is his or her personal and professional reputation. Volunteering to help people in the downtown area in a time of need is likely to enhance his reputation in the community; conversely, failure to participate could have negative consequences. Further, if compromising time with his family is a significant issue for Dr. Lester, he might consider ways to involve his family in the volunteer activity, thereby teaching his children important lessons about community and social responsibilities. Perhaps his wife and children could accompany him to the clinic on the night he works. Family members may be able to assist him, even if it is something as simple as visiting with people who are waiting to receive care or caring for children while their parents receive care.

CASE 3

The Managed Care Medicaid Proposal

As the dental director for the health department in your state, you have been working for some time to improve access to dental care for your medical assistance population. (Dental directors typically have a master's degree in public health, in addition to a degree in dentistry or dental hygiene.) Few dentists have signed up to participate in the program because of the low rate of reimbursement for dental benefits. Thus many Medicaid-eligible individuals have been unable to gain access to care. Further, as a result of the general economic problems the state faces, the legislature has been unwilling to raise the rate of reimbursement.

In fact, because of a recent budgetary shortfall, your state's Medicaid program dropped all dental coverage for adults, including emergency care, to maintain coverage for children through age 18. When you complain to the state commissioner of

CASE 3

The Managed Care Medicaid Proposal—cont'd

health, she points out that if you save money in the dental program for children, you may at least be able to restore emergency care for Medicaid-eligible adults. She suggests that you contact Medicaid Dent-Tell, a benefit company that has been providing a managed care plan for a state on the East Coast.

You learn the following: Medicaid Dent-Tell (a fictitious for-profit dental benefit company) contracted with an eastern state to provide school-based dental benefits to Medicaid-eligible children. The state reimbursed at a capitation rate of $4.50 per child per month. Medicaid Dent-Tell enrolled all Medicaid-eligible students in the public schools and hired dentists to go into the schools and do screening examinations and prophylaxis. Fluoride treatments were not routinely provided. Dentists stated that the portable equipment provided was inferior, because it did not have adequate suction equipment to prevent excessive swallowing and nausea. On the basis of the screening, notices were sent home to the parents of children who needed care and followed up with a second notice if parents failed to respond. The notices gave the name and address of the participating dentist closest to the family's residence, included information about the child's needs, and indicated which of the needed services would be covered under the plan. Medicaid Dent-Tell claims that the program is highly successful, that Dent-Tell has had little difficulty recruiting dentists to participate, and that Dent-Tell has effectively solved the access problems for the state.

The representative of Medicaid Dent-Tell indicates that the company is interested in expanding to other states. You realize that under such a plan you could provide care for the Medicaid-eligible children and still have money for adult services.

Would you support this plan? Why or why not?

ANALYSIS

This case points out the conflicts that may arise when dental care resources are limited, as they often are, and choices must be made between providing less-than-optimal care versus no care at all. The Medicaid-eligible population is by definition needy, so cost for dental (and medical) treatment is covered by the state. A continuing issue for those charged with managing Medicaid services is the justice-based question of how to divide a pie of limited size between competing services and among those eligible for coverage. As your state's dental director, you are charged with balancing the provision of all needed dental services to all eligible for coverage against the limited resources you have at your disposal.

Should you provide all needed dental care for children and use whatever remains for the elderly, do the opposite, or provide limited services to both populations? What level of limited service is acceptable? Also, what questions should you ask about the plan? For instance, you know how many individuals you need to cover. What percentage of the eastern state's children received care? If a fairly large number of dentists signed up, how many of the plan's patients were seen and what treatments were provided? At the end of the year, how much did the state pay the plan? How much did the plan pay the dentists? How many patients received treatment? In reality, the director probably will not get answers to these questions, but you should ask them.

The Professional-Patient Relationship

Professionals have duties both to prevent or remove harm and to provide benefit to their patients. By choosing the Medicaid Dent-Tell option, you have the opportunity to identify children in need of dental care and to inform their parents about the need to seek care and how to do so. This is the first part of fulfilling the obligations to remove harm and provide benefit, but it does not go far enough from an ethical standpoint. To identify needed services, without either providing them or offering a means to do so, falls short of the obligation to remove harm (treat disease). It also does not provide the full benefit at your disposal to your patients. But failing to opt for this approach will mean no services at all for the eligible elderly in your state, which would be a failure to live up to your ethical obligations to them.

More important is the obligation to design a plan that enables the population to get the needed care. This plan fails to take into account, or perhaps exploits, the shortcomings of the population it

Continued

CASE 3

The Managed Care Medicaid Proposal—cont'd

is intended to serve. Parents of economically and socially disadvantaged populations are highly unlikely to take advantage of a plan that requires them to (1) receive and understand the letter sent to them and (2) have the means and perseverance to make the necessary appointment, travel to the office, and perhaps pay some portion of the services not covered by the plan. Although the plan is "successful" in using resources and recruiting dentists, it is unlikely that patients will actually access needed services. Given that no care is provided, not even fluoride treatments, the dental director must ask whether this is an acceptable and responsible use of resources, even if it covers all eligible children.

The Professional-Society Relationship

As the state's dental director, your role-related obligations extend to the community (or society), in addition to whatever obligations you might have toward individual patients. Your title and job duties place you in a position that requires you to consider the good of the community, possibly even before the good of individual patients. Public policy decisions about the allocation of scarce resources generally rely on utilitarian calculations about what will yield the greatest proportion of benefit over harm for a particular community. In this case, the communities to be considered, in the order of their priority, are (1) the population eligible for state-supported dental services and (2) the state's population as a whole. The question you must answer as the state dental services director is whether it is better to provide some level of dental services to all eligible or to provide needed services to one subset of the eligible population at the exclusion of the rest of those eligible. If you cannot provide all needed services to everybody eligible, as is the case here and in most other states, what level of service would be minimally acceptable as a matter of ethical dental practice?

The Profession-Society Relationship

As is the case with any profession, dentistry has moral duties to the society in which its members practice. Those duties include meeting acceptable standards for the provision of dental services, not discriminating against particular groups of patients, and acting in ways that advance the oral health of the public. When faced with the problem of limited resources demonstrated by this case, what does the relationship between the dental profession and society tell us the state dental director ought to do? If you choose the Dent-Tell option, you need to enlist the services of sufficient numbers of dentists to provide the services involved. You may argue that your colleagues have some obligation to participate in programs that benefit those in need. But simple participation of dentists is not sufficient to satisfy the profession's obligations to society. Dentists must also live up to the standards of practice set by them as a profession. In this particular case, you must weigh whether the provision of limited treatments that are required by the state as part of the Dent-Tell program meets the standards of dental practice required by the profession of its members. In particular, you must weigh whether dental examination without further treatment and prophylaxis without fluoride treatments are acceptable as a matter of dental practice. If the choice is between offering this reduced level of dental services versus none at all, what is the ethically acceptable choice? Greater services for children could only be provided at the cost of denying all dental services to eligible adults. Which population ought to win out, or is the most humanely acceptable action to provide some, albeit less than optimal, care for all? How would you best serve justice while respecting your obligations to prevent and remove harm and do good? Is it appropriate for you to try to recruit your dental colleagues to participate in plans that fail to meet professional standards of care?

CASE 4

The Triage Proposal

As the dental director for the health department in your state, you have been working for some time to improve access to dental care for your public assistance population. (Typically a dental director has a master's degree in public health, in addition to a degree in dentistry or dental hygiene.) Few dentists have signed up to participate in the program because of the low rate of reimbursement for dental treatment. Thus many Medicaid-eligible individuals have been unable to gain access to care. Further, as a result of the general economic problems the state faces, the legislature has been unwilling to raise the rate of reimbursement.

In fact, because of a recent budgetary shortfall, your state's Medicaid programs dropped all dental coverage for adults, including emergency care, to maintain coverage for children through age 18. When you complain to the state commissioner of health, she points out that if you save money in the dental program for children, you may at least be able to restore emergency care for Medicaid-eligible adults. She suggests you consider some school-based dental health programs that would reduce the overall cost of care and suggests you talk to Dr. Harry Reagan, who has been running a triage program in the inner-city schools of your state capital.

Dr. Reagan describes the program. He says, "There is no way we can address all the dental needs of Medicaid-eligible children in this city. We have decided to go into the schools with a triage approach. The dentist does a very quick screening to identify children who need more extensive treatment. These are identified for later treatment by a mobile unit that comes to the school within a week or two." Meanwhile, a team of hygienists does fluoride treatments (without prophylaxis) and then seals the teeth of all program-eligible children. The mobile unit is supported by private contributions and staffed by volunteer dentists and one public health dentist. The unit provides emergency care, diagnostic and some additional preventive services (i.e., prophylaxis and space maintainers, because of the high rate of extraction), and routine restorative care (mostly amalgams).

Dr. Reagan says the program is effective because it is prevention oriented and treats those with the greatest need. He points out that initially the program offered the fluoride treatments and sealants to all schoolchildren for a fee. Medicaid paid the fee for those who were Medicaid eligible. Parents, especially single parents and families with both parents working, liked the program because their children could get preventive care without having to take the children out of school and without their taking time off from work. Although the program was successful, it was so heavily criticized by the dental community that organizers decided to limit the program to children on Medicaid. Despite this adjustment, the dental community still claims that the program does not meet standards of dental care. Dentists object to applying sealants without a complete diagnostic assessment (including radiographs), they think prophylaxis should precede fluoride treatments, and so on.

Dr. Reagan thinks they have not pushed the issue because it applies to a limited population and because Medicaid reimbursements are so low that local dentists are just as happy to avoid treating this population. On the other hand, Dr. Reagan doubts that the program could be expanded on a statewide basis without encountering formidable opposition from the dental community.

Should you advocate a similar program? Why or why not? How should you address the dental community and its complaints?

ANALYSIS

Like case 3, this case points out the ethical issues presented when resources are limited. But unlike case 3, in which it is proposed that the same minimum level of services be provided to all, this case suggests a different approach to justice. As in other aspects of health care, limited resources force decisions about how to fairly allocate what is available.

The Professional-Patient Relationship

As the state's dental director, you have an obligation to serve the best dental interests of your patients, who include all those who may receive state-supported dental care. Because there is not enough money to pay for the necessary dental care for all eligible citizens who need it, you must decide how best to accommodate your duties of justice while

Continued

CASE 4

The Triage Proposal—cont'd

also respecting your duties to prevent and remove harm and to provide benefit toward patients. So, while you know that the program cannot provide optimal care to all eligible patients, you must decide whether you can purchase sufficiently acceptable care that meets the obligation to avoid or remove harm. The provision of examinations followed by emergency dental services to those who need them seeks to remove and prevent harm. The provision of only prophylaxis, fluoride treatment, and sealants to everyone else should be seen as only marginally serving their best interests. In a climate of severely constrained resources, however, this may be the best you can hope to achieve.

The Professional-Society Relationship

Triage, or the process of treating those in greatest need first, is a common way of allocating scarce resources. Emergency cases receive priority, and others are treated in the order of urgency until treatment resources run out. In dealing with community needs, the dental professional has a duty to provide the best care possible. Under circumstances of limited resources, this may mean allocating care after assessing patient needs and then providing treatment so that all patients are eventually brought to a maintenance level. In this case, that means treating emergency cases first and then providing the level of services possible to the remaining patients consistent with the remaining level of resources. Although this approach may not yield the optimal results from the perspective of each individual patient, the dentist must take the community's good into account.

The Profession-Society Relationship

Your colleagues in the profession rightly question whether a triage program adequately meets the needs of Medicaid patients. The profession has a duty to ensure that the dental care provided by its members meets the needs of patients (doing that which is safe and effective, prevents or removes harm, and provides benefit) and lives up to the standard set by the profession. This is especially true for state-supported and state-endorsed programs meant to serve the public health. A quick examination followed by fluoride treatment and sealants, without prophylaxis, does not meet these standards in many dentists' minds. Although most dentists would not give a fluoride treatment without a prophylaxis, it does not mean that the treatment will be ineffectual.[5]

The question that you and your dental colleagues must ask yourselves is whether such cursory care that covers all eligible patients is worse than providing more adequate care for some, at the expense of failing to provide any care to some proportion of this population. A more general question is why such limited resources are available for dental services. Should you and the dental society lobby the state for a larger budget for such services? Why should you be content with the current division of the budgetary pie?

CASE 5

The Margo Stinson Case

Margo Stinson has worked as a dental hygienist for a periodontist for the last 18 years. She likes her work because she is able to arrange her schedule to accommodate her growing family. Margo and her husband, Tom, live next door to Stanley Freedman, who is the personnel manager for a manufacturing plant that employs about 700 semiskilled workers. In addition to his responsibilities for personnel management, he also purchases the medical and dental health benefits for his company. Seven months ago, the company signed a 3-year contract for dental benefits that provided company employees with a

CASE 5

The Margo Stinson Case—cont'd

list of dentists who agreed to participate in the plan. The plan cost the company $18.00 per month per employee, provided diagnostic and preventive services (with a limit of two prophylaxes per year) free of charge, and required a 50% copayment for restorative services and a one-time $500 reimbursement for orthodontic care. The company had published brochures informing employees of the benefits and listing all participating plan dentists.

Lately, Stan had been getting complaints from supervisors about the plan. Employees were requesting to take a half day off work to go to the dentist, and others were complaining about the long delays to get appointments with plan dentists or the long drive to gain accessibility to plan dentists. During an evening visit with Margo and Tom, Stan mentioned his frustration with dentists in the community. He said he thought his company was paying plenty for the dental benefit package. He mentioned that when he asked the benefit company why they had not signed up dentists who were more accessible, the company blamed the dentists for engaging in a conspiracy to blackball their plan and control the costs of dental services. Margo was stunned by the direct attack on the dental profession. She wondered what her role and responsibility was with respect to the issues Stan raised.

Does Margo have a responsibility to Stan? .To the patients covered by the plan? To the profession? Why or why not? What could Margo do?

ANALYSIS

Margo is in a tough spot. If she responds defensively to an attack on the profession, she may miss an important opportunity to enable Stan to help the company's employees secure dental care that better meets their needs. How prepared is Margo to address the various questions raised by the situation Stan finds himself in? Is it Margo's responsibility, as a dental hygienist, to know enough about the financing of dental benefit plans or the ways plans are marketed to benefit managers such as Stan to be able to counsel Sam? Actually, unless Margo knows some basics about the distinctions between medical and dental health needs of the population and some basics about the various methods for reimbursement of dental services, she cannot meet basic responsibilities she has to patients, to the public, and to the profession.

What basic information does Margo need? First, she needs to be clear about the following characteristics of dental disease, some of which are markedly different from medical illness and disease[6]:

- Dental disease does not heal without therapeutic intervention, so early treatment is the most efficient and least costly intervention.
- The need for dental care is universal and continuing, rather than episodic.
- The need for dental care is highly predictable and does not have the characteristics of an insurable risk.
- Patient cooperation and posttreatment maintenance are critical to the success of dental treatment and the prevention of subsequent disease.

Understanding Third-Party Reimbursement

Next, to help Stan evaluate why his plan is not working, Margo needs to be aware of the basic strategies for reimbursing employees for dental care and the advantages and disadvantages of each.[7]

1. *Direct reimbursement (DR)* is a self-funded dental benefit plan that reimburses employees according to the dollar amount spent on dental care, without regard to the type of treatment received. This method allows the patients to go to the dentist of choice. The design of the DR plan is selected by the employer to fit the employer's budget and therefore can vary widely among companies. For example, a plan may reimburse 100% of the first $200 of dental expenses and 80% of the next $1,000, resulting in a total annual maximum benefit of $1,000 per covered individual. A DR plan may also permit employees to pay their share of their dental expenses on a before-tax basis by establishing "flex" accounts. Though this plan is not as widely used as other plans, it is the American Dental Association's (ADA's) preferred method of financing dental treatment, and the ADA, as well as state dental societies, can assist companies in implementing a DR plan, or in estimating how different plans will affect costs. According

Continued

CASE 5

The Margo Stinson Case—cont'd

to an ADA estimate, approximately 1.5 million people (1% of the insured population) are covered by a DR plan.[8]

2. An *indemnity plan* is a fully insured or self-insured plan in which an assigned payment is provided for specific services, regardless of the actual charges made by the provider. Payment may be made to the enrollees or, by assignment, directly to dentists. Indemnity plans usually allow patients to go to the dentist of their choice. However, they reimburse based on a "usual, customary, and reasonable" (UCR) system. Thus UCR plans pay an established percentage of the dentist's fee or the plan administrator's "reasonable" or "customary" fee limit, whichever is less. The limits are the result of a contract between the plan purchasers and the third-party payer. Although these limits are called "customary," they may or may not accurately reflect the fees that area dentists charge. Forty-three percent of the insured population has this kind of plan.[9]
3. *Preferred provider organization (PPO)* programs are plans under which patients select a dentist from a network or list of providers who have agreed, by contract, to discount their fees. In PPOs that allow patients to receive treatment from a nonparticipating dentist, patients who choose a nonparticipating dentist are usually required to pay higher deductibles and copayments. PPOs can be fully insured or self-insured. PPOs are usually less expensive than comparable indemnity plans and are regulated under the appropriate insurance statutes in the company's state of domicile and operation. Thirty-one percent of Americans covered by a payment plan participate in a PPO.[9]
4. *Dental health maintenance organization (DHMO)* plans, or capitation plans, pay contracted dentists a fixed amount (usually on a monthly basis) per enrolled family or individual, regardless of utilization. In return, the dentists agree to provide specific types of treatment to the patient. The patient may be required to pay a copayment. Theoretically, the DHMO models typically offer the least expensive dental plans. Eighteen percent of the insured population participates in a DHMO.[9]

To be fully informed, Margo also needs to be aware of other dental plan features that may be available to employees.

1. *Discount/referral options* are arrangements in which employers direct employees to a limited number of providers who have agreed to discount their normal fees in exchange for the expectation of a larger patient pool. There is no reimbursement to the patient or to the provider. A third-party marketer will package and sell a discount program for a fee, in order to cover costs and profits. Approximately 7.5% of the insured population participates in this type of plan.[9]
2. *Point-of-service options* are arrangements in which patients with a managed care dental plan have the option of seeking treatment from an "out-of-network" provider. The reimbursement to the patient is usually based on a low table of allowances, with significantly fewer benefits than those provided by an "in-network" provider.
3. *Table of allowances* (sometimes called *schedule of allowances*) indemnity programs determine a list of covered services with an assigned dollar amount. The dollar amount represents how much the plan will pay for those services that are covered. Most often, it does not represent the dentist's full charge for those services. The patient usually pays the difference.

Then, much as Margo would empower a patient to reflect on his or her choices with respect to the use of a dental benefits package, she will need to empower Stan to ask better questions and make better choices when purchasing dental benefits on behalf of the company's employees.

Employer Issues

Benefit purchasers such as Stan are probably sincere when they say they want to purchase dental and medical plans that benefit the employee not only in the short term, but also in the long term. The challenge Stan faces in selecting among competing plans is the challenge we all face. How do we buy the best plan for the least money? How do we sort through the options? How do we figure out which is the best plan and the best deal?

CASE 5

The Margo Stinson Case—cont'd

First, Stan needs a clear view of what employees need. Because, as outlined previously, dental needs are predictable and depend on personal health habits, timely care-seeking behavior, and occupational safety, employees need a plan that encourages prevention and early intervention. Employees may need to be "insured" only against accidental dental injury or catastrophic illness, which is typically covered under workers' compensation and medical plans.

If Stan purchases a plan that reimburses dentists for diagnosis, prevention, restorations, crowns, and other procedures at cut rates, he can save the company (and patients) money in the short run, but he may be promoting a disease model rather than a health model of dentistry, which is unlikely to promote oral health and will likely be much more expensive in the long run. Also, if Stan purchases a plan that requires employees to switch providers, he may actually increase the overall cost of care to the patient. For example, the new dentist will need to conduct a diagnostic assessment even if records are transferred, travel time may be increased, rapport will need to be developed, and so on. Further, if fees are heavily discounted, the dentist is often encouraged by the plan to give scheduling priority to fee-for-service patients and use the PPO patients to fill down time, which usually cuts more heavily into work schedules. Costs that accrue to Stan's company include (1) time lost from work by employees whose dental problems grow more serious and more costly, and may result in compromised general health if neglected; (2) increased dissatisfaction with the company when increased needs for care are not covered by insurance; and (3) decreased quality of life, which often influences job performance. Thus it is in the interest of the employer to design a plan that promotes access to care and avoids rationing by inconvenience, as the current plan appears to do. A plan that reimburses at rates that are near or below the actual cost of providing services interferes with access and quality because dentists are prompted (by the low reimbursement rates) to think of these patients as filler for their schedule. A plan that pays a capitated rate for dental services encourages undertreatment, whereas a plan that pays for services at the dentist's usual fee for services or requires minimal copayments encourages overutilization. The designer of a plan needs to consider a plan that emphasizes preventive care and regular checkups, that allows patients freedom to choose their dentists, and that is flexible enough for smart treatment planning between patient and dentist.

The Benefits of Dental Coverage

But why provide any kind of dental benefit? Why not simply let employees take care of their own dental needs out of pocket? Why incur any expense in administering dental benefit programs? Dental benefit plans have been effective because they tend to reduce patients' inhibition to seeking care and encourage employees to take advantage of preventive care. Plans that encourage preventive care and early intervention are particularly important for employees at the lower end of the socioeconomic scale. In general, the dental benefits industry has been an asset for employees and the dental profession because of its influence on utilization.

Another thing Margo must realize is that Stan may not be completely free to select a plan or plans (some states require that employees have choices) that he thinks is best. Employees, through their union leaders, may direct the benefit purchaser to ratchet down costs, and employees may think their employer is willing to switch providers to secure lower costs. Capilouto[10] notes that "individuals are willing to switch medical plans in the face of relatively small increases in premium price. Dental insured, if faced with similar price differential, should act similarly." As pointed out earlier, frequent changes in providers or delivery systems disrupts the continuity of care and leads to a duplication of services. If a company is faced with an economic downturn, cutting costs by interrupting continuity of care could be costly in the long run. Stan's company may be better off switching to a direct reimbursement plan to have more control not only of the cost of care, but of the proportion of premium dollar that is returned to the employee in terms of direct benefit.

Employee Issues

Once a benefit plan has been selected, Stan has an obligation to educate employees about their benefit plan. For most employees the task of comparing plans is tedious, and often the plan documents are

Continued

CASE 5

The Margo Stinson Case—cont'd

written in language that obscures the plan's limitations and restrictions. Stan needs to educate patients about the plan(s) in simple language that anyone can understand. He needs to be held accountable for the ratio of premiums paid to payments made. After all, the benefit he is purchasing is something the employee has earned—it is part of the employee's compensation package. Stan has a moral and a fiduciary responsibility to see that the benefit is a real benefit and not an opportunity for third-party payers to realize higher profits. It is easy to manipulate plan descriptions to make a lesser plan appear better. It is easy to influence employee choice on the basis of relatively small cost savings. It is also easy to claim that you cannot provide desirable benefit packages with convenient providers because of the greediness of some dentists and the generally "unreasonable" cost of dental services. If Stan buys into strategies that befuddle the employee or shift blame for problems with care to the dentists, he may not only undermine the employees' trust in himself and his employer, he may also put the employer at risk for liability if an employee is harmed by the plan.

How Can Margo Empower Stan to Become a More Responsible Steward of the Employees' Compensation?

Employees trust Stan to use his power to bargain on their behalf for benefits. When thinking of cost containment, Stan needs to understand the ratio of premiums paid to payments made. For example, in 1986, $6.1 billion was paid in dental insurance premiums and $5.3 billion was paid to patients (13.4% went to administrative costs, etc.). By 1988, 19% went to administrative and other costs.[11] By 1996 some estimated administrative and other costs at approximately 27%, with some egregious instances where payout is less than 50%.[12] Stan also needs to consider variation based on the kind of plan he selects for employees. According to the National Association of Dental Plans in Dallas, Texas, in 1998 the percentage of each dollar going for dental care in DHMOs was 68.1%; in PPOs it was 81.3%; and in indemnity plans it was 80.2%. DR plans can raise that percentage to greater than 90%, depending on how the plan is administered. Finally, Stan needs to be aware that he and other employers cannot rely on regulation of the benefits industry because most states do not regulate on the loss ratio. Most employees would not choose to contribute a substantial proportion of their hard-earned dental benefits to a third-party payer's profits and administrative costs, especially if the choice of provider is restricted.

What Could Margo Do?

First, she needs to avoid responding defensively. Active listening, to learn as much as she can about the plan, would be most effective. She may want to express some empathy for the challenging job Stan has. If Stan feels understood, rather than challenged or criticized, he may be willing to rethink his problem and learn new information.

Although Stan's comments may suggest that he has misconceptions about (1) the distinction between medical and dental health benefits, (2) the reasons dentists have not signed up for the benefit program his company has purchased, (3) the real cost of the plan he has purchased and the benefit to employees, and (4) other alternatives that will put more benefits in the employees' pockets, Margo may wish to phrase these apparent misunderstandings as questions. For example, it is better to ask, "What is your understanding of the differences between purchasing dental and medical health benefits?" or "Has your carrier been willing to tell you the ratio of premiums paid to payments made?" or "What is the real cost of that dental benefit plan if employees need to take extra time to travel to plan dentists?" or "Have you asked any of the local dentists why they didn't sign up for your plan?"

Rather than try to answer all these questions herself, Margo may want to refer Stan to the American Dental Association's Council on Dental Benefit Programs. Recognizing the important role dental benefits have played in improving access to dental care for millions of Americans, the Council on Dental Benefit Programs has prepared brochures and other services to help employers of all sizes to design cost-effective, high-quality dental benefit plans for their employees.

Finally, the local or state dental association undoubtedly has persons available who could help Stan and other employers, union leaders, and concerned citizen groups to evaluate competing plans and to recommend plans that would be in the best interest of the employee and the company. Does Margo have an obligation to have some familiarity with alternative plans and the resources available to help the members of the public make informed choices?

CASE 6

The Dr. Ellis Case

Dr. Joan Ellis has always been a leader. She was active in community dentistry programs during dental school and served as class president her last 2 years. After dental school, she completed a general practice residency and earned a master's degree in dental public health in another state, while her husband completed specialty training in ophthalmology. After returning to her home state, she opened a general dentistry practice. On the basis of her public health background, she took a real interest in treating Medicaid recipients, although she realized she needed to limit the number of medical assistance patients if she were to maintain a viable practice. As did many dentists in the community, she recognized that the level of reimbursement for services barely covered overhead. Further, this population of patients often had trouble complying with the regimens thought necessary to maintain a successful practice. Cancellations and tardiness were just a few of the problems. More important, the time and effort required to complete the paperwork associated with reimbursement, together with denial of treatment Dr. Ellis thought essential, made working with this patient pool frustrating at best.

After exploring the problems associated with trying to lobby the legislature for increases in the reimbursement rate for dental benefits, Dr. Ellis decided that she would set aside one afternoon a week in which she would treat—free of charge—any Medicaid-eligible patients. By providing services free she avoided the frustration associated with completing paperwork, and by taking patients on a first come, first served basis (emergency cases excepted), she found she enjoyed the work more and served her patients better. Nonetheless, she realized she could not advocate this for everyone, and, even if she could, she was not sure it was a fair solution to the problems Medicaid-eligible people faced as they attempted to gain access to care. Over the years, she had served on a number of committees and boards that addressed access to care and dental disease prevention and oral health promotion. She was well versed in the issues and thought that access to care was impeded by the low rate of reimbursement for dental service. Although she did not agree with her colleagues, many of whom took the position that if society would not adequately reimburse they would not treat, she recognized that the profession had a responsibility to advocate for the disadvantaged. The profession had tried to influence the legislature. The legislature tended to view the profession's efforts as self-serving. Some viewed the profession as self-serving and unwilling to sacrifice anything for the welfare of others. Dr. Ellis was also aware that some states had successfully argued that inadequate reimbursement rates paid to dentists who participated in Medicaid programs severely hindered the ability of recipients to obtain necessary dental services and violated federal law.

Dr. Ellis has just been elected president of the state dental association. One of her primary goals is to improve access to care for the disadvantaged.

What strategies should she use?

ANALYSIS

Profession-Society/Community Issues

We have argued that the profession has a responsibility to put the oral health interests of society above the interests of the profession. But are there no limits to that responsibility? Does this mean that the profession must care for the underserved with little or no help from society at large? It does not. The provision of dental and medical care for the economically disadvantaged is a responsibility of the larger society. And society cannot shift a disproportionate share of that responsibility to the profession. Thus a state that designs a Medicaid dental plan that reimburses at rates that are near or below the actual cost of providing services may be in violation of federal law, because the plan has the effect of denying equal access to care. In a 1992 California case, the court found that the reimbursement rates set by California's Denti-Cal program were in violation of recipients' rights to equal access to dental care, statewide availability of care, timely receipt of care, and comparability of services in the Medi-Cal program (the state's Medicaid plan).[13] The trial judge ordered the state to increase fees from approximately 30% to 80% of the average amount billed. It took a class action suit, filed on behalf of Medicaid recipients of California, to bring about such a change in reimbursements, but such lawsuits have been successful in other states as well.

Continued

CASE 6

The Dr. Ellis Case—cont'd

Although the profession did not initiate these lawsuits, their success shows how society can be prompted to assume its share of the responsibility for promoting the oral health of the nation.

Dr. Ellis might develop a strategic plan to educate the public about the causes and prevention of dental disease and about the cost-benefit ratio of early intervention in dental disease. A good public education program might motivate the 40% of the population that does not regularly seek care or motivate the substantial number of people (35% to 40%) who have dental coverage, but do not use their benefit. Second, focus the profession on the underserved and on unmet need. One of the constants that ran through the health care reform debate during the Clinton administration was that it was intolerable to have 35 to 50 million (14% to 20% of the population) medically uninsured. (We do not know the proportion of the uninsured who are financially able to purchase care, but choose not to. There is no mandate to have health insurance as there is to have auto insurance.) But by comparison, only 40% of the population has dental benefits. There is an enormous unmet need. In estimating the need, it should not be assumed that people who do not have coverage do not get dental care. Indeed, many people do not see a dental benefit plan as much of a benefit and prefer to pay out-of-pocket. Nonetheless, it is reasonable to assume that an increase in dental benefit plans, especially of the type that keep administrative costs low, would enhance utilization of dental services. Also, patient expenditures tend to be greater (as much as 15% greater according to one study[14]) for those who have dental coverage. Third, challenge the state legislature to consider medical and dental benefits simultaneously when considering a package of primary health care benefits. Then challenge the state to provide adequate reimbursement for dental benefits—through class action suits, if efforts to persuade are ineffectual. Fourth, collaborate with the state and national professional associations to design alternative models for the delivery of dental care to the underserved, as well as to the employed. Consider how direct reimbursement plans enable employers to manage costs while preserving consumer sovereignty and eliminating interference in the caregiving partnership. Fifth, remind the profession of its public responsibilities. Like most of us, professions and professionals have a tendency to focus on self-interest, rather than the interests of society. Being a dental professional in the modern world means treating all patients equally and paying attention to epidemiologic, economic, and social elements of practice. Practicing dentistry means working in operatories, on committees, and in communities. The profession needs a cadre of professionals who are well trained to proactively engage legislatures, union leaders, employers, purchasers, and patients to buy benefits that are in the employee's interest.

REVIEW QUESTIONS

1. Given that dentistry possesses each of the essential attributes of a profession, what will be expected of you if you decide to become a dental professional?
2. Define and explain the following: direct reimbursement, an indemnity plan, preferred provider organization, dental health maintenance organization, discount/referral options, and the table of allowances.
3. List and explain the principle-based approach to bioethics, and list and describe three principles. Explain how they apply to ethical dilemmas in dental health care.
4. What is an advantage of professionalism? What is a disadvantage?
5. Respond to the questions posed in the case studies.

REFERENCES

1. Hall RH: The professions. In *Occupations and the social structure,* ed 2, Englewood Cliffs, NJ, 1975, Prentice-Hall.
2. Frankena W: *Ethics,* ed 2, Englewood Cliffs, NJ, 1975, Prentice-Hall.
3. Beauchamp TL, Childress JF: *Principles of biomedical ethics,* ed 4, New York, 1995, Oxford University Press.
4. Block LE, Freed JR: A new paradigm for increasing access to dental care: the Oregon Health Plan, *J Am Coll Dent* 63(1):30, 1996.
5. Johnston DW, Lewis DW: Three-year randomized trial of professionally applied topical fluoride gel comparing annual and biannual applications with/without prior prophylaxis, *Caries Res* 29:331, 1995.
6. Council on Dental Benefit Programs: *Policies on dental benefit programs,* Chicago, 1994, American Dental Association.
7. Council on Dental Benefit Programs: *Buyer's guide to dental benefits,* Chicago, 2001, American Dental Association.
8. Marshall JY, Director, ADA Dental Benefits Program: Personal communication, July 2001.
9. Valachovic RW et al: Trends in dentistry and dental education, *J Dent Educ* 65(6):539, 2001.
10. Capilouto E: Market forces driving health care reform, *J Dent Educ* 59(4):480, 1995.
11. Health Insurance Association of America: *Source book of health insurance,* Washington, DC, 1990, The Association.
12. Bramson JB, Feldman ME: A review of dental HMO expenses: where do the premium dollars really go? *J Am Dent Assoc* 127(1):118, 1996.
13. *Clark v Coye,* 1992 WL 370801 (E.D. Cal. Oct. 14, 1992).
14. Martens LV et al: Business trends in private general practice, *J Dent Res* 67:182, 1988 (abstract).

CHAPTER

17

THE LAW AND DENTAL PRACTICE: PROTECTING THE HEALTH OF THE COMMUNITY

Burton R. Pollack

Protecting the Health of the Community

Legislation designed to protect the public from unqualified health practitioners began in the early part of the nineteenth century. Before that time the principle of free enterprise enabled anyone to "treat" the sick and charge a fee for the service they provided. Many state legislatures believed that some form of qualification should be required to permit persons to engage in the practice of medicine and dentistry. Encouragement in general came from members of professional societies. Many leaders of the dental profession in the early and mid-nineteenth century were located in Baltimore. One was Dr. Shearjashub Spooner, who in speaking before the dental society in 1838 stated, "The dental profession should be protected by legislative enactment: every person before he be permitted to practice it, should serve a term of pupilage and pass an examination before a competent board of dentists."[1] Eleasar Parmly, another leader in the dental society, agreed. "If the legislature will do nothing more than merely to regulate the conditions by which members shall be admitted to practice . . . it would serve, at least, to draw a line of distinction, which the public would understand, between the regular members of the profession, and the quacks who disgrace it."[1] Chapin Harris, at the opening of the Baltimore College of Dental Surgery, stated, "Filled as the ranks of the profession are, with individuals who have never learned the first rudiments . . . it will doubtless require some time to effect the wished reformation, and [it] will only be accomplished [by fixing] a line of distinction between the competent and the incompetent. It is necessary that there should be some test of qualification by bodies qualified and regularly appointed for the duty." He later stated, "The community at large have experienced too much of the bad effects growing out of the ignorance of dental practitioners."[1] It was clear that the leaders in the profession were bent on having some form of regulation designed to protect the public from the unskilled, untrained, and unqualified.

Laws regulating the practice of dentistry

began in 1841 in Alabama. However, the law was rudimentary and only nominally regulated the practice of the profession. In 1868 Kentucky, New York, and Ohio specified, in detail, the requirements to practice the profession and gave power of enforcement to a government agency. Dr. J. Ben Robinson, in an article published in the *Journal of the American Dental Association,* reported the following:[2]

> The dentists of Kentucky, in a memorial to the legislature, in which they urged the enactment of a dental law stated their purpose as follows: "Your petitioners, therefore, respectfully pray your honorable body to protect the citizens of the Commonwealth of Kentucky from injury by incompetent dental practitioners, by such enactments as in your wisdom you may deem sufficient."

By 1913 all states and the District of Columbia, Puerto Rico, Hawaii, and Alaska had adopted dental regulatory legislation. However, challenges to these laws and those that regulated medical practice surfaced in many states, and in each the courts took the opportunity to point out that the purpose of the law was to protect the public's health.

An early case challenging a law limiting health practice to those who were qualified by law was brought before the Supreme Judicial Court of Massachusetts in 1835.[3] The court was to decide if a "bonesetter" fell within the law, and further, whether the law was constitutional. As to the first, the court found the following:

> A person who practises [practices] bonesetting and reducing sprains, swellings and contractions of the sinews, by friction and fomentation, but no other branch of the healing art, is a person practising [practicing] surgery, within the meaning of St. 1818, c. 113, § 1, which provides, that no person practising [practicing] physic or surgery shall be entitled to the benefit of law for the recovery of his fees, unless he shall have been licensed by the Massachusetts Medical Society or graduated a doctor in medicine in Harvard University.

The court, in deciding the law to be constitutional, went on to state the following:

> It appears to us, that *the leading and sole purpose of this act was to guard the public against ignorance, negligence and carelessness* in the members of one of the most useful professions, and that the means were intended to be adapted to that object. [Emphasis added.]

In 1889 a case that began in West Virginia was appealed to the U.S. Supreme Court.[4] It was a case in which a physician was found guilty of violating the law regulating medical practice. He challenged the law as to whether he met the conditions of the law in obtaining a license to practice, which had been denied, and whether the law was constitutional. In deciding, the court stated the following:

> The power of the state to provide for the general welfare of its people authorizes it to prescribe all such regulations as in its judgement will secure or tend to secure them against the consequences of ignorance and incapacity, as well as deception and fraud. . . . Due consideration, therefore, for the protection of society may well induce the state to exclude from practice those who have not such a license, or who are found upon examination not to be fully qualified.

As with physicians, challenges by dentists found their way into the courts. In 1889 the Supreme Court of Minnesota had the following to say about the state's law regulating dental practice:[5]

> The power rests on the right to protect the public against the injurious consequences likely to result from allowing persons to practice those professions who do not possess the special qualifications

essential to enable the practitioner to practice the profession with safety to those who employ him. The same reasons apply with equal force to the profession of dentistry, which is but a branch of the medical profession.

In concluding, the court stated the following:

The provisions and requirements of the law are undoubtedly rigorous. They ought to be, in any law aiming to protect the public against ignorance and incompetency in so important a profession as the medical profession, in any of its branches. We see nothing in the provisions of this law that was not clearly inserted by the legislature, in good faith, to effect the end in view. The law is valid.

In 1914 the Court of Appeals of New York was asked to rule on the validity of the law regulating dental practice.[6] In its ruling the court stated the following:

The general power of the state to exact proper skill and learning of those who follow pursuits involving the public health, safety, and welfare, and to prescribe appropriate tests therefore, cannot at this day be questioned. It has been exercised from time immemorial, and has been sustained by repeated decisions of the courts.

Cases in other states came to the same conclusion as the courts in Minnesota, New York, West Virginia, and Massachusetts. It is clear that all courts, when faced with ruling on whether state laws regulating medical and dental practice were constitutional, ruled in favor of their constitutionality based on the need of the state to protect the health and safety of the community from those who did not meet the rigid requirements to engage in practice.

Dental Law and Risk Management

Licensed health providers occupy a special place in society. The license granted them by the community enables them to pursue their profession in a virtual monopoly. Only those who are specially trained and who meet rigid qualifications and standards may hold themselves out to the community as providers of care and engage in practice defined by law. However, once having accepted the license, licensees are subjected to lifelong regulation by society as a whole and by individual patients whom they treat. The risks in practice are many. This section of the chapter examines the risks in dental practice and presents methods that enable practitioners to reduce and control them. This process is termed *risk management.*

After the crisis in medical and hospital malpractice in the early 1970s, risk management concepts borrowed from industry were adapted to the health field—particularly to hospitals. More recently, risk management principles have been applied to individual practice settings. These principles are designed primarily to protect the financial resources of an industry (e.g., hospital, private practitioner) from losses resulting from legal action. An effective risk management program includes the following:

1. Loss identification (exposure to legal claims)
2. Loss analysis (evaluation of loss experience)
3. Loss avoidance or reduction
4. Loss financing (financing claims exposure)

The following three activities available to a practitioner are associated with risk management:

1. Identifying areas of legal vulnerability (what risks have I assumed, or am I likely to assume?)
2. Instituting corrective or preventive measures (what risks can I eliminate or reduce?)

3. Purchasing liability insurance (what risk am I able to transfer to another to protect my financial assets?)

This section provides information related to the first two of these activities. The information presented is based on a thorough review of cases brought against dentists and opinions of courts deciding medical and dental malpractice suits. The text summarizes the areas of legal vulnerability associated with the practice of dentistry. The italicized risk management rules (i.e., recommendations, suggestions) represent corrective or preventive measures associated with the subject matter of the text. The amount of liability insurance purchased (the third listed activity) is a personal matter; practitioners must consider cost, scope of coverage, and amount of indemnification of losses that are desired on the basis of their ability to afford premium costs.

Risk management principles are applied to professional and general liability. General liability relates to negligence associated with injuries that result from the physical structures within the office. Employment practices liability insurance has become essential to any dentist employer. It is an outgrowth of the public concern for employee rights and the litigious society in which we now live. The insurance protects the employer from civil suits based on the employer's discrimination against an employee, his or her unlawful termination, and sexual harassment. However, no insurance is available to cover suits brought by government agencies for any violation of an employee's rights as protected by the law. Professional liability relates to injuries that result from the treatment of patients. For example, if a patient falls in the waiting room as a result of tripping over an electric cord, the incident comes under the general liability category. If the patient's tongue is lacerated during a crown preparation, the incident becomes one of professional liability. This chapter deals solely with professional liability. An effective risk management program does much to control the cost of malpractice insurance and to protect the reputation and resources of the practitioner.

This section also provides dentists, hygienists, dental assistants, and other office personnel with information about the legal risks of practice and methods designed to eliminate or reduce them. The goal is to enable the health practitioner to practice in a worry-free and claims-free environment. Because so much of risk management relates to law and the legal system, it is necessary to describe how the system works in the regulation of the health professions to fully understand both the risks in practice and the methods recommended to reduce or eliminate them.

COURTS AND LEGAL PRECEDENTS

What courts do is important to matters relating to the practice of dentistry, to public health, and to the lives of everyone in the United States. The foundation of U.S. law is English common law. The law in the United States springs from two distinct sources that in some cases overlap: case law and black letter law, described later in this section. Further, the organization of the courts plays an important role in establishing just what is the law.

COURTS

Courts are classified in many ways: as to their organization, whether lower or upper; their geographic jurisdiction, based on where they sit; their subject matter jurisdiction, criminal or civil; trial or appellate; and so on. For purposes of this chapter, lower and upper, that is, trial and appellate, are of concern. The issue is how legal precedent is set and how it affects the health professions in general and dental practice in particular.

Lower courts, also known as trial courts, are the courts of original jurisdiction. These courts are the first to hear and decide a case. Suits in which one party alleges that he or she suffered an injury resulting from the simple negligence or malpractice of another are heard in a lower court assigned that jurisdiction by the state, either by its constitution or through its court rules. The default setup is a jury trial with a judge and jury, although each side may affirmatively waive having a jury and have the judge sit alone (bench trial). Decisions made in the lower courts may be appealed to a higher (appellate) court should either party believe that (1) the procedure in the lower court violated procedure as established by appellate courts or court rules or (2) the judge, in the instructions to the jury, applied the wrong law, precedent case, or black letter law to guide the jury in arriving at a decision in the case, based on the facts as found by the jury. Juries decide the facts; the judge applies the law.

A major confusion for laypersons is that each state names its courts as it chooses, as does the federal government. For example, in New York the lower court of original jurisdiction is the Supreme Court; it is the first to hear an action brought against a dentist by a patient alleging negligence, malpractice, or breach of contract. There is one Supreme Court in each county of the state. The state is further divided geographically into four appellate jurisdictions and in each is an Appellate Division of the Supreme Court. The Appellate Divisions hear and decide appeals brought to them from the lower courts within their geographic jurisdiction. The highest court in the state is the New York Court of Appeals; it is the court of last resort in the state, and its decisions are binding on all courts of the state.

The lack of uniformity is evident in the given names of the courts in New Jersey and Illinois. In New Jersey the court of original jurisdiction is the Superior Court, one for each county in the state. The intermediate appellate court is the Superior Court, Appellate Division. The court of last resort in New Jersey is the Supreme Court. In Illinois the court of original jurisdiction is the Circuit Court, the intermediate appellate court is the Appellate Court of Illinois (District and Division), and the court of last resort is the Supreme Court. And so on for each state.

In the federal system the country is divided into 88 federal districts, each having at least one district court. The federal intermediate court is the U.S. Court of Appeals; at least one for each of the judicial circuits, of which there are 11. The highest court of the land, the court of last resort, is the U.S. Supreme Court consisting of eight justices and a chief justice. Any seven judges can hear a case, but five affirmative votes are needed to act on a case before the court. Decisions of the U.S. Supreme Court are binding on all courts in the United States.

When an appellate court decides a case, precedent law is established. All lower courts within the geographic jurisdiction of the appellate court are required to follow the precedent established by the appellate court. If the lower court does not and the case is appealed, the decision of the lower court will be reversed. If the case is not appealed, the decision of the lower court is final, notwithstanding the fact that in arriving at the decision precedent law was ignored. It is important to remember that only appellate courts establish precedent and that no one, not even the most experienced attorney, can predict with any degree of certainty how a judge or jury will decide a case. Fifty percent of all lawyers representing clients end up on the losing side and are proved wrong by either a judge or jury or by an appellate court.

Case Law

Case law, also known as court law, is that law established through decisions made by the courts. All appellate decisions are officially published and made available to all law libraries and included in electronic databases of legal publishing companies. Only the appellate courts make precedent law. The precedents they establish are known as case law. Except for cases decided in federal courts, case law is state specific. Only the jurisdiction in which the appellate court sits is affected by its case law. The decisions and opinions of the appellate courts are available within hours throughout the country. Case law may change with every decision reached by an appellate court. Attorneys must remain current on changes in case law that affect their fields of practice. It is not a simple task. Although appellate decisions are officially published, decisions of the lower courts are not. These are recorded in the court in which they are heard. Thousands of trial courts are scattered throughout the country. The result is that there is no simple way to collect national data on what takes place at the trial court level. For this reason it is not possible to obtain reliable data on what is taking place in the field of malpractice litigation. Only the insurance companies know, and they do not readily share information unless it suits them, and not all dentists have malpractice insurance.

Black Letter Law

Black letter law (BLL) is law written in black ink on white paper. These are laws that come from several sources: from elected officials serving in some form of formal organization (e.g., Congress, a state legislature, a city council) and from administrative agencies established by the elected body. Those laws adopted by Congress, a legislature, or any other elected body are called by different names: by Congress, acts of Congress; by a state legislature, statutes; and by lower jurisdictions, a variety of names (e.g., codes, ordinances). State BLL is state specific; therefore the BLL regulating the practice of dentistry in Vermont has no impact on dental practice in Ohio, although some laws might be common to both states.

CAVEATS IN RISK MANAGEMENT AND THE LAW

The United States has 51 jurisdictions: 50 states and the federal government. Each of the 50 states has exercised its right to regulate the health professions, including dentistry. In addition, Puerto Rico, the Virgin Islands, and the District of Columbia also regulate health practices. The federal government regulates some elements of health practice. Therefore 54 separate jurisdictions regulate the practice of dentistry. Except for federal regulations that apply to practitioners in all states, each jurisdiction has independent regulations. Except for some federal laws, there is no generic law in the United States. There are, however, legal principles that apply nationwide. For example, the legal principle of the statute of limitations is the same in all jurisdictions, but the statute may begin to run at different times and for different lengths of time in each individual jurisdiction.

The caveat is that for practitioners to know the specifics of the regulation of dental practice, they must be thoroughly familiar with local law. The same act may be legal in one state and illegal in another. As an example, in New York it is legal for a dental laboratory to select a shade for a crown. In Massachusetts it is illegal for a dentist to refer a patient to a laboratory for the purpose of selecting a shade. Therefore a dentist in New York who sends a patient to a dental laboratory for the selection of a shade is not in violation of the law, nor is the laboratory in violation of the state law. The same act performed by a dentist in Massachusetts would be in violation of the law.

Except for the purpose of presenting examples, this chapter describes generic legal principles and legal trends. It does not offer legal advice, although recommendations and suggestions are provided. Local attorneys, or government agencies, should be of assistance in determining the specific laws of the jurisdiction in which you conduct your practice.

Levels of Legal Risk

The artificial legal concept of "levels of legal risk" relates to the degree to which a dentist is willing to take a risk in the performance of a professional act. Refusing to treat a patient who does not follow the advice of a dentist presents the lowest level of legal risk to the dentist. However, if the dentist agrees to treat the patient although the patient did not comply with the dentist's advice, the risk is great. A good example of the concept relates to a dentist's advice that the patient have a thorough radiographic examination before treatment is begun. If the patient refuses and the dentist proceeds with the care, there is a risk that, because radiographs were not taken, an important pathologic condition was not discovered and as a result the patient suffered an injury. The dentist may lose a suit should the patient allege that the dentist was negligent in not discovering the condition. The dentist's defense is that the patient refused to have radiographs taken. Given the uncertainty of the outcome of jury trials, the dentist may lose the case. Therefore the lowest level of legal risk is to refuse to treat the patient. The highest level of legal risk is to treat a patient who refuses to follow advice. Under some circumstances, the dentist may be willing to take the risk after assessing the benefits of continuing to treat the patient. Patients who refuse to follow the advice of the dentist to seek specialty care or consultation present the same legal risk as those who refuse to submit to radiographs.

While you review the risk management rules, you should keep the concept of levels of legal risk in mind. Prudent dentists make certain that they are aware of the risks attached to any professional decision before acting. That is what this section of the chapter is all about: describing the risks.

Loss without Fault

Another artificial legal concept is "loss without fault." It evolved from a study I conducted in the early 1980s during the crisis in dental malpractice litigation. Four hundred cases in which a dentist was accused of malpractice were tracked from the initial service of suit papers to the closing of the case. The results were that in 80% of 400 cases brought against dentists, the insurance company, on the advice of a panel of dental experts and an attorney experienced in dental malpractice litigation, sought settlement before trial because it was apparent that the case could not successfully be defended. In only 20% of the cases the panel believed that the dentist was guilty of malpractice. In 60% of the cases in which settlement was sought, the dental experts were of the opinion that no negligence was present. This 60% represents "loss without fault"—no malpractice, but little or no chance of successfully defending the suit. Looking at the data from another perspective, of 400 cases alleging malpractice brought against dentists, in 80% there was no evidence of malpractice, but according to the expert panel in only 20% could the suit be successfully defended. Loss without fault is the foundation of much of risk management.

No hard evidence exists that malpractice claims against dentists are on the decline. Some speculate that the number of cases going to trial has diminished. More cases may be settled or withdrawn to explain the decline in cases going to trial. What is known is that in the past decade jury awards of money have shown a major increase.

REGULATION OF DENTAL PRACTICE

As stated previously, each of the jurisdictions has exercised its right to regulate dental practice. Except for federal regulation, the mechanism for regulation is similar. The elected body, the legislature, enacts legislation designed to regulate dental practice. Because the members of the electorate have neither the time nor the expertise to exercise control over the daily activities of the profession and the details of practice, they enact additional legislation (enabling legislation or statutory authority) establishing an administrative agency to further regulate the profession and grant to that agency the power to adopt administrative laws (rules and regulations) to carry out its mission.

Each state may vary the name of the administrative body and adopt any organizational structure to accomplish the goal of regulating the health profession, but the general regulatory structure is the same. In New York, for example, two administrative agencies regulate dentists and other health professionals: the state education department and the Board of Regents. The commissioner of education is empowered by legislative act to adopt regulations; the Board of Regents is empowered to adopt rules. In New York the State Board for Dentistry is not authorized to adopt rules or regulations for the purpose of regulating dental practice. It serves as an examining body, recommends licensure, and advises the Commissioner of Education, the Board of Regents, and the legislature on dental matters. It also serves as an administrative body to hear alleged violations of the rules and regulations and to recommend actions to be taken against the dentist to the State Education Department. By contrast, in Massachusetts one administrative agency regulates the practice of dentistry: the Massachusetts Board of Registration in Dentistry. It combines all the functions assigned to the three agencies in New York. Most other states, like Massachusetts, have only one administrative agency, although some of the regulatory functions may fall to other state agencies.

A combination of the statutes and the rules and regulations makes up the body of dental BLL, commonly referred to as the Dental Practice Act. However, in all jurisdictions, many other laws affect the practice of dentistry. These may be found in the public health law, the sanitary code, the education law, and others. The practitioner should be aware that the laws regulating dental practice are spread throughout the statutes and administrative laws of the state. In addition, a multitude of federal laws exercise control over dental practice. The old adage that ignorance of the law is no excuse should not be ignored.

The risk management principle is as follows: *Learn the laws of the jurisdiction in which you practice and the federal laws that apply to the practice of dentistry, and remain current on changes in the laws.* Although it is difficult, much can be learned by attending continuing education courses, reading journals and texts on the subject, and attending seminars. Also, annually request a copy of the current Dental Practice Act from the local licensing agency. If you are in doubt about a provision, consult the licensing agency or a local attorney.

LEGAL VULNERABILITY IN DENTAL PRACTICE

Legal vulnerability in dental practice may be divided into two broad categories: criminal and civil. Each broad category has subcategories, as shown in Fig. 17-1. The intentional torts listed on the chart are those most frequently associated with dental practice. False imprisonment, abuse of process, trespass to real property, conversion, interference with performance of a contract, and others are recognized in law but have little relevance in dental practice.

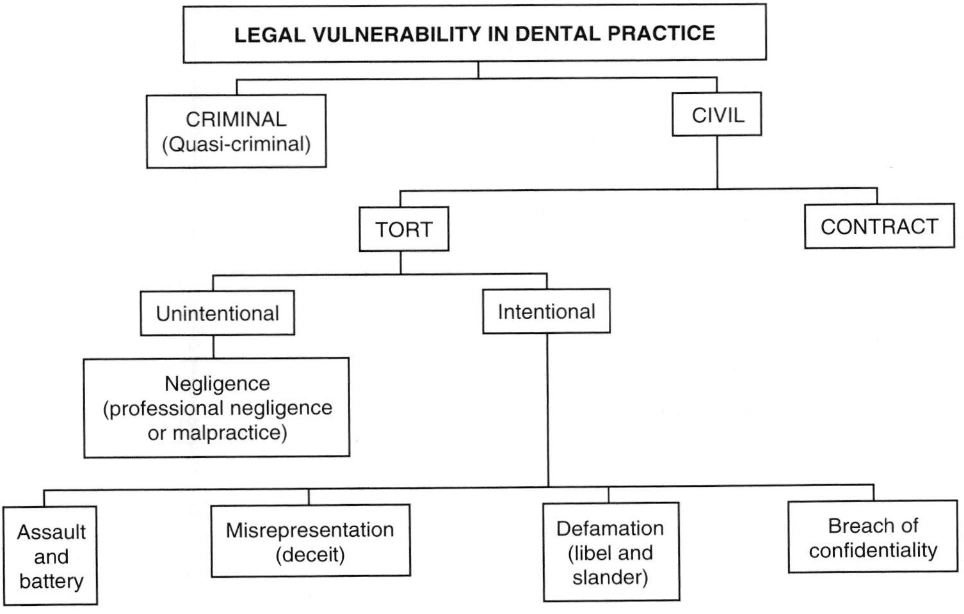

Fig. 17-1. Legal vulnerability in dental practice.

CRIMINAL AND QUASI-CRIMINAL VULNERABILITY

Violations of statutory law are termed *crimes.* They constitute acts that are deemed by the government to be against the public interest. They may be defined as misdemeanors or felonies. Violations of that part of the Dental Practice Act that is statutory, enacted by the legislature, also are classified as crimes and may include penalties such as loss or suspension of license, mandatory psychiatric counseling, drug rehabilitation, mandatory continuing education, fines, or even jail. If the legislature declares the violation a misdemeanor, the jail sentence may be less than if it classifies the violation a felony. In New York, for instance, aiding or abetting an unlicensed person to perform a service that requires a license is a class E felony, punishable by up to 3 years in jail. In other jurisdictions it may classified as a misdemeanor.

Violations of administrative laws (rules or regulations of administrative agencies, e.g., the state board, the state education department, the board of regents) are termed *quasi crimes.* Penalties may include all actions that are possible under crimes, except loss of personal freedom (jail). Because members of administrative boards and agencies are appointed rather than elected, the framers of the constitution believed that appointed individuals should not be granted the power to deprive anyone of liberty.

One of the major differences between a violation of a statute and that of an administrative law is the degree of evidence necessary to convict. In allegations of criminal behavior the state must prove "beyond a reasonable doubt" that the law was violated. For violations of administrative law the proof necessary is considerably less. (In civil actions the burden on the plaintiff is to prove by a "fair preponderance of the evidence" [more than 50%] that the defendant is guilty.)

In all dental practice acts, authority is granted to an administrative agency to impose punitive sanctions against a dentist who is found guilty of a violation. Therefore a dentist who is found guilty of violating the law regulating the prescription or the administration of controlled substances may have an additional action taken by the dental board, or if the violation occurs in New York, by the Board of Regents, against the license of the offender.

Professional liability insurance does not provide protection against either criminal or quasi-criminal allegations as it does in civil actions (those brought by a patient). Some malpractice policies may cover the defense of a claim against a dentist alleging a violation of the Dental Practice Act, but the policy will never indemnify the dentist for the payment of a fine. To do so is against strong public policy. However, if an allegation of negligence is attached to a violation of the law, either criminal or quasi-criminal, the defense of a civil suit based on an injury resulting from the alleged illegal act becomes more difficult because of trial practice procedures.

The risk management admonition is as follows: *Know the law, don't break it!*

THE DOCTOR-PATIENT CONTRACT

When the Doctor-Patient Relationship Begins

The legal foundation of the doctor-patient relationship is contract law. At the moment a dentist expresses a professional opinion to an individual who has reason to rely on the opinion, the doctor-patient relationship begins, and the doctor is burdened with implied warranties (duties). The fact that no fee is involved does not affect the relationship that attaches to the contract or the duties.

The example best demonstrating the moment the relationship begins and the duties attach is a situation in which a dentist gives a fellow party-goer dental advice at a social gathering. If the advice results in an injury, the dentist may be held liable for negligence. It is not a valid defense that no fee was charged or expected. The dentist would be held to the standard that patients should not be given dental advice unless and until an examination and a history are completed.

The risk management principle is as follows: *In social settings, never provide anyone, unless that person is a patient of record, with advice regarding the solution of dental problems.*

Must you accept anyone who comes to you for care? The answer is a qualified no. You may not refuse to treat a patient if the refusal is based in any way on race, creed, color, or national origin. With the effective date of the federal Americans with Disabilities Act of 1990, refusal to accept a patient on the basis of a disability is a violation of the law and brings with it severe penalties. Patients with acquired immunodeficiency syndrome (AIDS), who test positive for human immunodeficiency virus (HIV), or who have any communicable infectious disease fall into the category of disabled persons and may not be refused care if the refusal is based solely on the disability. The law declares that all health providers' offices are "places of public accommodation" and therefore subject to antidiscrimination laws. Local jurisdictions have followed the same course as Congress. Therefore in many jurisdictions a dentist's office is subject to the jurisdiction of the local human rights commission and the antidiscrimination policies that it enforces. For more on the care of patients who have AIDS or are HIV positive, see the section on histories later in this chapter.

As long as the person is not a patient of record, you may even refuse to provide emergency care, subject to the limitations stated previously. It may be unethical and immoral, but it is not illegal and cannot form the basis of a criminal or civil suit. However, remember that as soon as you express a professional judgment or perform a professional act the doctor-patient relationship begins, and duties begin to attach.

When the Doctor-Patient Relationship Ends

The relationship ends when any of the following takes place:

1. Both parties agree to end it.
2. Either the patient or the dentist dies.
3. The patient ends it by act or statement.
4. The patient is cured of the problem for which care was sought.
5. The dentist unilaterally decides to terminate the care.

The dentist's unilaterally terminating the relationship may support a claim of abandonment by the patient unless the dentist follows a procedure acceptable to the courts. Abandoning a patient before the agreed treatment is completed is unethical, and in some jurisdictions it is a violation of BLL.[7,8] In all jurisdictions abandonment may lead to a civil suit.

The major causes that contribute to a decision to terminate treatment before it is complete are as follows: (1) the patient has not fulfilled the payment agreement, (2) the patient has not cooperated in keeping appointments, (3) the patient has not complied with home care instructions, and (4) there has been a breakdown in interpersonal relationships. Any of these is ample justification for the dentist to terminate treatment.

A risk management rule is as follows: *Discontinue treatment of patients who do not cooperate in care, who become antagonistic, or who exhibit a litigious attitude.*

The recommended procedure to discontinue care without running the risk of a finding of abandonment by a court begins with a discussion of the problem with the patient as follows. (1) Advise the patient that it is in his or her best interest to seek care elsewhere. (2) Assure the patient that you will cooperate by making copies of the records available should the patient make the request in writing. (3) Let the patient know that you will be available to provide emergency care for a reasonable period of time. Note the conversation on the patient's record. Follow up the conversation with a certified letter, signed receipt requested, stating the aforementioned facts.

A risk management caveat is as follows: *Do not discontinue treatment at a time when the patient's health may be compromised.* (This decision is professional rather than legal.) It is best not to suggest any dentist the patient should see; instead, have the patient select the substitute practitioner.

EXPRESS TERMS

An express term is one in which both parties are in agreement. Putting the term in writing is not required to make it enforceable, although to prevent misunderstandings a written agreement is always preferred. Usually, the express terms define items such as the fee, the nature of the treatment, and the manner in which payments are to be made. The risk management principle is as follows: *When in doubt, write it out.* This may be done on separate forms or entered into the patient's record. It is best done on a separate form because the treatment record should contain only treatment notes and patient reactions to treatment.

GUARANTEES

Guarantees, or assurances of outcomes, made by the dentist or an employee constitute an express term in the agreement. In some jurisdictions guarantees attached to health care are illegal.[9] You may be held to a guarantee even if the treatment meets acceptable standards of care. A statement made by a dentist to the patient that the patient will be satisfied with the treatment is a guarantee. If the patient is not satisfied, the dentist has breached the contract despite the excellent quality of the service.

Therapeutic reassurances—statements whose purpose is to induce patients to accept care that is clearly in their best interest—are rare in dentistry, except in unusual situations and usually when related to oral surgery. Courts generally do not consider therapeutic reassurances guarantees.

The risk management rule is as follows: *Never guarantee a result.*

IMPLIED WARRANTIES (DUTIES) OWED BY THE DOCTOR

Attached to the doctor-patient relationship are additional duties that are implied, unless the express terms serve to void or modify them. They are enforceable although not written or stated. Over the years the courts have identified many of these implied duties. Some of the more important ones are included in the list that follows.

In accepting a patient for care, the dentist warrants that he or she will do the following:

1. Use reasonable care in the provision of services as measured against acceptable standards set by other practitioners with similar training in a similar community, and accepted as reasonable by the courts
2. Be properly licensed and registered and meet all other legal requirements to engage in the practice of dentistry
3. Employ competent personnel and provide for their proper supervision
4. Maintain a level of knowledge in keeping with current advances in the profession
5. Use methods that are acceptable to at least a respectable minority of similar practitioners in the community
6. Not use experimental procedures
7. Obtain informed consent from the patient before instituting an examination or treatment
8. Not abandon the patient
9. Ensure that care is available in emergency situations
10. Charge a reasonable fee for services based on community standards
11. Not exceed the scope of practice authorized by the license or permit any person acting under direction to engage in unlawful acts
12. Keep the patient informed of progress
13. Not undertake any procedure for which the practitioner is not qualified
14. Complete the care in a timely manner
15. Keep accurate records of the treatment rendered to the patient
16. Maintain confidentiality of information
17. Inform the patient of any untoward occurrences in the course of treatment
18. Make appropriate referrals and request necessary consultations
19. Comply with all laws regulating the practice of dentistry
20. Practice in a manner consistent with the code of ethics of the profession

The list generates a host of risk management rules. They are all important as principles of good risk management.

IMPLIED DUTIES OWED BY THE PATIENT

Patients, as well as doctors, are expected to comply with some rules of behavior relative to their care, without the rules being stated. In accepting care the patient warrants the following:

1. Home care instructions will be followed.
2. Appointments will be kept.
3. Bills for services will be paid in a reasonable time.
4. The patient will cooperate in the care.
5. The patient will notify the dentist or office in a timely manner of a change in health status.

Depending on the treatment, additional warranties may exist.

It is best to make the last duty part of the express written terms of the agreement. This can be done by placing the statement at the end of the history form and reminding the patient of the need to notify the office of a change in health status. If the patient breaches any of these duties, notes to that effect should be made in the patient's record.

For purposes of risk management: *If any of the warranties is broken by the patient, this should be noted on the patient's record, and consideration should be given to discontinuing the care of the noncompliant patient.*

RISK REDUCTION IN THE TRANSMISSION OF BLOOD-BORNE INFECTIOUS DISEASES

USE OF BARRIER TECHNIQUES

With the passage of the Americans with Disabilities Act of 1990, Congress has imposed its will on the courts, and by its declaration of a health provider's office as a "place of public accommodation" a dentist who refuses to treat a patient who has AIDS or is HIV positive is in violation of the law and subject to penalties. Not all patients are aware of their HIV status or know they have other blood-borne contagious diseases; therefore the use of barrier techniques in the treatment of all patients becomes increasingly important. In addition, many high-risk patients who are in need of dental care may decide not to disclose any information on their health history form relating to the presence of AIDS or HIV infection or their presence in groups that engage in high-risk behaviors for fear of being refused care. The result is that all patients must be treated as high-risk patients. It is clear that the provider of care is at greater risk of contracting AIDS from an infected patient than the healthy patient is of contracting AIDS from an infected health care worker.

The fact that the risk of contracting and transmitting AIDS in the dental office is low does not change the responsibility of the dentist to use appropriate barrier techniques. Hepatitis B represents a greater risk in dental practice, and, to ensure protection from transmission in the treatment of patients with hepatitis, barrier techniques must be employed.

As a further complication, it is virtually impossible for the dentist to identify, with any high degree of accuracy, patients who may engage in high-risk behaviors for either AIDS or HIV infection or patients with hepatitis. Therefore appropriate measures should be taken in the treatment of all patients to prevent the transmission of a blood-borne disease to other patients, to the staff in the office, or to the dentist and his or her family. As these measures relate to the use of barrier techniques, the legal issue is to what standard the dentist will be held. During the past several years the standard has seen dramatic changes.

Currently, dentists must use six basic infection control procedures to meet an acceptable standard of office practice:

1. All office personnel involved in the treatment of patients must wear protective eye shields.
2. All office personnel involved in the treatment of patients must wear surgical gloves.
3. All office personnel involved in the treatment of patients must wear surgical masks, and they must use splash shields when aerosol sprays are used or blood or saliva may splatter.
4. All instruments used in or near the oral cavity in the treatment of patients must be sterilized in a heat or heat-pressure sterilizer.
5. All touch or splash surfaces must be disinfected with an Environmental Protection Agency–registered hospital-grade disinfectant.
6. All contaminated, hazardous, and medical wastes must be disposed of in a manner consistent with local law.

In addition, some states have mandated the use of these and other barrier techniques in the treatment of all patients. Some have addressed the issue of hepatitis B carrier testing and regular monitoring of sterilization equipment.

Dentists should remain current with the latest Centers for Disease Control and Prevention (CDC) recommendations, Occupational Safety and Health Administration (OSHA) standards, American Dental Association (ADA) recommendations, and local law to determine what measures must be taken to prevent transmission of bloodborne diseases. Failure to meet the standards exposes the dentist to legal risk of action by a government agency for violation of the law and civil action by an individual (i.e., patient, staff) who contracted a bloodborne disease traced to the dentist's office. (For more information about the treatment of patients with transmissible diseases, see Chapter 9.)

Following are contact agencies from which information and their rules may be obtained:

- ADA: Council of Dental Therapeutics, 211 E. Chicago Ave., Chicago, IL 60611; telephone 800-621-8099, ext. 2522.
- CDC: Centers for Disease Control and Prevention, 1644 Freeway Park, Atlanta, GA 30333; telephone 404-639-1830.
- Local law: Either the state dental board, the department of health, or a local attorney.
- OSHA (by regional office):
    - Region I (CT, MA, ME, NH, RI, VT). 16-18 North St., 1 Dock Square Building, 4th Floor, Boston, MA 02109; telephone 617-565-1161.
    - Region II (NJ, NY, PR). 201 Varick St., 6th Floor, New York, NY 10014; telephone 212-337-2325.
    - Region III (DC, DE, MD, PA, VA, WV). Gateway Building, Suite 2100, 3535 Market St., Philadelphia, PA 19104; telephone 215-596-1201.
    - Region IV (AL, FL, GA, KY, MS, NC, SC, TN). 1375 Peachtree St., N.E., Suite 587, Atlanta, GA 30367; telephone 404-347-3573.
    - Region V (IL, IN, MI, MN, OH, WI). 230 S. Dearborn St., 32nd Floor, Room 3244, Chicago, IL 60604; telephone 312-353-2200.
    - Region VI (AR, LA, NM, OK, TX). 525 Griffin St., Room 602, Dallas, TX 75202; telephone 214-767-3731.
    - Region VII (IA, KS, MO, NE). 911 Walnut St., Room 406, Kansas City, MO 64106; telephone 816-374-5861.
    - Region VIII (CO, MT, ND, SD, UT, WY). Federal Building, Room 1576, 1961 Stout St., Denver, CO 80294; telephone 303-844-3061.
    - Region IX (AZ, CA, HI, NV). 71 Stevenson St., 4th Floor, San Francisco, CA 94105; telephone 415-995-5672.
    - Region X (AK, ID, OR, WA). Federal Office Building, Room 6003, 909 First Ave., Seattle, WA 98174; telephone 206-442-5930.

TORTS

A tort is a civil wrong or injury, independent of a contract, that results from a breach of a duty. The tort may be unintentional or intentional. An unintentional tort is one in which harm was not intended, as is the case in the tort of negligence. As the name implies, intentional torts contain the element of intended harm.

Negligence is an unintentional tort. If the negligence involves an act that is performed in a professional capacity, it is termed *professional negligence,* or *malpractice.* Thus if a dentist is accused of negligence in the performance of dental treatment, the allegation is one of professional negligence or malpractice. However, if the act is one in which the standard of care is able to be judged by laypersons, the allegation may be one of negligence, or simple negligence.

The intentional torts of major concern to the dentist include trespass to the person (commonly known as assault and battery), defamation, breach of confidentiality, and misrepresentation (deceit).

MALPRACTICE (PROFESSIONAL NEGLIGENCE) AND THE STANDARD OF CARE

Only malpractice related to dentistry is presented here. The New York courts have provided the most comprehensive definition of malpractice as it relates to physicians and dentists.[10] The following list includes some editorial changes and updating; important risk management concerns are italicized:

A doctor's responsibilities are the same whether or not he or she is paid for the services. By undertaking to perform a medical (dental) service, he or she does not—nor does the law require him or her to—guarantee a good result. He or she is liable only for negligence.

A doctor who renders a medical (dental) service is obligated to have that reasonable degree of knowledge and ability expected of doctors (or specialists) who do that particular (operation, examination) treatment in the community where he or she practices, or a similar community. (The trend in some jurisdictions, the most recent being New York for some of its appellate jurisdictions, is to apply a national standard. See the following section [A National Standard of Care?]).

The law recognizes that there are differences in the abilities of doctors, just as there are differences in the abilities of people engaged in other activities. To practice his or her profession, a doctor is not required to possess the extraordinary knowledge and ability that belongs to a few people of rare endowments, *but he or she is required to keep abreast of the times and to practice in accordance with the approved methods and means of treatment in general use.* The standard to which he or she is held is measured by the degree of knowledge and ability of the average doctor (or specialist) in good standing in the community where he or she practices (or in a similar community).

In the performance of medical (dental) services the doctor is obligated to use his or her best judgment and to use reasonable care in the exercise of his or her knowledge and ability. The rule requiring him or her to use his or her best judgment does not make him or her liable for a mere error in judgment, provided he or she does what he or she thinks is best after careful examination. The rule of reasonable care does not require the exercise of the highest possible degree of care; it requires only that he or she exercise that degree of care that a reasonably prudent doctor (or specialist) would exercise under the same circumstances.

If a patient should sustain an injury while undergoing medical (dental) care and that injury results from the doctor's lack of knowledge or ability, or from his or her failure to exercise reasonable care or to use his or her best judgment, he or she is responsible for the injuries that are the result of his or her acts.

Courts do not require that all dentists use the same modality of treatment. The standard can be met if a "respectable minority" of practitioners use the same treatment method. Therefore, for example, the Sargenti method in endodontic treatment and the Keyes technique in periodontal therapy may be acceptable to the courts as meeting the standard of reasonable care. It should be noted that the standard to which a dentist is held is the standard set by other dentists, not what a text, article, professional organization, or government agency recommends. These are hearsay, not available for cross-examination, and therefore may not be directly entered into evidence.

Additional risk management principles applied to malpractice prevention are the following:

1. Do not undertake treatment beyond your ability and training, even if the patient insists that you provide the care.
2. If, in your professional judgment, you believe that specialty care is required before the care you intend, do not undertake your treatment unless the patient follows your recommendation to obtain specialty care. This is of importance when the patient needs to receive periodontal therapy before the fabrication of crowns or fixed bridges.
3. If you recommend to the patient that specialty care is necessary and the patient refuses to follow your recommendation, the legal risk is increased if you undertake the care that, by your own admission, should have been provided by a specialist.
4. If you believe that certain tests or diagnostic procedures should be completed before you undertake treatment and the patient refuses, as in the case of the need for radiographs, the legal risk is markedly increased if you treat the patient without the diagnostic aid you recommend.

In items 2 through 4, the dentist has established a standard of acceptable care. By acceding to the patient's refusal to follow recommendations and treating the patient, even at the patient's request, the dentist has departed from the standard. This action presents a situation that is difficult to defend. Having the patient sign a statement to the effect that he or she is aware of the risk of noncompliance somewhat reduces the risk but does not completely eliminate it. A court might declare the statement exculpatory and void as against public policy. An exculpatory statement excuses an individual from liability for negligence. Agreements entered into by patients that relieve health practitioners from responsibility for negligent acts have not been enforced by the courts. When having to address the issue, courts have declared exculpatory clauses in doctor-patient agreements against public policy and therefore void.[11]

A National Standard of Care?

Establishing a standard of care to which a defendant dentist is held directly relates to who the court will permit to present testimony (the expert) as to the standard to which the defendant dentist is to be held. If the court limits the experts to those who practice in the community, be it local or even statewide, the standard would be "local," not "national." There is now a trend among the courts to apply a national standard of care. The trend is most evident when practitioners are certified by a specialty board. Under these circumstances a board-certified specialist from California may be permitted to present testimony as to the standard of care to which a board-certified specialist in the same specialty would be held in New York. Another somewhat disturbing effect of the trend is that there are two standards of care in those jurisdictions that accept a different standard of care for specialists than for generalists. The result is that a board-certified specialist would not be permitted to testify as to the standard of care of a generalist or non–board-certified specialist. Thus there are two standards of care in the community—one for generalists and another for board-certified specialists. A court in New York, in applying a national standard of care for board-certified radiologists, by permitting a board-certified radiologist from California who never practiced in New York to testify against a board-certified radiologist in New York, noted that the result is that a two-tiered level of care has been accepted.[12] The trend in the courts to apply a national standard to generalists is taking place but is progressing at a steady but slower rate.

Trespass to the Person (Assault and Battery)

The civil counterpart of the criminal act of assault and battery is trespass to the person. It constitutes a threat to harm (assault) and unauthorized touching (battery). Traditionally, lack of informed consent to care was treated as assault and battery. Recent decisions classify lack of informed consent as negligence or malpractice.[13] The change resulted in part from the recognition by the courts that, except in the most unusual cases, doctors do not intend to harm their patients, although the touching was not authorized by the patients. In some jurisdictions, if the consent is present but faulty, the rules of malpractice apply. If there is a total absence of consent, the case may be treated as trespass to the person.

Assault and battery cases not associated with lack of consent have occurred in dentistry. The use of force or unnecessary physical restraints in the treatment of uncooperative children has led to allegations of criminal assault and battery and civil trespass to the person. Dentists should be aware that if the allegation is criminal, professional liability insurance will not provide coverage. In some older professional liability policies, civil actions of assault and battery were covered. However, recent professional liability policies limit coverage to professional negligence.

The risk management principle applied to trespass to the person is as follows: *Avoid the use of physical force or unnecessary restraints in the treatment of patients, including children. If you feel that such measures are necessary, discuss the matter with the parents or guardian and have them present in the operatory.*

Risk management as it applies to consent is discussed later in the chapter.

Misrepresentation (Deceit)

Patients must be kept informed of their treatment status. This is one of the implied duties that the courts have attached to the doctor-patient relationship. If information is withheld that places a patient's health in jeopardy or deprives the patient of the legal right to bring suit against the practitioner, a legal action in deceit or fraudulent concealment may result. In the civil action of deceit and fraudulent concealment, the statute of limitations may be extended, and professional liability insurance may not provide coverage. In addition, a criminal action of fraud may also be alleged. The problems in dentistry most frequently associated with deceit and fraudulent concealment include the failure to inform the patient when an instrument breaks off in a root canal, when a root is fractured and the tip remains in the jaw, and when the dentist is aware that the success of the treatment will be compromised because of lack of cooperation by the patient. Informing the patient of an untoward event at the time it occurs defeats any future attempt by the patient to extend or toll (delay the beginning of) the statute of limitations. A note on the patient's record of the event and of the fact that the patient was informed should be made; if possible, the patient should be asked to initial or sign the entry. A more damaging situation would occur if the dentist assures the patient that all went well with a procedure, but in fact it did not—for example, a root tip was left in the bone or a file tip was left in the canal.

The risk management rules are as follows: *Never lie to patients about their treatments, and always keep them informed about their health status while in your care.*

Third-party payment coverage has led to many allegations of fraud and deceit. It is usually associated with passing off one metal for another in the fabrication of prosthetic appliances by substituting nonprecious for precious metals, with not collecting copayment fees from the patient, with substituting an approved-for-payment treatment for one that is not covered by the third party, or with predating care to ensure insurance coverage. Actions in criminal fraud also may result. Insurance companies are alert to such activities and are relentless in their pursuit of suspected dentists. The patient may also institute an action for the same act against the errant practitioner. Actions in fraudulent misrepresentation overlap actions in breach of contract. The choice is left to the plaintiff's attorney, and the one most damaging to the dentist's interests or most favorable to the success of the lawsuit will be selected.

The risk management rule is worth repeating and expanding: *Never lie to or deceive a patient or an insurance company.*

Defamation

The intentional tort of defamation is not of major concern in dentistry because most dentists are aware of the problem and its consequences.

The risk management admonition is as follows: *Keep your opinions about your patients to yourself unless the opinions are essential to successful treatment. Expressions about the mental health of a patient are particularly risky.*

Breach of Confidentiality

Breach of confidentiality was not known as a tort under English common law. It is a product of recent case law (law as stated by courts in deciding cases) and BLL (including statutes enacted by elected officials and administrative laws, rules, and regulations adopted by administrative agencies).[14] Confidentiality also is addressed in the code of ethics of the American Dental Association.[15]

Information obtained from the patient in the course of diagnosis or treatment must remain confidential. Unless the patient waives confidentiality, a breach may lead to a suit. Patients may waive confidentiality by their actions or words. It may also be waived by action of law, as in the case of the requirement to report certain communicable diseases to government health agencies. When a patient visits a specialist or another health practitioner at the dentist's request, the dentist is expected to inform that practitioner of the health status of the patient. In going to the specialist the patient, by his or her action, has waived confidentiality. A patient who seeks care from a group practice and is aware that the practitioners practice as associates has waived confidentiality. There are many other situations in which confidentiality is waived.

The risk management rule is as follows: *Never reveal any information about a patient to anyone without first obtaining permission from the patient—preferably in writing.* (See the following section on patient records.)

In some jurisdictions information related to sexual activity obtained from a minor must not be revealed to the parent without the minor's consent. Both criminal and civil actions may result from this specific form of breach of confidentiality. In the referral of a patient who has AIDS, is HIV positive, or has any other communicable infectious disease, should the referring dentist be of the opinion that such information is necessary in the treatment of the patient, no specific waiver is needed; however, to be on the safe side the matter should be discussed with the patient before the information is sent to the referred practitioner, and suitable notes should be entered on the patient's record.

Patient Records

Treatment records serve as documentation of the care the patients have received. They may be essential to the defense of a practitioner accused of negligence or malpractice.

One of the legal authorities in the field of medical malpractice and editor of a major text on the subject had the following to say about dental records: "Dentists seem to be among the worst record keepers. It is not unusual for the complete dental records to consist mainly or solely of a billing chart. Such scant records should be considered malpractice in and of themselves."[16]

The patient's dental record is considered by the courts as a legal document and must be treated as such. It serves many purposes in the judicial process. It contains information about the patient's complaint, health history, and basis for the diagnosis, and it reports all treatment rendered, the patient's reaction to treatment, and the results of the treatment. Case law requires that health practitioners keep accurate records of the diagnosis and treatment of their patients.[17] These records constitute an essential part of patient care. Treating a patient without maintaining accurate records is a serious departure from an acceptable level of care as defined by the courts. Some jurisdictions require that accurate records be kept as part of the rules and regulations of administrative health or licensing agencies.[18]

The outcome of many suits against dentists is decided on the content and quality of patient records. For the treating doctor the record is the only documentation of the course of treatment of the patient and the patient's reactions to the treatment. Memory alone is often viewed as self-serving, and, as often stated, "The shortest written word lasts longer than the longest memory." In cases in which the doctor and patient disagree on what took place and there is no written documentation of the event, the question of how much weight will be given to the oral statements may be determined in court by who makes the most credible witness. It can become a risky situation for the doctor.

In summary, failure to keep accurate records may constitute negligence and, in some jurisdictions, a violation of law. In addition, failure to keep accurate records markedly increases the chance of losing a malpractice suit.

The risk management rule is as follows: *Accurate and complete records must be maintained for each patient you treat or examine.*

RECORD OWNERSHIP

The right to ownership of the patient's treatment record has undergone considerable change during the past several decades. Courts have separated the physical record from the right of the patient to its contents. At one time doctors had the exclusive right to the possession of the record and its contents. Today, after many suits, the law has evolved so that the doctor is considered the custodian of the record and the patient has a property right in its contents.[19] Some jurisdictions have codified court decisions.

If the patient demands in writing to be sent a copy of the treatment record or demands that a copy be sent to another practitioner or to any other person or agency, the practitioner should comply with the request (in some jurisdictions, the practitioner must comply with the request), but, in either case, supply only copies. The term *record* includes the treatment record, radiographs, casts, results of tests, and consultation reports.

If the dentist believes that the patient, when demand is made for the record, intends litigation, the dentist should report the request to the insurance carrier after complying with the request. If no local law requires the dentist to comply with the request for copies of the record, the dentist should not comply unless the carrier approves in writing. If an attorney demands the record, the dentist should not comply without first informing the carrier. However, if the dentist does decide to comply, the attorney's demand should also include a written release from the patient. Should another dentist ask for a copy of the record, the original dentist should make certain that the request includes a written release from the patient.

Remember, in no case should the original records or radiographs be sent. The one exception is if the request is made by a court.

The risk management rules that are generated by the new view of the courts about the patients' rights to record ownership are as follows: *On the patients' written request for their records, comply but supply only copies. If you believe a patient intends to sue, before you comply contact your insurance carrier for advice.*

In some jurisdictions it is not required that a copy of the original records be given to a patient or to anyone designated by the patient. They require that only a summary of the treatment be provided. You are advised to check the local law. The risk management rule that the dentist retain the original of all patient records is underscored by what a California court said about a doctor's not producing the originals: "The inability of the physician to produce the original of the clinical record concerning his treatment of the plaintiff creates a strong inference of consciousness of guilt."[20]

FORM AND CONTENT

The changing law on ownership of patient records has had a profound effect on the form and content of the record. Keeping in mind that what is written on the record may be seen by the patient will serve as a guide to what should be entered on the record.

Financial information has no place on the treatment record. Separate records should be kept to record charges and payments.

The treatment record should be written in black ink or black ballpoint pen. It should be neat, well organized, and easily read. A sloppy record implies a sloppy dentist and has a negative effect on the jury and judge. Patient records, as all legal documents, should be legible and complete. There should be no blank spaces where information is supposed to be inserted. A decision by a New York court stated that a "patient record so sparse as to be accurate and meaningful only to the recording physician fails to meet the intent of the requirement to maintain records which accurately reflect the evaluation and treatment of the patient."[21] A later section of this chapter provides suggestions on the form and content of record keeping.

How long should patient records be retained? In many jurisdictions, laws specify the minimum time period for retention of patient treatment records. In New York, by rule, patient records are to be retained for at least 6 years, and records of a minor (below age 18) for at least 6 years, and until 1 year after the minor reaches age 21 years.[22] Failure to comply brings with it risk of allegations by a state agency of a violation of the law. On the civil side, practitioners are advised to keep the original treatment records for as long as possible. Although the statute of limitations runs for a specific period, the exceptions suggest that the records be kept for a period considerably longer than the statute. For example, in New York, an occurrence state (i.e., the statute of limitations begins to run from the time of the occurrence of the negligent incident), if you are accused of withholding information from a patient about a mishap in treatment, the courts may extend the statute on the basis of your fraudulent concealment. In Massachusetts, a discovery state (i.e., the statute of limitations does not begin to run until the patient discovered, or should have discovered, the act that produced the injury), the suit may begin many years after the patient completed treatment. Two thirds of the states have the discovery rule. The rest have the time-of-injury rule. But even in those states there are exceptions, which may include fraudulent concealment (noted previously), foreign body exception, and an exception for continuous treatment. In the case of minors, in many jurisdictions the statute on retention of records does not begin to run until the minor reaches majority. Therefore the records of minors must be kept for an extended period of time.

The appointment log, or book, is an integral and essential part of office records. It records appointments made for patients, either for consultation or treatment. It may serve the dentist well should the log accurately record not only the scheduled appointments but, in addition, late arrivals, canceled appointments, and no-shows. All entries on the log should be made in ink or ballpoint pen. Like the patient's treatment records, there should be no erasures obliterating original entries. Like the patient's treatment records, the appointment log should be kept for as long as possible—not discarded at the end of each year. Without records, it is virtually impossible to succeed in defending a suit.

The risk management rule is as follows: *Retain original patient treatment records, including radiographs, the appointment log, and all other documents related to the diagnosis and treatment of the patient, for as long as possible.*

RECORD-KEEPING RULES

1. Entries should be accurate, legible, and written in black ink or ballpoint pen.
2. In offices where more than one person is making entries, the entries should be signed or initialed. A sample of the initials and signatures of all persons who make entries on records should be maintained.
3. Entries that are in error should not be blocked out so that they cannot be read. Instead, a single line should be drawn through the entry and a note made above it stating "error in entry, see correction below." The correction should be dated at the time it is made.
4. Entries should be uniformly spaced on the form. There should be no unusual or irregular blank spaces. Always

write between the lines and never in the margins.

5. On health information forms there should be no blank spaces in the answers to health questions. If the question is inappropriate, draw a single line through the question, or record "not applicable" (NA) in the box. If the response is normal, write "within normal limits" (WNL).
6. Record all cancellations, late arrivals, and changes of appointments.
7. Document consents, including all risks and alternative treatments presented to the patient. Include any remarks made by the patient. Enter telephone conversations that relate to the care of the patient.
8. It is important to inform the patient of any adverse occurrences or untoward events that take place during the course of treatment and to note on the record that the patient was informed. If possible, have the patient initial or sign the entry.
9. Record all requests for consultations and their reports.
10. Document all conversations held with other health practitioners relating to the care of the patient.
11. All patient records should be retained for as long as possible.
12. If the practice is terminated, local law should be checked to determine the requirements on how, where, and in what form the records must be retained.
13. Guard confidentiality of information contained on the record.
14. Never surrender the original record to anyone, except by order of a court or to your own attorney. If you surrender the original record to your attorney, get a receipt.
15. Never tamper with a record once there is some indication that legal action is contemplated by the patient.
16. Keep patient records in a safe place (fireproof, waterproof, etc.).

WHAT NOT TO PUT ON THE TREATMENT RECORD

1. Financial information should not be kept on the treatment record. Use a separate financial form.
2. Do not record subjective evaluations, such as your opinion about the patient's mental health, on the treatment record unless you are qualified and licensed to make such evaluation. Record such observations on a separate sheet marked "Confidential—Personal notes." In most jurisdictions such notes are not discoverable, and the practitioner is not required to deliver them when a request is made for the records.
3. Do not record any correspondence with your professional liability insurance company, your attorney, or the attorney representing a patient on the treatment record. Record all such notes and any conversations with these individuals on a separate sheet marked "Confidential—Personal notes."

HISTORIES

MEDICAL HISTORY

An area of growing concern for dentists in malpractice liability relates to the health history. Major financial and professional losses have been caused by the dentist's failure to discover information about the patient's medical history. The primary cause of the problem is the design of the typical self-administered health history form and the manner in which the dentist deals with the completed form. The form used by most dentists has led to considerable difficulties. The most common has two columns in which patients may indicate whether they have a particular health problem. They are asked to place a checkmark in a "yes" or "no" box or to circle a "yes" or "no" word. In many cases there have been disputes at trial about who placed the checkmark or circle, notwithstanding the fact that the patient signed the form. Facts in dispute lead to problems for the defense attorney in the trial of a case. Questions have been raised as to whether a question on the health history form can ask if the patient has AIDS or is HIV positive. Currently there appears to be no problem related to asking the question provided it is asked of all patients and the answer is not used to refuse care to the patient. If the refusal to treat is based on other medical or dental considerations there would be no violation of any antidiscrimination laws.

The risk management rule is as follows: *If you use a self-administered health history form in which patients are to respond by marking a box, have them initial the appropriate box rather than using a checkmark.*

Other problems have arisen with the self-administered health history form. Did the patient understand the questions? Did the patient know the answer at the time the form was completed? Was the patient aware of the importance of the question to care? If the answer to any of these questions is no, the patient may leave a blank in place of an answer or may provide an answer that is not accurate. Blanks left on a completed history form may lead to difficulties: was the question ignored or was the answer negative? If a self-administered health form is used, there should be four columns instead of two, to avoid a possibility of blanks. The column headings should be "Yes," "No," "Don't Know," and "Don't Understand the Question."

Another problem is related to the manner in which the dentist follows up the self-administered health history. It is usual for the dentist to question the patient further, but the dentist usually limits the questioning to the positive answers on the form. Most forms are designed to alert the dentist solely to the positive answers. This process may lead to major errors. The patient may have misinterpreted or not understood the question and incorrectly answered in the negative. This has resulted in large malpractice losses. Several cases have been reported in which the dentist, using a "yes-no" form, failed to discover that the patient had a history of rheumatic fever and thus took no precautions in treatment. Do not leave it to patients to decide whether the answers to the questions on the health history are important to the success and safety of their care.

The risk management rule is as follows: *If you use a self-administered health history form and the choices to the patient are two—"yes" or "no"—follow up on the "no" answers as well as the "yes" answers to make certain the patient understood the questions, their importance in treatment, and the reason the questions were being asked.*

The best policy for the use of a self-administered health history form is not to use it. It leaves too much to chance in discovering medical problems that may compromise the successful and safe treatment of the patient. There is much more at stake than legal liability. When a history of rheumatic fever is not discovered, no matter who is at fault, the consequences to the patient and the dentist may be disastrous.

A more effective way to determine medical history is to have the history taken by someone who has been trained in the procedure and who has the background to interpret the responses—preferably, the treating dentist. If the history is elicited by someone other than the treating dentist, the dentist should review the history with the patient before treatment.

Another type of history-taking form is simple to design. Use a blank sheet of paper with a reminder list of the questions to be asked in the left margin. It is better to spend the extra time this takes than to have a patient, because of your negligence, suffer permanent injury as a result of the use of an inadequately designed form.

UPDATING THE MEDICAL HISTORY

Good dental practice requires that the patient's health history be updated at regular intervals. The frequency with which it should be done is a professional, not a legal, decision. The process is simple and effective: allow the patient to review the documented health history that was obtained at the last history-taking visit and ask if there are any changes. Make notes of the procedure and the patient's responses in the patient's record. An abbreviated history update form is simple to design. For example, the form may state the following: "I have reviewed the health history form completed on _____ , and I report the following: _____ ." If there has been no change, the patient writes "No change." If there is a change, the patient so indicates on the form. At times, depending on the nature of the change, the dentist may ask the patient to complete another full health history form.

The risk management rule is as follows: *Update the health history at appropriate intervals and document the process and responses.*

If you continue to use a self-administered health history form, place the following statement before the space for the patient's signature: "I understand and agree that in the event there is any change in my health status, I will notify your office at the earliest possible time." As an express term in the doctor-patient contract it places some of the burden on the patient but will not entirely relieve the doctor of the responsibility for updating the health status of the patient. Follow up on positive findings. It is essential to good patient care and to risk management concerns that positive findings in the medical history be followed up by consulting the patient's physician or another appropriate health provider or health facility. It is best to have consultant reports in writing. If this is inconvenient, information received by telephone should be noted on the patient's record.

The risk management rule is as follows: *Document all conversations with other health practitioners and health facilities that are or were involved in the treatment of your patient and from whom you received information. If you receive a written report, it should be placed in the patient's treatment folder.*

THE DENTAL HISTORY

The dental history presents fewer problems to the dentist than does the general health history. However, one issue not as yet addressed by the courts deserves attention. Dental disease is chronic, and almost everyone suffers from it. It does not begin when the patient comes to the dentist. Most patients change dentists several times throughout their lives. To have a complete picture of the etiology of the patient's current dental problem and the history of the treatment, it is essential that, in addition to the dental history obtained from the patient, the treating dentist should make every effort to obtain the records of the previous dentist(s). It is possible that the previous dentist's notes may assist in the treatment of the patient in areas such as an abnormal reaction to the administration of a drug, the level of patient cooperation, breaking of appointments, and delinquencies in the payment of fees. Not obtaining information that is available and that may be essential in the treatment of the patient may support an allegation of malpractice.

A good risk management practice is as follows: Whenever possible, obtain the records and radiographs of prior dentists and other health care providers who have treated your patient. Determine whether state law enables patients to secure copies of their records and radiographs, and, if such a law is present, use it to obtain the records rather than making a direct request. If you decide to make a direct request, make it in writing and include an authorization signed by the patient to release the records.

Examining the Patient and Completing a Treatment Plan

"Failure to diagnose" represents a growing area of legal vulnerability. A thorough clinical examination and radiographic review should be completed on each patient. The results should be recorded on the patient's record.

It is difficult to defend a case successfully when many of the questions on the form used to record the dental examination have been left blank. It is impossible to determine whether the blank indicates that the question was mistakenly omitted in the examination or if the result was within normal limits. If the form you use has questions that are not germane to your practice habits or are seldom answered, design your own form or purchase one that is more suited to your particular needs and habits of practice.

Many recent cases involve failure to diagnose periodontal disease. Periodontal issues present a major problem if there is no evidence that the patient was examined to determine periodontal needs, for example, pocket depth, plaque scores, bleeding points, mobility, or oral hygiene index. The answers to the following questions may become important if a suit alleging periodontal neglect is brought against the dentist: If periodontal disease was diagnosed, was the patient informed? Was the need for periodontal care neglected? Was a recommendation made for the patient to seek the services of a periodontist? In summary, was there failure to diagnose, failure to inform, failure to make a timely referral, or failure to treat? If the answer to any of the questions is positive, the dentist is at risk of an allegation of malpractice and is likely to lose the suit.

Issues related to the temporomandibular joint (TMJ) and surrounding tissues have become a target of litigation. The same questions raised about periodontal neglect apply equally to the joint, and the same risks in practice apply. The area of the joint should be examined and monitored during treatment. Problems may arise during orthodontic care, after the extraction of lower molars, and after procedures that require the jaws to remain open for long periods of time, such as the use of a rubber dam for an extended period of time during endodontic procedures. In a recent appellate court decision the court stated that all reversible and conservative forms of therapy to correct problems related to the TMJ should be ruled out as ineffective before surgery is performed. In that case, after multiple surgeries the patient, a 26-year-old woman, committed suicide.[23]

Acceptable dental practice includes presenting both a recommended treatment plan and a patient-accepted reasonable alternative. Either have the patient sign or initial the final plan or make a note of the patient's acceptance in the record.

Good risk management practice includes the following: *Complete a thorough dental examination and treatment plan before treatment is begun. The results should be accurately recorded, and all questions on the dental examination form should be answered. There should be documentation that the treatment plan was accepted by the patient.*

CONSENT

Legal problems related to lack of informed consent to dental care began to surface as a result of the explosion in medical malpractice in the early 1970s. The general principle that a doctor who treats a patient without the patient's express consent is guilty of an unauthorized touching, for which the doctor can be held liable to the patient in damages, began early in the twentieth century.[24] The fact that the patient needed the treatment and benefited as a result of the treatment did not relieve the doctor of liability. In the early years the civil claim was that the doctor was guilty of trespass to the person, or assault and battery. Today the courts have ruled that the legal action of malpractice is more appropriate, given the lack of intent to harm by the doctor. The legal procedure is different if the action is brought in trespass compared with actions brought in malpractice. In addition, many courts opined that the failure to obtain the consent of the patient before initiating treatment was a breach of the doctor-patient contract. Actions in contract law differ in procedure from both trespass actions and malpractice actions. The modern view is that if no consent was obtained the action may be in contract. However, if the consent was obtained but was faulty, as most of them are, the action in malpractice is more appropriate. The defendant dentist benefits if the action is in malpractice rather than in trespass or contract. In trespass and contract actions the patient-plaintiff is not required to produce an expert witness relating to the standard of professional care and whether the defendant dentist departed from the standard. In malpractice actions an expert testifying on behalf of the patient-plaintiff is required. Malpractice insurance policies rarely, if ever, cover allegations of breach of contract or trespass (assault and battery).

CONTENT OF CONSENT: WHAT AND HOW MUCH TO TELL

Having discussed the legal form of action, we now turn our attention to the content of the consent. As the years progressed since the first major case dealing with the consent to medical care, the courts turned their attention to the issue of whether the consent was informed: Was the patient given enough information on which to make an intelligent decision? The modern view is that the patient must be informed of all the following:

1. A description of the proposed treatment
2. The material or foreseeable risks
3. The benefits and prognosis of the proposed treatment
4. All reasonable alternatives to the proposed treatment
5. The risks, benefits, and prognosis of the alternative treatments

All these factors must be described to the patient in language the patient understands, and the patient must be given an opportunity to ask questions about the treatment and alternatives and to have the questions answered.

WHAT OF THE DESCRIPTION OF THE RISKS?

How much of the risk must be told to the patient for consent to meet the test of being informed? There is no agreement among state courts on which to present a bottom-line rule. In most states the patient must be given enough information about the risks to make an intelligent decision about whether to proceed with the proposed treatment. This is called the subjective prudent person rule. Another standard is whether a reasonable person in the patient's situation was given enough information to make an intelligent decision. This is called the objective reasonable person rule. In both rules the risks are termed *material* because they are material either to the patient or to the reasonable person. The third standard is the professional community standard; that is, what do other practitioners tell their patients about the risks when the same condition exists? These risks are termed *foreseeable.* As an example, in a state that follows the professional community standard, a dentist would not have to explain the risk of breaking an instrument in a canal during an endodontic procedure if it can be shown that few, if any, dentists in the community warn their patients of the possibility. In a reasonable-person state, whether objective or subjective, a dentist may not be required to inform an 80-year-old retiree of the possibility of permanent paresthesia after the extraction of an impacted lower third molar because the risk is not material to the patient or to any reasonable person in the same situation as the patient; the risk is not material. However, if the same dental situation is present when the patient is a trial lawyer, the risk becomes material and should be told to the patient before treatment is begun.

In material-risk states the patient-plaintiff is not required to present the evidence of an expert dentist. In foreseeable-risk states the patient-plaintiff is required to produce an expert witness for the judge or jury to determine the standard of disclosure of the professional community. Thus the burden on the patient-plaintiff in professional-community (foreseeable-risk) states is greater than that in reasonable-person (material-risk) states.

Many states have adopted statutes, administrative rules, or court procedural rules, superimposed on court decisions, that may have modified their courts' decisions. However, all fall within the standards described previously.

The prudent dentist will tell each patient both the foreseeable and the material risks. This approach will satisfy all court-imposed and BLL (i.e., statutes, administrative rules, and regulations) standards. Thus the dentist is advised to inform each patient faced with the extraction of an impacted lower third molar of the risk of permanent paresthesia regardless of who the patient is, the educational level, age, occupation, or whatever, no matter what the dentist believes other dentists tell their patients.

Another issue relating to what the patient should be told is the "common knowledge" doctrine. The patient should be aware of certain risks, by common knowledge, without having to be told by the dentist. All reasonable adults are expected to know that after the extraction of a tooth they will have some bleeding and, when the anesthetic wears off, some pain and possibly swelling. By contrast, no reasonable person would expect to have permanent loss of sensation of the lower lip after the extraction of an impacted lower wisdom tooth. However, the admonition is not to rely on common knowledge in describing the risks of the proposed procedure.

The risk management rules are as follows: *Tell the patient everything about what you recommend and the reasonable alternatives. Use language the patient understands. Give the patient an opportunity to ask questions, and provide answers. Document the entire process.*

FORM OF CONSENT: WRITTEN OR ORAL?

Consent to health care, like all agreements between parties, may be written or oral, and the terms may be expressed or implied. An expressed consent is one in which both parties agree, either orally or in written form. An implied consent is present either by the action of the parties or by law. Expressed and implied consents are discussed in the next section. Here we focus our attention on written and oral consents. As long as there is no dispute between the parties as to the details of the agreement, an oral agreement is effective and enforceable. Only when the parties disagree as to the details of the agreement does a written document become important. In general, laws that require agreements (contracts) to be written do not directly affect dental care. These include agreements relating to real property, contracts of sale over a specified amount, and contracts that cannot be completed within 1 year. They fall into a legal category called the "statute of frauds" and must be written to be enforceable. Oral agreements that involve orthodontic care and that extend for more than 1 year have been declared exceptions to the written rule. They are considered agreements per visit.

In a few situations the law requires that consent to health care be in writing and signed by the patient. Health facilities such as hospitals may require that the consent to treatment be written and signed by each patient. If you work in such a facility, you should comply with the rules and obtain the written and signed consent of each patient you treat in the facility. Failure to do so may compromise your legal position, and that of the institution, if a patient claims that you proceeded with treatment without valid consent. Other than institutional rules, few regulations require written consent to health care. Most refer to abortions, to donation of human organs, in New York to acupuncture, in some jurisdictions to HIV testing, and in others to surgical procedures. Recently a Pennsylvania court declared endodontic therapy surgical and thus held the procedure to the law requiring that the consent be in writing.[25] You should check the local law to determine whether, for the treatment you propose, consent must be written and signed. Also, you should check to see whether local law requires that you include specific information informing the patient about the treatment you propose.

As a general rule, despite the absence of any law requiring that consent be written, you should have documentation that a valid consent was obtained for a procedure that has high risks or is invasive. The best documentation is to have a written and signed consent to care that contains all the elements required for it to be valid. The problem is that without a written document there may be conflicting testimony as to exactly what the dentist informed the patient about the procedure and its attendant risks and exactly to what the patient agreed. In nonemergent situations where surgery is to be performed, it is best to allow patients to take consent forms home before signing, to allow the patient time to discuss the matter with family or friends. Your records should indicate that this was done and that the consent was discussed before treatment was begun.

FORM OF CONSENT: IMPLIED OR EXPRESSED?

In some dental practice situations implied consent may serve as an effective defense for the dentist. In simple, common, noninvasive procedures implied consent is likely to be supported by the courts. A routine dental examination is a good example of one in which the dentist does not have to rely on a written signed consent. Another situation is one in which the patient understands what is being done and makes no attempt to interrupt the procedure. In both situations consent is implied by the action of the party. However, if the procedure is invasive or the risks are great and likely to occur, written consent may prepare the patient for the possible consequences and serve to defuse a lawsuit.

In an emergency situation in which care must be rendered at once and consent of the patient could not be obtained, consent is implied by law, as compared with the previous situation in which consent is implied by the action of the party. Courts have applied the following test to support consent implied by law in an emergency situation: (1) consent would have been granted had the patient been able to do so; (2) a reasonable person in the patient's condition would have granted consent; and (3) an emergency was present in which treatment was necessary and time was of the essence to preserve the life or health of the victim. This legal theory is present in Good Samaritan situations; consent is implied by law.

WHO SHOULD OBTAIN CONSENT?

As a general rule the health provider is the person charged with obtaining consent to care. However, in practice, others associated with the office or institution in which the care is provided are assigned the responsibility to obtain consent. Two recent court cases, one in Pennsylvania and the other in New York, stated that anyone designated and trained by the provider may obtain a valid consent to care.[26,27] Despite the rulings, the dentist is advised to review the consent document with the patient; offer to answer any questions concerning the procedure and its risks, benefits, and alternatives; and note on the patient's record that this was done.

The risk management rule is as follows: *Before beginning any treatment procedure that requires consent, make certain that a valid consent was obtained.*

WHO MAY GRANT CONSENT?

As a general rule, only the recipient of care may grant a valid consent. As with all general rules, there are exceptions. The most obvious is that minors cannot grant valid consent for their health care. Only a minor's parent or legal guardian can grant a valid consent for the care of the minor—not the minor's adult sibling, not a neighbor, not even a grandparent who supports and pays for the care of the grandchild, and not the child's schoolteacher. However, the parent may grant to any of these people authority to consent to health care for the minor child. The authorization should be written and signed by the parent for the dentist to rely on the authorization.

The obvious question is, When does a minor become an adult? Most states set the majority age at 18 years. There are exceptions. The age at which a minor may grant a valid consent to health care may be established by state statute. It may be as low as 14 years. In addition, many states have defined an "emancipated minor" in contract law and extended it to include consent to health care. In general, an emancipated minor is one no longer dependent on parents for support. In addition, pregnant minors are emancipated, as are married minors. The net result is that emancipated minors may grant a valid consent to health care independent of parental consent. Who pays for the service has no effect on the consent to care. Payment for it is a separate issue; the parent may consent to the payment, but the emancipated minor must consent to the care.

In the case of divorced or separated parents, either may consent to the care of the child, unless there is a modification of the custody agreement. Again, payment is a separate issue, but it may be part of the custody agreement.

Keeping in mind that only the patient can grant a valid consent to health care, a husband cannot grant a valid consent to the care of his wife despite her inability to do so, nor can an adult for an elderly parent. In either case the spouse or adult child of the elderly parent must be appointed the legal guardian of the patient.

In the case of a mentally impaired adult, in some states consent granted by the parent may not be valid unless the parent is designated by the court as the patient's legal guardian. In others, a mentally impaired adult may be considered a minor and the rules of consent to the health care of minors apply. Check the local law of the state in which you practice.

TELEPHONE CONSENT

Telephone consent, properly executed, is acceptable to the courts. It must, however, contain all the elements that constitute a valid consent. In addition, it must be properly documented. In the case of a minor, the parent or guardian should be contacted by phone and told that a third party is listening on an extension. The parent should be told of the situation and the need for treatment, including all the facts that would be required to meet a valid consent. After the consent is obtained, appropriate notes should be made on the patient's chart, signed by the person who obtained the consent and countersigned by the third party.

SUMMARY OF CONSENT

A summary of consent as it relates to risk management is found in Box 17-1.

INFORMED REFUSAL

A new legal concept appears to be developing in the arena of malpractice litigation as an outgrowth of informed consent: informed refusal. In a medical malpractice case a woman was advised to undergo a Papanicolaou (Pap) smear. She did not follow the advice of her physician despite his repeated reminders over a period of several years. Later cervical cancer developed and the woman died. The physician was sued for failing to sufficiently inform the patient of the consequences of her refusal. Several members of the court, a minority, opined that the patient must be told of the possible consequences of refusal to make an intelligent decision in refusing a recommended course of treatment.[28] Thus the concept of informed refusal is gradually emerging.

If a practitioner recommends to a patient that surgery is the best course of treatment, the patient must be informed of the consequences of refusal. If the patient refuses the care and later has an injury because of not having the surgery performed, the practitioner may be liable to the patient in damages because the patient was not informed of the consequences of the refusal. The refusal, or the negligence of the patient to follow the advice of the practitioner, should be documented (along with the information that the patient was informed of the consequences of noncompliance) in the patient's record or on a form specially designed to record such information.

The risk management rule relating to the refusal of a patient to follow professional advice is as follows: *Document that the patient was informed about the best course of action to*

BOX 17-1

Consent: A Risk Management Guide

1. In general, the more invasive the procedure or the greater the risk, the more the requirements of a valid consent must be met; documentation that consent was obtained becomes important. For example, to obtain consent for an examination in which no invasive procedure is to be performed, it might be that implied consent by the actions of the patient is sufficient with little or no documentation on the patient's record. By contrast, in a situation where an invasive procedure is to be performed, all the requirements of a valid consent should be met, and documentation in the patient's record is essential.
2. The better the documentation, the less the legal risk. Written forms may be used, provided that the delivery of the form is linked to the patient's awareness by sufficient notes made on the patient's record, such as "Patient given handout number _____ to read, the proposed treatment and alternatives were discussed, and all the patient's questions were answered."
3. Make certain that the person from whom consent is obtained has legal standing to grant consent.
4. When consent for the treatment of a minor is obtained by telephone, it is best to follow up on the telephone conversation by sending a written consent in the mail to be signed by the parent or guardian and then returned to the office.
5. Check the local law to determine if written consent is required in situations related to specific treatment.
6. If you delegate to anyone in your office the responsibility to obtain consent from a patient, document that the person was trained in obtaining consent and that you reviewed the consent, discussed it with the patient, and answered all the patient's questions about the procedure.
7. Make certain that in obtaining the consent all elements to make the consent valid are included: a description of the procedure; why it is necessary; an estimate of the anticipated success; the prognosis if the procedure is not done; the foreseeable and material risks in having it done; and alternatives to the recommended procedure, including their risks, benefits, and prognoses. Present this in language the patient understands (use lay terms), and give the patient an opportunity to discuss all these topics with you. By describing the material risks and the foreseeable risks all bases are covered to satisfy any local law or court decision.
8. When the treatment includes an invasive procedure, it is best to allow the patient to take the consent form home before signing it.

take to preserve or improve his or her oral health and about the likely consequences if the advice is not followed.

Emergencies and the Good Samaritan Law

The Good Samaritan law, enacted in all states, provides immunity from suit for specified health practitioners who render emergency aid to victims of accidents. All such laws require that the aid be provided with no expectation of financial remuneration. Should an injury result from negligence, the victim is precluded by law from instituting a suit, provided there was no evidence of gross negligence. *Gross negligence* is defined as a wanton disregard for another's safety or the failure to exercise slight care. Immunity does not extend to acts performed in the office or in any health facility. The standard to which the Good Samaritan is held is based on education and experience. Not all states include dentists in the Good Samaritan law.

The risk management rule is as follows: *Determine whether the jurisdiction in which you practice includes dentists in the Good Samaritan law.* Be guided by the answer in rendering emergency aid at the scene of an accident, but keep in mind there are ethical responsibilities that attach to your role as a health professional.

An *emergency* is defined as any situation in which care must be provided at once to preserve the life or health of the patient. Because the interpretation is broad in most states, dental care may fall within the definition. In cases where a dental emergency exists and consent cannot be obtained because of a time constraint, consent to care is implied by operation of law.

The risk management rule in dealing with emergencies in which a minor is brought to the office by someone other than a parent is as follows: *Efforts should be made to obtain the consent of the parent before treatment is begun. These efforts should be accurately recorded on the record. If consent was obtained by telephone, the third party should sign the record following the note.*

One of the duties owed by the dentist to patients of record, by case law, and in some jurisdictions by BLL, is to make care available to patients in emergency situations. Generally the patient determines what constitutes an emergency.

The risk management rule in emergency situations for patients of record is as follows: *The availability of care is a 24-hour-a-day, 7-day-a-week responsibility.* If you are on vacation or otherwise unavailable, someone must cover for you, and that information must be made available to your patients. The most effective way to do this is with a message left on your answering machine or with a member of your staff who is available.

MISCELLANEOUS ISSUES

PACKAGE INSERTS

Inserts in drug packaging have been accepted into evidence in malpractice cases. Dentists and physicians have been found guilty of negligence for not following the warnings contained on the package inserts. Statements contained in the *Physicians' Desk Reference* (PDR) have also been admitted into evidence.[29]

The risk management rule is as follows: *Read all drug package inserts and the PDR before administering or prescribing a drug. Because inserts and the PDR are updated frequently, they should be consulted regularly.*

WHAT TO DO WHEN DOCTORS DISAGREE

Situations may arise in which the treating dentist and the patient's physician disagree on what prophylactic measures should be taken with a cardiac-compromised patient or other patient situations. The physician may recommend that no preventive measures be taken or that measures be taken that are not consistent with those the dentist believes are appropriate. If the physician's advice is followed and an injury results, it is difficult for the dentist to claim immunity on the basis of the physician's recommendation. The patient is a patient of the dentist, and the dentist operates on his or her own license. Dentists are not employees of physicians, nor are they required to carry out a physician's orders if they believe the orders are not consistent with the patient's needs. Whatever care is rendered by a dentist to the patient is interpreted as what the dentist, in her or his best judgment, thinks should be done.

If the dentist does not follow the advice of the physician and an injury occurs, the dentist will be judged on what other dentists in the community would do under similar circumstances and not on what the physician recommended. If the dentist's care meets acceptable community standards, there may be no liability.

If the patient demands that the physician's advice be followed by the dentist and the dentist believes that the advice is not in the best interests of the patient's health, the best course for the dentist to follow is to refuse to treat the patient, based on the principle of level of legal risk. When information about a patient's health is asked of the patient's physician, or a recommendation as to treatment is sought by the dentist, the request and the physician's response should be written. If the physician refuses to submit a written report, the dentist should enter statements made by the physician on the patient's record immediately after the conversation.

The risk management rule is as follows: *Exercise your own judgment when deciding on the dental care of the patient. Use advice by others, including physicians, as recommendations that you may either accept or reject. The final decision as to what is done is yours and the patient's.*

Associates and Employees

Several important legal issues are involved with associates and employees of the dentist. Those with an impact on legal vulnerability are discussed in this section. It is important for dentists to be aware that the more complex the arrangements of practice, the more exposure there is to legal entanglements.

Associations in practice may take many forms, some of which increase legal risk. The employer-employee relationship between dentists makes the employer-dentist individually or jointly liable for the negligent acts of the employee dentist. The legal doctrine for this transfer of liability to the employer, an innocent party, is known as respondeat superior (the person in the superior position, the employer, must answer for the acts of the one in the inferior position, the employee, to injured third parties). It is a form of vicarious liability (the substitution of an innocent party for a guilty one in the matter of liability to third parties). However, the employer may sue the employee for indemnification of the employer's losses. If both are insured by the same professional liability insurance company, complications may be avoided.

The same principle of respondeat superior applies to all employees of the dentist, including other dentists, hygienists, dental assistants, receptionists, and others. The employer-dentist is held liable for all acts performed by an employee in the course of conducting the business of the employer-dentist, even if the acts are specifically prohibited or illegal.

Another form of associate practice among dentists is the partnership. All partners are individually and jointly liable for the negligent acts of one partner. The choice of whom to sue is exercised by the plaintiff or the plaintiff's attorney. If a generalist, who is at low risk, has a partner who practices oral and maxillofacial surgery, which is of high risk, the generalist may be held liable for the negligent acts of the surgeon. It is not unusual for all partners to be joined in the suit. Vicarious liability is supported by the legal theory that all partners are united in interest (each benefits from the acts of others). To avoid serious complications, all should be covered by the same professional liability insurance company. From the standpoint of legal liability for negligent acts, practicing in a partnership agreement brings with it serious risks. In several cases, courts have stated that if the patient considers the practice to be a partnership, the courts will treat it as such, even if the agreement among a group of dentists is to practice as solo and independent practitioners. If they engage in sharing to the extent that the arrangement appears to be a partnership, they may take on the liability risks of a partnership.

The third form of association is the professional corporation. This relationship represents the lowest level of the transfer or sharing of legal risk. Except in unusual circumstances, innocent shareholders are not liable for the negligent acts of other shareholders. Only the guilty practitioner and the corporation are liable. However, all shareholders and the corporation should be insured by the same professional liability insurance company.

All states have enacted legislation to enable businesses to enter into a new form of legal entity, the limited liability company, designated as the LLC (or the L.L.C.). It has all the advantages of the traditional corporation as it relates to liability, or lack of shared liability of "innocent parties." Dentists may form an LLC, known as a professional limited liability company, or PLLC. Currently, two states permit a single dentist to form a PLLC: Texas and New York. In the future, other states may permit solo practitioners to form a PLLC. The advantage of an LLC over a corporation is that it is considerably less costly to form and maintain.

The independent contractor (IC) is the final form of association to be considered. With this arrangement, the principal hopes to avoid liability for the negligent acts of the IC. The courts examine, in detail, the arrangement between the parties before determining whether the principal is free from liability for the negligent acts of the IC. The matter of control of the ICs, who sets the hours for the IC, whose patients they are, who hires and pays auxiliary personnel, and who provides the equipment and supplies used by the IC are all questions that determine whether the IC is truly an IC or simply an employee in determining the liability of the principal (employer). Having the same professional liability insurance company prevents many complications. Recent court decisions have examined whether a dentist working with another under the cloak of an IC for the principal to avoid withholding a portion of the IC's earnings and the payment of unemployment and workers' compensation taxes was consistent with the law. The decisions reached clearly point out that such an arrangement is employer-employee. The rules to qualify as an IC are many and complex. The principal is at risk and will be penalized, not the bogus IC.[30]

The lowest level of legal risk in associateship practice is to practice as a professional corporation or as a professional limited liability company, and, in any form of joint practice, for all parties to be insured by the same professional liability insurance carrier. Before you agree to join another dentist or group as an IC, check the law.

The acts or statements made by nondentist employees present forms of legal risks to the employer-dentist other than those described previously. Employees of a dentist are treated by the courts as agents of the dentist when they are serving in the capacity for which they were employed. Thus if a receptionist, hygienist, or assistant assures a patient that after treatment the patient will be satisfied with the result or makes other such statements related to the services provided by the employer-dentist, an express guarantee has been made to which the dentist will likely be held.

The risk management advice is as follows: *Educate your employees to the precise role they are to play in communicating and dealing with patients. Supervise them carefully and monitor their activities at regular intervals. Remain current on changes in the law that affect dental auxiliaries.*

Interpersonal Relationships

A deterioration in good interpersonal relations between patient and dentist or between patient and staff still ranks as one of the leading causes of malpractice allegations. When a patient becomes angry, upset, or frustrated, instituting a lawsuit is one of the methods available for retaliation against the dentist or the dentist's staff. The resulting annoyance to the dentist may be reason enough to sue, regardless of the merits of the claim. For the patient, it works. For the dentist, it becomes a real problem involving time, effort, emotional distress, and at times dollars. Too often, efforts of the auxiliary staff made in the interest of shielding the dentist from complaints of difficult patients or patients with annoying problems result in a patient seeking redress through the courts. Most of these situations can be defused by an understanding and compassionate staff. The dentist must be accessible to patients, particularly to those with perceived problems. The judgment of the staff as to what is important to the patient should not be substituted for the patient's judgment of what is important.

The risk management advice is as follows: *Monitor the staff in their interpersonal relationships with patients. Listen to your patients. Make certain that patients with problems have access to you. Do not hide from your patients. Arrange for substitute care when you are absent for extended periods. If all efforts fail to restore a cordial relationship with a difficult patient, the safest course to follow is to discontinue treatment.*

Return of a Fee and Suing to Collect One

At one time, courts viewed the return of a fee by a doctor as an admission of wrongdoing. Today, it is viewed as an expression of good faith and interest in the welfare of the patient. If the return of a fee, or part of it, will appease a hostile patient and defuse a difficult situation, it is best to do so. With a patient who threatens to sue unless the fee is returned, and the dentist decides to return the fee, it is best to have the patient execute a release-from-liability form with acceptance of the returned fee. You should weigh the refusal to return the fee with the trauma and loss of time in defending a claim of malpractice; you might even lose the case.

At one time the return of a fee, no matter what the amount, by a health practitioner to a patient had to be reported to the National Practitioners Data Bank. On interpretation of the law by an administrative law judge, the reporting requirement was declared not to include private practitioners. Thus a dentist who returns a fee to a patient is not required to report it to the National Practitioners Data Bank.

One of the major causes of malpractice allegations is a response to an attempt by a doctor to collect a fee. Patients who are delinquent or who refuse to pay are inclined to claim poor quality of care as the reason. Should the doctor press to collect, especially through the courts, the patient is likely to countersue for malpractice. Weighing the risk of a countersuit in malpractice should be a guide before suing to collect the fee. If the dentist uses a collection agency to act on his or her behalf for fee collection, all correspondence sent to a patient should be reviewed. Usually there is more at stake for the practitioner than the fee.

The risk management advice is as follows: *Think of what might be prevented if a fee is returned and of the possible consequences if a suit is instituted to collect a fee. Do not let pride and principle interfere with making a practical decision. If you return a fee, insist that the patient execute a release-from-liability form.*

Current Targets in Malpractice Litigation

The traditional problems leading to allegations of malpractice are still with us: ill-fitting dentures and extraction of wrong teeth. The ill-fitting denture problem is often linked with statements made by the dentist that constitute guarantees of satisfaction or serviceability (see the section on guarantees earlier in this chapter). Most wrong-tooth extraction cases are the result of poor office practices and, in situations that involve oral and maxillofacial surgeons, with inadequate communication with the referring dentist.

Over the past several years new grounds of vulnerability have been discovered by patients and their attorneys. In addition, risks have increased because of the introduction of new and more sophisticated techniques into dental practice. New, fertile grounds of litigation include the following:

1. Failures in treating problems related to the TMJ
2. Failures associated with implants
3. Failure to diagnose, monitor, treat, or refer (particularly periodontal disease and TMJ dysfunctions)
4. Failure to obtain the informed consent of the patient by not informing the patient of the risk of failure and its consequences (particularly endodontics and orthodontics)
5. Failure to take necessary precautions (rubber dam, use of assistants, etc.) to prevent mechanical injuries to the patient, such as aspiration of foreign bodies (crowns and instruments) and lacerated soft tissues
6. Continuing to treat when the dentist is aware that the result will not be satisfactory, for example, in orthodontics when the patient is not cooperating in home care
7. Failure to identify a patient with a compromised medical history, such as rheumatic fever, heart murmur, or allergies
8. Failure to take precautions to protect a patient having a compromised medical condition, for example, to prevent subacute bacterial endocarditis
9. Performing a service at the insistence of the patient that is not in the best interest of the patient and will not produce acceptable results, such as treating periodontal disease that should be treated by a specialist; the same holds true in oral surgical cases
10. Not performing a service, at the insistence of the patient, that should be performed before certain treatment is undertaken, for example, radiographs before any treatment and periodontal care by a specialist before fabrication of fixed prostheses
11. Failure to inform the patient about the risk of paresthesia after surgical procedures
12. Failure to provide follow-up care after surgery, for example, abandonment

13. Failure to consult the patient's physician when the patient's health is compromised.

The risks are significantly increased for failure to maintain adequate records or remain current with new advances in the profession. Deteriorating interpersonal relationships between patient and dentist or patient and office staff and attempts by the dentist to collect the fee may be causes of the patient seeking redress in the courts.

What to Do and What Not to Do If You Are Sued

If a patient threatens you in writing with a suit, if you receive a letter threatening suit from an attorney representing a patient, or if you receive a summons, the following precautionary measures apply.

THINGS TO DO

1. At the earliest time after receiving the letter or summons, report it to your insurance carrier by telephone.
2. Make a copy of the papers and send the originals to your carrier; use certified mail, signed receipt requested. Include a copy of any envelope that contained the papers.
3. Write a summary of the treatment of the patient using the treatment record to refresh your memory. Include everything you recall, even if it is not on the record. Sign and date the summary.
4. Make a copy of the records, including radiographs, reports, and the summary. Lock the originals in a safe place.
5. Tell your staff about the suit and instruct them not to talk, without obtaining your permission, to anyone asking questions about the case.
6. Cooperate with your insurance carrier and the attorney assigned by it to your case.

THINGS NOT TO DO

1. Do not tell the patient or the patient's representative that you are insured.
2. Do not agree to or offer a settlement.
3. Do not agree to or offer to pay for a specialist's services without first consulting with your carrier or the attorney assigned to your case.
4. Do not alter your records in any way.
5. Do not lose or misplace any of your records.
6. Do not discuss the case, or the treatment of the patient, with anyone except representatives of your insurance company or the attorney assigned to your case.
7. Do not admit fault or guilt to anyone.
8. Do not contact any other practitioner about the case, even if the practitioner has written a report.
9. Do not agree to appoint or treat the patient-plaintiff during the course of the action.

On Being a Witness

In a case alleging malpractice a dentist may be a fact witness, an expert witness, or a defendant. However, some general rules apply to all who appear as a witness at trial: (1) dress properly; (2) do not be professionally arrogant; (3) face the jury when answering a question; (4) answer questions directly with either "Yes," "No," "I don't know," or "I don't understand the question; please repeat it"; (5) do not elaborate unless asked for a narrative; (6) do not be baited into an argument with either the lawyers or the judge; (7) wait before answering to give yourself time to think about the question and your answer and to give your lawyer time to object to the question; and (8) always tell the truth. A fact witness is at trial to recite the facts as the witness found them, not to render an opinion as to the standard to which the defendant dentist is held or to whether the defendant dentist departed from the standard. An expert witness is anyone who possesses special knowledge related to the issue at trial. Thus any dentist who is aware of the professional issues to be decided by the jury may qualify as an expert witness. The question is, How much weight will be given by the jury to the testimony of the expert? This depends on the credibility of the expert. An experienced practitioner in the field, who has contributed to texts and journals, has more credibility than one who recently graduated from dental school, so the jury is likely to give more weight to the opinion of the former than the latter. Cases often end up as a battle of the experts.

The defendant dentist as a witness has a greater burden at trial than either the fact witness or the expert. For the defendant dentist, much depends on the dentist's credibility before the jury. To be believed is the major issue. Not all that transpires between a dentist and a patient is recorded. Many facts in almost all cases are in dispute. Who the jury believes depends solely on who is more credible: the dentist or the patient. The credibility of the dentist depends on many factors, as stated in the general rules on how to be a witness. In addition, how the dentist conducts practice as described at the trial, the records kept by the dentist, and so on may influence the jury in assessing the credibility of the dentist. Many cases in which there is a legitimate question as to whether the dentist was guilty of malpractice are decided against the dentist on the basis of a lack of credibility, notwithstanding lack of evidence for the jury to find the dentist guilty of malpractice. One major caveat that all dentists named as defendants should be aware of is the following: tell your attorney everything you know about the case—hold back nothing—and do not distort the facts to make yourself look good. The most damaging thing that can take place at trial is for the attorney to be surprised by some damaging fact.

An Emerging Risk in Dental Practice (Not Related to Patient Care)

Employment practices litigation (allegations of discrimination, sexual harassment, or wrongful termination brought against an employer) is now the fastest growing area of commercial litigation. The Equal Employment Opportunity Commission reported settlements in employment practice–related claims in 1993 of $105 million, as compared with $35 million in 1991. The expectation is that future years' figures, when fully tabulated, will continue to set new records. Employees are becoming more litigious. Settlement and awards costs are skyrocketing. All employers in business, no matter how small, including dentists, can be the target of an employment practices liability lawsuit. Even an unintentional violation of the laws has the potential of placing the dentist's practice and future in financial jeopardy. Neither general liability, professional liability, nor workers' compensation policies will provide coverage for these claims.

Federal laws that relate to employment discrimination include the following:

1. Americans with Disabilities Act of 1990
2. Civil Rights Act of 1991
3. Age Discrimination in Employment Act of 1967
4. Older Workers Benefit Protection Act of 1990
5. Title VII of the Civil Rights Law of 1964

6. Equal Pay Act
7. Rehabilitation Act of 1973
8. Pregnancy Discrimination Act of 1978

Employment practices liability insurance coverage is available to dentists. Coverage may be provided for liability and defense costs for claims arising out of discrimination, sexual harassment, or wrongful termination brought by an employee, a former employee, or a prospective employee. Such practices may be criminal (in violation of the law) or civil (in violation of the civil rights of the person). It should be noted that policies of employment practices liability are limited to cover the dentist for cases brought by the employee, not by a government agency protecting the individual from such illegal practices.

SUMMARY STATEMENT ON RISK MANAGEMENT

Data obtained from January 1996 until December 2001 indicate that 64% of dental malpractice jury trials in New York were decided in favor of the defendant dentist.[31] If the judge and jury are convinced that the doctor acted in the best interest of the patient, notwithstanding the injury to the patient, they will probably decide that the doctor was free of culpability.

The best advice that an attorney can give to health practitioners to enable them to enjoy a professional life free from malpractice litigation brought by patients is to be careful and caring in all they do. It is advice that is simple and short, but goes a long way to prevent legal entanglements with patients and courts, should a lawsuit become a reality. Finally, the dentist should keep current on all laws that have an impact on dental practice and not break any of them. If in doubt, the dentist should consult an attorney before acting.

IN CONCLUSION ON SAFEGUARDING THE PUBLIC'S HEALTH

The extent and complexity of the laws regulating dentists and dental practice, compounded by the number of court decisions that have both interpreted the laws and decided cases on the subjects, and the fact that each jurisdiction has exercised its right to write its own laws regulating dentists and dental practice, may cause the reader to lose sight of the basic purpose of these laws and court decisions. The clear purpose was, and is, to protect the health of the community. To accomplish this goal, laws were adopted to grant the monopoly of holding oneself out as a dentist, and to financially profit from providing professional services, solely to those who could meet the standards required to obtain the license to engage in practice. Courts, in addition to interpreting the laws adopted by the community, punished practitioners who were negligent in their treatment of patients. In exchange for obtaining the monopoly of practice, the courts and the community, by way of adopting regulatory laws, have imposed on the licensees standards of conduct to which other citizens are not held. All of this has been done to protect the health of the community.

REVIEW QUESTIONS

1. In holding a dental employer liable to a patient injured by the negligence of a dental hygienist, what legal principles are applied by the courts?

2. Dentists A and B are partners in practice. While A is away on an extended vacation, a new patient enters the practice. During the patient's first visit, B commits a negligent act that injures the patient. The patient has a choice of suing both A and B jointly, A alone, or B alone. Given the facts in the case, on what legal basis will a suit against A, either separately or jointly with B, be permitted by the courts?
3. A minor is taken to the office of an orthodontist by his grandmother, who believes that the child is in need of orthodontic care. The treatment plan, the fee, and the schedule of payments are explained to the child's grandmother in writing. She signs the agreement, stating that the child lives with her and that she pays for all his expenses, including his medical care. She further states that his parents are divorced and that her daughter, the child's mother, has custody, but is unable to care for him. His father cannot be located. Unfortunately, during the course of the treatment the child is injured through the negligence of the orthodontist. The grandmother sues the orthodontist on behalf of the child. The mother suddenly appears on the scene, claiming the orthodontist did not have consent to treat the child. Do you think the consent given by the grandmother was valid? If not, why not? If yes, on what do you base your decision?
4. A dentist performs an endodontic procedure for a patient. During the filing of the canal the tip of the instrument breaks, and, despite several attempts to remove it, the dentist is unsuccessful. The dentist does not inform the patient, but goes on to complete the procedure, allowing the instrument tip to remain in the canal. Ten years pass, and the patient is now under the care of another dentist. The patient complains of pain in the area of the tooth that has been endodontically treated. The new dentist, on examination of the area, discovers a large area of infection at the apex of the root of the tooth. She informs the patient that it was caused by the instrument tip that was allowed to remain in the canal. The statute of limitations for malpractice actions in the state is 3 years from the date the incident took place that caused the injury. The patient, in our hypothetical case, enters suit against the original dentist 10 years after she left his practice. This dentist asks the judge to whom the case is assigned to dismiss the case on the grounds that the statute of limitations has expired. Do you think the judge will dismiss the case or let it continue? On what basis would the judge's decision be made?
5. A patient is referred to an endodontist by a general dentist, who indicates on his written referral form that the tooth needing treatment is the upper right first molar. The endodontist completes the treatment successfully and without incident. Three months later the patient goes to his physician complaining of pain in the left side of his tongue. On examination the physician discovers a large eroded lesion and refers the patient to an oncologist. Based on a biopsy of the lesion it is diagnosed as squamous cell carcinoma; however, by this time it has metastasized to other organs of the body. One year later the patient dies as a result of the spread of the carcinoma. The spouse of the de-

ceased enters suit against the endodontist, claiming that had he discovered the lesion during the course of his treatment her husband would have survived for a longer period of time. The question before the jury is whether the endodontist had a duty to go beyond the specific referral and complete a soft tissue examination of the entire mouth. What do you think, and why?

REFERENCES

1. *A history of the American Dental Association 1859-1959,* Chicago, 1959, American Dental Association.
2. Robinson JB: The American Association of Dental Examiners, *J Am Dent Assoc* 58, June 1859.
3. *Hewitt v Charier,* 33 Mass. 353, 16 Pick. 353.
4. *Dent v State of West Virginia,* 129 U.S. 114.
5. *State v Vandersluis,* 42 Minn. 129.
6. *People v Griswold,* 213 N.Y. 92.
7. Section 2F of the Principles of Ethics and Code of Professional Conduct of the American Dental Association, April 2000.
8. In New York, Rules of the Board of Regents, Part 29, Section 29.2 (a), (1).
9. In New York, Section 29.2 (a), (6) of the Rules of the Board of Regents, Part 17.
10. Modified from *Pattern jury instructions. Civil,* vol 1, 2:150. *Malpractice,* Rochester, NY, Lawyers Cooperative Publishing, 1996.
11. *Porubiansky v Emory University et al,* 275 S.E. 163p aff'd 282 S.E. 902.
12. *Riley v Weiman,* 528 N.Y.S.2d 925.
13. *Murriello v Crapottay,* 51 A.D.2d 1049, and Dries v. Gregor, 424 N.Y.S.2d 561.
14. In New York, Rules of the Board of Regents, Part 29, Section 29.1 (b), (8).
15. Section 1.B.2. of the Principles of Ethics and Code of Professional Conduct of the American Dental Association, April 2000.
16. Louisell DW, Williams H: *Medical malpractice,* New York, 2000, Matthew Bender.
17. *Schwarz v Board of Regents of the State of New York,* 453 N.Y.S.2d 836.
18. In New York, Rules of the Board of Regents, Part 29, Section 29.2 (a), (3).
19. Application of Susan Striegel, 399 N.Y.S.2d 584.
20. *Thor v Boska,* 38 Cal. App.3rd 558 Cal Rptr 296.
21. *Schwarz v Board of Regents of the State of New York,* 453 N.Y.S.2d 836.
22. Rules of the Board of Regents, Part 29, Section 29.2 (a), (3).
23. *Lawrence Coert, and the Estate of Sandra Coert v Federal Insurance Company and Doran Ryan, DDS,* 430 N.W.2d 379
24. *Mohr v Williams,* 95 Minn. 261. (1905).
25. *Perkins v Desipio, DDS,* 736 A.2d 608.
26. *Bulman v Myers,* 467 A.2d 1353.
27. *Hoffson v Orentreich,* NYLJ, June 21, 1989, p. 22, col. 5.
28. *Truman v Thomas,* 155 Cal. Rptr. 752.
29. *LeBeuf v Atkins,* 621 P.2d 787, 28 Wash. App. 50.
30. *In the Matter of Mark Slovin, DDS, PC, v Thomas F. Hartnett, as Commissioner of Labor,* 158 A.D.2d 824.
31. *New York medical malpractice,* vol XV, issue 4, December 2001, East Islip, NY, Moran.

APPENDIX

THE ORGANIZATION OF HEALTH-RELATED ACTIVITIES AT THE FEDERAL LEVEL OF GOVERNMENT

Lester E. Block

Although the department most closely associated with public health–related activities is the Department of Health and Human Services (DHHS), there are currently 13 other departments in the executive branch of government. The other 13 are the Departments of Agriculture, Commerce, Defense, Education, Energy, Housing and Urban Development, Interior, Justice, Labor, State, Transportation, Treasury, and Veterans' Affairs. Although DHHS is the primary department that addresses issues of public health concern and develops and implements public health–related policy programs, virtually all the other departments are also engaged in various levels of public health–related activities.[1] Fig. A-1 shows the organizational structure of the federal government.

DEPARTMENT OF DEFENSE

The Department of Defense (DOD) is responsible for maintaining the health of members of the armed forces and their dependents.

DEPARTMENT OF VETERANS' AFFAIRS

The Department of Veterans' Affairs (VA) maintains a large network of facilities that provide health services to eligible veterans. The Veterans Administration was established as an independent agency in 1930 for the purpose of consolidating and coordinating federal agencies created for or concerned with administration of laws providing benefits to veterans. In March 1989 legislation

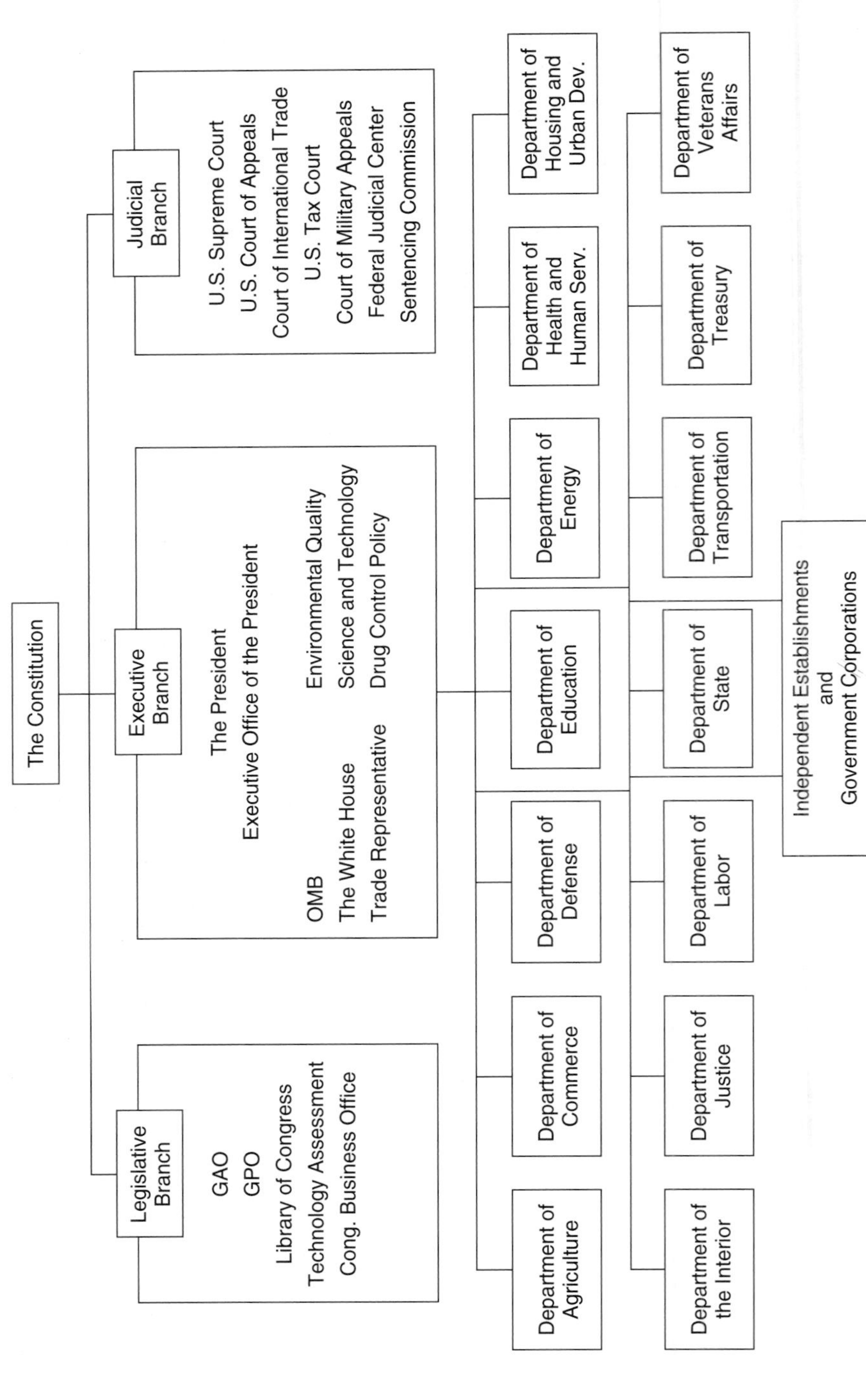

Fig. A-1. Organizational structure of the federal government. (From Illinois Center for Instructional Technology Accessibility, University of Illinois at Urbana-Champaign. Available at http://cita.rehab.uiuc.edu/images/image-longdesc-008:gif)

elevated it to cabinet-level status as the Department of Veterans' Affairs.[2]

The difference between the DOD and the VA is that the DOD primarily serves current and retired members of the armed forces, whereas the VA serves those with some service-connected disability who have honorably left the service.[3] The VA provides some dental care to eligible patients through its system of hospitals.[4,5]

DEPARTMENT OF JUSTICE

The Department of Justice, along with another governmental agency, the Federal Trade Commission, has the responsibility for the enforcement of the federal antitrust laws, which have in more recent years been applied to health care providers. Although not often thought of by the public or even by public health practitioners as public health related, the impact of the Department of Justice and the Federal Trade Commission on the public's health is significant. The Department of Justice in addition supervises the activities of the Bureau of Prisons. The Bureau of Prisons' Health Services Division has oversight for all dental, medical, and psychiatric programs, as well as for environmental, occupational, and food and nutrition services, in federal prisons.

DEPARTMENT OF AGRICULTURE

The Department of Agriculture, although not often considered an important public health agency, has, with its responsibility for the inspection of various food products, a major role in protecting the public's health.

DEPARTMENT OF TRANSPORTATION

The Department of Transportation is responsible for automobile, highway, and airline safety.

DEPARTMENT OF THE TREASURY

The Department of the Treasury is responsible for the manufacturing and labeling of alcohol and tobacco products and the health of members of the Coast Guard.

SOCIAL SECURITY ADMINISTRATION

The Social Security Administration, although not officially a department, administers a national program of contributory social insurance whereby employees, employers, and the self-employed pay contributions that are pooled in special trust funds. When earnings stop or are reduced because of death, retirement, or disablement, monthly cash earnings are paid to partially replace the earnings the family has lost. The responsibility for the administration of the Medicare program was transferred from the Social Security Administration to the Health Care Financing Administration (HCFA) (now called the Centers for Medicare and Medicaid Services [CMS]). Medicare is a health insurance program for the elderly, disadvantaged, and physically and mentally challenged. In 1995 the Social Security Administration was transferred from the DHHS to independent agency status in the executive branch of the federal government. The Social Security Administration is headed by a commissioner appointed by the president with the advice and consent of the Senate.[1,6,7]

DEPARTMENT OF HEALTH AND HUMAN SERVICES (DHHS)

DHHS has four major agencies under its jurisdiction: the Administration on Aging, the Administration for Children and Families, the Centers for Medicare and Medicaid Services (CMS), and the Public Health Service (Fig. A-2). The DHHS budget is second only to that of the Department of Defense.[3,8] DHHS is the largest grant-making agency in the federal government, and its Medicare program is the nation's largest health insurer. The following three agencies are considered DHHS Human Services Operating Divisions.

Administration on Aging

The Administration on Aging (AOA) is the principal agency designated to carry out the provisions of the Older Americans Act of 1965.

Administration for Children and Families

The Administration for Children and Families (ACF) is responsible for federal programs that promote the economic and social well-being of families, children, individuals, and communities and is responsible for the Head Start program, which provides educational, social, medical, dental, nutritional, and mental health services to preschool children from low-income families.

Centers for Medicare and Medicaid Services (CMS) (Formerly the Health Care Financing Administration [HCFA])

In June 2001, the name of the Health Care Financing Administration (HCFA) was changed to the Centers for Medicare and Medicaid Services (CMS). The Secretary of Health and Human Services had initially suggested that the new name be the Medicare and Medicaid Administration (MAMA), but he said that women found that acronym insulting and it reinforced an image of paternalism/materialism at a time when President Bush is interested in Medicare beneficiaries taking more responsibility for their health plan.[9,10] The CMS is responsible for the oversight of the federal portion of the Medicaid program and has full responsibility for the Medicare program and related federal medical care quality control staffs. CMS also administers the Utilization and Quality Control Peer Review Organization Program, which reviews services provided to Medicare patients to ensure that services are medically necessary, provided in the appropriate settings, and meet professionally recognized standards of quality health care.[1] CMS also administers the new Children's Health Insurance Program through approved state plans. CSM serves about 70 million elderly, disabled, and poor Americans through Medicare and Medicaid, approximately one fourth of the U.S. population. The two largest federal health care programs are Medicare and Medicaid, which account for about 80% of annual federal health care expenditures (which totaled $335 billion in fiscal year 1995). The remaining federal health care–related expenditures were divided mostly among the eight Public Health Service agencies

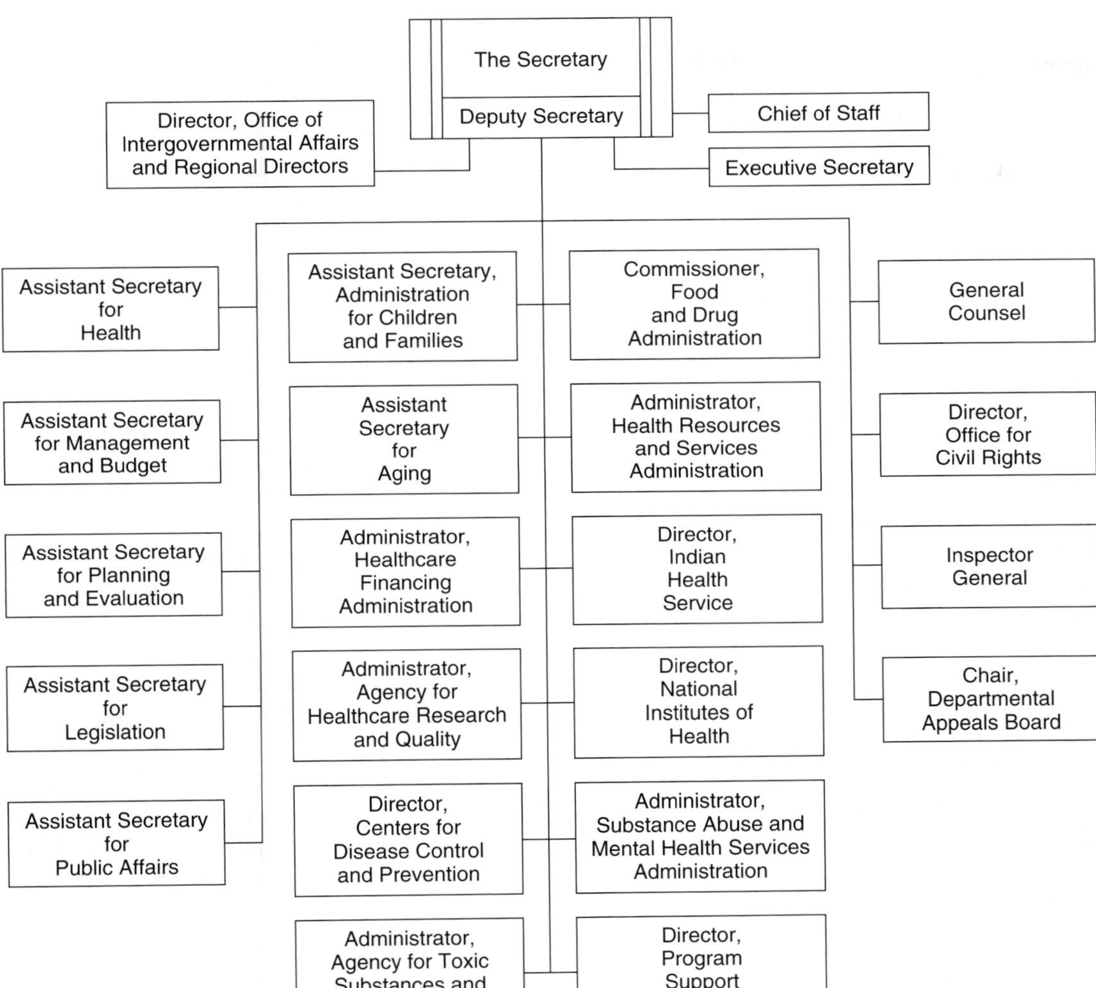

Fig. A-2. The Department of Health and Human Services. (Note that the Assistant Secretary for Health's office is more commonly called the Office of Public Health and Science.) (From Office of the Federal Register, National Archives and Records Administration, General Services Administration: *United States government manual 2000-2001*, Washington, DC, 2000, US Government Printing Office, p 227.)

($22.4 billion), the VA ($17.3 billion), the DOD ($10 billion), and the Environmental Protection Agency ($7.3 billion).[11]

In January 2001, CMS sent a letter to state Medicaid directors urging the states to ensure that they are working to address a "growing and dangerous health problem," that being "a lack of enforcement of existing (Medicaid) requirements." The letter requested states to produce action plans for ensuring children's access to dental services under Medicaid.[12]

Public Health Service

It should be noted that the Public Health Service (PHS) is not synonymous with the U.S. Public Health Service Commissioned Corps discussed in Chapter 1. The Public Health Service includes the following eight operating divisions: the Agency of Health Care Policy and Research, the Agency for Toxic Substances and Disease Registry, the Centers for Disease Control and Prevention, the Food and Drug Administration, Health Resources and Services Administration, the Indian Health Service, the National Institutes of Health, and the Substance Abuse and Mental Health Services Administration.[1,13]

In 1995 there was a significant reorganization of the PHS. Previously, the Assistant Secretary of Health was in charge of the PHS. In the reorganization, the Office of the Assistant Secretary (OASH) was significantly downsized and changed to the Office of Public Health and Science.[14] The OASH still reports to the Secretary of DHHS but is now responsible for the coordination of interagency activities and no longer has authority over the eight operating divisions or the PHS, which now report directly to the Office of the Secretary. Although the current DHHS organizational chart does not indicate the existence of the PHS, it is still considered a functional entity.[15] After the 1995 reorganization, the U.S. Surgeon General also served as the Assistant Secretary of Health. Since President Bush took office in January 2001, the Surgeon General no longer serves in that capacity.

The 1995 reorganization appears to have decreased the influence of public health and the public health staff within DHHS and strengthened the influence of the social services staff. It has been suggested that because a good part of the blame for the failure of health care reform was placed by the Clinton administration on high-level public health staff in the department who had worked for its passage, the downsizing of the OASH and the cutting back of power was in part an act of retribution.

Since the formation of the PHS, which was created in 1789 to provide for "the temporary relief and maintenance of sick or disabled seamen," the federal government's role in regard to the health of its citizens has greatly expanded. From the singular role of responding to the health care needs of the many merchant seamen who arrived ill and unattached in American port cities, cities that had little capacity to take care of them, the PHS has grown to prominence as a federal enterprise dedicated to promoting and protecting the public's health.[16]

Three different sets of congressional committees authorize laws governing federal public health–related activities. These committees establish overall spending ceilings and appropriate moneys annually for program operations. The House Commerce Committee and the Senate Labor and Human Resources Committee establish many overall policies of the eight PHS agencies through the Public Health Service Act. The House and Senate budget committees set overall annual spending ceilings for all government agencies, including the PHS. The House and Senate appropriations committees and their related subcommittees approve annual spending under these ceilings.[17]

Although public health and politics are often better kept separate, the reality is that the political environment in a society has a major impact on the value placed on the public's health and the funding and role of public health agencies within that society. When in 1994, for the first time in more than 40 years, the Republicans gained a majority in both Houses of Congress, one of their clear goals was to downsize government and limit the regulatory powers, activities, and functions of federal agencies. Between 1994 and 1996 the Republican-controlled Congress, with the acquiescence of the Clinton administration, began to change the PHS and other federal agencies in significant ways. The first true casualty was the Office of Technology (OTA), which was eliminated. The OTA was a small nonpartisan agency created by Congress in 1972 to advise the legislative branch on important issues involving science and technology. In lieu of this agency, Congress will have to depend on getting this kind of information from private sources, which may not provide as unbiased a perspective.[11]

The PHS is charged with the responsibility of promoting health standards, ensuring that the highest level of health care is available for all U.S. citizens, and cooperating with other nations on health projects. It has always been charged with the following:[18]

1. The physical diagnosis of the entire population
2. Setting goals for protecting and improving the nation's health
3. Devising and initiating programs to achieve those goals
4. Measuring whether these goals have been met

The Public Health Service includes eight operating divisions:[1,13,19]

1. The Agency for Healthcare Research and Quality (AHRQ) was established by the Omnibus Budget Reconciliation Act of 1989 as the successor to the National Center for Health Services Research and Health Care Technology Assessment. The agency is the federal government's focal point for health services research. It develops and disseminates scientific and policy information about the quality, effectiveness, and cost of health care.
2. The Centers for Disease Control and Prevention (CDC) is the federal agency charged with protecting the public health of the nation by providing leadership and direction in the prevention and control of diseases and other preventable conditions and responding to public health emergencies. Among its 11 major operating components are the National Center for Injury Prevention and Control, the National Center for Chronic Disease Prevention and Health Promotion, the National Center for Infectious Diseases, the National Center for Health Statistics, and the Public Health Practice and Promotion Office. The oral health activities of the CDC are located primarily within the Division of Oral Health, which is located in the National Center for Chronic Disease Prevention. The Division of Oral Health, which contains the Program Services Branch and the Surveillance, Investigations, and Research Branch, has the responsibility for supporting state and local oral disease prevention programs, promoting oral health nationally, and fostering applied research to enhance oral disease prevention.[20] Among the CDC's oral health–related activities are dental infection control, community water fluoridation, oral health surveillance,

oral pharyngeal cancer and tobacco-related issues, and support for state and oral health programs.[21]

In early 1996 the CDC announced a reorganization of its dental program, which was indicative of the continuing diminution of the organizational status of dental public health programs throughout the country at the federal, state, and local levels. In this announced reorganization, what was formerly the Division of Oral Health was to lose its divisional status and become the Oral Health Program (OHP). The OHP would be located in the Division of Cancer Prevention and Control (DCPC), which is located in the National Center for Chronic Disease Prevention and Health Promotion (NCCDPHP). At the announcement of this change the director of NCCDPHP[22] stated that he believed that this transfer would "strengthen current oral health activities," a view that was not held by organized dentistry and most dental public health practitioners, who believed that the administrative demotion of the dental program would be deleterious to the public's dental health.[23] Shortly after the announcement, the American Dental Association went to Congress, alerting key members to the shifting emphasis in government health programs at the expense of dental health. This effort bore fruit and the OHP was restored to divisional status in early 1997.[24] This is an example of the necessity for the teamwork described in Chapter 1 between public health agencies and nongovernmental organizations to achieve the goal of optimal oral health for the public. In addition to the Division of Oral Heath, NCCDPHP contains the following seven divisions: Adult and Community Health, Adolescent School Health, Cancer and Prevention Control, Diabetes Translation, Nutrition and Physical Activity, Reproductive Health, and the Office of Smoking and Health.

3. The Agency for Toxic Substances and Disease Registry (ATSDR) carries out health-related responsibilities in regard to the various laws relating to sites and the substances found at those sites and other forms of uncontrolled releases of toxic substances into the environment. The agency functions to protect the public and workers from exposure or the adverse health effects of hazardous substances.
4. The Food and Drug Administration (FDA) is responsible for protecting the health of the nation against impure and unsafe foods, drugs, cosmetics, and other potential hazards.
5. The Indian Health Service (IHS) focuses on the goal of raising the health status of Native Americans and Native Alaskans. It provides a comprehensive health services delivery system for both groups.
6. The National Institutes of Health (NIH) is the principal biologic research agency of the federal government; its mission is to use science in the pursuit of knowledge to improve health. Among its 29 institutes and centers are the National Cancer Institute; the National Heart, Lung, and Blood Institute; and the National Institute of Dental and

Craniofacial Research (NIDCR). NIDCR supports and conducts clinical and laboratory research designed to understand, treat, and prevent the infections and inherited and acquired craniofacial-oral-dental diseases and disorders that compromise millions of human lives. NIDCR staff conduct basic, clinical, and epidemiologic research. The two divisions in NIDCR are the Division of Extramural Research and the Division of Intramural Research. In addition, there are four offices: Science Policy and Analysis, Communication, International Health, and Information Technology. The CDC has recently joined with the NIDCR to establish the Dental, Oral, and Craniofacial Data Resource Center. The Center's main function will be to assemble data and other information needed to support research, program evaluation, and policy development for these and other PHS agencies. It is hoped that the data generated will show how the states and the nation are progressing in meeting the nation's *Healthy People 2010* objectives discussed in Chapter 1.[25] NIDCR has recently developed a three-part plan to eliminate craniofacial, oral, and dental health disparities that focuses on research, research capacity, and information dissemination. The goals of the plan are to address health disparities, build a more diverse workforce, and facilitate the transfer of research advances for adoption by the public and care providers.[26] There has been concern on the part of a group of leading dental educators in regard to the suggestion by the former NIH director that the number of institutes receiving independent appropriations be cut from 24 to 6. The group indicated that the public would suffer if the National Institute of Dental and Craniofacial Research were to disappear and a small number of "mega-chiefs" were to set the entire NIH agenda.[27]

7. The Substance Abuse and Mental Health Services Administration (SAMHSA) provides national leadership to ensure that knowledge, based on science and state-of-the-art practice, is effectively used for the prevention and treatment of addictive and mental disorders. SAMHSA includes the Centers for Substance Abuse Prevention, Substance Abuse Treatment, and Mental Health Services.
8. The Health Resources and Services Administration (HRSA) has leadership responsibility in the PHS for general health services and resource issues relating to access, quality, and cost of care. Its mission is to improve the nation's health by ensuring equal access to comprehensive, culturally competent, quality health care for all. It supports states and communities in their efforts to plan, organize, and deliver care, especially to underserved-area residents, migrant workers, mothers and children, the homeless, and other special-need groups.[1] HRSA, at over $3 billion, has the second highest annual budget of any PHS agency.[28]

   There are four bureaus within HRSA. The Bureau of Primary Health Care serves as a national focus to help ensure the availability and delivery of health care services in areas with health professional shortages and to those with special needs. The Bureau of Primary Health Care's mission is to ensure that underserved and vulnerable people get the health care they need. The Bureau of Primary Health Care administers the National Health Service Corps Program, which recruits and places health care practitioners for areas with health professional shortages and for minority and women's programs, immigration health services, and community and migrant health programs.

The Bureau of Health Professions provides national leadership in ensuring a health professions workforce that meets the health care needs of the public. The Bureau of Health Professions works to increase the diversity of the health care workforce and its distribution and ensure health care workforce quality, and it provides national leadership in coordinating, evaluating, and supporting the development and utilization of the nation's health care personnel.[26] Among the agencies within the Bureau of Health Professions are the Center for Public Health and the Divisions of Medicine and Dentistry, Health Professions, Diversity, and Quality Assurance.[29] The Bureau of Health Professions operates the National Practitioner Data Bank and the Vaccine Injury Compensation Program, and it supports through grants health profession training institutions, among which are grants to support dental public health residencies.

The HIV/AIDS Bureau is responsible for implementing the Ryan White Care Act.

The Maternal and Child Health Bureau develops, administers, directs, coordinates, monitors, and supports federal policy and programs concerning health and health care–related systems for the nation's mothers and children.[1,18] The Maternal and Child Health Bureau contains the Division of Child, Adolescent and Family Health; the Division of Services for Children with Special Health Needs; the Division of Perinatal Systems and Women's Health; the Division of Research, Training and Education; and the Division of State and Community Health.

Activities related to dental care in the Public Health Service can be found primarily in the following: (1) Centers for Disease Control and Prevention; (2) Health Resources and Services Administration, Bureau of Health Professions; (3) National Institutes of Health, National Institute of Dental and Craniofacial Research (NIDCR), which carries out support programs of basic and clinical dental research; and (4) Agency for Healthcare Research and Quality.[3,30,31]

DEPARTMENT OF HEALTH AND HUMAN SERVICES REGIONAL OFFICES

Ten regional offices of the DHHS serve all DHHS agencies. The following are the locations and states within the jurisdiction of each region:[1]

Number of Region	States in Jurisdiction	Location of Regional Office
1	CT, MA, ME, NH, RI, VT	Boston, MA
2	NJ, NY, Puerto Rico, Virgin Islands	New York, NY
3	DC, DE, MD, PA, VA, WV	Philadelphia, PA
4	AL, FL, GA, KY, MS, NC, SC, TN	Atlanta, GA
5	IL, IN, MI, MN, OH, WI	Chicago, IL
6	AR, LA, NM, OK, TX	Dallas, TX
7	IA, KS, MO, NE	Kansas City, KS
8	CO, MT, ND, SD, UT, WY	Denver, CO
9	AZ, CA, HI, NV, American Samoa, Guam, Territories of the Pacific	San Francisco, CA
10	AK, ID, OR, WA	Seattle, WA

REFERENCES

1. Congressional Quarterly: *Federal regulatory directory,* ed 10, Washington, DC, 2001, Congressional Quarterly Press.
2. Office of Inspector General: *Inspector General semiannual report Oct 1, 1989-March 31, 1990,* no RC550-0568, Washington, DC, 1990, Department of Veterans' Affairs.
3. Wilson FA, Neuhauser D: *Health services in the United States,* ed 2, Cambridge, MA, 1985, Ballinger.
4. Deputy Assistant Secretary for Planning and Management Analysis: *Geographic distribution of VA expenditures fiscal year 1990 state, county, and congressional district,* Washington, DC, 1991, Department of Veterans' Affairs.
5. Floyd D, Director of Dental Policy and Planning, Department of Veterans' Affairs, Washington, DC: Personal communication, July 10, 1991.
6. Office of the Federal Register: *US government manual, 2000/2001,* Washington, DC, June 1, 2000, National Archives and Records Administration.
7. Eldridge G, editor: *Government research directory,* ed 14, Detroit, 2001, Gale Group, Inc.
8. Greene JC: Federal programs and the profession, *J Am Dent Assoc* 92:689, 1976.
9. Pear R: Medicare agency changes name in an effort to emphasize service, *New York Times* 150(51,785):A23, June 15, 2001.
10. Bureau of National Affairs: HCFA renaming only first of series of agency mission reforms officials say, *BNA's Health Care Policy Report* 19(24):960, 2001.
11. Inglehart J: Health policy report politics and public health, *N Engl J Med* 334(3):1203, 1996.
12. Palmer C: Medicaid Dental Care urged HCFA's call for action plan to ensure child oral health stirs debate, *ADA News* 32(6):12, March 19, 2001.
13. Brandt E: The federal contribution to public health. In Scutchfield FD, Keck CW, editors: *Principles of public health practice,* Albany, NY, 1997, Delmar.
14. US Department of Health and Human Services: Office of Public Health and Science organizational chart, March 11, 1996.
15. US Department of Health and Human Services: Organizational chart, March 13, 1996.
16. Pickett G, Hanlon JJ: Philosophy and purpose of public health. In *Public health administration and practice,* ed 9, St Louis, 1990, Mosby.
17. Congressional Quarterly: *Washington information directory, 2000/2001,* Washington, DC, 2000, Congressional Quarterly.
18. Sommer A: Viewpoint on public health's future, *Public Health Rep* 110:657, 1995.
19. *Federal yellow book,* Washington, DC, Spring 2001, Monitor.
20. National Center for Chronic Disease Prevention and Health Promotion, Centers for Disease Prevention and Control: Improving Oral Health: Preventing unnecessary disease among all Americans, Feb 15, 2002. Available at http://www.cdc.gov/nccdphp/oh/ataglanc.htm.
21. Division of Oral Health Centers for Disease Control and Prevention: Division of Oral Health, National Center for Chronic Disease Prevention and Health Promotion, Feb 2, 2001. Available at http://www.health.gov/nhic/NHICScripts/Entry.cFm?HRCode=HR2306.
22. Marks JS: Letter from Director National Center for Chronic Disease Prevention and Health Promotion, Department of Health and Human Services, Atlanta: Personal communication, Feb 28, 1996.
23. Wyatt S: Division of Cancer Prevention and Control, Centers for Disease Control and Prevention, Department of Health and Human Services, Atlanta: Personal communication, Feb 20, 1996.
24. Palmer C: CDC oral health division to return, *ADA News* 17(21):1, 1996.
25. CDC, NIDCR join to create the Dental Oral and Craniofacial Center to catalogue and analyze data, *ADA News* 32(4):12, Feb 19, 2001.

26. NIDCR to implement health disparities plan, *NIDCR Research Digest* 2001, pp 1-2.
27. Goldhaber P et al: The growing family of NIH institutes, *Science* 292:1835, June 8, 2001 (editorial).
28. Sumaya CV: Oral health for all: the HRSA perspective, *J Public Health Dent* 56(1):S35, 1996.
29. U.S. Department of Health and Human Services Administration: Bureau of Health Professions: program and overview, Feb 13, 2002. Available at http://bhpr.hrsa.gov/program.html.
30. Agency for Health Care Policy and Research: *AHCPR purpose and programs,* Public Health Service no OM90-0096, Rockville, MD, 1990, US Department of Health and Human Services.
31. *Forward plan for health, FY1977-1981,* DHEW pub no (05) 76-50024, Washington, DC, 1975, US Department of Health, Education, and Welfare.

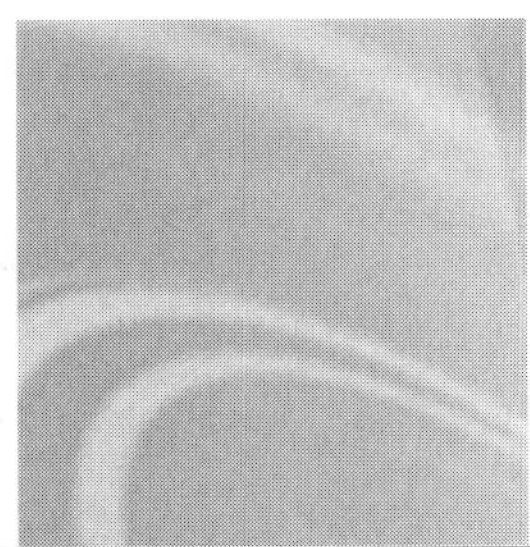

INDEX

Page references followed by t indicate tables; b, boxes; f, figures.

O